Physical Metallurgy

Physical Metallurgy

KM HARRIS

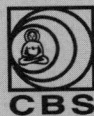

CBS Publishers & Distributors Pvt Ltd

New Delhi • Bengaluru • Chennai • Kochi • Kolkata • Mumbai
Hyderabad • Jharkhand • Nagpur • Patna • Pune • Uttarakhand

Disclaimer
Science and technology are constantly changing fields. New research and experience broaden the scope of information and knowledge. The author has tried his best in giving information available to him while preparing the material for this book. Although all efforts have been made to ensure optimum accuracy of the material, yet it is quite possible some errors might have been left uncorrected. The publisher, the printer and the author will not be held responsible for any inadvertent errors or inaccuracies.

Physical Metallurgy

ISBN: 978-81-239-2652-0

Copyright © Publisher

First Edition: 2016
Reprint: 2017

All rights reserved. No part of this book may be reproduced or transmitted in any form or by any means, electronic or mechanical, including photocopying, recording, or any information storage and retrieval system without permission, in writing, from the author and the publisher.

Published by Satish Kumar Jain and produced by Varun Jain for
CBS Publishers & Distributors Pvt Ltd
4819/XI Prahlad Street, 24 Ansari Road, Daryaganj, New Delhi 110 002, India.
Ph: 23289259, 23266861, 23266867   Website: www.cbspd.com
Fax: 011-23243014   e-mail: delhi@cbspd.com; cbspubs@airtelmail.in.
Corporate Office: 204 FIE, Industrial Area, Patparganj, Delhi 110 092
Ph: 4934 4934   Fax: 4934 4935   e-mail: publishing@cbspd.com; publicity@cbspd.com

Branches
- **Bengaluru:** Seema House 2975, 17th Cross, K.R. Road, Banasankari 2nd Stage, Bengaluru 560 070, Karnataka
  Ph: +91-80-26771678/79   Fax: +91-80-26771680   e-mail: bangalore@cbspd.com
- **Chennai:** 7, Subbaraya Street, Shenoy Nagar, Chennai 600 030, Tamil Nadu
  Ph: +91-44-26680620, 26681266   Fax: +91-44-42032115   e-mail: chennai@cbspd.com
- **Kochi:** Ashana House, No. 39/1904, AM Thomas Road, Valanjambalam, Ernakulam 682 016, Kochi, Kerala
  Ph: +91-484-4059061-65   Fax: +91-484-4059065   e-mail: kochi@cbspd.com
- **Kolkata:** 6/B, Ground Floor, Rameswar Shaw Road, Kolkata-700 014, West Bengal
  Ph: +91-33-22891126, 22891127, 22891128   e-mail: kolkata@cbspd.com
- **Mumbai:** 83-C, Dr E Moses Road, Worli, Mumbai-400018, Maharashtra
  Ph: +91-22-24902340/41   Fax: +91-22-24902342   e-mail: mumbai@cbspd.com

Representatives
- Hyderabad 0-9885175004   • Jharkhand 0-9811541605   • Nagpur   0-9021734563
- Patna   0-9334159340   • Pune   0-9623451994   • Uttarakhand 0-9716462459

Printed at India Binding House, Noida, UP, India

Preface

Metallurgy is the art of working metals, comprehending the whole process of separating them from other matters in the ore, smelting, refining and parting them; sometimes in a narrower sense, only the process of extracting metals from their ores. Metallurgy is a domain of materials science that studies the physical and chemical behaviour of metallic elements, their intermediate compounds, and their mixtures, which are called alloys. It is also the technology of metals: the way in which science is applied to their practical use.

Physical metallurgy is the science of making useful products out of metals. Metal parts can be made in a variety of ways, depending on the shape, properties, and cost desired in the finished product. The desired properties may be electrical, mechanical, magnetic or chemical in nature; all of them can be enhanced by alloying and heat treatment. The cost of a finished part is often determined more by its ease of manufacture than by the cost of the material. This has led to a wide variety of ways to form metals and to an active competition among different forming methods, as well as among different materials. Large parts may be made by casting. Thin products such as automobile fenders are made by forming metal sheets, while small parts are often made by powder metallurgy (pressing powder into a die and sintering it). Usually a metal part has the same properties throughout. However, if only the surface needs to be hard or corrosion-resistant, the desired performance can be obtained through a treatment that changes only the composition and strength of the surface.

This reference textbook on physical metallurgy summarises the various metallurgical principles for engineers and contains 26 chapters. Chapter 1 is devoted to basic structure of materials as various properties of materials are related with structure. Chapter 2 deals with strengthening mechanism of materials and discusses grain boundary strengthening, solid solution strengthening, dispersion strengthening and precipitation hardening. Chapter 3 concentrates on phase diagrams which indicate the phases existing in the system at any temperature and composition. Chapter 4 brings to light heat treatment of stainless steel and discusses its stages of heat treatment. Chapter 5 is devoted to heat treatment of steel. Heat treatment is a group of industrial and metalworking processes used to alter the physical, and sometimes chemical properties of a material. Chapter 6 acquaints the readers with heat treatment of tool steel which refers to a variety of carbon and alloy steels that are particularly well-suited to be made into tool. Chapter 7 discusses corrosion technology of metals—the basic cause of corrosion is the instability of metal in its refined form. Chapter 8 concentrates on cast iron which usually refers to grey iron, but also identifies a large group of ferroalloys, which solidify with a eutectic. Chapter 9 is devoted to powder metallurgy which is that branch of fabrication which is concerned with the production of finished, or semi-finished products from basic materials in the form of powders. Chapter 10 deals with aluminium alloys in which aluminium is the predominant metal and typical alloying elements are copper, magnesium, manganese, silicon, and zinc. Chapter 11 focuses on cast iron alloys which have low values of impact resistance, corrosion resistance and temperature resistance. Chapter 12 deals with copper and copper alloys and constitute one of the major groups of commercial metals. These alloys are widely used because of their excellent electrical and thermal conductivity, outstanding resistance to corrosion, and ease of fabrication, together with good strength and fatigue resistance. Chapter 13 acquaints the readers with titanium alloys which are metallic materials and contain a mixture of titanium and other chemical elements. Chapter 14 brings to light die casting alloys which are normally nonferrous. Chapter 15 concentrates on grain refinement of light alloys which offers number of advantages in foundry operations and in subsequent mechanical and thermal processing and surface finishing stages. Chapter 16 deals with fracture which is the separation of an object or material into two, or more pieces under the action of stress. Chapter 17 is devoted to fatigue which is the progressive and localised structural damage that occurs when a material is subject to cyclic loading. Chapter 18 concentrates on forming processes with metals. Chapter 19 focuses on joining materials and discusses joining processing such as adhesive bonding, soldering and brazing, welding and fastening systems. Chapter 20 is devoted to mechanical and nondestructing tests which are important to use in design. The main purpose of this test is to check whether material meets the specifications or not. Chapter 21 deals with metallography which is the general study of metals and their behaviour, with particular reference to their microstructure and macrostructure. Chapter 22 acquaints the readers with pyrometry which measures the temperatures of objects without touching them. Chapter 23 brings to light electrical properties of materials. Modern technology would be unthinkable without magnetic materials and magnetic phenomena. Considering this chapter 24 concentrates on magnetic properties of materials. Chapter 25 is devoted to optical properties of materials. Various aspects of properties such as optical constants, absorption and emission of light of materials are discussed in detail. Chapter 26 focuses on thermal properties of materials which are important whenever heating and cooling devices are designed.

Glossary and index have been provided at the end for quick reference. Diagrams, figures and tables supplement the text. All the topics have been covered in a cogent and lucid style to help the reader grasp the information quickly and easily.

It may not be wrong to hold that the present reference textbook on *Physical Metallurgy* is a complete treatise on this subject. It is essential reading for all students for B.Tech (Metallurgical/Mechanical/Electrical/Chemical/Civil/Environmental Engineering). Besides students, the book will prove useful to industrialists and consultants in material sciences and nanosciences.

The reference textbook also caters to the requirement of the syllabus prescribed by various Indian universities for undergraduate students pursuing engineering, and allied courses. It has been prepared with meticulous care, aiming at making the book error-free. Constructive suggestions are always welcome from users of this book.

KM Harris

Contents at a Glance

Preface   v

1. **Basic Structure of Materials**   1–30
2. **Strengthening Mechanism of Materials**   31–48
3. **Phase Diagrams**   49–74
4. **Heat Treatment of Stainless Steel**   75–82
5. **Heat Treatment of Steel**   83–153
6. **Heat Treatment of Tool Steel**   154–171
7. **Corrosion Technology of Metals**   172–215
8. **Cast Iron**   216–236
9. **Powder Metallurgy**   237–266
10. **Aluminium and Aluminium Alloys**   267–275
11. **Cast Iron Alloys**   276–289
12. **Copper and Copper Alloys**   290–306
13. **Titanium Alloys**   307–313
14. **Die Casting Alloys**   314–317
15. **Grain Refinement of Light Alloys**   318–324
16. **Fracture**   325–337
17. **Fatigue**   338–354
18. **Forming Processes with Metals**   355–370
19. **Joining Materials**   371–395
20. **Mechanical and Nondestructive Tests**   396–410
21. **Metallography**   411–429
22. **Pyrometry**   430–458
23. **Electrical Properties of Materials**   459–468
24. **Magnetic Properties of Materials**   469–484
25. **Optical Properties of Materials**   485–501
26. **Thermal Properties of Materials**   502–512

Glossary   513–517
References   519
Index   521–527

Contents

Preface   v

Contents at a Glance   vii

1. Basic Structure of Materials   1–30

Introduction   1
Atoms and Molecules   1
    Atomic Structure   1
    Quantum Numbers   3
    Size of Atoms   5
    Bonds   6
    States of Matter   10
Crystals   10
    Packing Factor   11
    Structure and Properties   12
    Interatomic Forces in Crystals   13
    Liquids   16
Surfaces   17
    Friction   18
Metals as Crystalline   21
    Growth of Metal Crystals   21
Block Slip Model   22
    Slip Planes   24
Dislocations   25
    Crystal Defects   26
    Movement of Dislocations   27
    Dislocation Multiplication   29

2. Strengthening Mechanism of Materials   31–48

Introduction   31
Strengthening Mechanisms in Metals   32
    Work Hardening   32
    Solid Solution Strengthening/Alloying   32
    Precipitation Hardening   33
Grain Boundary Strengthening   34
    Theory   34
    Subgrain Strengthening   35
    Hall-Petch Relationship   36
    Grain Refinement   37
Solid Solution Strengthening or Hardening   38
    Amount of Solute   38

Atomic Size Difference	38
Nature of Distortion	38
Dispersion Strengthening or Hardening	39
Age (Precipitation Hardening)	40
Heating (Solutionising)	40
Quenching	41
Ageing	41
Martensitic Transformation	44
Composite Materials	44
Fibre Reinforced Materials	45
Laminated Materials	46
Disperse Materials	46
Strengthening Mechanisms in Amorphous Materials	46
Polymer	46
Glass	47
Applications and Current Research	47
Molecular Dynamics Simulations	48

3. Phase Diagrams   49–74

Introduction	49
Gibbs' Phase Rule	50
Definitions	50
Simple One-component	52
Assumptions	54
Derivation of the Phase Rule	55
Binary Phase Diagrams	55
Lever Rule	57
Thermal Analysis—Heating and Cooling Curves	69
Time–Temperature Transformation Curves	72

4. Heat Treatment of Stainless Steel   75–82

Introduction	75
Properties	75
Applications	76
Architectural	76
Types of Stainless Steel	76
Comparison of Standardised Steels	78
Stainless Steel Finishes	79
Heat Treatment of Stainless Steel	79
Stages of Heat Treatment	79

5. Heat Treatment of Steel   83–153

Introduction	83
Iron–Iron Carbide Equilibrium Diagram	83
Various Phases in Diagram	84

Critical Temperatures	88
Solidification and Microstructures of Slowly Cooled Steels	89
Microstructures of Hypoeutectoid Steels	89
Microstructures of Hypereutectoid Steels	91
Estimation of Carbon from Microstructures	93
Non-equilibrium Cooling of Steels	93
Widmanstatten Structures	94
Property Variation with Microstructure	95
Classification and Applications of Steels	96
On the Basis of Carbon	97
On the Basis of Alloying Elements and Carbon	99
On the Basis of Deoxidation	99
On the Basis of Grain Coarsening Characteristics	101
On the Basis of Method of Manufacture	101
On the Basis of Depth of Hardening	102
On the Basis of Form and Use	102
Transformation Products of Austenite	103
Transformation of Austenite to Pearlite	103
Transformation of Austenite to Bainite	104
Transformation of Austenite to Martensite	105
Isothermal Transformation Diagram	108
Determination of TTT Diagram	108
Critical Cooling Rate	111
Continuous Cooling Transformation (CCT) Diagrams	112
Determination of CCT Curves	112
Heat Treatment of Steel	112
Cooling Media	115
Austenitic and Ferritic Grain Size in Steels	117
Grain Size Control	117
Grain Size Measurement	119
Comparision Method	119
Heyn's Intercept Method	124
Jefferies Planimetric Method	124
Conventional Annealing (Full Annealing)	125
Process of Annealing	125
Types of Annealing	126
Bright Annealing	126
Box Annealing	126
Isothermal (Cycle) Annealing	127
Spheroidise Annealing	127
Subcritical Annealing	128
Normalising	129
Process	129
Hardening	130
Conventional Hardening	130

Timed Quench (Interrupted Quench)	131
Martempering (Marquenching)	133
Ausforming	134
Retention of Austenite	134
Effects of Retained Austenite	136
Elimination of Retained Austenite	136
Cold Treatment (Subzero Treatment)	136
Plastic Deformation	137
Tempering	137
Purpose	137
Process	138
Secondary Hardening	140
Temper Brittleness (Embrittlement)	140
Quench Cracks	140
Other Heat Treatments	141
Patenting	142
Isoforming	143
Hardenability of Steel	143
Maximum Hardness	143
Hardenability	143
Jominy End-Quench	145
Ideal Diameter	145
Safety Considerations	146
Materials	146
Procedure	147
Analysis	148
Case Hardening	148
Processes	149
Applications	152
Induction Hardening	152

6. Heat Treatment of Tool Steel   154–171

Introduction	154
AISI-SAE Grades	154
Water-Hardening Grades	154
Air-Hardening Grades	155
Cold-Working Grades	155
Shock Resisting Grades	156
High Speed Grades	156
Hot-Working Grades	156
Special Purpose Grades	156
Hardening and Tempering	157
Theoretical Aspects	157
How Hardening and Tempering is Done in Practice	159

Dimensional and Shape Stability	164
Distortion During the Hardening and Tempering of Tool Steel	164
How can Distortion be Reduced?	166
Subzero Treatment	166
Surface Treatment	167
Nitriding	167
Nitrocarburising	167
Ion Nitriding	167
Case Hardening	168
Hard Chromium Plating	168
Surface Coating	168
Testing Mechanical Properties of Tool Steel	168
Hardness Testing	168
Tensile Strength	170
Impact Testing	170
Some Words of Advice to Tool Designers	171
Choice of Steel	171
Design	171
Heat Treatment	171

7. Corrosion Technology of Metals   172–215

Introduction	172
Consequences of Corrosion	172
Chemistry of Corrosion	173
Factors that Control the Corrosion Rate	174
Corrosion Prevention	175
Conditioning the Metal	175
Conditioning the Corrosive Environment	176
Electrochemical Control	177
Dry Corrosion	177
Formation of an Oxide Layer	178
Passivation	178
Anodising	178
Dry Corrosion Reactions	179
Pilling-Bedworth Ratio	179
Application	179
Formation and Growth of Films	180
Growth of Nonporous Films	180
Growth of Porous Films	180
Growth Laws	181
Parabolic Law	181
Logarithmic Law	182
Cubic Law	182
Linear Law	182

Effect of Temperature	183
Action of Hydrogen	184
Hydrogen Embrittlement	184
Hydrogen Attack	185
Wet Corrosion	185
Description of a Wet Corrosion Process	185
Crucial Mechanisms Determining Corrosion Rates	186
Corrosion Prevention Measures	187
Expressions and Measures of Corrosion Rates	187
Basic Properties that Determine if Corrosion is Possible and How Fast Material can Corrode	189
Electrochemical Theory of Wet Corrosion: Fundamentals	189
Galvanic Corrosion	192
Galvanic Series	194
Preventing Galvanic Corrosion	194
Lasagna Cell	196
Galvanic Compatibility	196
Polarisation	196
Concentration Cell Corrosion	198
Metal Ion Concentration Cells	199
Oxygen Concentration Cells	200
Active-Passive Cells	200
Stray-Current Corrosion	200
Detection of Stray Currents	201
Stray Currents in Transit Systems	201
Nature of Stray Currents	202
Uniform Corrosion	203
Pitting Corrosion	203
Mechanism	203
Susceptible Alloys	204
Environment	204
Pitting and Crevice Corrosion of Stainless Steel	204
Stress Corrosion Cracking	206
Metals Attacked	207
Polymers Attacked	207
Crack Growth	208
Prevention	208
Season Cracking	208
Ammonia	209
Materials	209
Caustic Embrittlement	209
Cause	209
Prevention	209
Corrosion Fatigue	209

Erosion-Corrosion	210
Mass Transport Control	210
Phase Transport Control	210
Cavitation	210
Intergranular Corrosion	211
Selective Corrosion	212
Corrosion/Selection of Materials	212
General Principles	213

8. Cast Iron   216–236

Introduction	216
Production of Cast Iron	216
Factors Influencing Microstructure	216
Amount of Total Carbon	217
Amount of Silicon	217
Amount of Phosphorus	217
Amount of Sulphur	218
Amount of Manganese	218
Cooling Rate	218
Types of Cast Iron	220
Grey Cast Iron	220
Types of Grey Cast Iron	221
Alloying Elements	224
White Cast Iron	225
Cooling of a Hypoeutetic Cast Iron with 3 per cent Carbon	226
Cooling of an Eutectic Cast Iron	226
Cooling of a Hypereutectic White Cast Iron	227
Malleable Cast Iron	228
Types of Malleable Cast Iron	230
Ductile Cast Iron	231
Mottled Cast Irons	232
Chilled Cast Irons	232
Alloy Cast Irons	234
Ni-Hard	234
Ni-Resist	235
Silal and Nicrosilal	235
Heat Treatment of Cast Irons	235
Stress Relieving	235
Annealing	235
Hardening and Tempering	236
Surface Hardening	236

9. Powder Metallurgy   237–266

Introduction	237

    Methods   237
        Powders Preparation   238
        Mixing   241
        Compacting   241
        Sintering   245
    Advantages and Disadvantages of Powder Metallurgy (P/M)   249
        Advantages of Powder Metallurgy   249
        Disadvantages of Powder Metallurgy   250
    Characterisation and Testing of Metal Powders   250
        Chemical Composition   251
        Shape, Size and Distribution   251
        Particle Porosity and Microstructure   252
        Other Properties   253
    Manufacture of Some Typical Powder Metallurgy (P/M) Components   256
        Oil Impregnated Porous Bearings (Self-lubricating Bearings)   256
        Cemented Carbides   257
        Cermets   258
        Cemented Carbide Tipped Tools (Sintered Carbide Cutting Tools)   258
        Diamond Impregnated Tools   259
        Production of Refractory Metals   260
        Electrical Contact Materials   261
        Sintered Metal Friction Materials   262
    Types of Metals and Applications   263
        Porous Metals   263
        Alloys with Excessively High Melting Temperatures   263
        Alloys of Metals which are Mutually Insoluble in the Liquid State   264
        Alloys with Poor Casting Qualities   264
        Alloys Containing Insoluble Constituents Required in a Fine Dispersion   265
        Alloys Not Readily Machinable in Their Finished Form and Yet Required to be more Dimensionally Accurate   266

10. Aluminium and Aluminium Alloys   267–275

    Introduction   267
    Engineering Uses of Aluminium Alloys   267
        Aluminium Alloys Versus Types of Steel   267
        Heat Sensitivity Considerations   268
        Household Wiring   269
        Alloy Designations   269
        Applications   272
    Heat Treating of Aluminium and Aluminium Alloys   273
    Ingot Preheating Treatments (Homogenising)   273
        Annealing   273
        Precipitation Hardening   274

11. Cast Iron Alloys   276–289

Introduction	276
Production of Cast Iron Alloys	276
Types	276
Heat Treating Iron Castings	279
Steps in Heat Treating	279
Annealine Treatments	279
Stress-relieving Treatment	279
Normalising Treatments	280
Austempering	280
Martempering	281
Spheroidal Graphite Cast Iron	281
Steps in Production of SG Iron	281
Properties of SG Cast Iron	282
Effect of Alloying Elements on the Properties of Ductile Iron	283
Magnesium Treatment	284
Factors that Affect the Properties of the SG Cast Iron	285
Applications of SG Iron	286
Heat Treatment of SG Cast Iron	286
Austenitising Ductile Cast Iron	287
Annealing Ductile Cast Iron	287
Normalising Ductile Cast Iron	288
Quenching and Tempering Ductile Cast Iron	288
Austempering Ductile Cast Iron	289

12. Copper and Copper Alloys   290–306

Introduction	290
Classification of Copper Alloys	291
Solid Solution Alloys	291
Age-hardenable Alloys	291
Insoluble Alloying Elements	292
Deoxidisers	292
Copper–Zinc Alloys: The Brasses	292
Designation System of Brasses	294
Bronze	295
Composition	295
Properties	296
Uses	296
Phosphor Bronze	297
Industrial Uses	297
Musical Instruments	297
Variants	297
Aluminium Bronze	297
Compositions	298

Material Properties	298
Applications	298
Wrought Phosphor Bronzes	299
Wrought Copper–Nickel Alloys and Nickel Silvers	299
Copper–Nickel–Zinc Alloys	300
Beryllium Copper	302
Properties	302
Uses	302
Alloys	303
Heat Treating of Copper and Copper Alloys	304
Homogenising	304
Annealing	304
Stress Relieving	305
Precipitation Hardening	305

13. Titanium Alloys 307–313

Introduction	307
Transition Temperature	307
Classification of Titanium Alloys	307
Properties	308
Grades	308
Heat Treating of Titanium and Titanium Alloys	309
Alloy Types and Response to Heat Treatment	309
Stress Relieving	310
Annealing	310
Solution Treating and Ageing	312

14. Die Casting Alloys 314–317

Introduction	314
Aluminum Alloys	314
Zinc Alloys	314
Zinc-Aluminum (ZA) Alloys	316

15. Grain Refinement of Light Alloys 318–324

Introduction	318
Grain Refinement Methods	319
Aluminium Alloys	319
Magnesium Alloys	321
Environmental Considerations	323
Theories of Grain Refinement	323
Summary	324

16. Fracture 325–337

Introduction	325
Fracture Strength	325

Types of Fracture	326
Brittle Fracture	326
Ductile Fracture	326
Crack Separation Modes	327
Fracture Mechanics	328
Linear Elastic Fracture Mechanics	328
Nonlinear Elasticity and Plasticity	332
Engineering Applications	332
Appendix: Mathematical Relations	333
Griffith's Criterion	333
Irwin's Modifications	333
Elasticity and Plasticity	334
Fracture Toughness	334
Crack Growth as a Stability Problem	335
Transformation Toughening	336
Conjoint Action	336
Stress–Corrosion Cracking (SCC)	337

17. Fatigue   338–354

Introduction	338
Fatigue Life	338
Characteristics of Fatigue	338
High-Cycle Fatigue	339
Low-Cycle Fatigue	341
Fatigue and Fracture Mechanics	342
Factors that Affect Fatigue Life	342
Design Against Fatigue	343
Fatigue Failure	343
Stages in Fatigue Failure	344
Effect of Mean Stress	349
Cumulative Damage	351
Factors Affecting the Fatigue Properties of Metals	351
Materials and Fatigue Resistance	353

18. Forming Processes with Metals   355–370

Introduction	355
Casting	355
Sand Casting	356
Die Casting	357
Casting and Grain Structure	359
Manipulative Processes	360
Cold Working	360
Hot Working	368
Machining	369

19. Joining Materials — 371–395

Introduction — 371
Adhesive — 371
    Types of Adhesives — 371
    Application of Adhesion — 373
    Mechanisms of Adhesion — 373
    Failure of the Adhesive Joint — 373
    Design of Adhesive Joints — 374
    Testing the Resistance of the Adhesive — 374
Soldering — 375
    Applications — 375
    Solders — 375
    Flux — 376
    Basic Soldering Techniques — 377
    Solderability — 379
    Desoldering and Resoldering — 379
    Lead-free Electronic Soldering — 380
    Soldering Defects — 380
    Tools — 380
Brazing — 380
    Common Techniques — 382
Welding — 386
    Processes Involved in Welding — 386
    Welds in Steel — 388
    Welds in Aluminium — 390
    Welds in Copper — 391
    Corrosion of Welds — 392
    Weldability — 392
    Safety Issues — 392
Fastener — 393
    Fastening Systems — 393
    Rail Fastening System — 394

20. Mechanical and Nondestructive Tests — 396–410

Introduction — 396
Hardness — 397
    Brinell Test — 397
    Vickers Machine — 397
    Rockwell Test — 399
    Shore Scleroscope — 399
    Ductility — 399
Tensile Test — 400
    Stress–Strain Curve — 400
    Commercial Results — 402

	Proof Stress	402
	Elongation	402
	Compression Test	403
	Type of Fracture	404
	Speed of Loading	405
	Effect of Previous Deformation	406
	Fracture	406
	Notched Bar Tests	409
	Fracture Mechanics and Fracture Toughness	410
21.	**Metallography**	**411–429**
	Introduction	411
	Preparing Metallographic Specimens	411
	Analysis Techniques	412
	Design, Resolution and Image Contrast	412
	Bright and Dark Field Microscopy	413
	Polarised Light Microscopy	413
	Differential Interference Contrast Microscopy	413
	Oblique Illumination	413
	Scanning Electron and Transmission Electron Microscopes	414
	X-ray Diffraction Techniques	414
	Quantitative Metallography	414
	Metallographic Examination	415
	Slag Content	415
	Alloy Identification	415
	Heat Treatment	416
	Composite Artefacts	416
	Nonferrous Alloys	416
	Fabrication Techniques	416
	Alternative Approaches	416
	Methods of Examination	417
	Micrography	417
	Electron Microscope	421
	Macrography	423
	Measurement and Control	424
	Cooling	429
22.	**Pyrometry**	**430–458**
	Introduction	430
	Principle of Operation	431
	Applications	432
	Tuyère Pyrometer	432
	Pyrometry of Gases	432
	Advantages of Pyrometers	432
	Fast Response	432

No Adverse Effects	433
Measuring Moving Objects	433
Measuring Objects which are Difficult to Access by Contact Measuring Devices	433
Physical Principles	434
Spectral Intensity	434
Wavelength of Maximum Intensity	435
Total Intensity	435
Properties of Real Objects	435
Emissivity of Various Materials	437
Determining the Emissivity of an Object	439
Choosing the Spectral Range	440
Emissivity Errors	440
Atmospheric Windows	441
Spot Size and Measuring Distance	442
Fixed Optics	443
Optics with Variable Focus	443
Filling Up the Spot Size	443
Measuring Through Openings	444
Pyrometer	444
Construction and Function	444
Pyrometer Types	445
Narrow Band Pyrometers	445
Broad Band Pyrometers	445
Total Band Pyrometers	445
Two-Colour Pyrometer	445
Bright Flames Flame Pyrometers	446
Non-Luminous Flames	447
Four-Colour Pyrometer	447
Infrared Radiation Thermometers/Pyrometers	447
Digital Pyrometers: State-of-the-Art-Technology	449
Advantages of Digital Signal Conversion	450
Fibre Optics Pyrometer	450
Sighting and Viewing Devices	452
Linearisation	453
Calibration	453
Optics, Lenses and Window Material	453
Window Materials	454
Sources of Interference	455
Trouble-Shooting	456
Accessories	457

23. Electrical Properties of Materials — 459–468

Introduction	459
Electrical Resistance	459

Applications of Resistance Materials	462
Superconductivity	463
Magnetism	464
Ferromagnetism	464
Paramagnetism	464
Diamagnetism	464
Magnetostriction	466
Piezoelectricity	466
Photoconductivity	467
Thermoelectricity	467
Seebeck Effect	467
Peltier Effect	467

24. Magnetic Properties of Materials   469–484

Introduction	469
Magnetic Phenomena and Their Interpretation	471
Diamagnetism	472
Paramagnetism	473
Ferromagnetism	475
Antiferromagnetism	476
Ferrimagnetism	477
Applications	479
Electrical Steels (Soft Magnetic Materials)	479
Permanent Magnets (Hard Magnetic Materials)	481
Magnetic Recording	482

25. Optical Properties of Materials   485–501

Introduction	485
Optical Constants	486
Absorption of Light	490
Emission of Light	495

26. Thermal Properties of Materials   502–512

Introduction	502
Interpretation of the Heat Capacity by Various Models	505
Thermal Conduction	507
Thermal Expansion	510
Glossary	513–517
References	519
Index	521–527

Chapter 1

Basic Structure of Materials

INTRODUCTION

The physical metallurgy deals with the nature, structure and properties of metals and alloys. The various properties of materials are related with structure. The structures are of many types such as crystal structure, macrostructure and microstructure, etc. All these affect the properties of metals and alloys, and hence, it is necessary to study these structures.

ATOMS AND MOLECULES

All matter is made up of atoms. A material that is made up of just one type of atom is called an element. Hydrogen, carbon, copper and iron are examples of elements. An atom is the smallest particle of an element that has the characteristics of that element. We can thus talk of a copper atom or an iron atom. Atoms themselves are made up of other particles which are not characteristics of the element but are basic building blocks out of which all atoms are constructed. Each atom is composed of a nucleus, which is positively charged, and electrons, which are negatively charged. We can think of an atom as being a very small nucleus which contains virtually all the mass of the atom, surrounded by a cloud of electrons which occupies most of the space of the atom.

The term molecule is used to describe groups of atoms which tend to exist together in a stable form. Thus, for instance, hydrogen tends to exist in a stable form as a combination of two hydrogen atoms rather than as just individual atoms. Some molecules may exist as combinations of atoms from a number of different elements. Water, for example, consists of molecules each of which is make up of two hydrogen atoms and an oxygen atom.

Atomic Structure

The atom consists of a positively-charged nucleus surrounded by negatively charged electrons. Attractive forces occur between the electrons and the nucleus (opposite charges attract) and repulsive forces occur between the electrons (like charges repel). For such forces to result in stable atoms, Bohr proposed a model for atomic structure in which electrons move in fixed orbits round the nucleus, like planets orbiting the sun. Only certain orbits are possible and only in these orbits is there stability. With this model, electrons in orbits close to the nucleus have stronger forces of attraction holding them in orbit than electrons which are in orbits further out.

The force of attraction between oppositely-charged particles is inversely proportional to the square of the distance between their centres; in other words, if the radius of the orbit is doubled then the force is reduced to a quarter of its value. Thus, electrons in close orbits are much more difficult to remove from: an atom than those in further out orbits.

Elements differ from each other in the charge carried by the nucleus. Since the charge is carried by protons this is the same as saying they differ according to the number of protons. Atoms of the same element all having the same number of protons and this number is specific to that element. The atomic number of an element is the number of protons in its atoms. An atom will normally carry no net charge and thus the number of electrons will be characteristic of the element concerned. Hydrogen has just one election, carbon has twelve. The Bohr Model proposed that the electrons existed in orbits, these sometimes being referred to as shells. The innermost orbit, sometimes called the K shell, can hold just two electrons before it is full, the second orbit out, called the L shell, requires eight electrons to be full. Thus hydrogen with just one electron has this electron in the innermost orbit—the K shell (Fig. 1.1). This K shell for hydrogen is only partially occupied. Helium has two electrons. These both occupy the K shell and fill it. Lithium has three electrons. Two of the electrons occupy and fill the K shell and the remaining electron is in the L shell which is thus only partially filled. Carbon with six electrons has two filling the K shell.

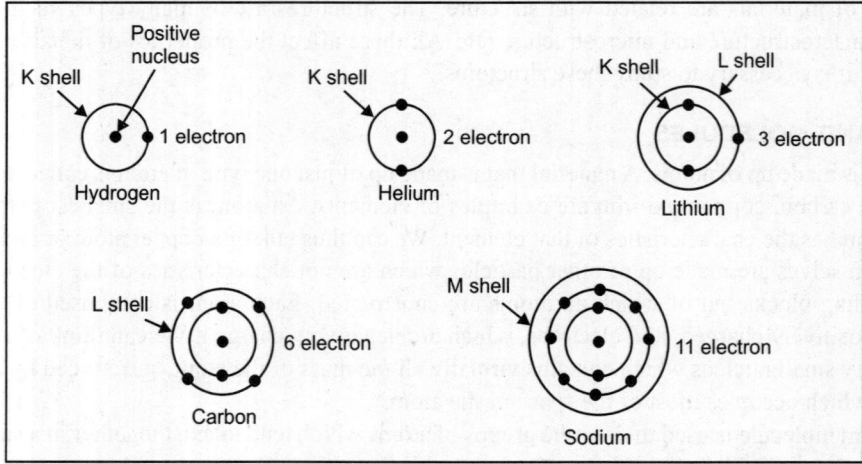

Fig. 1.1. Simple atomic model.

Table 1.1 shows how the shells are occupied, according to this Bohr Model of the atom for elements with atomic numbers up to eighteen.

Table 1.1. Bohr model shells.

Atomic number	Element	Electronic configuration		
		K	L	M
1	Hydrogen	1	–	–
2	Helium	2	–	–
3	Lithium	2	1	–
4	Beryllium	2	2	–
5	Boron	2	3	–
6	Carbon	2	4	–

(Contd ...)

		Electronic configuration		
Atomic number	Element	K	L	M
7	Nitrogen	2	5	–
8	Oxygen	2	6	–
9	Fluorine	2	7	–
10	Neon	2	8	–
11	Sodium	2	8	1
12	Magnesium	2	8	2
13	Aluminium	2	8	3
14	Silicon	2	8	4
15	Phosphorus	2	8	5
16	Sulphur	2	8	6
17	Chlorine	2	8	7
18	Argon	2	8	8

Elements with full outer shells, e.g. helium with its full K shell and neon with its full K and L shells, are ones which are generally referred to as inert. They do not combine with other elements to form compounds. In comparison, elements with just one electron in their outer shell are particularly active, combining readily with other elements to form compounds—lithium with one electron in the L shell and sodium with one electron in the M shell are examples of such elements. In forming compounds, i.e. bonds with other elements, the aim appears to be to achieve full outer shells. Thus helium is inert because it already has a full outer shell and does not form compounds because it would be impossible for it to do this and still achieve a full outer shell. Sodium, on the other hand, could achieve a full outer shell by donating its one outer shell electron to another element. Chlorine just happens to need one electron to complete a shell and thus sodium forms a compound with chlorine, sodium chloride (NaCl) or common salt, with the result that both sodium and chlorine then achieve the desired full outer shell state. Another way this state can be achieved is by two atoms sharing electrons. Hydrogen atoms combine with themselves to give a molecule, H_2, with each atom sharing an electron with the other so that each then has a full shell.

Therefore, elements are characterised by different numbers of electrons, with these electrons occupying a shell structure around the nucleus. Only electrons outside full shells take part in interactions between atoms, the aim of such interactions being to achieve full shells.

The valency of an element is equal to either the number of electrons in the outermost shell or the number of electrons needed to fill the shell. Thus, sodium has a valency of one since it has just one electron in its outermost shell. Chlorine is just one electron short of a complete shell and so also has a valency of one. Oxygen has two electrons in the K shell and six in the L shell. As it needs two further electrons to complete its outermost shell it has a valency of two. Carbon has two electrons in the K shell and four electrons in the L shell. This means it has a valency of four.

Quantum Numbers

The above discussion has been in terms of the Bohr Model of the atom. This model has long since been supplanted but the concept of shells still applies to modern atomic models. Each electron has four quantum numbers, denoted by n, l, m_l and m_s, with each electron in an atom having its own characteristic set of quantum numbers (Pauli exclusion principle). n is called the principal quantum number and can have an integer value of 1,2,3,4, etc. l is called the angular momentum quantum number and can have an integer value in the range 0 to $(n-1)$; m_l is the magnetic quantum number and can have an integer value in the range 0 to ± 1; m_s is the spin quantum number and can have the value $+\frac{1}{2}$ or $-\frac{1}{2}$.

Consider the situation with n equal to 1. A consequence of this value is, since $(n-1)$ is zero, that l is 0. Because l is zero then m_l is zero. Since m_s can be either $+\frac{1}{2}$ or $-\frac{1}{2}$, then there are just two possible combinations of quantum numbers that can occur with n equal to one. This means that for the $n = 1$, or K shell, there are just two possible electrons.

Consider the situation with n equal to 2, the condition for the L shell. l can have the values 0 or 1, ml the value 0, –1 or +1, and m_s $+\frac{1}{2}$ or $-\frac{1}{2}$.

The possible combinations of quantum numbers for $n = 2$ are thus:

l	m_l	m_s	
0	0	$+\frac{1}{2}$	} 2s Subshell
0	0	$-\frac{1}{2}$	
1	0	$+\frac{1}{2}$	
1	0	$-\frac{1}{2}$	
1	1	$+\frac{1}{2}$	} 2p Subshell
1	1	$-\frac{1}{2}$	
1	–1	$+\frac{1}{2}$	
1	–1	$-\frac{1}{2}$	

There are therefore, a total of eight possible combinations of quantum numbers for the $n = 2$ shell and this shell can accommodate eight electrons. The shell is considered to be made up of two subshells, the s shell where $l = 0$ and the p shell where, $l = 1$.

If n equals 3, the condition for the M shell, then the quantum numbers give eighteen possible combinations for the shell. These can be considered to be in three subshells: the $3s$ with two possible configurations, the $3p$ with six possibilities and the $3d$ with ten. The s shell is where, $l = 0$, the p shell where, $l = 1$ and the d shell where, $l = 2$.

Table 1.2 shows the electronic configurations of elements with atomic numbers up to eighteen.

Table 1.2. Electronic configuration of elements.

		Electronic configuration				
		K $n = 1$	L $n = 2$		M $n = 3$	
Atomic number	Element	1s	2s	2p	3s	3p
1	Hydrogen	1	–	–	–	–
2	Helium	2	–	–	–	–
3	Lithium	2	1	–	–	–
4	Beryllium	2	2	–	–	–
5	Boron	2	2	1	–	–
6	Carbon	2	2	2	–	–
7	Nitrogen	2	2	3	–	–
8	Oxygen	2	2	4	–	–

(Contd ...)

		Electronic configuration				
		K n = 1	L n = 2		M n = 3	
Atomic number	Element	1s	2s	2p	3s	3p
9	Fluorine	2	2	5	–	–
10	Neon	2	2	6	–	–
11	Sodium	2	2	6	1	–
12	Magnesium	2	2	6	2	–
13	Aluminium	2	2	6	2	1
14	Silicon	2	2	6	2	2
15	Phosphorus	2	2	6	2	3
16	Sulphur	2	2	6	2	4
17	Chlorine	2	2	6	2	5
18	Argon	2	2	6	2	6

Size of Atoms

An atom is not something with a firm boundary. If you think of the Bohr Atom model as being similar to the solar system then the edge of the atom might be compared with the orbit of the outer planet, i.e. Pluto. However, modern views of the atom lead to a less-defined picture with an electron only having a certain probability that it can be found at a certain distance from the nucleus, there no longer being the certainty that it will be in some particular well-defined orbit. The size of the atom might then be defined by the boundary, within which there is a 90 per cent or perhaps 99 per cent chance of finding the outer electron. Another way is by specifying the boundary in terms of how close atoms are packed in solids. Thus, the radius of an atom would be half the distance between centres of atoms when they are packed together in some crystal structure. With such a method of specifying size, account must be taken of whether the structure has the atom as an ion rather than as a neutral atom. Removing an electron from an atom, to give a positive ion, will reduce the effective size of the atom while adding an electron, to give a negative ion, will increase the size.

Table 1.3 shows the sizes generally specified for some common atoms.

Table 1.3. Sizes of atoms.

Element	Atomic number	Atom radius (nm)
Aluminium	13	0.143
Cadmium	48	0.150
Carbon	6	0.071
Chlorine	17	0.107
Chromium	24	0.125
Cobalt	27	0.125
Copper	29	0.128
Hydrogen	1	0.046
Iron	26	0.124

(Contd ...)

6 Physical Metallurgy

Element	Atomic number	Atom radius (nm)
Lead	82	0.175
Magnesium	12	0.160
Manganese	25	0.112
Molybdenum	42	0.136
Nickel	28	0.125
Nitrogen	7	0.071
Oxygen	8	0.060
Phosphorus	15	0.109
Sodium	11	0.186
Tin	50	0.158
Titanium	22	0.147
Tungsten	74	0.137
Vanadium	23	0.132
Zinc	30	0.133

Bonds

The way in which atoms join together, or molecules join together, is called bonding. The following are the different types of bonding (Fig. 1.2) that can occur; the type of bonding existing within a material determines many of its properties.

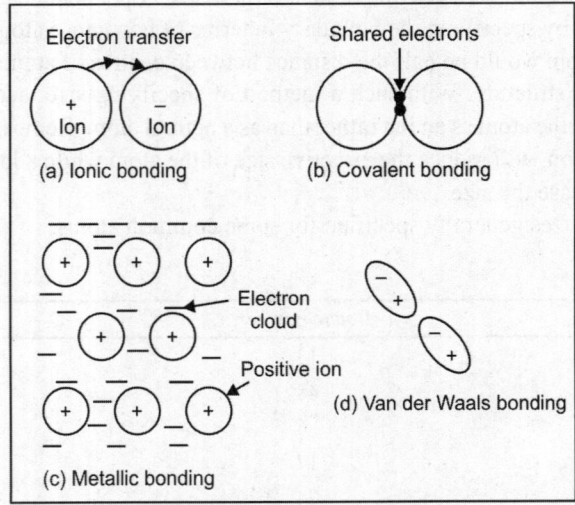

Fig. 1.2. Types of bonds.

Ionic bonding

An individual atom is electrically neutral, having as much positive charge as negative charge. However, if an atom loses an electron it must then have a net positive charge. It is then referred to as an ion—in this case, a positive ion. If an atom gains an extra electron it ends up with a net negative charge, becoming a negative ion. In an ionically bonded material an atom of one element gives an electron to an atom of another element. One element then consists of positive ions and the other of negative ions. Unlike-charged bodies attract each other thus, there is a force of attraction between the atoms of the two constituent elements in the material.

Sodium chloride, common salt, is an example of an ionic bonded material. In order for the sodium and the chlorine atoms to assume the 'full shell' configuration for their atoms the sodium has to lose an electron and the chlorine gain one. The transfer of an electron from a sodium atom to a chlorine atom enables this to happen and provides a bond between the atoms [Fig. 1.2(a)]. Sodium chloride exists as a vast structure of sodium and chlorine ions rather than just as a single pair of ions. In such an array like-charged ions repel each other and unlike-charged ions attract each other. Thus sodium ions repel sodium ions, chlorine ions repel chlorine ions, but sodium and chlorine ions attract each other. A stable structure results because sodium and chlorine ions alternate and the attractive forces are just enough to overcome the repulsive forces.

With ionic bonding there is no directionality of forces and hence no directionality of bonding. Materials with this form of bonding have high melting and boiling points since the bond is a very strong one.

Covalent bonding

Ionic bonding is not possible with some elements because the energy required to remove electrons in outer shells is too great. An alternative way by which atoms of such elements can realise the 'full shell' configuration is by sharing electrons with neighbours. Thus a hydrogen molecule involves two hydrogen atoms, each atom having just one electron, sharing a pair of electrons [Fig. 1.2(b)]. This type of bond, called a covalent bond, can be thought of as two positive ions held together by the pair of electrons located between them, each ion being attracted to the electrons.

An atom may share electrons with more than one other atom, if by doing so it can achieve the 'full shell' configuration. Thus, for example, carbon needs four electrons to obtain a 'full shell', whereas chlorine requires only one. Thus the compound carbon tetrachloride, CCl_4, consists of a carbon atom bonded by covalent bonds to four chlorine atoms. Each chlorine atom shares one of the carbon electrons and the carbon atom obtains a share in one electron from each of the four chlorine atoms (Fig. 1.3). A convenient way of representing such bonds is by a line linking atoms, each line representing a pair of electrons being shared.

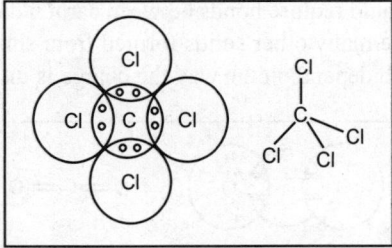

Fig. 1.3. The carbon tetrachloride molecule

The atoms in some molecules can have bonds involving more than one pair of shared electrons. Where two pairs are shared the bond is said to be a double bond, where three pairs a triple bond. Oxygen molecules are composed of two oxygen atoms with two pairs of shared electrons [Fig. 1.4(a)]. Carbon dioxide molecules consist of a carbon atom with two oxygen atoms, the bonds between each oxygen atom and the carbon being double bonds.

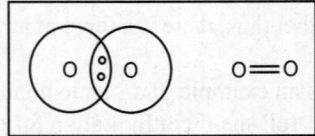

Fig. 1.4. The oxygen molecule.

Covalent bonds are directional bonds, the bond only occurring in the direction of the shared pair, or pairs, of electrons. These directions are determined by the repulsive forces that occur between the pair involved in the bond and other electrons in the outer shell of the atoms. Covalent bonds are very strong bonds. Diamond is an example of a material formed as a result of covalent bonds, the bonds being between carbon atoms, with each atom forming bonds with four other atoms.

Metallic bonding

Metals have atoms from which electrons are readily released. Thus, for example, copper with an atomic number of 29 has full K, L and M shells and just one electron in the N shell. This odd electron is only very loosely attached to the copper atom. In solid copper these electrons become detached from the atoms leaving a positive copper ion. The electrons that have been detached do not combine with any ion but remain as a cloud of negative charge floating between the ions. The result is bonding, the positive ions being held together by their attraction to the cloud or negative charge in which they are embedded [Fig. 1.2(c)]. Such bonds are not directional and are, in general, weaker than ionic or covalent bonds.

Because the metal ions are not bonded directly to each other but to the electron cloud, a metallic solid can be formed from a mixture of two or more metallic elements, the result being called an alloy. Because of this form of bonding it is not necessary for the constituents of an alloy to be present in fixed proportions, as is necessary with compounds and structures formed by ionic or covalent bonding.

Van der Waals bonding

Carbon dioxide has a molecule formed by a carbon atom bonding with covalent bonds to two oxygen atoms (Fig. 1.5). Since the molecule has electrons already participating in a molecular bond there are no electrons available to participate in further bonds. One might imagine from this that solid carbon dioxide would not be possible since it would require bonds between carbon dioxide molecules. However, solid carbon dioxide is possible, as are many other solids formed from similar molecules. Molecular solids are held together by forces which depend on the way the charge is distributed within a molecule.

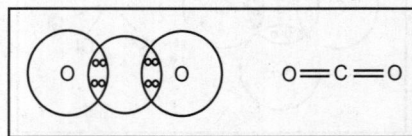

Fig. 1.5. The carbon dioxide molecule.

The water molecule consists of two hydrogen atoms with bonds to an oxygen atom, as shown in Fig. 1.6. The electrons tend to be more concentrated at the oxygen end of the molecule than the hydrogen ends, which can be conceived as essentially bare protons. The result is what is termed an electric dipole.

Forces can occur between such dipoles such that bonding can occur when the dipoles align themselves to result in unlike-charged ends in close proximity (Fig. 1.7). Such bonding forces are much weaker than ionic, covalent or metallic bonds.

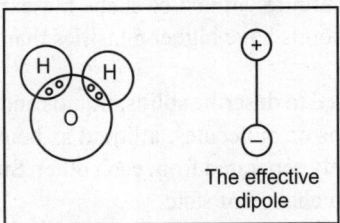

Fig. 1.6. The water dipole.

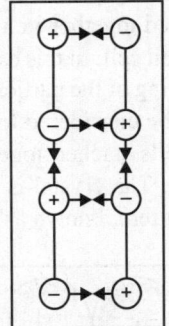

Fig. 1.7. Bonding between dipoles.

It is also possible to have dipole forces used for bonding where molecules are not permanent dipoles like the water molecule. The hydrogen atom can be considered to consist of a single electron orbiting a proton. At some point we can conceive the electron being at a particular position and the hydrogen atom being a dipole orientated in a particular direction. This instantaneous dipole can exert forces on neighbouring hydrogen atoms.

It will attract the unlike charge and repel the like charge with the result that a neighbouring hydrogen atom becomes a dipole orientated in such a way that it is attracted to the initial dipole. A pond then occurs. This form of bond is called a van der Waals bond. Such bonds are much weaker than ionic, covalent or metallic bonds.

A comparable effect occurs when a charged piece of plastic is brought close to a small piece of (uncharged) paper—the paper becomes attracted to the plastic. This is because the charge on the paper becomes redistributed as a result of the presence of the plastic; the charge of the same sign as that on the plastic being repelled to the remote parts of the paper while the opposite sign is attracted to the nearer ends of the paper.

The result is that there is a smaller distance between the unlike charges and a greater distance between like charges. Hence a net attractive force occurs.

Ionic, covalent and metallic bonds are termed primary bonds, while the bonds resulting form either permanent or induced dipoles are called secondary bonds. Primary bonds are much stronger than secondary bonds.

States of Matter

Materials can be classified as having three possible states: gas, liquid or solid. Solids have definite shapes and volumes. Liquids have definite volumes but can alter their shape to take up the shape of a containing vessel. Gases have no definite volume or shape but expand until they fill any container in which they are placed. In general, solids have higher densities than their liquids and these in turn have higher densities than their gases.

A simple model which can be used to describe solids, liquids and gases is to consider a solid as being a well-packed arrangement of atoms or molecules, a liquid as being a jumbled heap of such particles and a gas as being the particles widely separated from each other. Such a model can explain the changes in density occurring when there is a change of state.

CRYSTALS

The form of crystals and the way in which they grow can be explained if matter is considered to be made up of small particles which are packed together in a regular manner, as in Fig. 1.8. The dotted lines in Fig. 1.8 enclose what is called the unit cell. In this case the unit cell is a cube. The unit cell is the geometric figure which illustrates the grouping of the particles in the solid. This group is repeated many times in space within a crystal, which can be considered to be made up, in the case of a simple cubic crystal, of a large number of these unit cells stacked together. Figure 1.9 shows that portion of the stacked spheres that is within the unit cell. The crystal is considered to consist of large numbers of particles arranged in a regular, repetitive pattern, known as the space lattice.

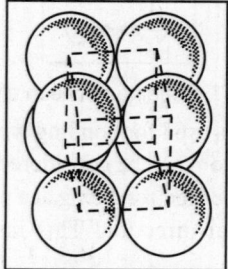

Fig. 1.8. A simple cubic structure.

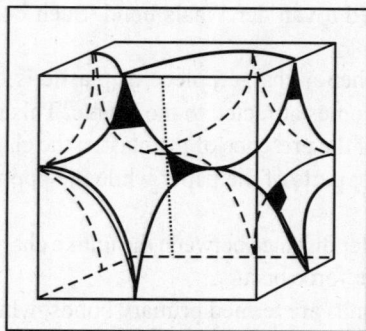

Fig. 1.9. The simple cubic structure unit cell.

It is this regular, repetitive pattern of particles that characterises crystalline material. A solid having no such order in the arrangement of its constituent particles is said to be amorphous.

The simple cubic crystal shape is arrived at by stacking spheres in one particular way (Fig. 1.8). By stacking spheres in different ways, other crystal shapes can be produced. With the simple cubic unit cell the centres of the spheres lie at the corners of a cube. With the body-centred cubic unit cell the cell is slightly more complex than the simple cubic cell in that it has an extra sphere in the centre of the cell. The face-centred cubic cell is another modification of the simple cubic cell, having spheres at the centre of each face of the cube. Another common arrangement is the hexagonal close packed structure.

Packing Factor

An important feature of the different forms of crystal structure is the amount of free space within the structure. This affects the movement of foreign atoms to within the structure and the ease with which the structure can deform, The fraction of a unit cell that is occupied by atoms is called the packing factor. The larger the packing factor the greater the fraction of the unit cell occupied and so the smaller the amount of free space.

Consider the simple cubic structure unit cell shown in Fig. 1.9. Within the unit cell there is effectively one atom (this figure being obtained by counting up the volumes of the pieces of atom considered to lie within the unit cell). If the radius of an atom is r then the total volume occupied by the atoms in the unit cell is $1 \times \frac{4\pi r^3}{3}$. The length of a side of the unit cell is $2r$ and its total volume is $(2r)^3$. Hence the

$$\text{Packing fraction} = \frac{1 \times \frac{4\pi r^3}{3}}{(2r)^3}$$

$$= 0.52$$

This means that 52 per cent of the unit cell is occupied, the remaining 48 per cent being free space. For the face-centred cubic structure, the number of atoms within the unit cell is four and hence the occupied volume is $4 \times \frac{4\pi r^3}{3}$. The unit cell has a face diagonal of length $4r$ and hence a side of length L given by (using Pythagoras theorem):

$$(4r)^2 = L^2 + L^2$$

$$L = \frac{4r}{\sqrt{2}}$$

Hence the volume of the unit cell is $(4r/\sqrt{2})^3$.

$$\text{Packing fraction} = \frac{1 \times \frac{4\pi r^3}{3}}{(4r/\sqrt{2})}$$

$$= 0.74$$

Thus compared with the simple cubic structure the face-centred cubic structure is more closely packed.

Table 1.4 shows the packing factors for the different unit cells. The hexagonal close-packed and the face-centred cubic structures are therefore the most close-packed structures. Metallic solids tend to form the most densely packed structures although some will give the other structures because of the existence of some directionality in the way the atoms bond together.

Table 1.4. Packing fractions.

Unit cell structure	Packing fraction
Simple cubic	0.52
Face-centred cubic	0.74
Body-centred cubic	0.68
Hexagonal close-packed	0.74

Structure and Properties

The way in which atoms, or molecules, are packed together in a material is called the structure of that material. Sodium chloride—common salt is composed of sodium ions, positive, and chlorine ions, negative. These are arranged in the simple cubic structure illustrated in Figure 1.9. A single crystal of sodium chloride, however, consists of large numbers of sodium and chlorine ions all bonded together by ionic bonds, in this cubic form into an enormous structure. Figure 1.10 illustrates part of this structure. Such a structure is three-dimensional in the sense that ions are held in place by bonds in three dimensions.

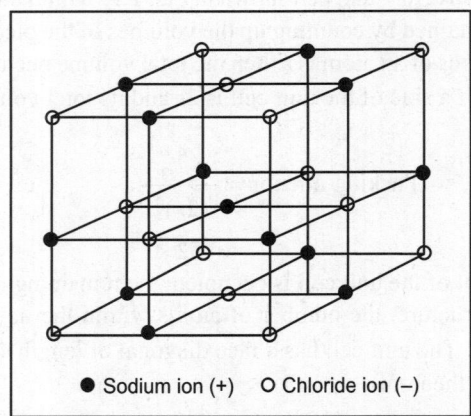

Fig. 1.10. Part of a giant structure—sodium chloride crystal—showing the position of the ions.

Diamond is an example of a crystal structure based solely on carbon atoms. Each atom is bound, by covalent bonding, to four other carbon atoms in a tetrahedral arrangement. Figure 1.11 illustrates this arrangement and shows how an enormous three-dimensional structure can be built up. The strength of these bonds between the carbon atoms and the uniform arrangement in which each atom is held in its place in the structure makes diamond a very hard material.

Graphite—the lead in pencils—is, by contrast, a very soft material. It is because layers of graphite can be easily removed that it finds a use as pencil lead. Graphite also, like diamond, consists only of carbon atoms. However, the way in which the carbon atoms are arranged in the solid is different and it is because of this difference that carbon has different properties in graphite and in diamond. Figure 1.12 shows the structure of graphite.

It can be considered to be a 'layered' structure since the atoms are strongly bonded together with covalent bonds, in two-dimensional layers, with only very weak bonds, Van der Waal bonds, between the atoms in different layers.

Basic Structure of Materials 13

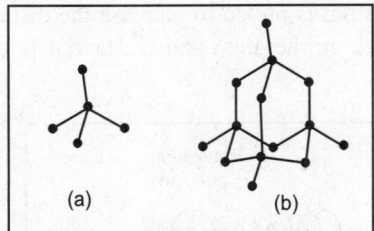

Fig. 1.11. (a) The bonding arrangement for the carbon atoms in diamond, and (b) part of the three-dimensional structure of diamond.

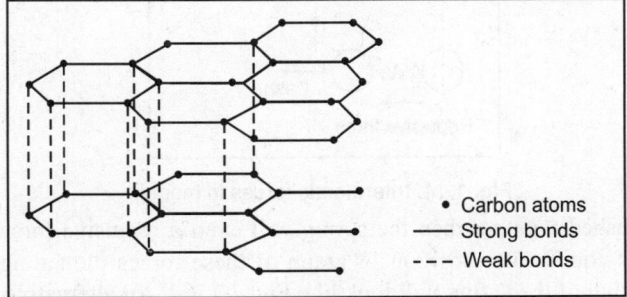

Fig. 1.12. The layered structure of graphite.

The way in which atoms, or molecules, are packed together thus markedly affects the properties.

Interatomic Forces in Crystals

A simple model for a crystal, whatever the form of the crystal, is that of an orderly array of spheres to represent the atoms with the spheres linked one with another by springs to represent the interatomic bonds. Figure 1.13 shows such a model. To move one atom aside from its equilibrium position means stretching or compressing springs.

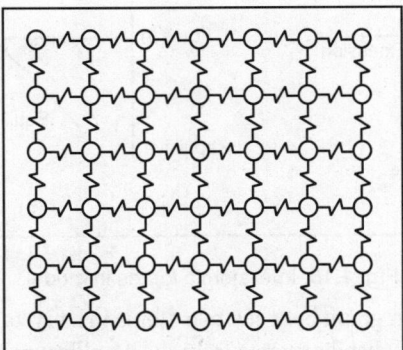

Fig. 1.13. Simple model of a crystal.

For simplicity, consider the stretching and compressing of just one spring (Fig. 1.14). Assuming that the spring obeys Hooke's law then the forces required to extend or compress it are proportional to the extension or compression. If one atom is pulled to increase the distance between the atoms then the spring will exert an attractive force on the atom and endeavour to attract it back to its equilibrium position.

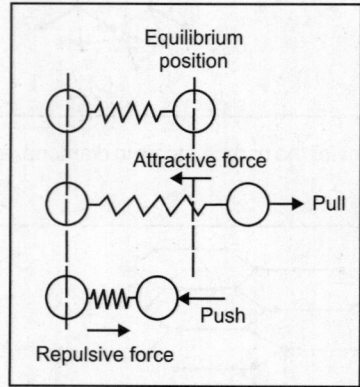

Fig. 1.14. Interatomic forces in model.

If the atoms are pushed together then the spring will exert a repulsive force in an endeavour to restore the atom to its equilibrium position. A graph of these forces plotted against the amount of stretching or compressing of the spring will look like Fig. 1.15(a). An alternative way of drawing this graph is shown in Fig. 1.15(b). At the equilibrium position the force acting on an atom is zero. If the separation of atoms is increased there is an attractive force which increases as the separation increases. If the separation of the atoms is decreased there is a repulsive force which increases as the separation is decreased.

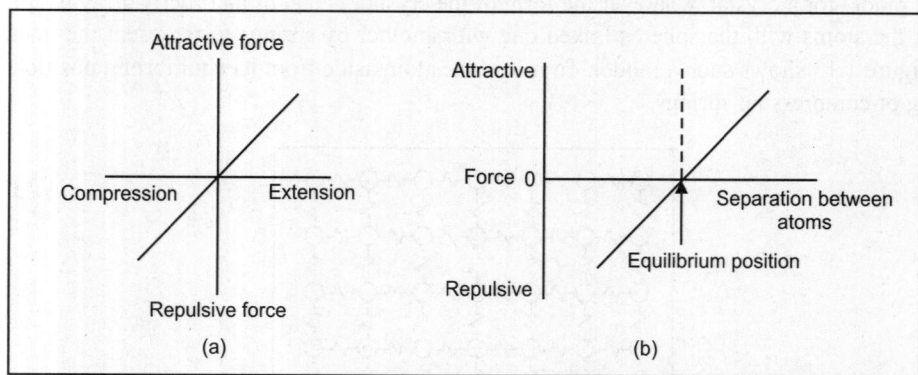

Fig. 1.15. Interatomic forces in model.

In general the force-separation graph between two atoms in a crystal is considered to have the form shown in Fig. 1.16. This, at small displacements from the equilibrium position, is rather like the result derived from a consideration of the simple balls and springs model.

Consider stretching the simple model of the crystal is shown in Fig. 1.13. Figure 1.17 shows the edges of two planes of atoms which are at right angles to the stretching forces.

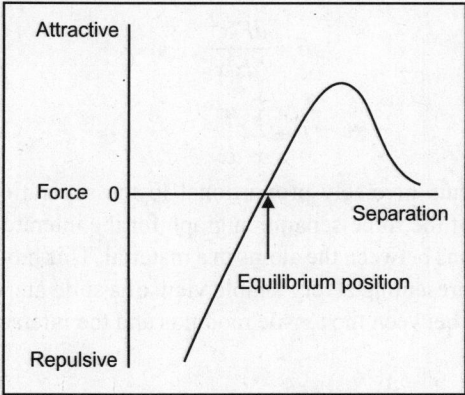

Fig. 1.16. Interatomic forces in a crystal.

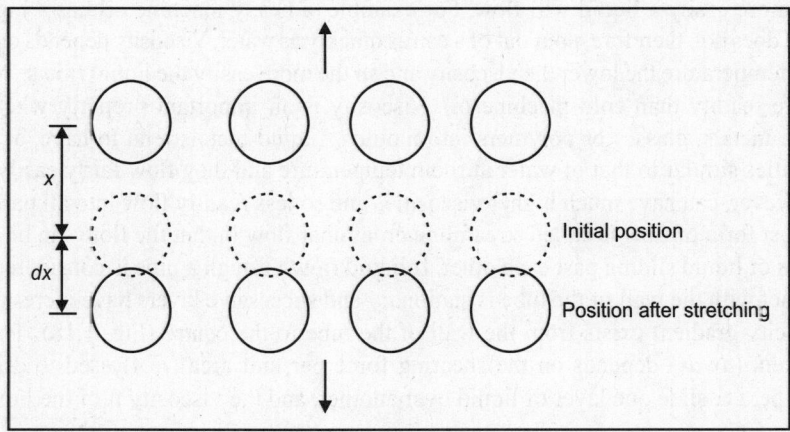

Fig. 1.17. Stretching the crystal model.

If the cross-sectional area of the material is A and the atomic separation is x, then the number of atoms in such an area: is A/x^2. The action of stretching causes each pair of atoms across the plane to resist being stretched. If the attractive force between each pair of atoms is dF when the material is stretched by an amount dx, then:

$$\text{Total resisting force} = \frac{A}{x^2}dF$$

and so

$$\text{Stress} = \frac{\text{Force}}{\text{Area}} = \frac{dF}{x^2}$$

Strain = Extension per unit length

$$= \frac{dx}{x}$$

The tensile modulus (Young's modulus) E is stress/strain, hence:

$$E = \frac{dF/x^2}{dx/x}$$

$$E = \frac{1}{x}\frac{dF}{dx}$$

The tensile modulus is thus inversely proportional to the separation of the atoms and directly proportional to the gradient of the force-separation graph for the interatomic forces. The modulus is a characteristic of the interactions between the atoms in a material. This model of a crystalline solid must, however, be taken as only representing a very simple view of a solid and so the above result is only an indication of the relationship between the tensile modulus and the interactions between the atoms.

Liquids

A characteristic of liquids is that they can be made to flow. Some liquids flow more easily than others and the property used to describe the ease with which a liquid flows is called viscosity. The lower the viscosity the more easily a liquid will flow. For example, a heavy machine oil has a higher viscosity than water and does not, therefore, pour out of a can as quickly as water. Viscosity depends on temperature; the higher the temperature the lower the viscosity and so the more easily the liquid flows. Warm machine oil flows more readily than cold machine oil. Viscosity is an important property when it comes to pouring liquid metals, glasses or polymers into moulds. Liquid metals tend to have, at their melting points, viscosities similar to that of water at room temperature and they flow fairly easily. Glasses and polymers, however, can have much higher viscosities and so less readily flow into all parts of a mould.

The simplest form of flow is called streamline or laminar flow in that the flow can be considered in terms of layers of liquid sliding past each other. If liquid flow through a pipe is considered, the layer of liquid in contact with the wall of the tube is stationary and successive layers have increasing velocities so that a velocity gradient exists from the wall of the tube to the centre (Fig. 1.18). The size of this velocity gradient (dv/dx) depends on the shearing force per unit area (F/A) used to drive the liquid through the pipe, i.e. slide one layer of liquid over another, and the viscosity η of the liquid.

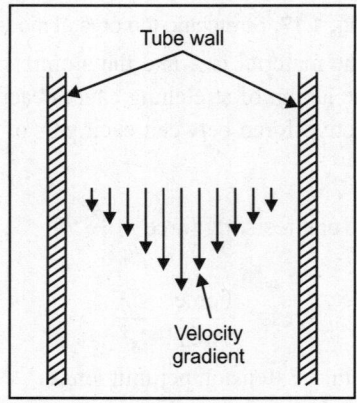

Fig. 1.18. Viscous flow.

A liquid consists of large numbers of molecules in random motion; the higher the temperature the greater the average molecular speed. When there is laminar flow there is an orderly velocity in a particular direction, superimposed on top of the random molecular velocity, such that molecules in one layer have an orderly velocity slightly greater than that in the adjacent layer (Fig. 1.19). The random motion of the molecules carries them across the layers in both directions. This means that the layer with the faster orderly velocity will lose some of its molecules and gain some of the molecules from the slower moving layer. The net result is that its molecules will have a lower average orderly velocity. We can think of this faster moving layer of liquid being dragged back by the existence of the adjacent slower moving layer. It is this drag which we call viscosity.

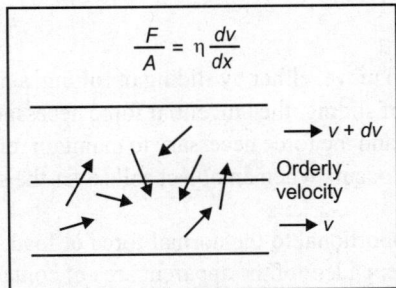

Fig. 1.19. Molecular motion with laminar flow.

We can explain the decrease in viscosity resulting from an increase in temperature by considering that a higher temperature means a higher average random molecular speed—more molecules move per second from one layer to another. Not only do molecules in a slower moving layer move into a faster moving layer but molecules in a faster moving layer move into a slower moving layer. The effect of this movement between layers being increased is that a greater number of molecules are accelerated by the pressure used to move the liquid. An increased rate of flow means a lower viscosity.

The viscosity of many liquids is independent of the velocity gradient in the liquid. This means that the velocity gradient is proportional to the applied pressure. If the pressure is doubled the velocity gradient is doubled. The liquid flows no more easily with a high velocity gradient than with a low velocity gradient. Such liquids are called Newtonian liquids. There are however liquids, notably polymers, which decrease in viscosity when the velocity gradient increases. Non-drip paints are such liquids. In the tin the paint has a high viscosity. When it is being brushed onto a surface, i.e. a velocity gradient is occurring, the viscosity decreases and the paint flows quite easily. When the brushing ceases, i.e. the velocity gradient is reduced, the paint becomes more viscous and so does not so readily flow and drip.

Polymers are long chain molecules. These long chains become easily tangled with each other. The paint in the tin consists of tangled molecules and because of this does not flow easily. When the paint is brushed the act of brushing aligns many molecules so that their chains point in the same direction. This allows them to slide more easily over one another and so the viscosity decreases.

SURFACES

Molecules in the bulk of a liquid are surrounded by other molecules and are subjected to attractive forces which are roughly the same in all directions. At the surface of the liquid, however, the molecules have no liquid molecules above them, only below resulting in a net attractive force downwards into the liquid on surface molecules. If the surface of a liquid is to be increased more molecules have to be moved into the surface against the attractive force. Energy is thus required to increase surface area. This is referred to as the free surface energy. The free surface energy is defined as the energy required to produce unit area of surface. It has the symbol γ and units of J/m². Water, at room temperature, has a free surface energy of about 0.070 J/m². The free surface energies of liquid metals, however, are much higher, e.g. molten aluminium 0.50 J/m² and molten iron 1.50 J/m². In the same way that liquids have free surface energies, so also do solids. Atoms in the bulk of a solid are subject to attractive forces in all directions while those in the surface are subject to only inward-directed forces. Thus to increase the surface area of a solid requires energy. This is discussed later in connection with the propagation of cracks through solids. When a crack propagates, new solid surfaces are produced and this requires energy.

Friction

When one object moves or tends to move, either by sliding or rolling, against another the force opposing this is called friction. In the case of sliding, the tangential force necessary to start relative movement of the objects is called static friction and the force necessary to maintain relative motion is called kinetic or dynamic friction. Rolling friction occurs when an object rolls over the surface of another object. There are two basic laws of friction:

1. The frictional force is proportional to the normal force or load.
2. The frictional force is independent of the apparent area of contact between the sliding surfaces.

A consequence of the first law is that for any particular pair of surfaces the ratio of frictional force to normal force is a constant. This constant is called the coefficient of friction (μ).

$$\mu = \frac{\text{Frictional force } F}{\text{Normal force } N}$$

The second law uses the term 'apparent area of contact' in relation to the sliding surfaces. This is because when two surfaces are in contact the real contact between them occurs at only a limited number of discrete points. No matter how smooth a surface, on a molecular scale it is very irregular. Hence contact tends to occur at only the peaks of the surface irregularities (Fig. 1.20). The real area of contact is only a very small fraction of the apparent area of contact. It is these small, real, contact areas that have to carry the load between the surfaces.

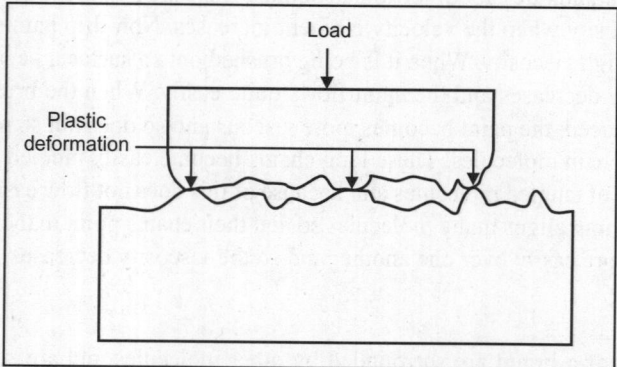

Fig. 1.20. Real contact points between surfaces.

Because the real area of contact between surfaces is so small the pressures at the contact points will be very high, even under light loading. In the case of metals, this pressure will generally be high enough to cause appreciable plastic deformation. The greater the load the more the material will deform and so the greater will the real area of contact become. The points of contact crush down plastically until the area of contact is sufficiently large to support the load at the yield pressure. The true area of contact A is, given by:

$$A = \frac{\text{Normal force } N}{\text{Yield pressure } p}$$

The yield pressure is equal to the indentation hardness value obtained for the metal as a result of a hardness test such as the Brinell test. A consequence of the above equation is that the true area of contact is proportional to the normal force and hence the second law of friction could be written as: the frictional force is proportional to the real area of contact between the sliding surfaces.

The pressures at the real points of contact between two surfaces are very high and as a consequence strong adhesion takes place between the two surfaces at these points. With metals the process is cold welding. When the surfaces slide over each other these junctions between the surfaces must be sheared. The frictional force thus arises from the force to shear junctions and the force required to plough the asperities of one surface through those of the other surface. In general this 'ploughing' term is relatively small and most of the frictional force is due to the shearing of junctions. Thus, to a reasonable approximation:

$$\text{Shear strength} = \frac{\text{Fractional force } (F)}{\text{True area } (A)}$$

$$= \frac{\mu N}{N/p}$$

Hence,
$$\mu = \frac{\text{Shear strength}}{\text{Yield pressure}}$$

The shear strength concerned in the above equation is that of the softer material of a sliding pair. Thus for a low coefficient of friction, and hence low frictional forces, a low yield strength and high yield pressure, i.e. hardness, is required. Such a combination would appear to be impossible since metals with a high hardness have a high shear strength. If, however, a hard metal is coated with a thin layer of soft metal, the load can be borne by the hard metal, since the asperities would penetrate the soft layer, but the greatest area of contact would be with the soft layer. Consequently, an increase in load may produce only a very small change in the real area of contact with the hard surface. The result is a low coefficient of friction. Thus surface coatings and surface treatments can be used to give low frictional forces. To keep frictional forces low between plain bearing surfaces the materials used are generally compounded to give either small particles of a hard phase embedded in a soft matrix or softer phase material dispersed throughout a hard matrix. With the hard particles within the soft matrix it is considered that the hard particles support the load while the sliding takes place within a thin smeared film of the softer material. There is some doubt as to whether this is actually the mechanism that occurs. Materials based on this principle are the white metals. In the case of the softer materials being dispersed throughout the hard matrix, when sliding occurs the soft material becomes smeared over the surface and the result is similar to that produced by a soft metal layer being used to coat a hard surface. Copper-lead alloys are examples of this type of material.

Frictional forces involve only the surface layers of materials. However, most metals exposed to air become coated with an oxide film or adsorbed gas. In addition the surfaces may be coated with a layer of dirt. All such layers affect the frictional forces. Lubricants are used to interpose films between moving surfaces so that friction is reduced. The lubricant film reduces the number and area of the metallic junctions between the sliding surfaces.

The wear of surfaces can be explained in terms of the adhesion occurring between the points of real contact between surfaces. The term 'wear' is used for the unintentional removal of material from two rubbing surfaces. Four different forms of wear situation can be considered to exist.

1. When the junctions between the surfaces are weaker than the sliding materials, shearing occurs at the interface and there is little transfer of metal from one surface to the other, i.e. little wear occurs. An example of this is a tin-base alloy sliding on steel.
2. When the junctions are stronger than one of the metals but weaker than the other, shearing takes place a small distance within the softer material. Wear of the softer material thus occurs and eventually a film of softer material builds up on the harder surface. An example of this is a lead base alloy sliding on steel.
3. When the junctions are stronger than both metals, shearing will take place mainly in the softer of the two metals but some fragments of the harder metal may be ploughed out. An example of this is copper sliding on steel.
4. When both the sliding surfaces are the same, the process of deformation and sliding causes the junction material to work harder. As a consequence of this shearing occurs within both the metals and considerable wear can occur.

Rolling friction is considered to mainly occur as a result of the energy lost by the elastic deformation and recovery of the surface over which the rolling occurs. It is an elastic hysteresis effect. The surface becomes elastically deformed as the ball begins to roll over it and after the ball has passed the surface recovers but the deformation of the surface is greater than the energy released when it recovers. The result is an energy loss, this being the rolling friction loss. In the above discussion it has been assumed that plastic deformation of the surface does not occur as the ball rolls over it, e.g. a permanent groove being produced. In such a case energy would be needed for the plastic deformation. When a ball bearing rolls in its race, only elastic deformation occurs and since for the steels involved the hysteresis losses are very small the rolling resistance is very small. Typically the rolling coefficient of friction is about 0.001. This is not the only source of friction with a ball and roller bearing since the balls are surrounded by a cage to keep them apart and prevent them rubbing on each other. Friction between the balls and the cage can be greater than that between the balls and the race, hence the use of a lubricant to reduce it. The material used for the cage must also be one that has a low coefficient of friction with respect to the steel used for the ball bearings.

With metals sliding on metals the true area of contact between them is proportional to the normal force and so the frictional force is proportional to the normal force. Hence the coefficient of friction, the ratio of frictional force to normal force, is a constant and independent of the value of the normal force. With polymers, sliding on metals or polymers this is not generally true. Polymers deform visco-elastically and the true area of contact depends on time as well as the normal force. A consequence of this is that the frictional force is proportional to (normal force), where, x has a value of about three-quarters, and hence a coefficient of friction that tends to decrease with increasing load.

Table 1.5 gives typical values of the kinetic coefficient of sliding friction.

Table 1.5. Kinetic coefficients of friction.

Materials involved	Coefficient of kinetic friction
Mild steel on mild steel	0.5
White metal on steel	0.5
Copper-lead alloy on steel	0.2
Phosphor bronze on steel	0.4
Nylon on nylon	0.3
Nylon on steel	0.2
PTFE on PTFE	0.05
Bronze impregnated with PTFE on steel	0.05

METALS AS CRYSTALLINE

Metals are crystalline substances. The term grain is used to describe the crystals within the metal. A grain is merely a crystal without its geometrical shape and flat faces because its growth was impeded by contact with other crystals. Within a grain the arrangement of particles is just as regular and repetitive as within a crystal with smooth faces. A simple model of a metal with its grains is given by the raft of bubbles on the surface of a liquid. The bubbles pack together in an orderly and repetitive manner but if 'growth' is started at a number of centres then 'grains' are produced. At the boundaries between the 'grains' the regular pattern breaks down as the pattern changes from the orderly pattern of one 'grain' to that of the next 'grain'.

The grains in the surface of a metal are not generally visible. They can be made visible by careful etching of the surface with a suitable chemical. The chemical preferentially attacks the grain boundaries. Examples of the different forms of crystal structure adopted by metallic elements are shown in Table 1.6.

Table 1.6. Crystal structure adopted by metallic elements.

Body-centred cubic	Face-centred cubic	Hexagonal close-packed
Chromium	Aluminium	Beryllium
Molybdenum	Copper	Cadmium
Niobium	Lead	Magnesium
Tungsten	Nickel	Zinc

Growth of Metal Crystals

Figure 1.21 shows the various stages that can occur when a metal solidifies. Crystallisation, whether with metals or any other substances, occurs round small nuclei, which may be impurity particles. The initial crystals that form have the shape of the crystal pattern into which the metal normally solidifies, e.g. face-centred cubic in the case of copper.

However, as the crystal grows it tends to develop spikes. The shape of the growing crystal thus changes into a 'treelike' growth called a dendrite. As the dendrite grows so the spaces between the arms of the dendrite fill up.

Outward growth of the dendrites ceases when the growing arms meet other dendrite arms. Eventually the entire liquid solidifies. When this happens there is little trace of the dendrite structure, only the grains into which the dendrites have grown.

22 Physical Metallurgy

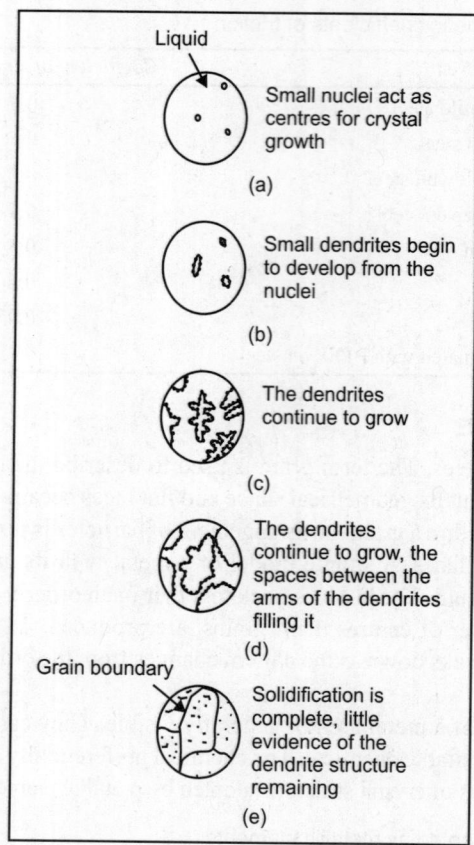

Fig. 1.21. Solidification of a metal.

Why do metals tend to grow from the melt as dendrites? Energy is needed to change a solid, at its melting point, to a liquid without any change in temperature occurring; this energy is called latent heat. Similarly, when a liquid at the fusion point (i.e. the melting point) changes to a solid, energy has to be removed, no change in temperature occurring during the change of state; this is the latent heat. Thus, when the liquid metal in the immediate vicinity of the metal crystal face solidifies, energy is released which warms up the liquid in front of that advancing crystal face. This slows, or stops, further growth in that direction. The result of this action is that spikes develop as the crystal grows in the directions in which the liquid is coolest. As these warm up in turn, so secondary, and then tertiary, spikes develop as the growth continues in these directions in which the liquid is coolest.

BLOCK SLIP MODEL

A simple theory to explain the elastic and plastic behaviour of metals is tile 'block slip' theory, where a metal is considered to be made of blocks of atoms which can move relative to each other. When a stress is applied to the metal, blocks of atoms become displaced (Fig. 1.22). When the yield stress is reached there is movement of large blocks of atoms as they slip past each other, the plane along which this movement occurs being the slip plane.

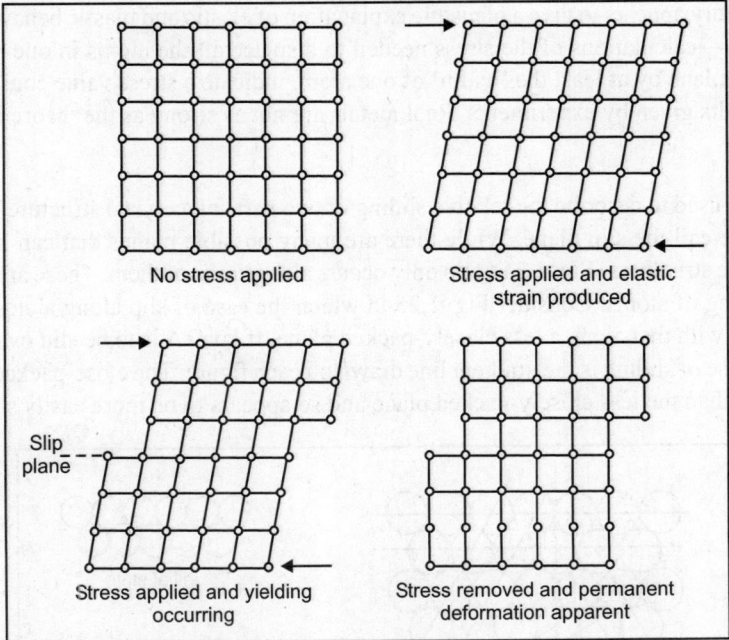

Fig. 1.22. 'Block slip' model showing plastic behaviour of metals under stress.

Metals are composed of many crystals. A crystal within a metal is just a region of orderly packed atoms. Such a region is generally referred to as a grain. The surfaces that divide the different regions of orderly packed atoms are termed grain boundaries. When plastic deformation occurs in a metal, movement occurs along slip planes and the result is rather like Fig. 1.23. Slip occurs only in those planes which are at suitable angles to the applied stress.

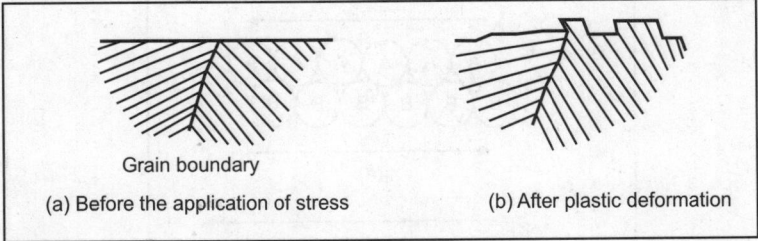

Fig. 1.23. Grain boundary (a) Before the application of stress, and (b) after plastic deformation.

The result is that the surface of the metal shows a series of steps due to the different movements of the various planes of atoms. These can be seen under a microscope. The slip lines do not cross over from one grain to another; the grain boundaries restrict the slip to within a grain. Thus the bigger the grains the more slippage that can occur; this would show itself as a greater plastic deformation. A fine grain structure should therefore have less slippage and so show less plastic deformation, i.e. be less ductile. A brittle material is thus one in which each little slip process is confined to a short run in the metal and not allowed to spread, a ductile material is one in which the slip process is not confined to a short run in the metal and does spread over a large part of the metal.

While this theory appears to give a plausible explanation of elastic and plastic behaviour there is one big disadvantage—calculations of the stress needed to displace all the atoms in one plane relative to those in the next plane by at least the 'width' of one atom, indicate a stress value considerably greater than the real results given by experiments. Real metals are not as strong as the theoretical model.

Slip Planes

The term 'slip' is used to describe the relative sliding of two parts of a crystal structure on either side of a plane which we call the slip plane. While there are many possible planes that can be considered to exist in crystalline structures (Fig. 1.24), slip only occurs along some of them. These are the planes with the closest packing of atoms. Consider Fig. 1.25 in which the ease of slip along a close-packed plane can be compared with that along a less closely-packed plane. If layer A is to be slid over layer B then a measure of the ease of sliding is the gradient line drawn on each figure. The close-packed plane involves a lower gradient than the less closely-packed plane and so appears to be more easily slid.

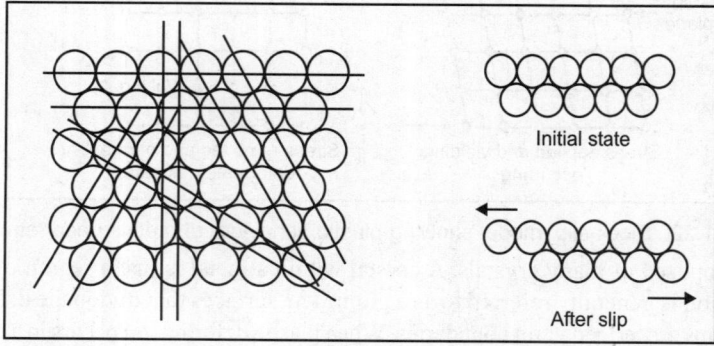

Fig. 1.24. Some of the possible planes in a regularly-packed array of atoms.

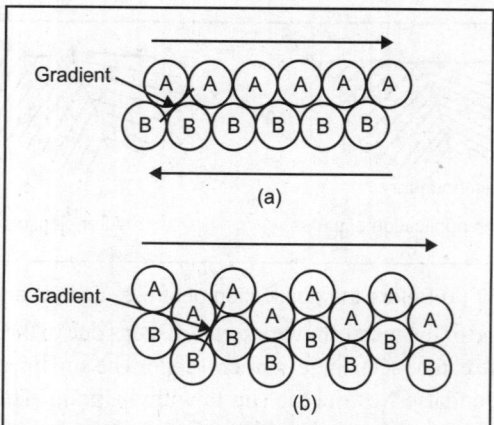

Fig. 1.25. Ease of sliding with different planes, (a) close-packed plane, and (b) less closely-packed plane.

Figure 1.26 shows the hexagonal close-packed structure. It has just a single slip plane though there are three directions in which slip can occur. The face centred cubic system has four slip planes, each having three slip directions. The body centred cubic system has more slip planes and directions than the other systems but because it is less well packed materials with, this form of structure tend to be harder and less ductile.

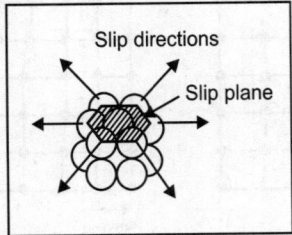

Fig. 1.26. The slip plane and slip directions for a hexagonal close-packed structure.

DISLOCATIONS

The 'block slip' model has atoms perfectly arranged in an orderly manner within the metal. If, however, we consider the arrangement to be imperfect then permanent deformations can be produced with much less stress. When you have a large carpet which is perfectly flat on the floor, it requires quite an effort to slide the entire carpet and make it move across the floor.

But if there is a ruck in the carpet (Fig. 1.27), then the carpet can be slid over the floor by pushing the ruck along a bit at a time and considerably less effort is required. This is the type of movement which is considered to take place within a metal, the 'ruck' in the crystal being a dislocation of atoms due to imperfect packing of the atoms within the metal. Figure 1.28 illustrates the movement that occurs when stress is applied and permanent deformation occurs. The dislocation moves through the array of atoms without wholesale movement of planes of atoms past each other; it is a bit-by-bit process like the ruck in the carpet.

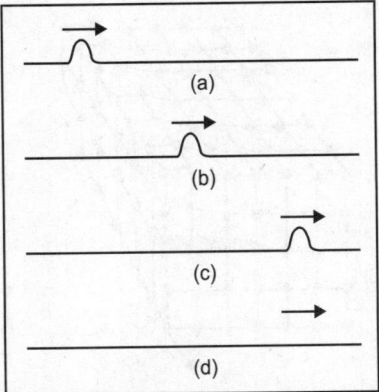

Fig. 1.27. Movement of a ruck across a carpet.

Figure 1.29 shows the form of a screw dislocation and its movement through the array of atoms under the action of stress. With an edge dislocation the line of dislocation is at right angles to the slip plane; with a screw dislocation the line of dislocation is parallel to the slip plane. In practice, dislocations are often neither straight lines, at right angles to, or parallel to, the slip plane but curved lines, which can, however, be considered to be a combination of edge and screw dislocations.

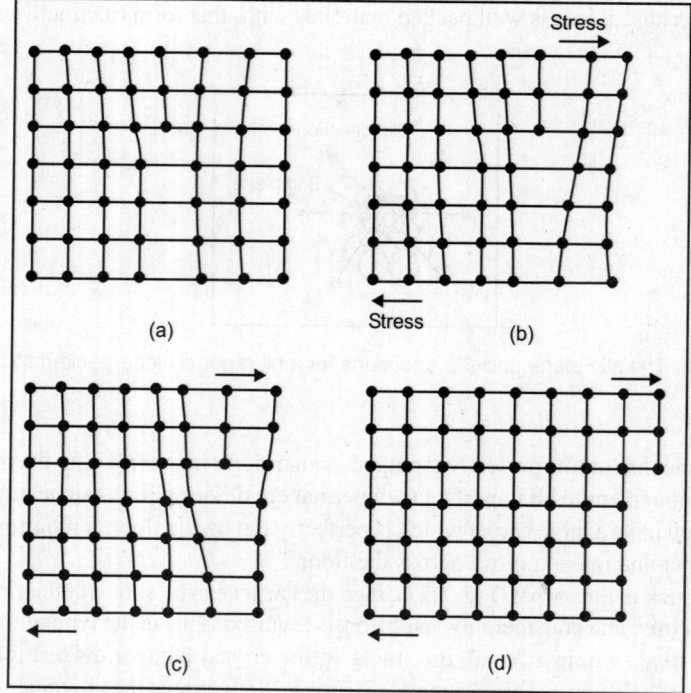

Fig. 1.28. Movement of a dislocation through an atomic array under the action of stress.

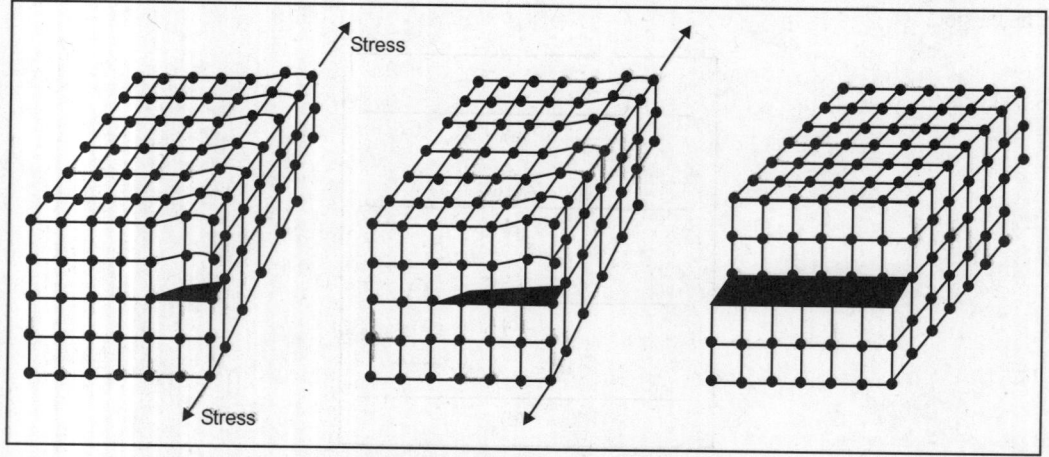

Fig. 1.29. Principle of the screw dislocation.

Crystal Defects

The dislocations referred to above, i.e. edge and screw dislocations, are line defects in the crystal structure. Line defects are long in one direction while measuring only a few atomic diameters at right angles to their length. Another form of defect is a point defect.

Point defects are only of the order of an atomic diameter in all directions. Such defects take the form of:
1. A vacancy in the crystal structure as a result of a missing atom [Fig. 1.30(a)].
2. An atom displaced from its normal position to a position within the lattice of the other atoms [Fig. 1.30(b)], this being called a self-interstitial defect, or onto the surface of the crystal.
3. A foreign atom, whether an impurity atom or a deliberate alloying addition, substituting for one of the crystal atoms [Fig. 1.30(c)], this being called a substitutional atom defect.
4. A foreign atom occupying a vacant site within the crystal lattice [Fig. 1.30(d)], this being called an interstitial atom defect.

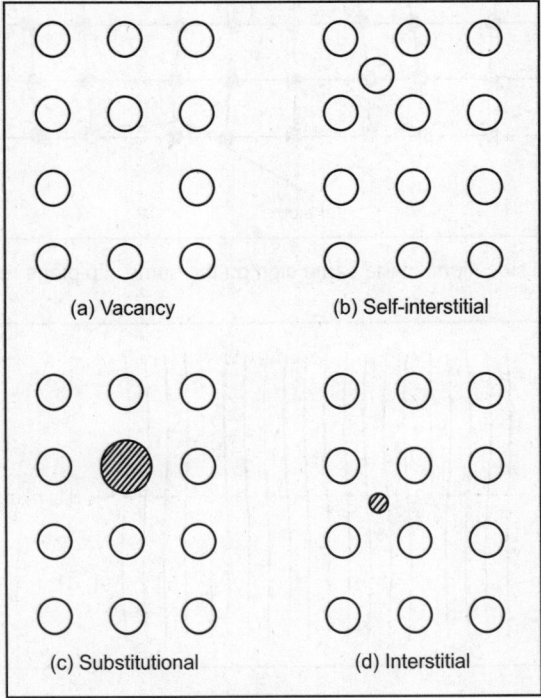

Fig. 1.30. Point defects.

Movement of Dislocations

What happens when two dislocations come close to each other during their movement through a metal? As Fig. 1.31 shows, the atoms on one side of the slip plane are in compression and on the other side in tension. When two dislocations come together the regions of compression can impinge on each other and so hinder the movement of the dislocations. If the movement is such as to bring the compression region against the tension region of another dislocation then it is possible for the two dislocations to annihilate each other (Fig. 1.32). In general, the more dislocations a metal has, the more the dislocations get in the way of each other and so the more difficult it is for the dislocations to move through the metal. More stress is needed to cause yielding.

The movement of dislocations through a metal is also hindered by the grain boundaries. The more grain boundaries there are in a metal the more difficult it is to produce yielding of that metal. More grain boundaries occur when the grain size in a metal is small.

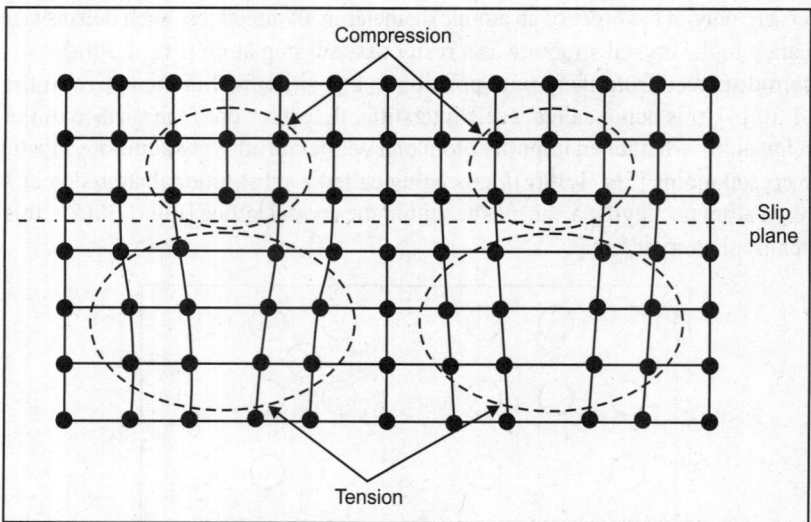

Fig. 1.31. Two dislocations of the same sign on the same slip plane repel each other.

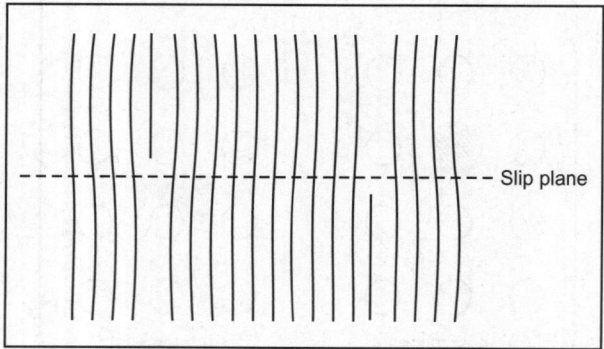

Fig. 1.32. Two edge dislocations of opposite sign on the same slip plane can move together and annihilate each other.

The movement of dislocations is hindered by anything that destroys the continuity of the atomic array. The presence of 'foreign' atoms can distort the atomic array of a metal and so hinder the movement of dislocations. Thus possible ways of increasing the yield stress of a metal are by:
1. Increasing the number of dislocations.
2. Reducing the grain size.
3. Introducing 'foreign' atoms.

Work hardening occurs as a result of a material being plastically deformed, the result being a higher yield stress. This occurs because the dislocation density is increased by plastic deformation and so there is more interaction between dislocations.

Dispersion hardening increases the yield stress of a material by producing a dispersion of fine particles throughout the material. These hinder the movement of dislocations, hence increasing the yield stress. One form of dispersion hardening is called precipitation hardening. With this the dispersion of fine particles is produced as a result of a specific form of heat treatment applied to the material to cause a precipitation to occur within the material.

The alloying of metals involves the introduction of foreign atoms into the crystal lattice. These produce interstitial and substitutional point defects which hinder the movement of dislocations, hence increasing the yield stress. This is referred to as solution hardening.

Dislocations can annihilate each other if they are of opposite sign and move together along the same slip plane, as in Fig. 1.32. However, this does not occur too frequently at room temperature. At higher temperatures another annihilation mechanism can occur. This is because at higher temperatures diffusion of atoms can become significant. This leads to what is called dislocation climb when an edge dislocation moves in a direction at right angles to its slip plane. The result of such movement is that more edge dislocations of opposite sign can annihilate each other (Fig. 1.33).

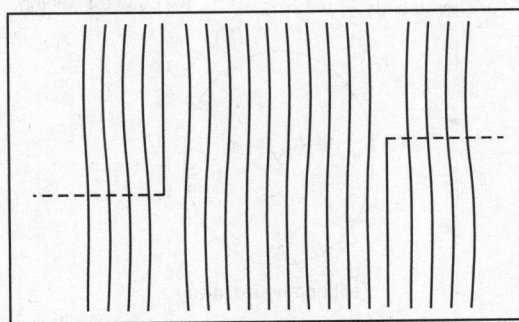

Fig. 1.33. Two edge dislocations of opposite sign can climb to be on the same slip plane and then annihilate each other.

If a work hardened material is heated to about 0.3 to 0.4 times its melting temperature (in degrees kelvin), some diffusion occurs and dislocations become rearranged and the number reduced. At this temperature there is no change in grain size. The result of such changes is that residual stresses are released, recovery being said to occur, and there is a slight reduction in yield stress. At higher temperatures recrystallisation occurs. New grains of low dislocation density are produced. The result is a marked decrease in yield stress. The heat treatment which allows recrystallisation to occur with a consequent decrease in yield stress is called annealing.

The effects of diffusion and consequent annihilation of dislocations as a result of dislocation climb is particularly evident in the behaviour of metals when subjected to a load for a long period of time at a high temperature. The strain increases steadily with time.

Dislocation Multiplication

The number of dislocations piercing a unit area of a polycrystalline material is of the order of 10 to a 100 million per square centimetre. These occur as a result of fabrication processes. However, if the material is subject to plastic deformation this dislocation density increases to as much as a million per square centimetre. A possible mechanism for this multiplication is called the Frank-Read source, these being the names of the people who originally postulated such a source.

Consider the dislocation shown in Fig. 1.34(a). The movement of the ends of the dislocation are hindered, by other dislocations or possibly foreign atoms. Thus, when a stress is applied the ends of the dislocation cannot move. The result is that the dislocation bows out, as in Fig. 1.34(b).

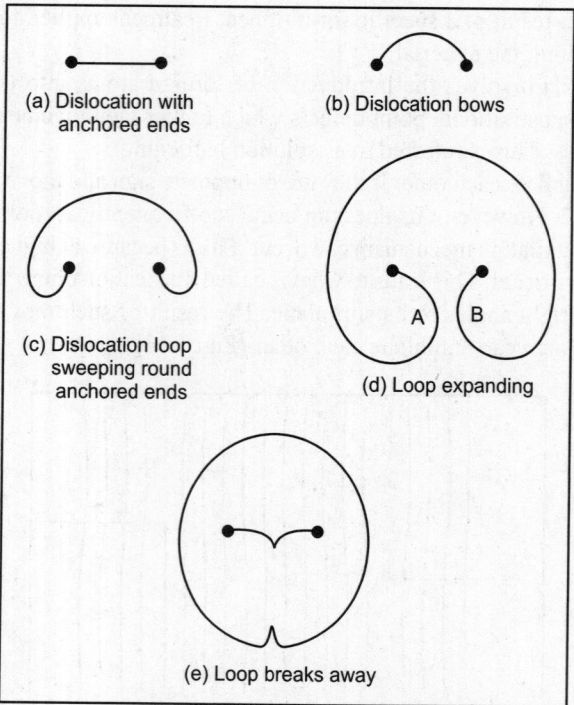

Fig. 1.34. The Frank-Read source.

Initially the bowed dislocation has a large radius. However, as the stress increases the radius decreases until the minimum radius is reached when the dislocation forms a semicircle. This is the condition of maximum stress. Beyond that point the radius decreases and the stress required to keep the dislocation expanding decreases. The dislocation forms a loop which grows by sweeping round the fixed ends until eventually the two sides meet to form a complete loop. When this occurs the portions of the dislocation A and B annihilate each other and the final result is an expanding dislocation loop which is free of the points anchoring the ends of the initial dislocation and the original pinned dislocation. This can continue multiplying.

Chapter 2

Strengthening Mechanism of Materials

INTRODUCTION

Methods have been devised to modify the yield strength, ductility, and toughness of both crystalline and amorphous materials. These strengthening mechanisms give engineers the ability to tailor the mechanical properties of materials to suit a variety of different applications. For example, the favourable properties of steel result from interstitial incorporation of carbon into the iron lattice. Brass, a binary alloy of copper and zinc, has superior mechanical properties compared to its constituent metals due to solution strengthening. Work hardening (such as beating a red-hot piece of metal on anvil) has also been used for centuries by blacksmiths to introduce dislocations into materials, increasing their yield strengths.

Plastic deformation occurs when large numbers of dislocations move and multiply so as to result in macroscopic deformation. In other words, it is the movement of dislocations in the material which allows for deformation. If we want to enhance a material's mechanical properties (i.e. increase the yield and tensile strength), we simply need to introduce a mechanism which prohibits the mobility of these dislocations. Whatever the mechanism may be, (work hardening, grain size reduction, etc.) they all hinder dislocation motion and render the material stronger than previously.

The stress required to cause dislocation motion is order of magnitude lower than the theoretical stress required to shift an entire plane of atoms, so this mode of stress relief is energetically favourable. Hence, the hardness and strength (both yield and tensile) critically depend on the ease with which dislocations move.

Pinning points, or locations in the crystal that oppose the motion of dislocations, can be introduced into the lattice to reduce dislocation mobility, thereby increasing mechanical strength. Dislocations may be pinned due to stress field interactions with other dislocations and solute particles, or physical barriers from grain boundaries and second phase precipitates. There are four main strengthening mechanisms for metals, the key concept to remember about strengthening of metallic materials is that it is all about preventing dislocation motion and propagation; you are making it energetically unfavourable for the dislocation to move or propagate. For a material that has been strengthened, by some processing method, the amount of force required to start irreversible (plastic) deformation is greater than it was for the original material.

In amorphous materials such as polymers, amorphous ceramics (glass), and amorphous metals, the lack of long range order leads to yielding via mechanisms such as brittle fracture, crazing, and shear band formation. In these systems, strengthening mechanisms do not involve dislocations, but rather consist of modifications to the chemical structure and processing of the constituent material.

Unfortunately, strength of materials cannot infinitely increase. Each of the mechanisms elaborated below involves some trade off by which other material properties are compromised in the process of strengthening.

STRENGTHENING MECHANISMS IN METALS

Work Hardening

The primary species responsible for work hardening are dislocations. Dislocations interact with each other by generating stress fields in the material. The interaction between the stress fields of dislocations can impede dislocation motion by repulsive or attractive interactions. Additionally, if two dislocations cross, dislocation line entanglement occurs, causing the formation of a jog which opposes dislocation motion. These entanglements and jogs act as pinning points, which oppose dislocation motion. As both of these processes are more likely to occur when more dislocations are present, there is a correlation between dislocation density and yield strength,

$$\Delta\sigma_y = Gb\sqrt{\rho\perp}$$

where, G is the shear modulus, b is the Burgers vector, and $\rho\perp$ is the dislocation density.

Increasing the dislocation density increases the yield strength which results in a higher shear stress required to move the dislocations. This process is easily observed while working a material. Theoretically, the strength of a material with no dislocations will be extremely high ($\tau = G/2$) because plastic deformation would require the breaking of many bonds simultaneously, at moderate dislocation density values of around 10^7–10^9 dislocations/m^2, the material will exhibit a significantly lower mechanical strength. Analogously, it is easier to move a rubber rug across a surface by propagating a small ripple through it than by dragging the whole rug. At dislocation densities of 10^{14} dislocations/m^2 or higher, the strength of the material becomes high once again. It should be noted that the dislocation density can't be infinitely high because then the material would lose its crystalline structure.

Solid Solution Strengthening/Alloying

For this strengthening mechanism, solute atoms of one element are added to another, resulting in either substitutional or interstitial point defects in the crystal (Fig. 2.1). The solute atoms cause lattice distortions that impede dislocation motion, increasing the yield stress of the material. Solute atoms have stress fields around them which can interact with those of dislocations. The presence of solute atoms impart compressive or tensile stresses to the lattice, depending on solute size, which interfere with nearby dislocations, causing the solute atoms to act as potential barriers to dislocation propagation and/or multiplication.

The shear stress required to move dislocations in a material is:

$$\Delta\tau = Gb\sqrt{c}\varepsilon^{3/2}$$

where, c is the solute concentration and ε is the strain on the material caused by the solute.

Increasing the concentration of the solute atoms will increase the yield strength of a material, but there is a limit to the amount of solute that can be added, and one should look at the phase diagram for the material and the alloy to make sure that a second phase is not created.

In general, the solid solution strengthening depends on the concentration of the solute atoms, shear modulus of the solute atoms, size of solute atoms, valency of solute atoms (for ionic materials), and the symmetry of the solute stress field. Note that the magnitude of strengthening is higher for non-symmetric stress fields because these solutes can interact with both edge and screw dislocations whereas symmetric stress fields, which cause only volume change and not shape change, can only interact with edge dislocations.

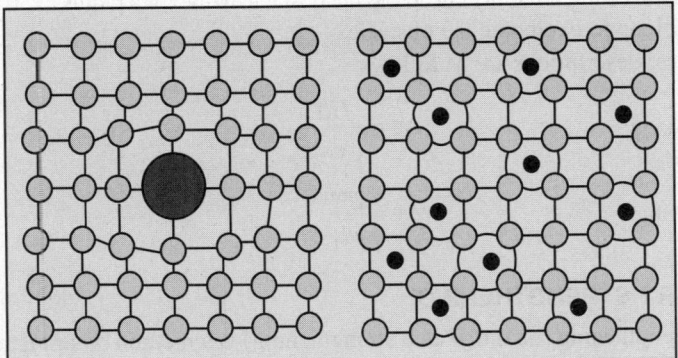

Fig. 2.1. This is a schematic illustrating how the lattice is strained by the addition of substitutional and interstitial solute. Notice the strain in the lattice that the solute atoms cause. The interstitial solute could be carbon in iron for example. The carbon atoms in the interstitial sites of the lattice creates a stress field that impedes dislocation movement.

Precipitation Hardening

In most binary systems, alloying above a concentration given by the phase diagram will cause the formation of a second phase. A second phase can also be created by mechanical or thermal treatments. The particles that compose the second phase precipitates act as pinning points in a similar manner to solutes, though the particles are not necessarily single atoms.

The dislocations in a material can interact with the precipitate atoms in one of two ways (Fig. 2.2). If the precipitate atoms are small, the dislocations would cut through them.

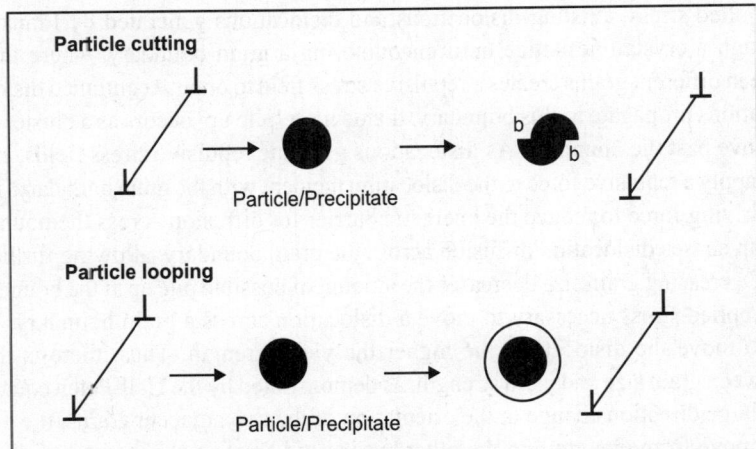

Fig. 2.2. This is a schematic illustrating how the dislocations can interact with a particle. It can either cut through the particle or bow around the particle and create a dislocation loop as it moves over the particle.

As a result, new surfaces (b in Fig. 2.2) of the particle would get exposed to the matrix and the particle/matrix interfacial energy would increase. For larger precipitate particles, looping or bowing of the dislocations would occur which results in dislocations getting longer. Hence, at a critical radius of about 5 nm, dislocations will preferably cut across the obstacle while for a radius of 30 nm, the dislocations will readily bow or loop to overcome the obstacle.

The mathematical descriptions are as follows:

For particle bowing:
$$\Delta\tau = \frac{Gb}{L-2r}$$

For particle cutting:
$$\Delta\tau = \frac{\gamma\pi r}{bL}$$

GRAIN BOUNDARY STRENGTHENING

Grain-boundary strengthening (or Hall-Petch strengthening) is a method of strengthening materials by changing their average crystallite (grain) size. It is based on the observation that grain boundaries impede dislocation movement and that the number of dislocations within a grain have an effect on how easily dislocations can traverse grain boundaries and travel from grain to grain. So, by changing grain size one can influence dislocation movement and yield strength. For example, heat treatment after plastic deformation and changing the rate of solidification are ways to alter grain size.

Theory

In grain-boundary strengthening the grain boundaries act as pinning points impeding further dislocation propagation. Since the lattice structure of adjacent grains differs in orientation, it requires more energy for a dislocation to change directions and move into the adjacent grain. The grain boundary is also much more disordered than inside the grain, which also prevents the dislocations from moving in a continuous slip plane. Impeding this dislocation movement will hinder the onset of plasticity and hence increase the yield strength of the material.

Under an applied stress, existing dislocations and dislocations generated by Frank-Read Sources will move through a crystalline lattice until encountering a grain boundary, where the large atomic mismatch between different grains creates a repulsive stress field to oppose continued dislocation motion. As more dislocations propagate to this boundary, dislocation 'pile up' occurs as a cluster of dislocations are unable to move past the boundary. As dislocations generate repulsive stress fields, each successive dislocation will apply a repulsive force to the dislocation incident with the grain boundary. These repulsive forces act as a driving force to reduce the energetic barrier for diffusion across the boundary, such that additional pile up causes dislocation diffusion across the grain boundary, allowing further deformation in the material. Decreasing grain size decreases the amount of possible pile up at the boundary, increasing the amount of applied stress necessary to move a dislocation across a grain boundary. The higher the applied stress to move the dislocation, the higher the yield strength. Thus, there is then an inverse relationship between grain size and yield strength, as demonstrated by the Hall-Petch equation. However, when there is a large direction change in the orientation of the two adjacent grains, the dislocation may not necessarily move from one grain to the other but instead create a new source of dislocation in the adjacent grain. The theory remains the same that more grain boundaries create more opposition to dislocation movement and in turn strengthens the material.

Obviously, there is a limit to this mode of strengthening, as infinitely strong materials do not exist. Grain sizes can range from about 100 μm (0.0039 inch) (large grains) to 1 μm (3.9×10^{-5} inch) (small grains). Lower than this, the size of dislocations begins to approach the size of the grains. At a grain size of about 10 nm (3.9×10^{-7} inch), only one or two dislocations can fit inside of a grain (Fig. 2.3). This scheme prohibits dislocation pile-up and never results in grain boundary diffusion. The lattice resolves the applied stress by grain boundary sliding, resulting in a decrease in the material's yield strength.

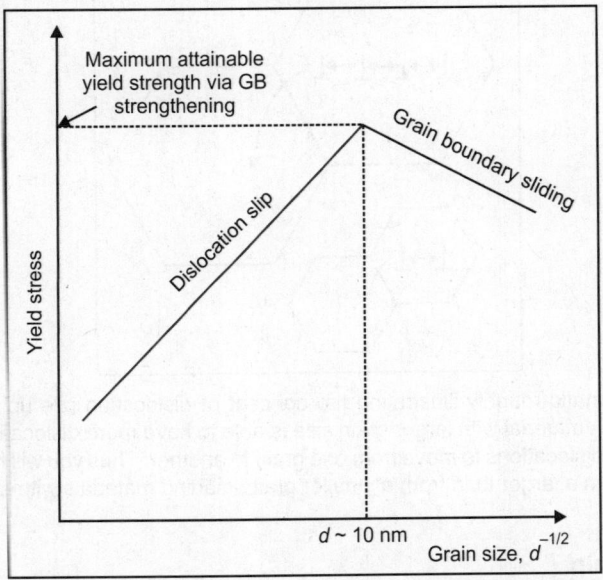

Fig. 2.3. Hall-Petch Strengthening is limited by the size of dislocations. Once the grain size reaches about 10 nanometres (3.9×10^{-7} inch), grain boundaries start to slide.

To understand the mechanism of grain boundary strengthening one must understand the nature of dislocation-dislocation interactions. Dislocations create a stress field around them given by:

$$\sigma \propto Gb \ln\left(\frac{r}{r_0}\right)$$

where, G is the material's shear modulus, and b is the Burgers vector. If the dislocations are in the right alignment with respect to each other, the local stress fields they create will repel each other. This helps dislocation movement along grains and across grain boundaries. Hence, the more dislocations are present in a grain, the greater the stress field felt by a dislocation near a grain boundary:

$$\tau_{\text{felt}} = \tau_{\text{applied}} + n_{\text{dislocation}} \tau_{\text{dislocation}}$$

Subgrain Strengthening

A subgrain is a part of the grain that is only slightly disoriented from other parts of the grain. Current research is being done to see the effect of subgrain strengthening in materials. Depending on the processing of the material, subgrains can form within the grains of the material. For example, when Fe-based material is ball-milled for long periods of time (e.g. 100+ hours), subgrains of 60–90 nm are formed. It has been shown that the higher the density of the subgrains, the higher the yield stress of the material due to the increased subgrain boundary. The strength of the metal was found to vary reciprocally with the size of the subgrain, which is analogous to the Hall-Petch equation. The subgrain boundary strengthening also has a breakdown point of around a subgrain size of 0.1 nm, which is the size where any subgrains smaller than that size would decrease yield strength (Fig. 2.4).

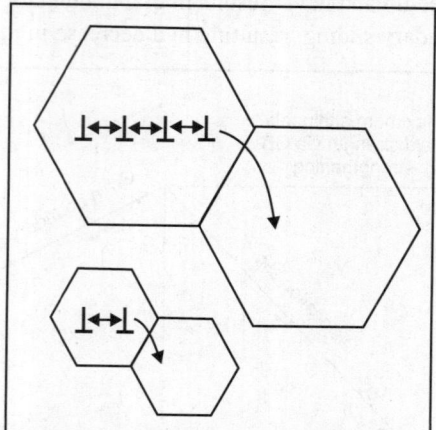

Fig. 2.4. This is a schematic roughly illustrating the concept of dislocation pile up and how it affects the strength of the material. A material with larger grain size is able to have more dislocation to pile up leading to a bigger driving force for dislocations to move from one grain to another. Thus you will have to apply less force to move a dislocation from a larger than from a smaller grain, leading materials with smaller grains to exhibit higher yield stress.

Hall-Petch Relationship

There is an inverse relationship between delta yield strength and grain size to some power, x.

$$\Delta \tau \propto \frac{k}{d^x}$$

where, k is the strengthening coefficient and both k and x are material specific. The smaller the grain size, the smaller the repulsion stress felt by a grain boundary dislocation and the higher the applied stress needed to propagate dislocations through the material (Table 2.1).

Table 2.1. Hall-Petch constants.

Material	σ_o [MPa]	k [MPa m$^{1/2}$]
Copper	25	0.11
Titanium	80	0.40
Mild steel	70	0.74
Ni$_3$Al	300	1.70

The relation between yield stress and grain size is described mathematically by the Hall-Petch equation:

$$\sigma_y = \sigma_0 + \frac{k_y}{\sqrt{d}}$$

where σ_y is the yield stress, σ_o is a materials constant for the starting stress for dislocation movement (or the resistance of the lattice to dislocation motion), k_y is the strengthening coefficient (a constant unique to each material), and d is the average grain diameter.

Theoretically, a material could be made infinitely strong if the grains are made infinitely small. This is impossible though, because the lower limit of grain size is a single unit cell of the material. Even then, if the grains of a material are the size of a single unit cell, then the material is in fact amorphous, not crystalline, since there is no long range order, and dislocations cannot be defined in an amorphous material. It has been observed experimentally that the microstructure with the highest yield strength is a grain size of about 10 nm (3.9×10^{-7} inch), because grains smaller than this undergo another yielding mechanism, grain boundary sliding. Producing engineering materials with this ideal grain size is difficult because only thin films can be reliably produced with grains of this size.

Reverse or inverse Hall-Petch relation

The Hall-Petch relation predicts that as the grain size decreases the yield strength increases. The Hall-Petch relation was experimentally found to be an effective model for materials with grain sizes ranging from 1 millimetre to 1 micrometre. Consequently it was believed that if average grain size could be decreased even further to the nanometer length scale the yield strength would increase as well. However, experiments on many nanocrystalline materials demonstrated that if the grains reached a small enough size, the critical grain size which is typically less than 100 nm (3.9×10^{-6} inch), the yield strength would either remain constant or decrease with decreasing grains size. This phenomenon has been termed the reverse or inverse Hall-Petch Relation. A number of different mechanisms have been proposed for this relation. As suggested by Carlton they fall into four categories: (i) dislocation based, (ii) diffusion based, (iii) grain boundary shearing based, and (iv) two phase based.

Other explanations that have been proposed to rationalise the apparent softening of metals with nanosized grains include poor sample quality and the suppression of dislocation pile-ups.

Many of the early measurements of a reverse Hall-Petch effect were likely the result of unrecognised pores in samples. The presence of voids in nanocrystalline metals would undoubtedly lead to their having weaker mechanical properties.

The pile-up of dislocations at grain boundaries is a hallmark mechanism of the Hall-Petch relationship. Once grain sizes drop below the equilibrium distance between dislocations, though, this relationship should no longer be valid. Nevertheless, it is not entirely clear what exactly the dependency of yield stress should be on grain sizes below this point.

Grain Refinement

Grain refinement, also known as inoculation, is the set of techniques used to implement grain boundary strengthening in metallurgy. The specific techniques and corresponding mechanisms will vary based on what materials are being considered.

One method for controlling grain size in aluminium alloys is by introducing particles to serve as nucleants, such as Al-5 per cent Ti. Grains will grow via heterogeneous nucleation; that is, for a given degree of undercooling beneath the melting temperature, aluminium particles in the melt will nucleate on the surface of the added particles. Grains will grow in the form of dendrites growing radially away from the surface of the nucleant. Solute particles can then be added (called grain refiners) which limit the growth of dendrites, leading to grain refinement. TiB_2 is a common grain refiner for Al alloys; however, novel refiners such as Al_3Sc have been suggested.

One common technique is to induce a very small fraction of the melt to solidify at a much higher temperature than the rest; this will generate seed crystals that act as a template when the rest of the material falls to its (lower) melting temperature and begins to solidify. Since a huge number of minuscule seed crystals are present, a nearly equal number of crystallites result, and the size of any one grain is limited (Table 2.2).

Table 2.2. Typical inoculants for various casting alloys.

Metal	Inoculant
Cast iron	FeSi, SiCa, graphite
Mg alloys	Zr, C
Cu alloys	Fe, Co, Zr
Al-Si alloys	P, Ti, B
Pb alloys	As, Te
Zn alloys	Ti
Ti alloys	Al-Ti intermetallics

SOLID SOLUTION STRENGTHENING OR HARDENING

Since no two elements have the same atomic diameter, solute atoms will be either smaller or larger in size than the solvent atoms. Due to the difference in atomic size, lattice distortion is produced when one element is added to the other. Smaller solute atoms will produce a local tensile stress field and larger solute atoms will produce a local compressive stress field in the crystal. In both the cases, the stress field of a moving dislocation interacts with the stress field of the solute atom. This increases the stress required to move the dislocation through the crystal.

The increase in strength produced due to the addition of solute element to the solvent depends on the following factors.

Amount of Solute

Higher the amount of solute, more will be the local distortion in the lattice and more will be the obstacles to the moving dislocations and higher will be the strength and hardness. The increase in strength is proportional to $C^{1/2}$, where, C is the solute concentration. For dilute solutions, increase in strength with concentration is approximately linear.

Atomic Size Difference

As the atomic size difference between the solute and solvent increases, the intensity of stress field around solute atoms also increases. This increases the resistance to the motion of dislocations thereby increasing hardness and tensile strength. Therefore, more the atomic size difference, higher is the hardness and tensile strength.

Nature of Distortion

The nature of distortion produced by solute atoms also affects the hardness and tensile strength. Spherical distortion produced by substitutional solute atoms is much less effective than the non-spherical distortion produced by interstitial solute atoms. This is shown in Fig. 2.5.

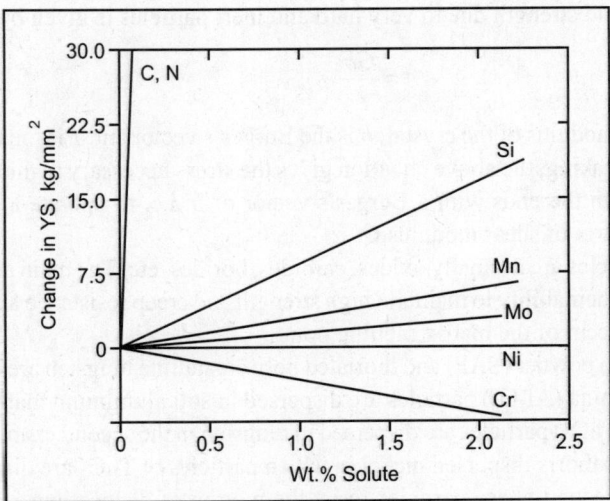

Fig. 2.5. The variation of yield stress of iron with different solute additions.

Figure 2.5 shows that the elements Cr, Ni, Mo, Mn and Si are less effective in increasing the YS of iron than the elements like C and N. This is due to the fact that C and N form interstitial solid solutions and produce tetragonal distortion in the lattice whereas the other elements form substitutional solid solutions and produce spherical distortion.

Ordered solid solutions are more harder and stronger than disordered solid solutions. In some cases, they may even be brittle. However disordered solid solutions, in general are ductile. If the solid solubility is exceeded, the lattice strains will be relieved and hardness (and TS) will decrease.

DISPERSION STRENGTHENING OR HARDENING

Here the resistance to the motion of dislocations is increased by introducing finely divided hard particles of second phase in the soft matrix. The increase in hardness and TS is due to the interaction of the stress field around the particles with the stress field of a moving dislocation and also due to physical obstruction by the hard particles to the moving dislocations.

The extent of strengthening or hardening produced depends up on the amount of second phase particles, characteristics and properties of second phase and particle size, shape and distribution. As the amount of second phase increases, hardness increases. For a given amount of second phase, the hardness and TS depend on the particle size, shape and distribution. Too fine and too coarse particles have less hardening and strengthening effect. The distance between the particles, i.e. the inter-particle distance depends on their size. Finer the particles lesser is the inter-particle distance because the particles come closer to each other.

Coarser the particles more is the inter-particle distance. Therefore, maximum hardening/strengthening is observed at some intermediate spacing of particles, not too less and not too more. Amongst the round, disc and needle shaped particles, needle shaped particles have better hardening and strengthening effect. For better and uniform properties, the distribution of particles should be uniform. The optimum properties are usually observed at a concentration of particles from 2 to 15 per cent (by volume), their size between 0.01 and 0.1 μm, and a spacing of 0.1 to 1.0 between particles.

The increase in yield strength due to very hard and inert particles is given by:

$$\tau = \frac{Gb}{l} \qquad \ldots (2.1)$$

where, G is the shear modulus of the crystal, b is the Burger's vector and l is the mean spacing between the particles. Truly speaking, the above equation gives the stress necessary to move a dislocation line of length 1 pinned at both the ends with a Burger's vector of b, i.e. to operate a Frank-Reed source of length 1 through a matrix of shear modulus G.

The dispersed particles are normally oxides, carbides, borides, etc. The main advantage of dispersion hardened materials is their ability to maintain high strength and creep resistance at elevated temperatures of the order of 80 per cent of the matrix melting point.

Sintered aluminium powder (SAP) and thoriated poly crystalline tungsten are the common examples of this type. Hard alumina (Al_2O_3) particles are dispersed in soft aluminium matrix in the first example and thorium dioxide (ThO_2) particles are dispersed in tungsten in the second example. The other familiar example of this type is thoria dispersed nickel in which particles of ThO_2 are dispersed in nickel. In all the above examples, second phase particles resist the motion of dislocations increasing the strength. The common method of manufacturing dispersion hardened materials is powder metallurgy. The powders of the required shape, size and distribution are mixed in the right proportion, compacted and sintered at the correct temperature.

AGE (PRECIPITATION HARDENING)

Some of the alloys show increase in hardness with time at room temperature or after heating to slightly higher temperatures. This type of hardening is called age (or precipitation) hardening and is observed in alloys such as Al – 4.5% Cu, Al – 6% Zn – 2.5% Mg, Cu – 2% Be, Ni – 17% Cu – 8% Sn, Ti– 6% Al – 4% V, etc. The conditions for age or precipitation hardening to occur in any alloy system are:

1. The solubility of solute in the solvent must decrease with decrease in temperature.
2. The precipitate that separates out from the matrix should be coherent. Coherent precipitation means that the solute atoms concentrate to a degree sufficient to give the composition of second phase. There is no true interface between the precipitate particle and the surrounding matrix. Since the solute atoms are of different size from the solvent atoms, large amount of elastic distortion, is observed around the precipitate particle.

These coherent precipitate particles are powerful obstacles to the motion of dislocations. This is because the large elastic distortion of the matrix around the particles interacts strongly with the stress field of dislocations. In some systems like Mg-Pb, Al-Mn and Al-Mg decrease in solubility is observed with decrease in temperature, but the precipitate is not coherent and hence the alloys from these systems cannot be hardened by the above process.

The general steps involved in age/precipitation hardening are explained below for a typical system of which the equilibrium diagram is shown in Fig. 2.6.

Heating (Solutionising)

The alloy is heated to a temperature between the solvus and eutectic temperature such as T, so that it forms a single phase solid solution, i.e. $\alpha + \theta \rightarrow \alpha$. The alloy is held at this temperature for sufficient period for complete homogenisation.

Strengthening Mechanism of Materials

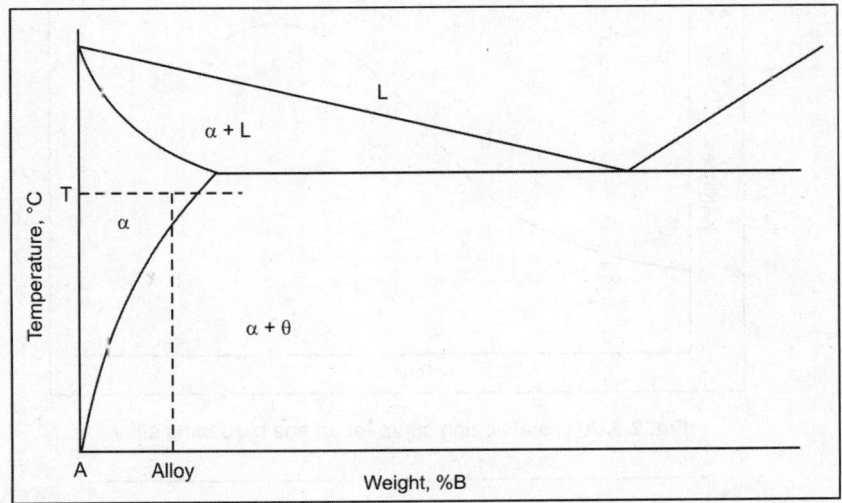

Fig. 2.6. A typical equilibrium diagram showing decrease in solubility with decrease in temperature.

Quenching

It is rapidly cooled to room temperature, usually in water, to obtain a supersaturated solid solution (α'). The alloy now is in solution treated condition and its hardness will be relatively low, but is higher than that of the annealed (slowly cooled) condition. The alloy can be easily cold rolled under this condition.

Ageing

In some of the systems solution treated alloy shows increasing hardness with time at room temperature (i.e. natural ageing). In others, increase in hardness with appreciable rate is not observed at room temperature and hence such alloys are aged at elevated temperatures to increase the kinetics of precipitation (i.e. artificial ageing). In artificial ageing, the ageing temperature is roughly between 15 to 25 per cent of the temperature difference of room temperature and solutionising temperature. Over ageing decreases the hardness and hence ageing is ordinarily stopped as soon as the optimum hardness is obtained. A typical ageing curve is shown in Fig. 2.7.

In reality, the ageing curve is not smooth as shown in Fig. 2.7. The curve may show more than one maxima. This is due to the existence of several intermediate precipitates (GP zones, i.e. Guinier-Preston zones). Another factor which influences the form of ageing curve is the heterogeneous precipitation. In heterogeneous precipitation, precipitation does not occur at the same rate throughout the entire solid solution. It starts first and is completed first at grain boundaries and at slip lines that may have been developed by quenching stresses or by cold working before the ageing treatment. Under this situation, at a given time, different regions of the sample are ageing at different rates and therefore are at different stages of the ageing process. This also gives more than one maxima on the ageing curve. The kinetics of ageing process is influenced by the following factors.

Temperature of ageing

The effect of temperature of ageing on peak hardness value and the time to reach the peak hardness is shown schematically in Fig. 2.8.

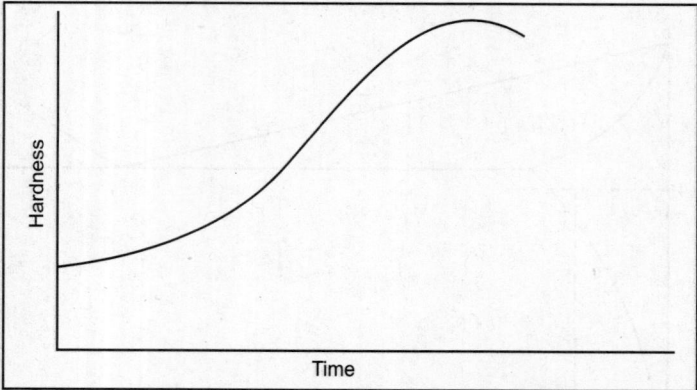

Fig. 2.7. A typical ageing curve for an age hardening alloy.

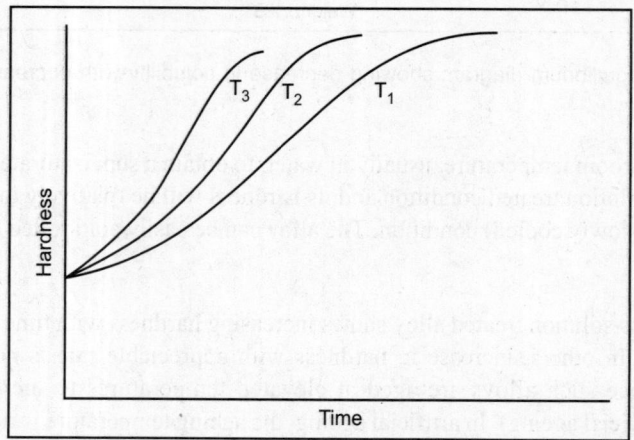

Fig. 2.8. Effect of ageing temperature on peak hardness.

The peak hardness and the time to reach the peak hardness both decrease with increasing temperature of ageing.

Cold work on α′

In some of the alloys with cold working or straining on solution treated alloy, the kinetics of precipitation increases. The peak hardness value increases and the time to reach the peak hardness decreases with increase in the degree of cold work as shown schematically in Fig. 2.9.

Alloy composition

The alloy composition should be such that the response to precipitation hardening should be good. For this purpose the solute concentration should not be too less and also should not exceed the solubility limit, e.g. for Al-Cu system, the solubility limit is 5.65 per cent Cu at 548°C (eutectic temperature) and hence an alloy with 4.0 to 4.5 per cent Cu is suitable for this purpose. The effect of composition of alloy on kinetics of ageing is shown schematically in Fig. 2.10.

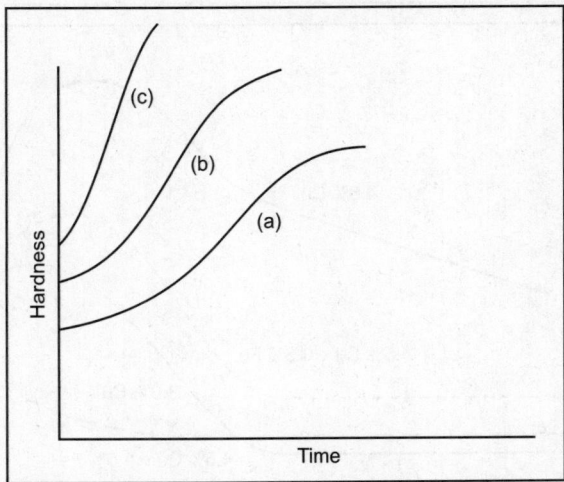

Fig. 2.9. Effect of cold work on ageing curves: (a) without cold work, (b) with intermediate degree of cold work, and (c) with high degree of cold work.

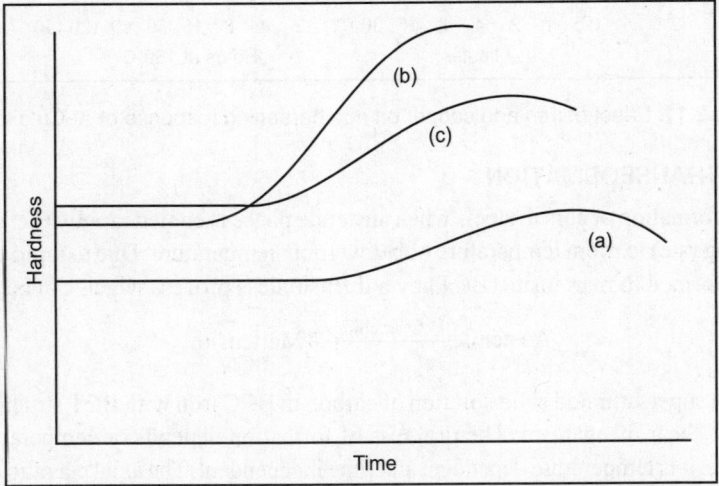

Fig. 2.10. Effect of alloy composition on ageing curves. (a) Alloy composition too less in solute, (b) alloy composition near the solubility limit, and (c) alloy composition greater than solubility limit.

Impurity and homogeneity

Impurities also affect the kinetics of precipitation, e.g. in Al-alloys, the iron content, should be less. The deleterious effect of iron on properties of Al–4.5 per cent Cu alloy is shown in Fig. 2.11.

The response to precipitation hardening of Al-4.5 per cent Cu alloy with 1.0 per cent Fe is almost similar to that of Al-1.5 per cent Cu alloy with no Fe. This is due to the fact that iron combines with Cu and Al and forms Al-Cu-Fe compound. This compound is insoluble and hence the Cu that can dissolve in Al during solution treatment gets, reduced. Non-homogeneity of alloy composition decreases the response to precipitation hardening.

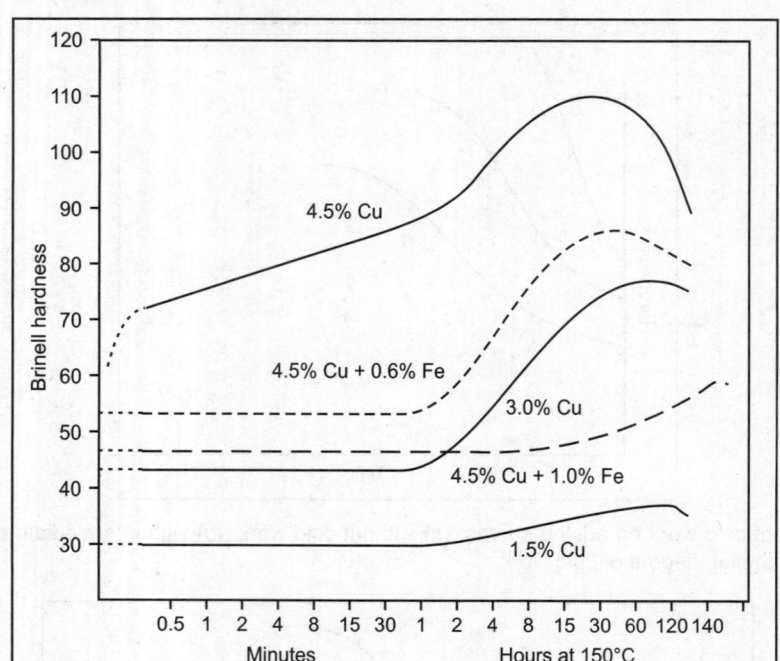

Fig. 2.11. Effect of iron and copper on age hardening response of Al-Cu alloys.

MARTENSITIC TRANSFORMATION

Martensitic transformation occurs in steels when austenite phase is cooled rapidly (i.e. cooled exceeding the critical cooling rate) to room temperature of below room temperature. Due to rapid cooling, austenite (FCC) gets transformed to martensite (BCT) by a diffusionless process which can be shown as below:

$$\text{Austenite (FCC)} \xrightarrow{\text{Quenching}} \text{Martensite (BCT)}$$

Martensite is a supersaturated solid solution of carbon in BCC iron with BCT structure and is formed from austenite by shear mechanism. The progress of formation depends on temperature and does not depend on time, i.e. it is temperature dependent and time independent. The axial c/a ratio of the martensite, i.e. BCT lattice depends on the carbon in the austenite before it transforms to martensite. Martensite is a hard phase and its hardness depends on the carbon in the austenite or steel. Because of the formation of BCT structure from FCC structure, the lattice gets distorted and the intense stress field around the carbon atoms in martensite effectively hinders the motion of dislocations. Martensitic transformation is very important for controlling the properties of steels. The other commercially important system in which martensitic transformation is observed is copper-aluminium system (aluminium bronzes) in which the high temperature β phase transforms to martensite on rapid cooling.

COMPOSITE MATERIALS

A composite material is a combination of two or more chemically unlike materials with distinct boundaries between them. Such materials have their own specific properties and are usually different from their individual material properties. The properties such as strength, resistance to heat, or some other property of composite materials are better than the properties of the individual materials from which they are made. Modern living demands materials with excellent properties and the specific requirements are increasing day by day from the modern society. Such demands can be met by producing materials using anyone or more methods in combination from the methods discussed already this chapter. However, when these methods fail to give the required properties, we combine different materials to obtain the desired properties, i.e. we produce composite material.

For example, the varied requirements of materials to be used in certain applications such as space vehicles, air crafts, rockets, high pressure vessels, building construction, etc. can be best satisfied by composite materials, and often, only by them. Composite materials made artificially are called man-made composites. Nature also produces composite materials. Some of the examples of natural composites are wood, bamboo and bone. Wood and bamboo consist of cellulose and lignin whereas, bone consists of collagen and apatite.

Composite materials can be divided into three main classes:
1. Fibre reinforced materials.
2. Laminated materials.
3. Disperse materials.

Fibre Reinforced Materials

Here the fibres of high strength materials are introduced into the soft and ductile matrix. The strength of soft and ductile matrix gets increased by high strength fibres. The resulting composite material will have high stiffness, high specific strength (specific strength = UTS/density), elevated temperature strength and high fracture toughness. Fibres mainly bear the load and the matrix transfers and distributes the external load to the fibres. Also, die matrix protects the fibres from external actions and imparts certain physico-chemical properties, such as resistance to corrosion and oxidation, electrical and thermal conductivity, etc.

The strength of fibrous composite materials depends on the factors such as:
1. The mechanical properties of the matrix and fibres.
2. The volume concentration of fibres.
3. Their distribution and orientation.
4. The firmness of bond at the matrix-fibre interface (i.e. the bond strength).
5. The thermal stability of fibres in the matrix.

The properties of composite materials at elevated temperatures may get affected by the reactions occurring between the matrix and fibres. This may result in dissolution or softening of fibres and may also form brittle layer at the interfaces.

The fibres can be of metals or nonmetals. The common metallic fibres which are used in composite materials are of boron, beryllium, molybdenum, tungsten, steel and stainless steel and the nonmetallic fibres are of carbon, glass, silica, alumina, silicon carbide and aramide. The aramide is an aromatic polyamide fibre with a very rigid molecular structure and is marketed under the trade name *Kevlar*. Whiskers (thread like single crystals) of silicon carbide, boron carbide and aluminium oxide also have been used in place of fibres.

The matrix can also be metallic or non metallic. The common metallic matrices are of aluminium, copper, titanium alloys, nickel alloys, and the non-metallic matrices are of unsaturated polyesters and epoxy resins.

Fibre reinforced composites find large number of applications in diversified fields. This is because of high specific strength of these materials, and the possibility of obtaining the desired combination of properties by proper selection of the matrix and fibres, and by variation of concentration and orientation of the fibres. To site a few, fibre glass (glass fibres reinforced by plastic matrix) is, used for helmets, car and jeep bodies, scooter bodies and similar applications. Nylon and steel fibres are used in plastic matrix for vehicle tyres. Carbon fibres reinforced with plastic are used in aerospace applications. The materials in which fibres are reinforced with plastic are called 'fibre reinforced plastics (FRP). Boron fibre reinforced aluminium composites are used in the manufacture of aircraft parts. Reinforced cement concrete (RCC) consists of steel rods in cement concrete and is used in construction work.

Laminated Materials

Here the composite material consists of two or more layers of unlike components. Examples are laminated plywood, Alclad aluminium alloy, copper clad stainless steel and titanium clad steel. Thermostatic controls consisting of a bimetallic strip of copper and nickel used to control temperatures in ovens and furnaces is also a composite material of this type. The properties of these composites and fibre reinforced composites are highly sensitive to direction of loading with respect to the direction of lamillae or fibres.

Disperse Materials

Here the particles of one material are distributed as a mechanical mixture into the other (base). This is the same as dispersion hardening or strengthening. Some of the examples of such composites are sintered aluminium powder (SAP), thoriated tungsten and thoria dispersed nickel, which have been already described in dispersion hardening. The other example is the strengthening of nickel alloy by hafnium dioxide particles. This alloy is nontoxic but has slightly less heat resistance as compared to the alloy strengthened by thorium dioxide particles.

Large number of methods are available for the production of composite materials. Some of the important methods are unidirectional solidification, infiltration of the molten metal, plasma spraying, electroplating, diffusion bonding and powder metallurgy.

In addition to the above methods, materials can be strengthened by thermo-mechanical and maraging treatments. Metals can also be strengthened by irradiation, particularly by fast neutrons which will introduce defects in the crystals giving somewhat similar effect to that of strain hardening.

STRENGTHENING MECHANISMS IN AMORPHOUS MATERIALS

Polymer

Polymers fracture via breaking of inter- and intra molecular bonds; hence, the chemical structure of these materials plays a huge role in increasing strength. For polymers consisting of chains which easily slide past each other, chemical and physical cross linking can be used to increase rigidity and yield strength. In thermoset polymers (thermosetting plastic), disulphide bridges and other covalent cross links give rise to a hard structure which can withstand very high temperatures. These cross-links are particularly helpful in improving tensile strength of materials which contain lots of free volume prone to crazing, typically glassy brittle polymers.

In thermoplastic elastomer, phase separation of dissimilar monomer components leads to association of hard domains within a sea of soft phase, yielding a physical structure with increased strength and rigidity. If yielding occurs by chains sliding past each other (shear bands), the strength can also be increased by introducing kinks into the polymer chains via unsaturated carbon-carbon bonds. Increasing the bulkiness of the monomer unit via incorporation of aryl rings is another strengthening mechanism. The anisotropy of the molecular structure means that these mechanisms are heavily dependent on the direction of applied stress. While aryl rings drastically increase rigidity along the direction of the chain, these materials may still be brittle in perpendicular directions. Macroscopic structure can be adjusted to compensate for this anisotropy.

For example, the high strength of Kevlar arises from a stacked multilayer macrostructure where aromatic polymer layers are rotated with respect to their neighbours. When loaded oblique to the chain direction, ductile polymers with flexible linkages, such as oriented polyethylene, are highly prone to shear band formation, so macroscopic structures which place the load parallel to the draw direction would increase strength.

Mixing polymers is another method of increasing strength, particularly with materials that show crazing preceding brittle fracture such as atactic polystyrene (APS). For example, by forming a 50/50 mixture of APS with polyphenylene oxide (PPO), this embrittling tendency can be almost completely suppressed, substantially increasing the fracture strength.

Glass

Many silicate glasses are strong in compression but weak in tension. By introducing compression stress into the structure, the tensile strength of the material can be increased. This is typically done via two mechanisms: thermal treatment (tempering) or chemical bath (via ion exchange).

In tempered glasses, air jets are used to rapidly cool the top and bottom surfaces of a softened (hot) slab of glass. Since the surface cools quicker, there is more free volume at the surface than in the bulk melt. The core of the slab then pulls the surface inward, resulting in an internal compressive stress at the surface. This substantially increases the tensile strength of the material as tensile stresses exerted on the glass must now resolve the compressive stresses before yielding.

$$\sigma_{y=\text{modified}} = \sigma_{y,0} + \sigma_{\text{compressive}}$$

Alternately, in chemical treatment, a glass slab treated containing network formers and modifiers is submerged into a molten salt bath containing ions larger than those present in the modifier. Due to a concentration gradient of the ions, mass transport must take place. As the larger cation diffuses from the molten salt into the surface, it replaces the smaller ion from the modifier. The larger ion squeezing into surface introduces compressive stress in the glass's surface. A common example is treatment of sodium oxide modified silicate glass in molten potassium chloride.

APPLICATIONS AND CURRENT RESEARCH

Strengthening of materials is useful in many applications. One main application of strengthened materials is for construction. In order to have stronger buildings and bridges, one must have a strong frame that can support high tensile or compressive load and resist plastic deformation. The steel frame used to make the building should be as strong as possible so that it does not bend under the entire weight of the building. Polymeric roofing materials would also need to be strong so that the roof does not cave in when there is build-up of snow on the rooftop.

Research is also currently being done to increase the strength of metallic materials through the addition of polymer materials such as bonded carbon fibre reinforced polymer.

Molecular Dynamics Simulations

The use of computation simulations to model work hardening in materials allows for the direct observation of critical elements that rule the process of strengthening materials. The basic reasoning derives from the fact that, when examining plasticity and the movement of dislocations in materials, a focus on the atomistic level is many times not accounted for and the focus rests on the continuum description of materials. Since the practice of tracking these atomistic effects in experiments and theorising about them in textbooks cannot provide a full understanding of these interactions, many turn to molecular dynamics simulations to develop this understanding.

The simulations work by utilising the known atomic interactions between any two atoms and the relationship $F = ma$, so that the dislocations moving through the material are ruled by simple mechanical actions and reactions of the atoms. The interatomic potential usually utilised to estimate these interactions is the Lennard–Jones 12:6 potential. Lennard–Jones is widely accepted because its experimental shortcomings are well-known. These interactions are simply scaled up to millions or billions of atoms in some cases to simulate materials more accurately.

Molecular dynamic simulations display the interactions based upon the governing equations provided above for the strengthening mechanisms. They provide an effective way to see these mechanisms in action outside the painstaking realm of direct observation during experiments.

Chapter 3
Phase Diagrams

INTRODUCTION

For a given substance, it is possible to make a phase diagram which outlines the changes in phase. Generally temperature is along the horizontal axis and pressure is along the vertical axis, although three-dimensional phase diagrams can also account for a volume axis. Curves representing the 'fusion curve' (liquid/solid barrier), the 'vapourisation curve' (liquid/vapour barrier), and the 'sublimation curve' (solid/vapour barrier) can be seen in the diagram (Fig. 3.1). The area near the origin is the sublimation curve and it branches off to form the fusion curve (which goes mostly upward) and the vapourisation curve (when goes mostly to the right). Along the curves, the substance would be in a state of phase equilibrium, balanced precariously between the two states on either side.

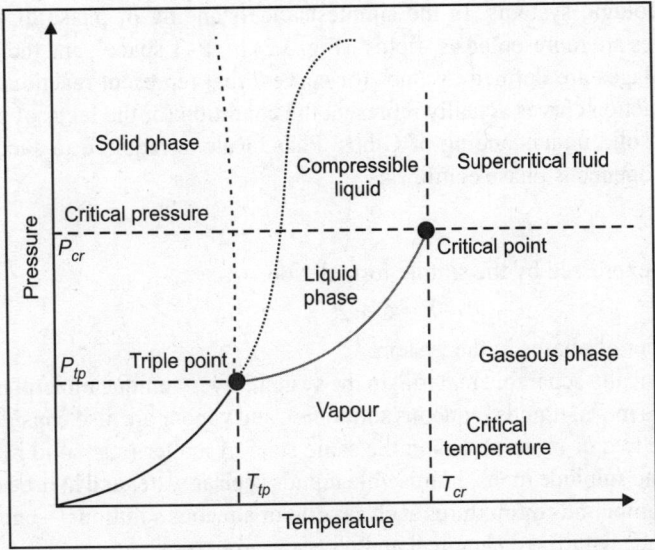

Fig. 3.1. A simple phase diagram.

The point at which all three curves meet is called the triple point. At this precise temperature and pressure, the substance will be in a state of equilibrium between the three states, and minor variations would cause it to shift between them.

Finally, the point at which the vapourisation curve 'ends' is called the 'critical point'. The pressure at this point is called the 'critical pressure' and the temperature at this point is the 'critical temperature'. For pressures or temperatures (or both) above these values, essentially there is a blurry line between the liquid and gaseous states. Phase transitions between them do not take place, although the properties themselves can transition between those of liquids and those of gases. They just do not do so in a clear-cut transition, but metamorph gradually from one to another.

GIBBS' PHASE RULE

Minerals are the monitors of the physical and chemical conditions under which they are formed. The occurrences of minerals, their parageneses (stable associations), types of reactions, and compositional variation (e.g. zoned minerals) all provide important information about geologic history and processes. Of particular importance to geologists are:
1. Estimates of pressure and temperature (geothermobarometry).
2. Estimates of other physico-chemical conditions such as acidity (pH) and oxidation state (eH).
3. Partial pressures of gases (e.g. fugacities of H_2O, CO_2, etc.).
4. Partitioning of major and trace elements between phases (e.g. minerals, melts and/or fluids) to characterise and quantify petrogenetic processes.
5. Use of minerals in geochronology and thermochronology.

Gibbs' Phase Rule provides the theoretical foundation, based in thermodynamics, for characterising the chemical state of a (geologic) system, and predicting the equilibrium relations of the phases (minerals, melts, liquids, vapours) present as a function of physical conditions such as pressure and temperature. Gibbs' Phase Rule also allows us to construct phase diagrams to represent and interpret phase equilibria in heterogeneous geologic systems. In the simplest understanding of phase diagrams, stable phase (mineral) assemblages are represented as 'fields' (Fig. 3.2) in 'P–T space', and the boundaries between stable phase assemblages are defined by lines (or curves) that represent reactions between the phase assemblages. The reaction curves actually represent the condition (or the locus of points in P–T space) where $\Delta G_{rxn} = 0$. A solid understanding of Gibbs' Phase Rule is required to successfully master the applications of heterogeneous phase equilibria.

Definitions

Gibbs Phase Rule is expressed by the simple formulation:
$$P + F = C + 2,$$
where, P is the number of phases in the system.

A phase is any physically separable material in the system. Every unique mineral is a phase (including polymorphs); igneous melts, liquids (aqueous solutions), and vapour are also considered unique phases. It is possible to have two or more phases in the same state of matter (e.g. solid mineral assemblages, immiscible silicate and sulphide melts, immiscible liquids such as water and hydrocarbons, etc.). Phases may either be pure compounds or mixtures such as solid or aqueous solutions—but they must 'behave' as a coherent substance with fixed chemical and physical properties.

C is the minimum number of chemical components required to constitute all the phases in the system.

For historical reasons, geologists normally define components in terms of the simple oxides (e.g. SiO_2, Al_2O_3, CaO, etc.). If two possible components always occur in the same proportions in multiple phases in a system, these can be combined into a single component (remember, we are always trying to define the minimum number of components required to make all the phases in the system). Consider the reaction:

$$CaMg(CO_3)_2 + 2SiO_2 = CaMgSi_2O_6 + 2CO_2$$
Dolomite + 2 Quartz = Diopside + 2 Carbon Dioxide

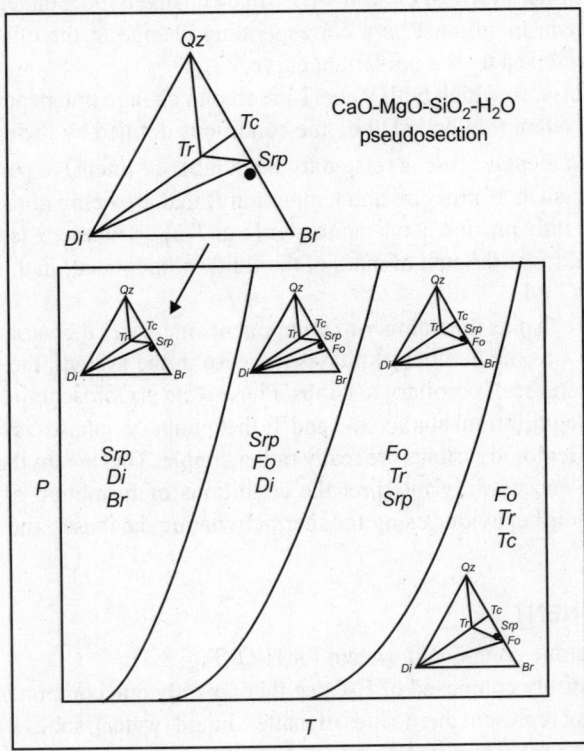

Fig. 3.2. Diagram of simple Gibbs' Phase Rule.

Normally we would pick the four components: CaO, MgO, SiO_2, and CO_2 based on the simple oxides. However, because Ca and Mg are in a 1:1 ratio in both dolomite and diopside (and not present in quartz or carbon dioxide), we can consider this a ternary system with components: $CaMgO_2$, SiO_2, and CO_2.

In some geologic systems it is convenient to define the components in terms of end-member compositions (e.g. binary systems such as carbonates, $CaCO_3$–$MgCO_3$; alkali feldspars, $NaAlSi_3O_8$–$KAlSi_3O_8$, etc.). In some cases, a given mineral assemblage may be represented by a subset of the whole system if fewer components are needed to define the compositions of the observed mineral assemblage—this is known as a degenerate system.

A good example of this can be seen on a ternary (3 component) chemographic projection if the phases of interest plot in a co-linear fashion (i.e. requiring only two components to define the phase compositions in what is otherwise a three component system).

F is the number of degrees of freedom in the system (also referred to as the variance of the system). For geologic applications, this generally refers to the number of variables (e.g. pressure and temperature)

that can be independently changed without altering the state of the system (i.e. the number of phases and their compositions are constant). Three common types of equilibria are possible:
1. Invariant equilibria, in which neither P or T can be changed; on a phase diagram, this is represented as a singular invariant point
2. Univariant equilibria, in which either P or T can be changed independently, but to maintain the state of the system, there must be a corresponding change in the other variable; on a phase diagram this is referred to as a univariant curve.
3. Divariant equilibria, in which both P and T are free to change independently without changing the state of the system (but bounded by the conditions defined by the univariant equilibria).

The integer in the Gibbs phase rule is related to the number of intensive parameters (i.e. those that are independent of mass; such as pressure and temperature) that are being considered. Note that many phase diagrams consider only one intensive parameter (e.g. T-X_{fluid}, where, T is intensive, and the mole fraction of fluid is related to the amount of mass of the fluid components); in this case, the Gibbs Phase Rule would be: $P + F = C + 1$.

It is generally the case that as the number of components increase, the variance of the system must also increase. Conversely, as the number of phases increase in the system, the variance of the system must correspondingly decrease. A corollary to Gibbs' Phase Rule is Goldschmidt's Mineralogical Phase Rule: for a given rock in equilibrium at a fixed P and T, the number of phases is less than or equal to the number of components. Geologic systems are really rather simple. This means that we have a reasonable expectation that we can successfully interpret the conditions of formation of rocks in their natural settings, and to model their behaviour using the thermodynamic databases and programs presented at the end of this module.

SIMPLE ONE-COMPONENT

Let's consider the simple one component system for H_2O (Fig. 3.3):
1. The system is entirely composed of H_2O, so there is only one component present.
2. The phases present represent three states of matter: liquid (water), solid (ice), and vapour (steam). All have distinct physical properties (e.g. density, structure or lack of, etc.) and chemical properties (e.g. $\Delta G_{formation}$, molar volume, etc.) so they must be considered distinct phases.
3. Note that there is only one point on this diagram where all three phases coexist in equilibrium—this 'triple point' is also referred to as an invariant point; because P and T are uniquely specified, there are zero degrees of freedom.
4. Each of the curves represents a chemical reaction that describes a phase transformation: solid to liquid (melt/crystallisation), liquid to vapour (boiling/condensation), solid to vapour (sublimation/deposition). There are three univariant curves around the invariant point; it is always the case that for a C-component system, there will always be C+2 univariant curves radiating around an invariant point. This relationship is further explained in the unit on the method of Schreinemakers. There is only one degree of freedom along each of the univariant curves: you can independently change either T or P, but to maintain two coexisting phases along the curve the second variable must change by a corresponding fixed amount.
5. There are three distinct areas where only ice, liquid, or vapour exit. These are divariant fields. T and P are both free to change within these fields and you will still have only one phase (a bit hotter or colder, or compressed or expanded, but nonetheless the same phase).

6. The end of the 'boiling curve', separating the liquid to vapour transition, is called the 'critical point'. This is a particularly interesting part of the phase diagram because beyond this region the physico-chemical properties of water and steam converge to the point where they are identical. Thus, beyond the critical point, we refer to this single phase as a 'supercritical fluid'.

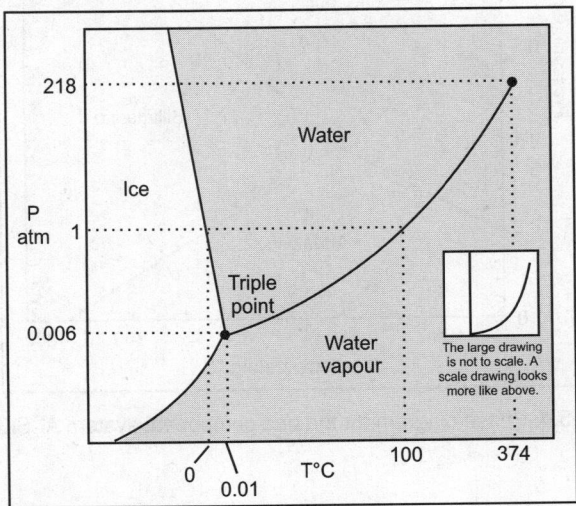

Fig. 3.3. Phase diagram for the one component system H_2O. This diagram is not to scale; a scale version looks like the thumbnail in the white box.

Now, let's consider a simple one component system that describes the mineral phases in the aluminosilicate system (Fig. 3.4):

1. The entire system is defined by one component: Al_2SiO_5 (i.e. all the phases can be completely made of this one component).
2. There are three solid phases shown in this diagram: the polymorphs of Al_2SiO_5 and alusite, kyanite and sillimanite.
3. There is only one unique place on this diagram where all three phases can coexist in equilibrium—the invariant point at 3.8 Kb and 500°C; at this point there are zero degrees of freedom.
4. There are three univariant reactions on this diagram, each representing the phase transitions: andalusite = sillimanite, andalusite = kyanite, and kyanite = sillimanite. In each of these reactions, either pressure or temperature can be changed independently, but for the state of the system to remain the same (i.e. two solid phases coexisting in equilibrium), the other variable must change by a fixed amount to maintain the assemblage on the univariant curve—so there is one degree of freedom. In a later section, we will see that the univariant curves represent the condition where, $\Delta G_{rxn} = 0$ (i.e. the intersection of the 'free energy surface' with the Pressure-Temperature plane represented by the phase diagram).
5. There are three divariant fields in which only a single mineral phase is stable. Within these fields pressure and temperature may be changed independently without changing the state of the system—thus there are two degrees of freedom in the divariant fields.

These principles extend to the more complicated binary, ternary and multi-component systems.

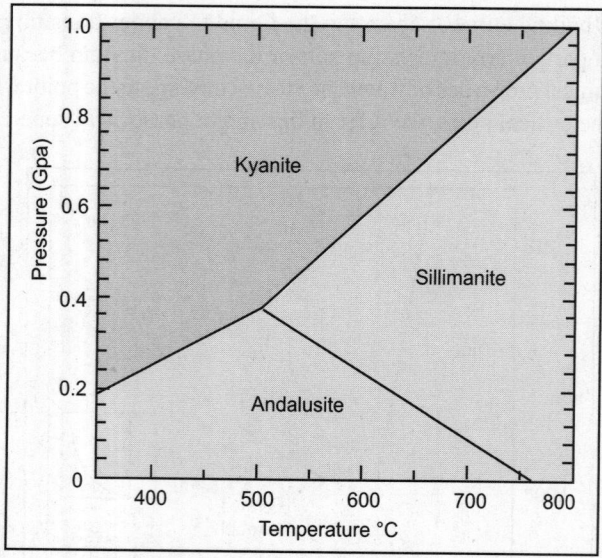

Fig. 3.4. Phase diagram for the one component system Al_2SiO_5.

Assumptions

There are a number of important assumptions that must be considered when applying Gibbs' Phase Rule:
1. The relationships described by the Gibbs' Phase Rule apply the concepts of equilibrium thermodynamics. It is assumed that geologic systems have enough time to naturally equilibrate. It is also assumed that geologic systems are 'closed' systems—that is the mass of the system remains essentially constant, and the system is free to consume or liberate energy to do work.
2. For geologic systems, heat and work are considered to be the major contributors to the system's energetics—that is, 'P-V work' is the dominant source of energy consumed/liberated by the system. We do not consider the effects of external fields (e.g. electrical, magnetic, gravitational), and we do not consider surface energy or boundary effects.
3. No kinetic effects are considered. This may present problems with an equilibrium thermodynamics approach if metastable phases are present in the system. In natural settings it is common for a given mineral to exist under physical conditions that exceed its predicted stability limits. A good example is the persistence of kyanite into the sillimanite stability field. This particular reaction: (i) has a very small ΔG_{rxn} (and thus, a small 'driving force' to make the reaction go), and (ii) the polymorphic reaction is of the 'reconstructive' kind, and requires the breaking and reforming of strong covalent bonds. The presence of metastable phases may complicate matters in trying to determine the equilibrium conditions for stable mineral assemblages, but they are essential indicators of changing physical conditions that allow us to interpret pressure-temeperature-time paths.
4. In some cases, surface reactions (e.g. sorption, catalysis) may operate in geological environment and contribute to the overall energetics of the system. Surface energies are not included in the Gibbs phase rule formulation.

5. Gibbs' Phase Rule cannot be applied indiscriminately. It is important to obtain the best possible characterisation of the identity, composition and structural state of the phases present. For example, complex materials such as mixed layer silicates may cause problems, or minerals that exhibit a range of structural states (e.g. the alkali feldspars). An overview of analytical techniques that are used to characterise minerals, melts and fluids can be found at the companion website on geochemical instrumentation and analysis.
6. Recognising these assumptions and limitations, the Gibbs Phase Rule still provides a powerful way to analyse and interpret geological systems. Although geologic systems are dynamic and often in a state of disequilibrium, the equilibrium approach demonstrates what the state of the system would be given sufficient time and energy to achieve that equilibrium. It also provides information on the phase changes or reactions that would be expected in a system that is thrown out of equilibrium due to changes in physical conditions. Thus a knowledge of the sequence of possible reactions provides important information about 'pathways' in geologic systems that allow interpretations of tectonic environments, petrogenetic processes, and the evolution of geologic systems.

Derivation of the Phase Rule

It is important to recognise that the simple formulation of Gibbs' Phase Rule is derivative from fundamental thermodynamic principles. The Gibbs–Duhem equation establishes the relationship between the intensive parameters temperature (T) and pressure (P) and the chemical potential of all components (μ_i) in the system:

$$dG = Vdp - Sdt + \Sigma N_i d\mu_i$$

This means that there are:
1. $C + 2$ independent variables that describe the system: P, T and one each for the chemical potential for all components.
2. P independent equations (of the Gibbs–Duhem form) that describe the energetics of the system—one equation for each phase.

In mathematical terms, the variance (F) is determined by the difference between (C+2) variables and (P) equations. Thus,

$$F = C + 2 - P \text{ or as originally written, } P + F = C + 2$$

BINARY PHASE DIAGRAMS

Other much more complex types of phase diagrams can be constructed, particularly when more than one pure component is present. In that case concentration becomes an important variable. Phase diagrams with more than two dimensions can be constructed that show the effect of more than two variables on the phase of a substance. Phase diagrams can use other variables in addition to or in place of temperature, pressure and composition, for example the strength of an applied electrical or magnetic field and they can also involve substances that take on more than just three states of matter (Fig. 3.5).

One type of phase diagram plots temperature against the relative concentrations of two substances in a binary mixture called a binary phase diagram (Fig. 3.6). Such a mixture can be either a solid solution, eutectic or peritectic, among others. These two types of mixtures result in very different graphs. Another type of binary phase diagram is a boiling point diagram for a mixture of two components, i.e. chemical compounds. For two particular volatile components at a certain pressure such as atmospheric pressure, a boiling point diagram (Fig. 3.7) shows what vapour (gas) compositions are in equilibrium with given liquid compositions depending on temperature. In a typical binary boiling point diagram, temperature is plotted on a vertical axis and mixture composition on a horizontal axis.

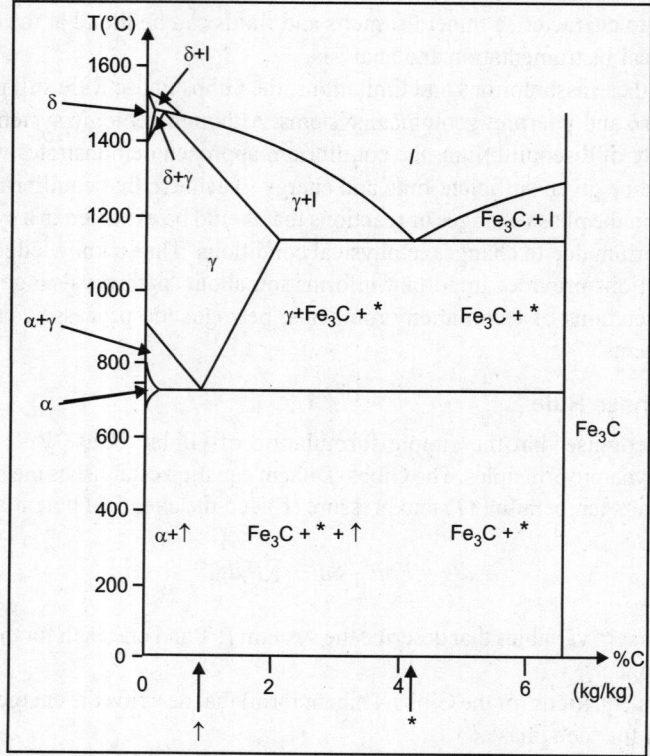

Fig. 3.5. The iron–iron carbide (Fe–Fe$_3$C) phase diagram. The percentage of carbon present and the temperature define the phase of the iron carbon alloy and therefore its physical characteristics and mechanical properties. The percentage of carbon determines the type of the ferrous alloy: iron, steel or cast iron.

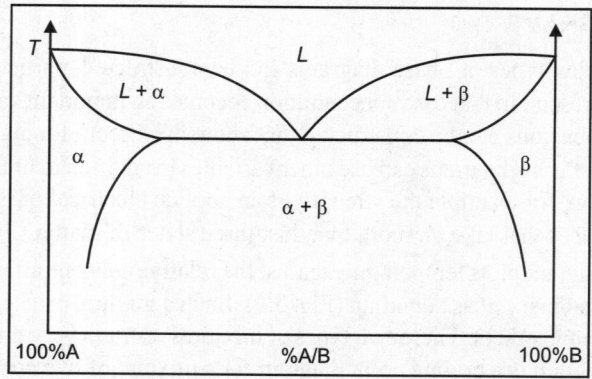

Fig. 3.6. A phase diagram for a binary system displaying a eutectic point.

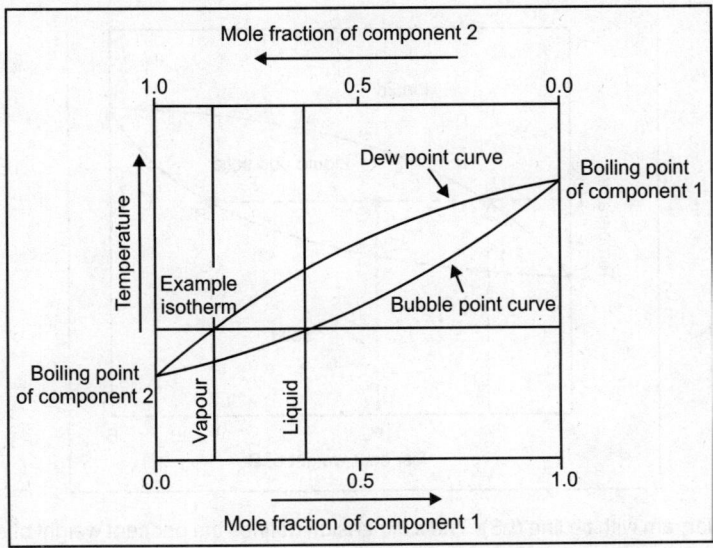

Fig. 3.7. Boiling point diagram

A simple example diagram with hypothetical components 1 and 2 in a non-azeotropic mixture is also shown in Fig 3.7. The fact that there are two separate curved lines joining the boiling points of the pure components means that the vapour composition is usually not the same as the liquid composition the vapour is in equilibrium with. In addition to the above mentioned types of phase diagrams, there are thousands of other possible combinations. Some of the major features of phase diagrams include congruent points, where a solid phase transforms directly into a liquid. There is also the peritectoid, a point where two solid phases combine into one solid phase during cooling.

The inverse of this, when one solid phase transforms into two solid phases during heating, is called the eutectoid. A complex phase diagram of great technological importance is that of the iron-carbon system for less than 7 per cent carbon. The x-axis of such a diagram represents the concentration variable of the mixture. As the mixtures are typically far from dilute and their density as a function of temperature is usually unknown, the preferred concentration measure is mole fraction. A volume based measure like molarity would be unadvisable.

Lever Rule

The lever rule is a tool used to determine weight percentages of each phase of a binary equilibrium phase diagram. It is used to determine the per cent weight of liquid and solid phases for a given binary composition and temperature that is between the liquidus and solidus.

Calculations

Before any calculations can be made a tie line is drawn on the phase diagram to determine the percent weight of each element; on the phase diagram to the right it is line segment LS (Fig. 3.8). This tie line is drawn horizontally at the compositions temperature from the liquid to the solidus. The per cent weight of element B at the liquidus is given by w_l and the per cent weight of element B at the solidus is given by w_s.

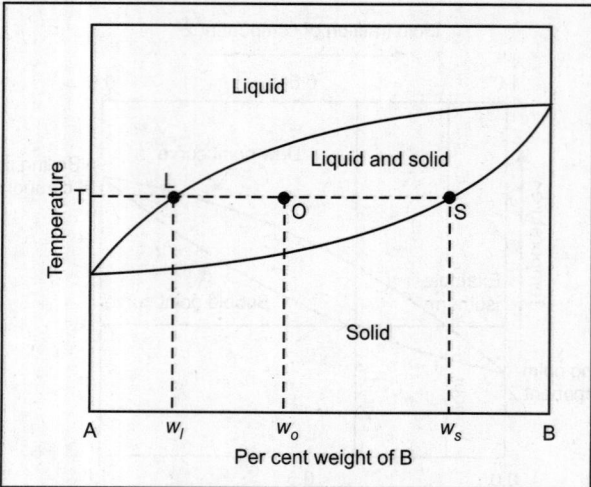

Fig. 3.8. A phase diagram with tie line (LS). The x dimension defines the per cent weight of elements A and B. The per cent weight of solid and liquid can then be calculated using the following lever rule equations:

$$\text{Per cent weight of the solid phase} = X_s = \frac{w_o - w_l}{w_s - w_l}$$

$$\text{Per cent weight of the liquid phase} = X_l = \frac{w_s - w_o}{w_s - w_l}$$

where, w_o is the per cent weight of element B for the given composition.

Thus, binary combinations of elements are relatively easy to investigate and can be recorded on a simple two-dimensional graphical system but ternary combinations are more difficult to investigate and recording involves a three-dimensional system of graphical construction while quaternary or more complex systems are almost invariably too complex for such treatment. For these reasons, a wide range of diagrams of binary systems is available but the information on ternary systems is comparatively limited and on quaternary systems almost nonexistent.

Equilibrium diagrams are invaluable in giving a clear picture of the stable interrelationship between elements in the solid state and, in conjunction with other information, they supply the basis of the metallurgical approach to all fabrication processes including casting, mechanical working, heat treatment, powder metallurgy and welding.

However, it is easiest to approach the idea of an equilibrium diagram from the relationship between two elements fully soluble in each other in the solid state. Copper and nickel are metals of this type, copper melting at 1083°C and nickel at 1455°C. With ranges of full solid solubility, where all factors such as size of atom, type of bond, valency and type of structure formed are favourable, the melting of an alloy tends to occur at a temperature approximately proportionate to the arithmetical average of the quantities of the elements present in the alloy related to their respective melting temperatures, but complete melting does not occur at a fixed temperature as with a pure metal. Melting tends to take place over a range of temperatures: therefore the temperature at which melting is about to begin and the temperature at which all melting is just completed must be found. These temperatures are called the 'solidus' and 'liquidus' respectively. Figure 3.9 shows how these temperatures vary for alloys of differing proportions of copper and nickel; the compositions are recorded on the abscissa and the temperatures on the ordinate. The lower of the two lines joining points A and B is the of plot the solidus temperatures and the upper line the plot of the liquidus temperatures. Below these lines the alloys exist as a single phase of solid solution containing proportions of the elements equal to the proportions in which they are present as a whole (i.e. the elements are uniformly distributed throughout each other). Above the lines a single liquid solution of uniform composition exists.

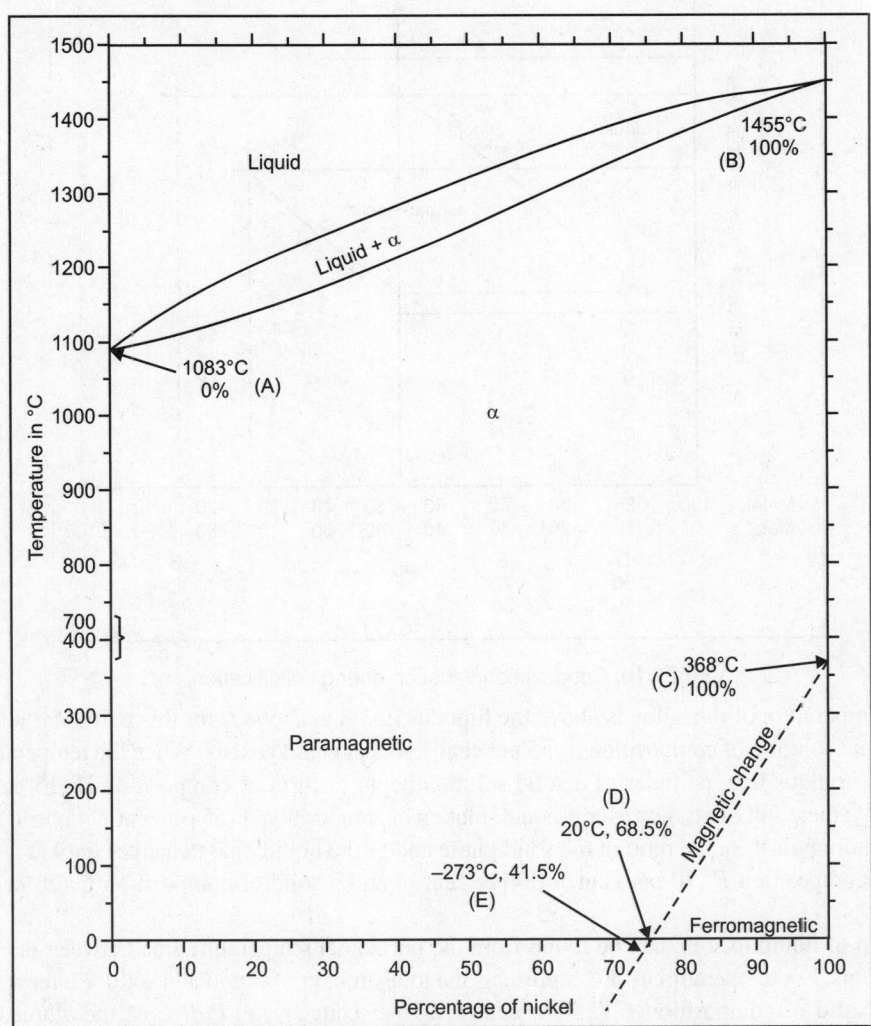

Fig. 3.9. Binary equilibrium diagram: copper–nickel.

Between the lines a rather complicated state is represented and a mixture of liquid of one composition exists around a solid of a differing composition, the proportions of liquid and solid and their compositions depending on the particular temperature and basic composition, as explained below. The only change which occurs with falling temperature once solidification is complete is a magnetic change and that only occurs within a certain composition range, as indicated by the dotted line DC.

To understand what is represented between the liquidus and solidus lines, let us consider an enlarged section of a diagram as shown in Fig. 3.10. In this the vertical solid line AA represents an alloy of x and y (55 per cent x, 45 per cent y).

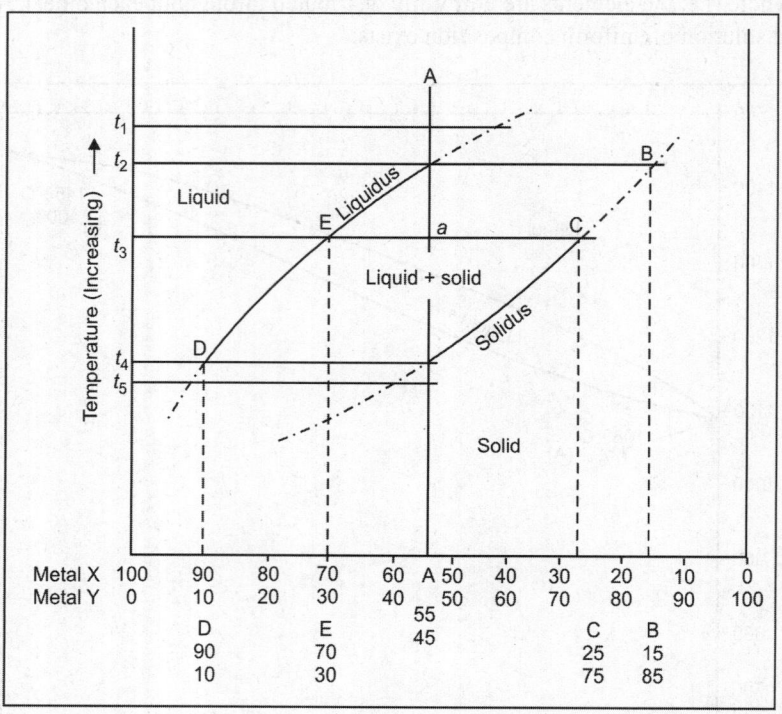

Fig. 3.10. Composition variation during solidification.

If the temperature of this alloy is above the liquidus line (i.e. above t_2 for this particular alloy) then a single liquid solution of composition A (55 per cent x, 45 per cent y) exists. When the temperature falls to t_2 on the liquidus line, particles of a solid solution begin to form of composition B (15 per cent x, 85 per cent y); there still exists, however, a liquid solution of composition A (55 per cent x, 45 per cent y). As the temperature falls to t_3, the ratio of the solid phase and of the liquid phase changes until at t_3 we have a liquid of composition E (70 per cent x, 30 per cent y) and a solid of composition C (25 per cent x, 75 per cent y).

The ratio of liquid to solid can be found from the horizontal temperature line between the liquidus and the solidus. For temperature t_3, EC represents the total amount of liquid and solid, Ea represents the amount of solid of composition C (25 per cent x, 75 per cent y), i.e. Ea/EC of the whole, and aC represents the amount of liquid of composition E (70 per cent x, 30 per cent y), i.e. aC/EC of the whole.

If the temperature continues to fall, the amount of liquid decreases as more solid is deposited from it. At temperature t_4 the liquid is almost completely gone and what little remains is of composition D (90 per cent x, 10 per cent y). Meanwhile the amount of solid has increased in quantity and changed in composition until it has attained the main composition A (55 per cent x, 45 per cent y). Finally when the temperature reaches t_e solidification is complete and at and below this temperature we have a solid solution of the same composition as the original liquid [i.e. composition A (55 per cent x, 45 per cent y)]. With rising temperatures the sequence is reversed, liquid of composition D (90 per cent x, 10 per cent y) begins to form at temperature t_4 and complete melting takes place at t_2.

If solubility of two elements in each other is still possible but tends to take place under less favourable conditions (such as the atom size factor being near the limit), then a simple uniform relationship will no longer exist and the diagram will be distorted. Since copper and gold are fully soluble in each other although their atom size factors are near to the limit, so their equilibrium diagram is as shown in Fig. 3.11. The diagram is distorted in the region of the liquidus and solidus lines, while compounds tend to form in certain conditions in the solid state as shown.

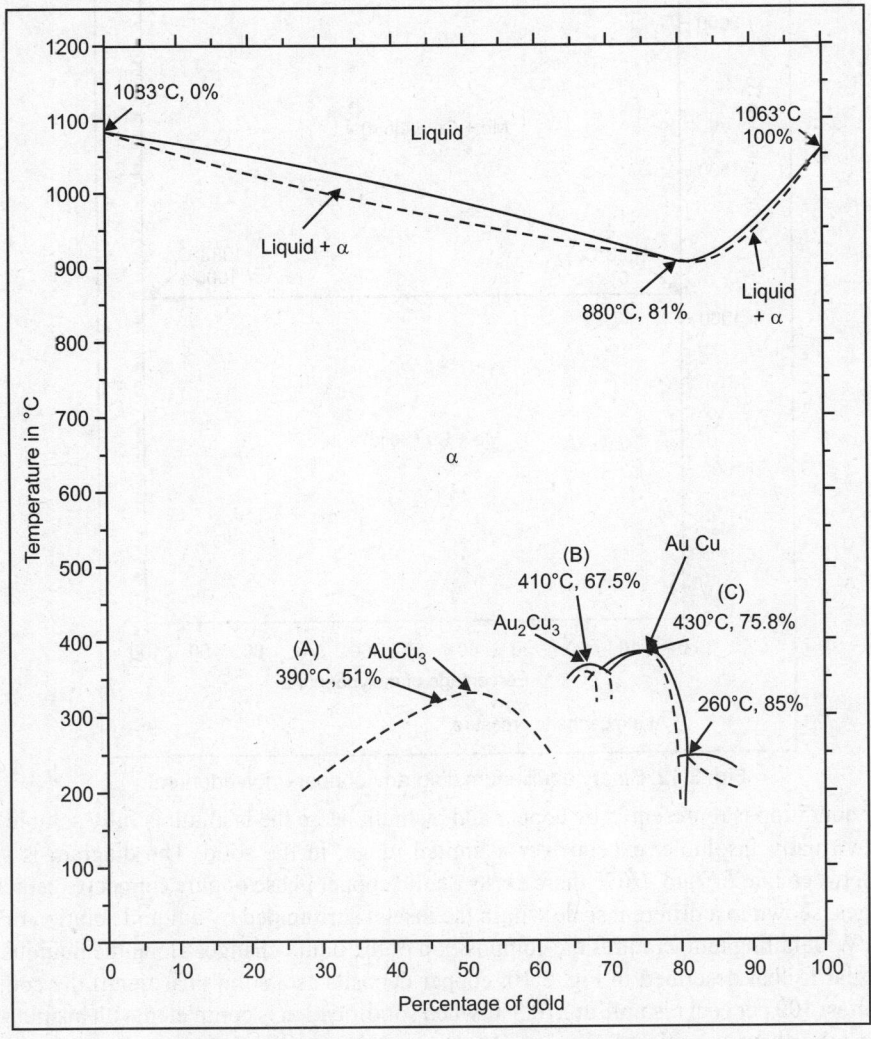

Fig. 3.11. Binary equilibrium diagram: copper–gold.

In contrast to copper-nickel and copper-gold alloys, copper and molybdenum (Mo) are virtually insoluble in each other in all proportions under all conditions, therefore the diagram is as shown in Fig. 3.12. Below *AB* both are solid and present as separate phases, above *AB* the copper is liquid and the molybdenum solid. Above *CD* (2325°C, the melting point of molybdenum) the molybdenum is liquid and the copper a vapour because the boiling temperature of copper is 2310°C.

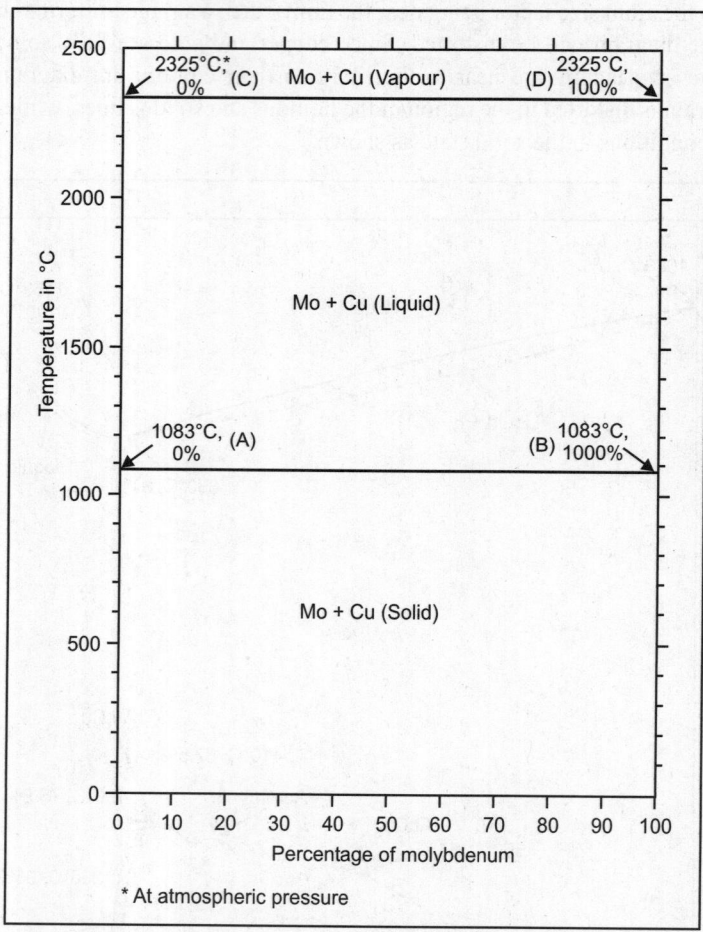

Fig. 3.12. Binary equilibrium diagram: copper–molybdenum.

Another condition is represented by copper and bismuth. Here the bismuth is fully soluble in liquid copper but virtually insoluble, except over a limited range, in the solid. The diagram is shown in Fig. 3.13. Between line *EF* and *ABCF* there exists a solid copper phase of pure copper (except in certain limited ranges, shown to a different scale within the insets) surrounded by a liquid solution of bismuth and copper. With falling temperatures the composition of the liquid changes along the liquidus line in a manner similar to that described in Fig. 3.10, copper deposits as a solid phase until the composition becomes almost 100 per cent bismuth at 270.3°C when solidification is completed with bismuth forming as a separate solid phase around the copper grains. There is a slight variation in the mode of solidification at 99.8 per cent bismuth, when a eutectic is formed.

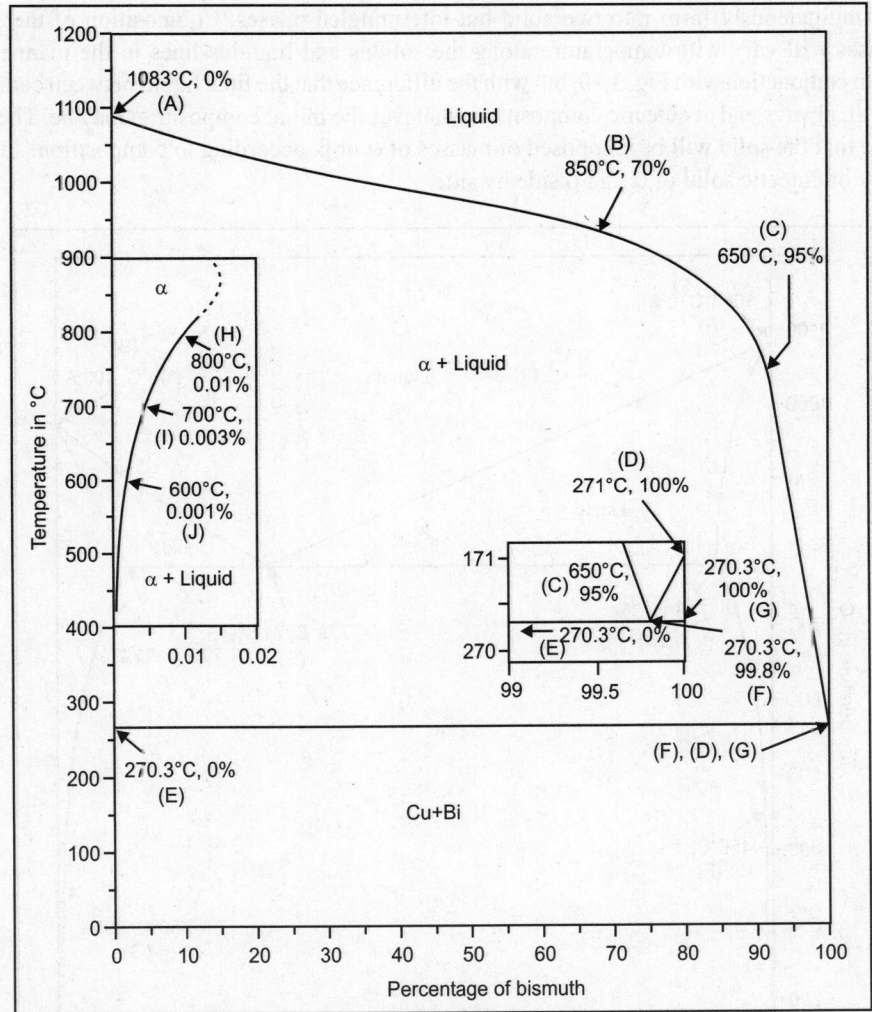

Fig. 3.13. Binary equilibrium diagram: copper–bismuth.

When full liquid solubility is possible with complete solid insolubility or very limited solid solubility then a eutectic relationship may exist. The nature of eutectic behaviour is the simultaneous solidification of two mutually insoluble solid phases from a liquid solution at a fixed temperature in fixed proportions.

These conditions exist for copper and silver which possess limited solid solubility in each other but are fully soluble in the liquid state, are illustrated in Fig. 3.14. In the figure ADB is the liquidus and $ACDEB$ the solidus. The area ACF represents the limited solution conditions (α phase) of silver in copper while BEG represents the conditions for the limited solid solution of copper in silver (β phase). Below $FCDEG$ the two phases α and β exist side by side.

Area ADC shows the conditions giving solid α phase in a liquid solution and area DBE those giving solid β phase in liquid solution. D is the eutectic point at 779°C with a 71.5 per cent silver content and **it can be seen from the diagram that, under these conditions, the solution will solidify at a fixed temperature** and will simultaneously form into two solid but intermingled phases. Composition of the solid and liquid phases will vary with temperature along the solidus and liquidus lines in the manner already described in conjunction with Fig. 3.10, but with the difference that the final liquid between compositions *C* and *E* will, always end at eutectic composition whatever the initial composition may be. The result of this will be that the solid will be composed of masses of α or β, according to composition, surrounded by a matrix of eutectic solid of α and β side by side.

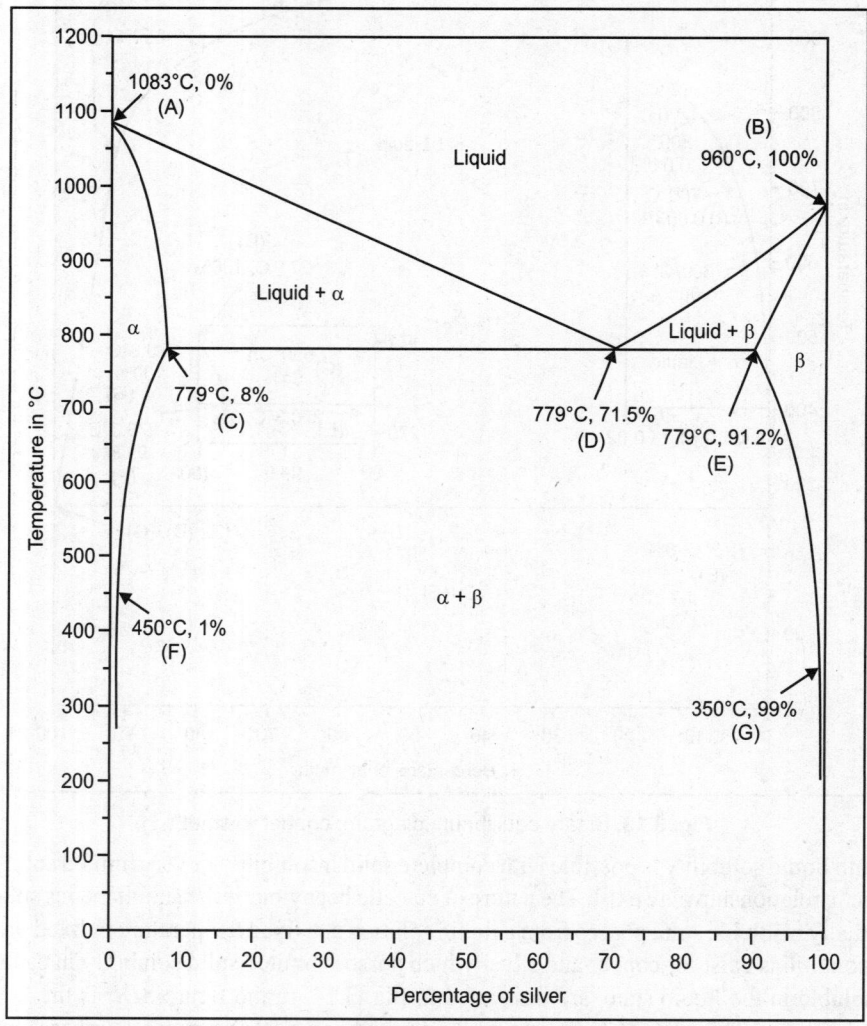

Fig. 3.14. Binary equilibrium diagram: copper–silver.

One other liquid–solid binary relationship needs description. This is the peritectic reaction in which a solid phase, forming from a cooling liquid, reacts at a particular temperature with the remaining liquid to form another single solid phase of composition intermediate between that of the first solid phase and the liquid. This is illustrated, for copper and tin, in Fig. 3.15 which shows the copper–tin diagram up to

32 per cent Sn. The peritectic point is at C where solid phase α of composition B (13.5 per cent Sn) reacts with tin–rich liquid of composition D (25.5 per cent Sn) to form a solid phase β containing 22 per cent Sn. If the total tin content is in excess of proportion B but below that of C (i.e. between 13.5 and 22 per cent) then α phase will exist surrounded by β immediately the temperature starts to fall below 798°C, all liquid having disappeared.

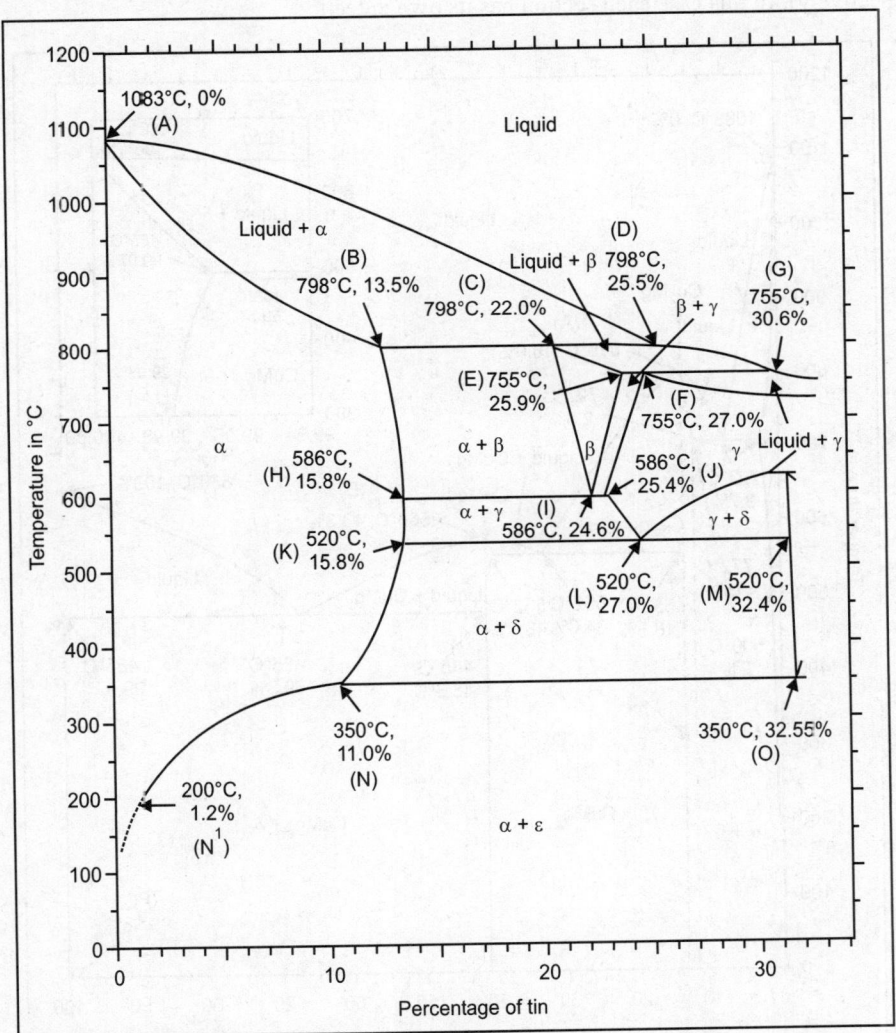

Fig. 3.15. Biliary equilibrium diagram: copper–tin (up to 32 per cent tin).

On the other hand, if composition is over that of C but less than D (i.e. between 22 and 25.5 per cent) then all the α will convert to β which will exist with a liquid phase whose composition will follow down the liquidus line DG as the temperature falls. At 755°C (Points E, F and G) another peritectic reaction occurs. In this alloy system, if the alloy composition is below 13.5 per cent or above 30.6 per cent Sn, β does not form at all under equilibrium conditions.

Many variations and combinations of these modes of behaviour are to be found in other systems. The formation of a compound may break a diagram up into two parts, since the compound will behave as a separate constituent. If more than one compound can form, then the diagram may be correspondingly divided. Copper and magnesium are examples of a binary combination which can form two compounds by which the diagram (Fig. 3.16) is divided into three at points A and B (compounds Cu_2-Mg and Cu-Mg_2 respectively). In this case each section has its own eutectic.

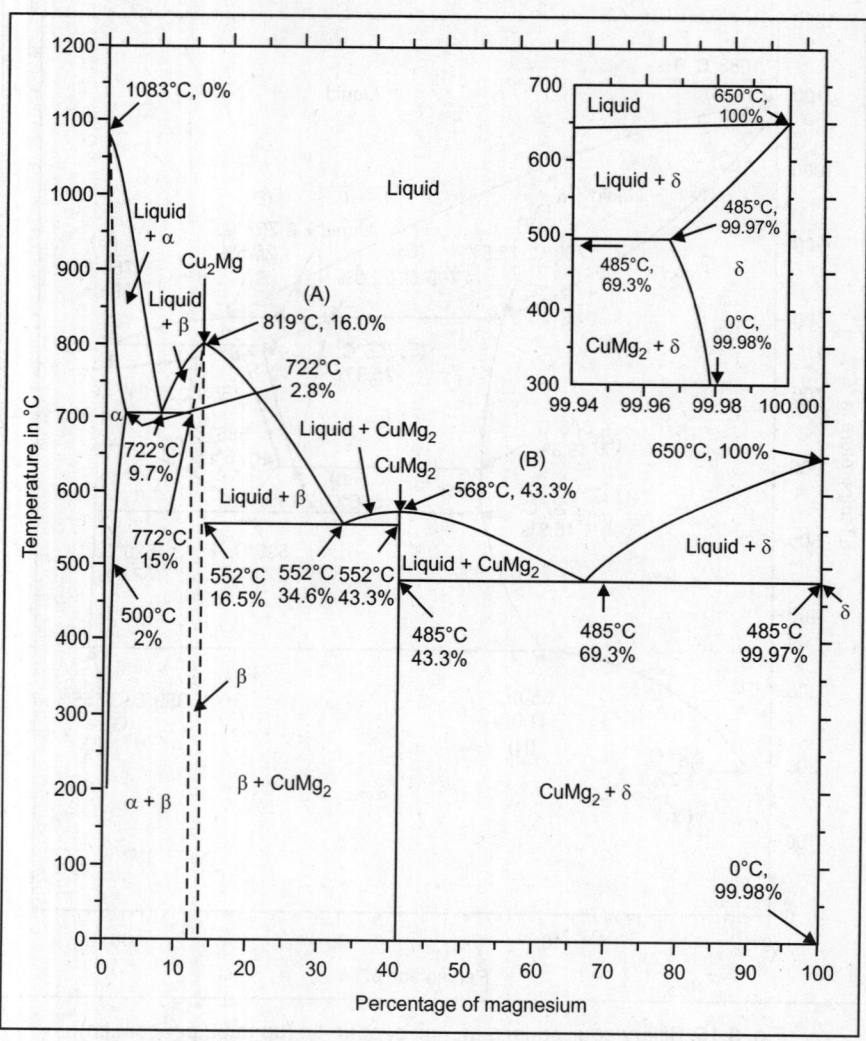

Fig. 3.16. Binary equilibrium diagram: copper–magnesium.

Behaviour in the solid state can be subject to variations similar to those between the liquid and solid, as a glance at Fig. 3.15 will show, and the form of the diagram makes them readily recognisable.

For example, in Fig. 3.15 two eutectoids are shown at I and L respectively. A eutectoid is formed when a single solid phase breaks up on cooling into two different phases at a fixed composition and temperature. In a like manner a peritectoid can be formed when two solid cooling phases combine at fixed composition and temperature to form a third single solid phase of intermediate composition. This is observable in the copper-silicon system, shown in Fig. 3.17, at point A where, α and β combine to form κ phase.

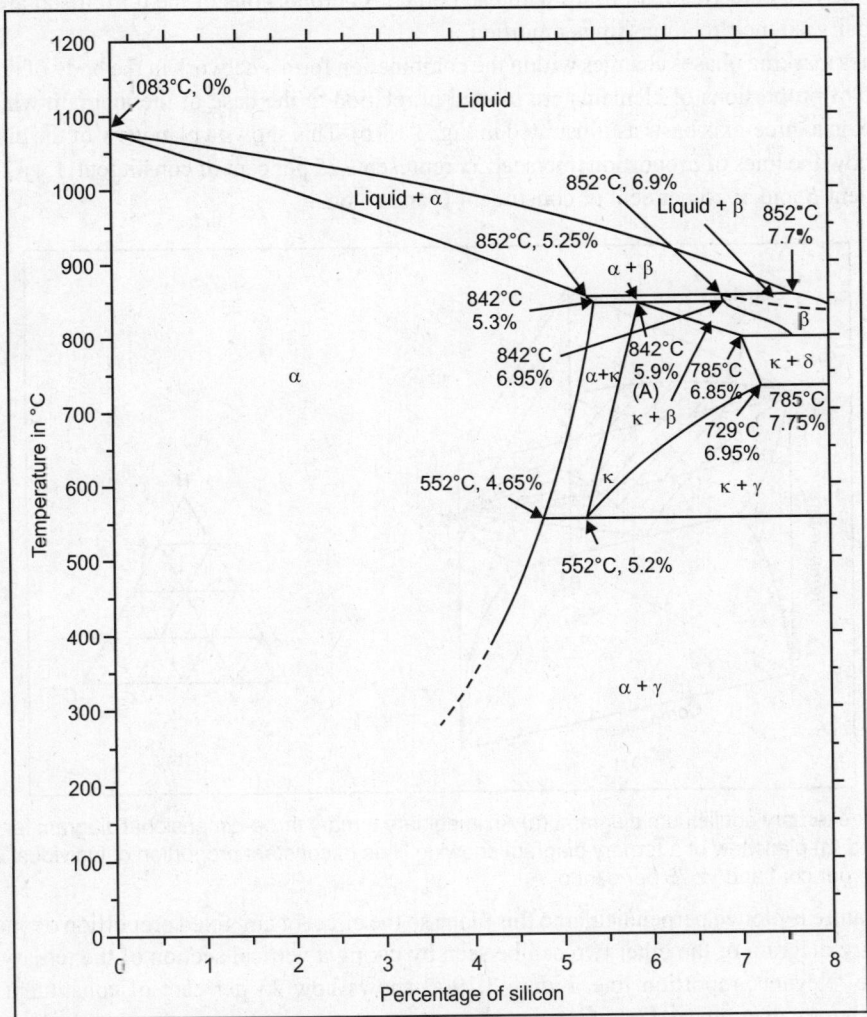

Fig. 3.17. Binary equilibrium diagram: copper–silicon.

All the diagrams which have been used for illustration are taken from binary systems based on copper so that it can be seen that the different modes of behaviour are not confined to one individual metal but can appear in any combination of metals which gives rise to the appropriate condition.

Ternary diagrams are not so easy to illustrate but they can be pictured as three-sided prisms bounded on each side by binary diagrams with bases originating from a common end plane, each edge of a prism representing a pure metal.

68 Physical Metallurgy

The profile of the top surface of the ternary diagram, the liquidus, will be shaped according to the interaction of each binary pair with the third element and in a like manner, solid phases will interrelate within the body. In Fig. 3.18(a) is illustrated an imaginary ternary diagram of metals A, B and C. Metals A and B are fully soluble in each other, metals A and C have a simple eutectic relationship and metals B and C also have a eutectic relationship with each other. As proportions of the third metal are added to the other pairs, so their relationship is modified.

The lines marking phases changes within the combination form a network in the body of the diagram the effects of proportions of elements are plotted in relation to the base of the diagram which can be divided up on a three-axis basis as illustrated in Fig. 3.18(b). This shows a plan view of the diagram and indicates how the lines of proportion intersect; xx represents 25 per cent of constituent A, yy 25 per cent of constituent B and zz 25 per cent of constituent C and so on.

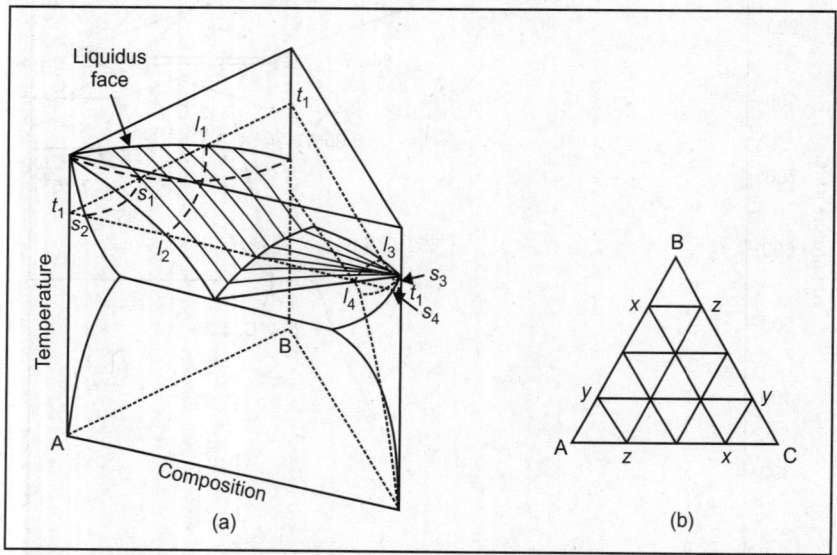

Fig. 3.18. The ternary equilibrium diagram. (a) An imaginary ternary three-dimensional diagram for metals A, B and C, and (b) plan view of a ternary diagram showing lines of constant proportion of individual elements, e.g. xx is 25 per cent and yz 75 per cent of A.

Temperature is plotted perpendicular to this plane so the effect of any fixed proportion of one element on the binary diagram of the other two can be seen by taking a vertical section of the ternary diagram through the relevant proportion line. Figure 3.19(a) shows how 25 per cent of constituent B might modify the binary diagram of A and C to that shown on a vertical section yy.

It is sometimes helpful to see the effect of the constituents on each other at a particular temperature level, so a horizontal section, called an isotherm, can be taken at the appropriate temperature level giving a diagram similar to that shown in Fig. 3.19(b) which corresponds to the temperature level $t_1 t_1 t_1$ in Fig. 3.18(a).

An example of an actual ternary diagram is shown in Fig. 3.20(a) and 3.20(b). Figure 3.20(a) shows the general diagram and Fig. 3.20(b) shows typical isothermal sections. Diagrams for greater numbers of constituents have been prepared but they are too complicated for consideration here.

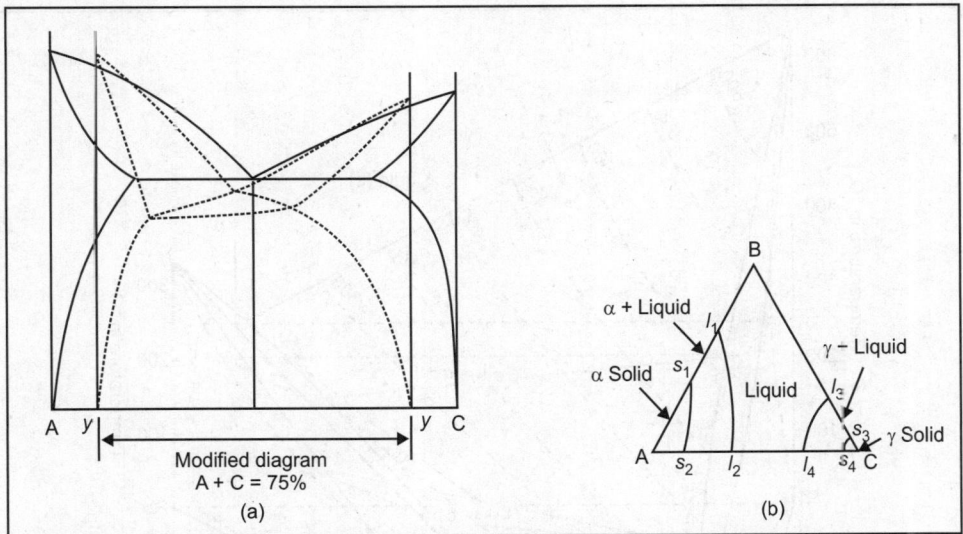

Fig. 3.19. Use of ternary equilibrium diagrams. (a) effect of 25 per cent B on relationship of A and C (section yy), and (b) state of alloys at temperature t_1.

THERMAL ANALYSIS—HEATING AND COOLING CURVES

If the equilibrium diagram is to be used, there must be some method for correlating the composition of a piece of metal of uncertain but suspected composition with the diagram. Much can be done by microscopical examination but the most useful means may be by thermal analysis. The use of this depends on the fact that if a substance is being heated or cooled through a phase change then, at the temperature of the change, there will be a difference in the absorption or dispersion rate of thermal energy because the thermal characteristics of the phases will differ. If a marked amount of latent heat has to be absorbed or given up, then a marked arrest point will appear on the temperature-time curve for the metal.

On the other hand, if there is no noticeable latent heat change involved, then a change of gradient may be the only sign of the phase change and considerable care may be required if it is to be observed. Under normal atmospheric pressure, these temperature inflections will always take place at the exact temperature of the phase change, provided that sufficient time is allowed for the change to take place and that the rate of heating or cooling is not so rapid that superheating or undercooling is caused.

Thermal analysis offers the only reliable means for plotting the liquidus temperature of an alloy of known composition and, hence, for constructing an equilibrium diagram. It is neither the only method nor the best method for verifying or examining solid phase change effects. Having obtained an equilibrium diagram, thermal analysis may be used to verify the composition of a piece of alloy metal known to be composed of metal of the type for which the diagram applies. Note that this is not a means for analysing an alloy of unknown composition, but simply for confirming the absence or presence and quantity of an element in an alloy whose composition is known or suspected within fairly close limits. The limits of composition, within which thermal analysis can be attempted, will depend on how much is known of the nature and complication of the particular alloy system.

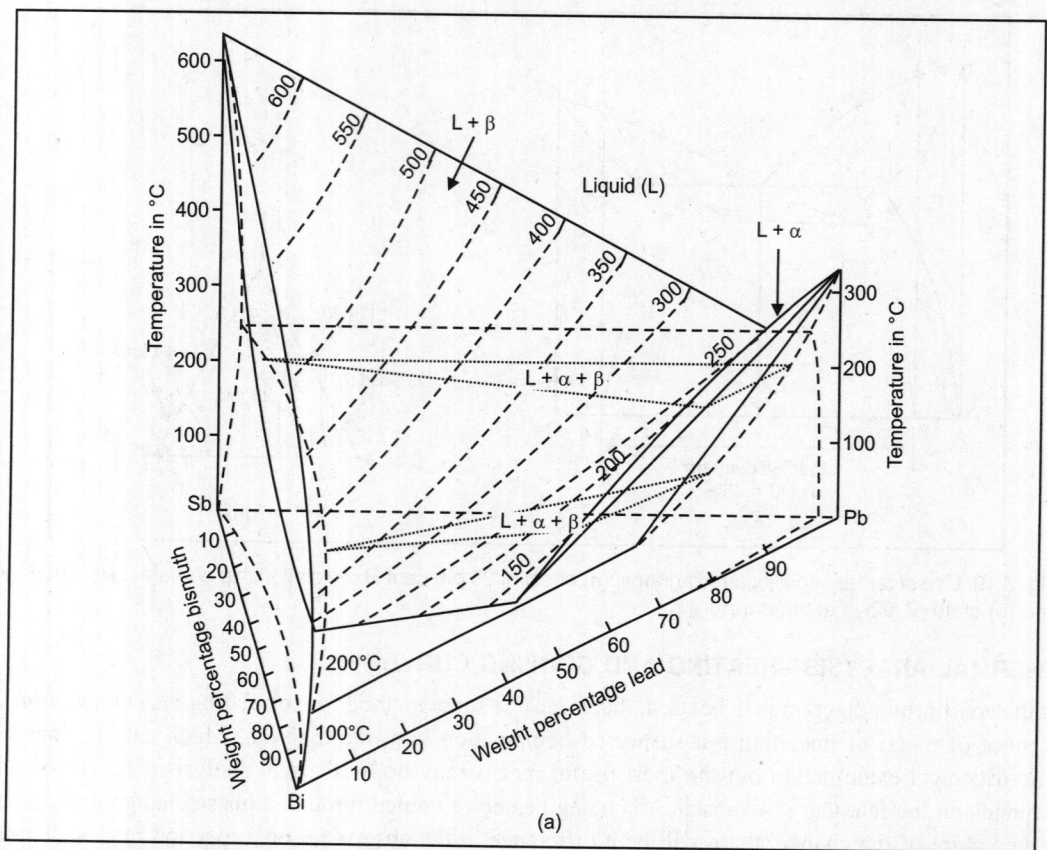

Fig. 3.20(a). A typical ternary equilibrium diagram—Temperature-composition diagram of the system lead–bismuth–antimony.

Thermal analysis is usually performed on a small sample of the metal which, if the metal is not to be melted, has a hole drilled into its interior (or cast in, if the metal is being melted) to carry a thermocouple. The thermocouple is carefully packed into the hole so that any change of temperature of the metal immediately influences the thermocouple. A small furnace of a type which can be heated to the necessary temperature at a reasonably controlled rate and then can be cooled at a rate sufficiently low to prevent excessive undercooling is used to give the heating and cooling conditions for the specimen.

A heating and cooling curve for the furnace will be of the general type indicated in Fig. 3.21(a) but this will be modified within the metal sample and might be as shown in Fig. 3.21(b), which shows two types of 'arrest' points and their characteristics during heating and cooling. Under ideal conditions the level of their arrests would be the same on both curves but it is difficult to keep the heating rate down to a sufficiently slow and yet uniform rate.

So the heating curve may be less reliable, possibly giving slightly elevated readings. Cooling is more uniformly controllable since it is dependent on the insulation of the furnace in relation to the uniformity of atmospheric temperature and so may give more reliable results. A curve of the type shown in Fig. 3.21(b) may be difficult to interpret, if the changes are slight and closely spaced, and so a special method of recording is used.

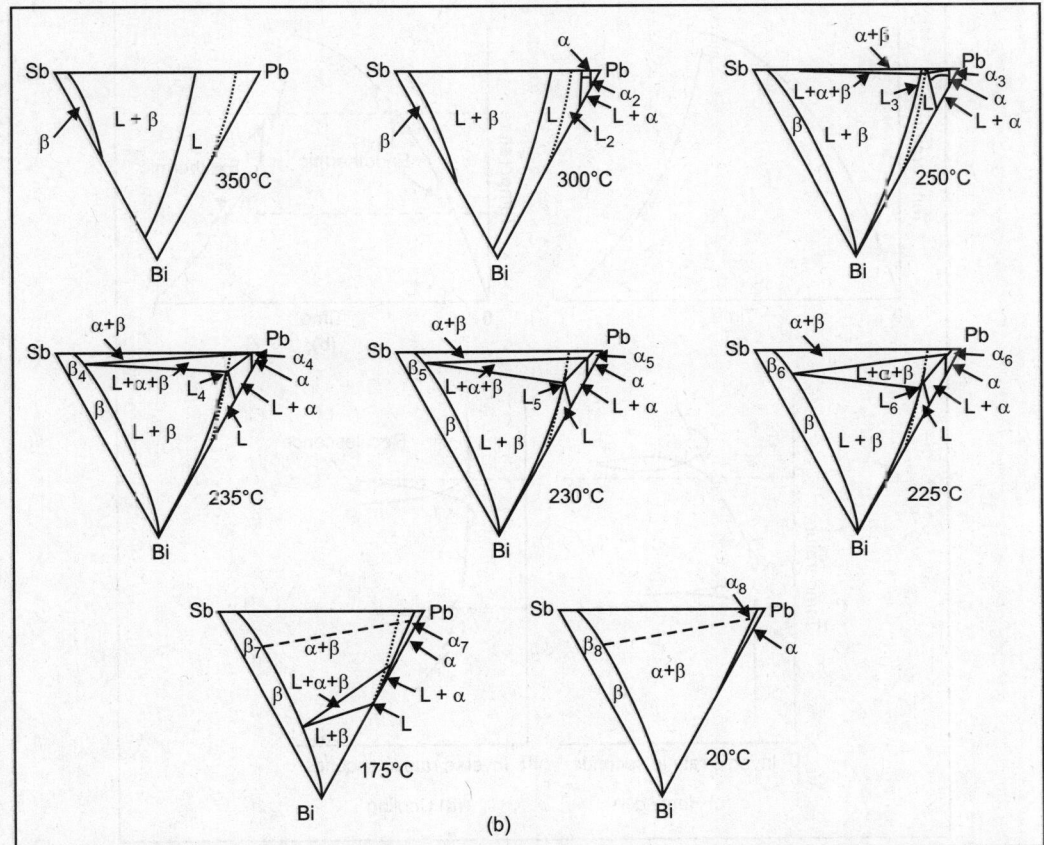

Fig. 3.20(b). A typical ternary equilibrium diagram—Isotherms of the system lead–bismuth-antimony.

This is the so-called 'inverse-rate' curve which is plotted as the times taken for temperature changes of a constant amount of increment and decrement. Such curves for the furnace have a smooth uniform shape but sharp peaks appear at the change points for the specimen, as shown in Fig. 3.21(c). If cooling is a little rapid, the phase change temperature may be depressed below the true temperature by an appreciable amount; an effect known as 'undercooling'. If in such circumstances the exothermal reaction is strong, then a phenomenon known as 'recalescence' may occur. In the latter case the temperature falls below the change temperature before transformation begins and then tends to rise again towards the true value as transformation proceeds [Fig. 3.21(c)].

For the most accurate results another system of thermal analysis recording is sometimes employed, although it entails more complicated work in setting up. This is the 'differential' method using a neutral test piece, which shows no phase changes in the relevant range, as a reference body alongside the test specimen in the furnace. In this case any temperature differences which may appear between the two bodies as a result of phase changes in the test specimen are noted and then plotted against the temperature of the reference body.

Figure 3.22(a) shows a series or idealised cooling curves for differing alloys of cadmium and bismuth related to the equilibrium diagram shown in Fig. 3.22(b).

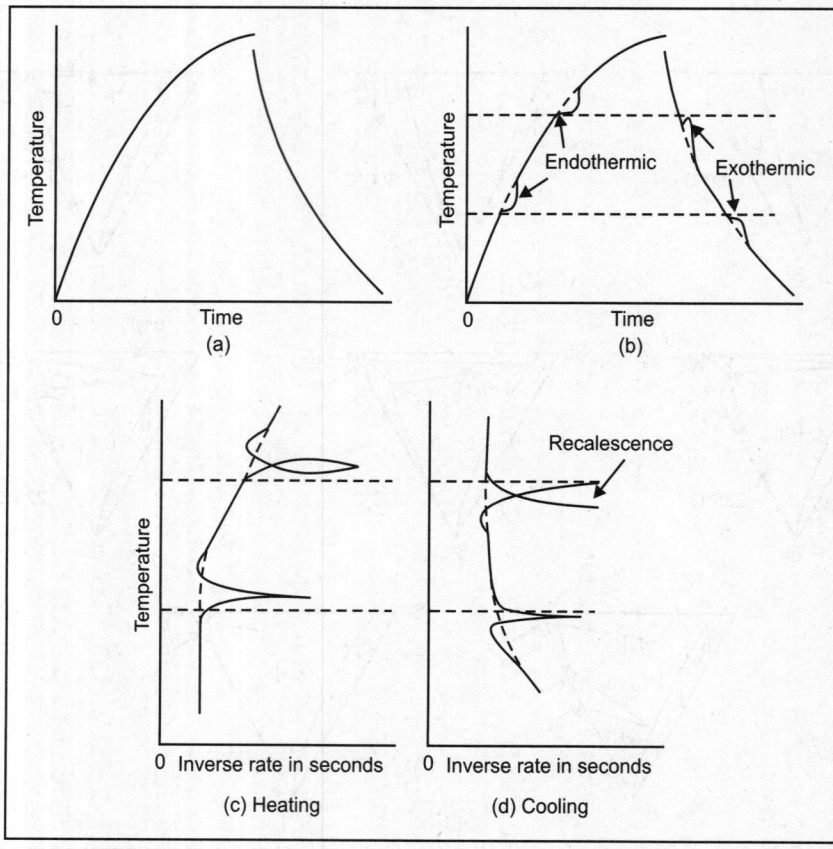

Fig. 3.21. Heating and cooling curves. (a) Furnace heating and cooling curves, (b) heating and cooling curves of an alloy in the furnace, (c) Phase changes cause steps according to the nature and magnitude of the energy change involved, and (d) inverse rate curves.

TIME–TEMPERATURE TRANSFORMATION CURVES

A hint has already been given that the information which can be obtained from an equilibrium diagram is liable to be limited. One cannot tell from an equilibrium diagram alone whether or not a particular alloy's mechanical properties can be enhanced by heat treatment. This difficulty arises because the diagram shows the stable condition but does not indicate if the rate and mode of development of the stable condition are sufficiently slow to be controllable. It is here that time-temperature-transformation curves begin to serve their purpose.

The name is almost self-explanatory since the diagram records the times required for metal, which has been heated to a 'critical' temperature (i.e. a temperature high enough to cause the metal structure to change completely to another structure typical of the elevated temperature), to revert completely or 'transform' to the lower temperature structure after being quenched to a constant or 'isothermal' temperature low enough for the change to take place. The method of operation is to take a series of specimens of the same composition, heat them long enough at elevated temperature to ensure the formation of a homogeneous high temperature phase (usually a solid solution from two or more phases), then quench them in an isothermal bath (molten lead or salts are often employed) at the relevant temperature.

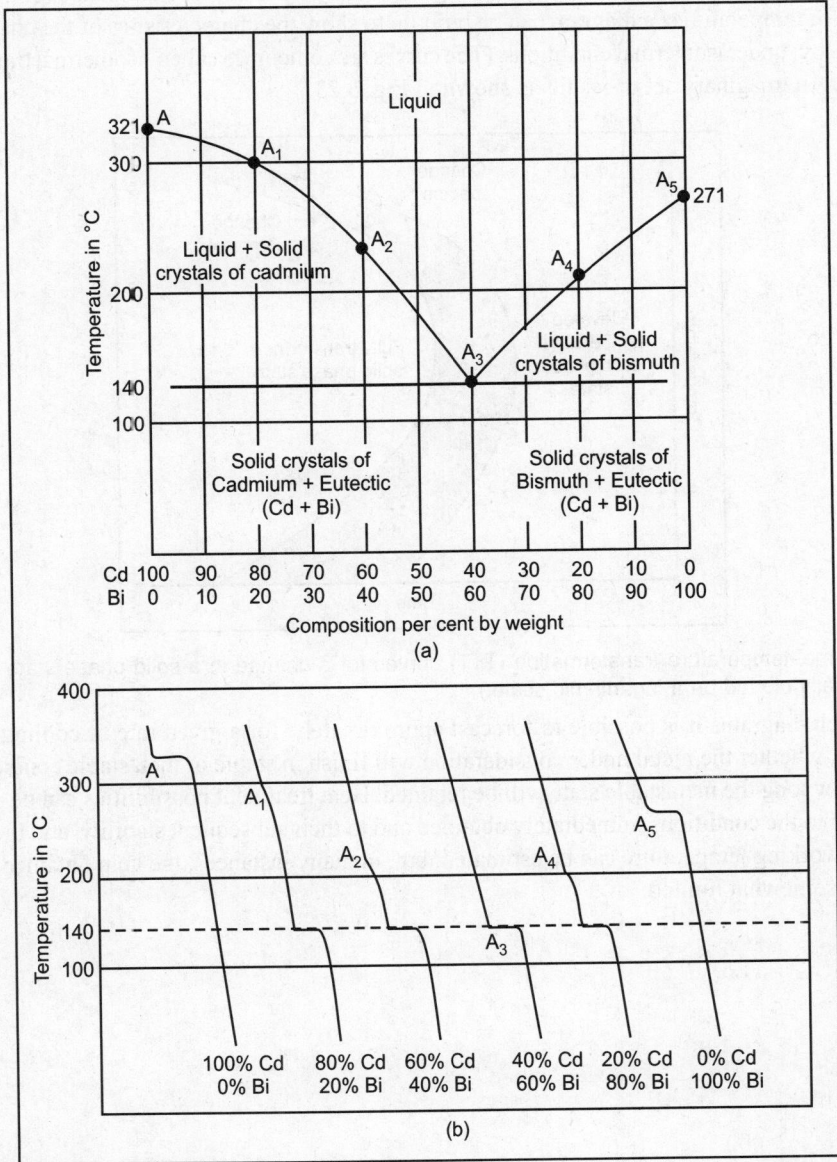

Fig. 3.22. Correlation of equilibrium diagram with cooling curves: (a) equilibrium diagram of the cadmium–bismuth system, and (b) time–temperature cooling curves for a series of alloys between cadmium and bismuth.

At regular intervals of time, decided by trial and error, single specimens are taken out and rapidly quenched to room temperature. These specimens are subsequently sectioned and examined under the microscope to find, (i) with which specimen the structure begins to change to its stable form, and (ii) with which specimen the change is just complete. Each specimen represents a time interval which can be plotted on a graph. With a sufficiently large number of specimens, examined over a sufficiently wide range of temperatures, a diagram can be built up to show the characteristics of the change, for the particular alloy; under isothermal conditions. (The curves are sometimes called 'isothermal transformation diagrams'.) An imaginary set of results is shown in Fig. 3.23.

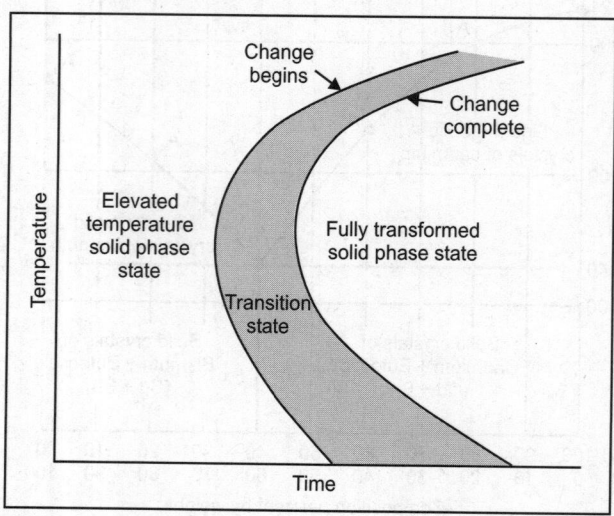

Fig. 3.23. Time–temperature transformation (TTT) curves for a change in a solid phase state of a metal. (Time is usually plotted on a logarithmic scale.)

From such diagrams it is possible to forecast approximately, for a given rate of cooling to a given temperature, whether the metal under consideration will finish in stable or metastable condition and, if the latter, how long the metastable state will be retained. Heat treatment possibilities can be assessed in relation both to the conditions immediately obtained and to their subsequent stability, and the influence of elevated working temperature can be estimated; but, in many instances, the help obtained from TTT diagrams is somewhat limited.

Chapter 4
Heat Treatment of Stainless Steel

INTRODUCTION

In metallurgy stainless steel, also known as inox steel or inox from French 'inoxydable', is defined as a steel alloy with a minimum of 10.5 or 11 per cent chromium content by mass. Stainless steel does not stain, corrode, or rust as easily as ordinary steel, but it is not stain-proof. It is also called corrosion-resistant steel or CRES when the alloy type and grade are not detailed, particularly in the aviation industry. There are different grades and surface finishes of stainless steel to suit the environment the alloy must endure. Stainless steel is used where both the properties of steel and resistance to corrosion are required.

Stainless steel differs from carbon steel by the amount of chromium present. Unprotected carbon steel rusts readily when exposed to air and moisture. This iron oxide film (the rust) is active and accelerates corrosion by forming more iron oxide. Stainless steels contain sufficient chromium to form a passive film of chromium oxide, which prevents further surface corrosion and blocks corrosion from spreading into the metal's internal structure. Passivation only occurs if the mixture of chromium is high enough, or if the manufacturer performs this last step.

PROPERTIES

High oxidation-resistance in air at ambient temperature is normally achieved with additions of a minimum of 13 per cent (by weight) chromium, and up to 26 per cent is used for harsh environments. The chromium forms a passivation layer of chromium(III) oxide (Cr_2O_3) when exposed to oxygen. The layer is too thin to be visible, and the metal remains lustrous. The layer is impervious to water and air, protecting the metal beneath. Also, this layer quickly reforms when the surface is scratched. This phenomenon is called passivation and is seen in other metals, such as aluminium and titanium. Corrosion-resistance can be adversely affected if the component is used in a non-oxygenated environment, a typical example being underwater keel bolts buried in timber.

When stainless steel parts such as nuts and bolts are forced together, the oxide layer can be scraped off, causing the parts to weld together. When disassembled, the welded material may be torn and pitted, an effect known as galling. This destructive galling can be best avoided by the use of dissimilar materials for the parts forced together, for example bronze and stainless steel, or even different types of stainless steels (martensitic against austenitic), when metal-to-metal wear is a concern. Nitronic alloys reduce the tendency to gall through selective alloying with manganese and nitrogen. In addition, threaded joints may be lubricated to prevent galling.

APPLICATIONS

Stainless steel's resistance to corrosion and staining, low maintenance, relatively low cost, and familiar luster make it an ideal material for many applications. There are over 150 grades of stainless steel, of which fifteen are most commonly used. The alloy is milled into coils, sheets, plates, bars, wire, and tubing to be used in cookware, cutlery, hardware, surgical instruments, major appliances, industrial equipment (for example, in sugar refineries) and as an automotive and aerospace structural alloy and construction material in large buildings. Storage tanks and tankers used to transport orange juice and other food are often made of stainless steel, due to its corrosion resistance and antibacterial properties. This also influences its use in commercial kitchens and food processing plants, as it can be steam-cleaned and sterilised and does not need paint or other surface finishes.

Stainless steel is used for jewelery and watches with 316L being the type commonly used for such applications. It can be re-finished by any jeweler and will not oxidise or turn black.

Some firearms incorporate stainless steel components as an alternative to blued or parkerised steel. Some handgun models, such as the Smith and Wesson Model 60 and the Colt M1911 pistol, can be made entirely from stainless steel. This gives a high-luster finish similar in appearance to nickel plating. Unlike plating, the finish is not subject to flaking, peeling, wear-off due to rubbing (as when repeatedly removed from a holster), or rust when scratched. Some automotive manufacturers use stainless steel as decorative highlights in their vehicles.

Architectural

Stainless steel is used for buildings for both practical and aesthetic reasons. Stainless steel was in vogue during the art deco period. The most famous example of this is the upper portion of the Chrysler Building. Some diners and fast-food restaurants use large ornamental panels and stainless fixtures and furniture. Owing to the durability of the material, many of these buildings retain their original appearance.

The forging of stainless steel has given rise to a fresh approach to architectural blacksmithing in recent years.

Type 316 stainless is used on the exterior of both the Petronas Twin Towers and the Jin Mao Building, two of the world's tallest skyscrapers.

The Parliament House of Australia in Canberra has a stainless steel flagpole weighing over 220 tons. The aeration building in the Edmonton Composting Facility, the size of 14 hockey rinks, is the largest stainless steel building in North America.

TYPES OF STAINLESS STEEL

There are different types of stainless steels: when nickel is added, for instance, the austenite structure of iron is stabilised. This crystal structure makes such steels virtually non-magnetic and less brittle at low temperatures. For greater hardness and strength, more carbon is added. With proper heat treatment, these steels are used for such things as razor blades, cutlery, and tools.

Significant quantities of manganese have been used in many stainless steel compositions. Manganese preserves an austenitic structure in the steel as does nickel, but at a lower cost.

Stainless steels are also classified by their crystalline structure:
1. Austenitic, or 300 series, stainless steels make up over 70 per cent of total stainless steel production. They contain a maximum of 0.15 per cent carbon, a minimum of 16 per cent chromium and sufficient nickel and/or manganese to retain an austenitic structure at all temperatures from the cryogenic region to the melting point of the alloy. A typical composition

of 18 per cent chromium and 10 per cent nickel, commonly known as 18/10 stainless, is often used in flatware. 18/0 and 18/8 are also available. Superaustenitic stainless steels, such as alloy AL-6XN and 254SMO, exhibit great resistance to chloride pitting and crevice corrosion due to high molybdenum content (>6 per cent) and nitrogen additions, and the higher nickel content ensures better resistance to stress-corrosion cracking versus the 300 series. The higher alloy content of superaustenitic steels makes them more expensive. Other steels can offer similar performance at lower cost and are preferred in certain applications. Low-carbon versions, for example 316L or 304L, are used to avoid corrosion problems caused by welding. Grade 316LVM is preferred where biocompatibility is required (such as body implants and piercings). The 'L' means that the carbon content of the alloy is below 0.03 per cent, which reduces the sensitisation effect (precipitation of chromium carbides at grain boundaries) caused by the high temperatures involved in welding.
2. Ferritic stainless steels generally have better engineering properties than austenitic grades, but have reduced corrosion resistance, due to the lower chromium and nickel content. They are also usually less expensive. They contain between 10.5 per cent and 27 per cent chromium and very little nickel, if any, but some types can contain lead. Most compositions include molybdenum; some, aluminium or titanium. Common ferritic grades include 18Cr-2Mo, 26Cr-1Mo, 29Cr-4Mo, and 29Cr-4Mo-2Ni. These alloys can be degraded by the presence of σ chromium, an intermetallic phase which can precipitate upon welding.
3. Martensitic stainless steels are not as corrosion-resistant as the other two classes but are extremely strong and tough, as well as highly machinable, and can be hardened by heat treatment. Martensitic stainless steel contains chromium (12–14 per cent), molybdenum (0.2–1 per cent), nickel (less than 2 per cent), and carbon (about 0.1–1 per cent) (giving it more hardness but making the material a bit more brittle). It is quenched and magnetic.
4. Precipitation-hardening martensitic stainless steels have corrosion resistance comparable to austenitic varieties, but can be precipitation hardened to even higher strengths than the other martensitic grades. The most common, 17–4 PH, uses about 17 per cent chromium and 4 per cent nickel. The Lockheed-Martin Joint Strike Fighter is the first aircraft to use a precipitation-hardenable stainless steel — Carpenter Custom 465 — in its airframe.
5. Duplex stainless steels have a mixed microstructure of austenite and ferrite, the aim usually being to produce a 50/50 mix, although in commercial alloys the ratio may be 40/60. Duplex stainless steels have roughly twice the strength compared to austenitic stainless steels and also improved resistance to localised corrosion, particularly pitting, crevice corrosion and stress corrosion cracking. They are characterised by high chromium (19–28 per cent) and molybdenum (up to 5 per cent) and lower nickel contents than austenitic stainless steels. Duplex grades are characterised into groups based on their alloy content and corrosion resistance. Lean duplex refers to grades such as UNS S32101 (LDX 2101), S32304, and S32003. The standard duplex is 22 per cent chromium with S31803/S32205 known as 2205 being the most widely used. Super duplex refers to 25 per cent chromium grades such as S32760 (Zeron 100), S32750 (2507), and S32550 (Ferralium). Hyper duplex refers to higher chromium grades such as S32906. The properties of duplex stainless steels are achieved with an overall lower alloy content than similar-performing super-austenitic grades, making their use cost-effective for many applications.

Comparison of Standardised Steels

Comparison of standardised steels is shown in Table 4.1.

Table 4.1. Comparison of standardised steels.

EN-standard Steel no. k.h.s DIN	EN-standard steel name	SAE grade	UNS
		440A	S44002
1.4112		440B	S44003
1.4125		440C	S44004
		440F	S44020
1.4016	X6Cr 17	430	S43000
1.4408	G-X 6 CrNiMo 18–10	316	
1.4512	X6CrTi 12	409	S40900
		410	S41000
1.4310	X10CrNi 18–8	301	S30100
1.4318	X2CrNiN 18–7	301LN	N/A
1.4307	X2CrNi 18–9	304L	S30403
1.4306	X2CrNi 19–11	304L	S30403
1.4311	X2CrNiN 18–10	304LN	S30453
1.4301	X5CrNi 18–10	304	S30400
1.4948	X6CrNi 18–11	304H	S30409
1.4303	X5CrNi 18–12	305	S30500
	X5CrNi 30–9	312	
1.4541	X6CrNiTi 18–10	321	S32100
1.4878	X12CrNiTi 18–9	321H	S32109
1.4404	X2CrNiMo 17–12–2	316L	S31603
1.4401	X5CrNiMo 17–12–2	316	S31600
1.4406	X2CrNiMoN 17–12–2	316LN	S31653
1.4432	X2CrNiMo 17–12–3	316L	S31603
1.4435	X2CrNiMo 18–14–3	316L	S31603
1.4436	X3CrNiMo 17–13–3	316	S31600
1.4571	X6CrNiMoTi 17–12–2	316Ti	S31635
1.4429	X2CrNiMoN 17–13–3	316LN	S31653
1.4438	X2CrNiMo 18–15–4	317L	S31703
1.4539	X1NiCrMoCu 25–20–5	904L	N08904
1.4547	X1CrNiMoCuN 20–18–7	N/A	S31254

Stainless steel grades

There are a number of different systems for grading stainless and other steels.

Stainless steel in 3D printing

Some 3D printing providers have developed proprietary stainless steel sintering blends for use in rapid prototyping. Currently available grades do not vary significantly in their properties.

Stainless Steel Finishes

Standard mill finishes can be applied to flat rolled stainless steel directly by the rollers and by mechanical abrasives. Steel is first rolled to size and thickness and then annealed to change the properties of the final material. Any oxidation that forms on the surface (scale) is removed by pickling, and a passivation layer is created on the surface. A final finish can then be applied to achieve the desired aesthetic appearance.

HEAT TREATMENT OF STAINLESS STEEL

Stainless steels are often heat treated; the nature of this treatment depends on the type of stainless steel and the reason for the treatment. These treatments, which include annealing, hardening and stress relieving, restore desirable properties such as corrosion resistance and ductility to metal altered by prior fabrication operations or produce hard structures able to withstand high stresses or abrasion in service. Heat treatment is often performed in controlled atmospheres to prevent surface scaling, or less commonly carburisation or decarburisation.

Stages of Heat Treatment

Annealing

The austenitic stainless steels cannot be hardened by thermal treatments (but they do harden rapidly by cold work). Annealing (often referred to as solution treatment) not only recrystallises the work hardened grains but also takes chromium carbides (precipitated at grain boundaries in sensitised steels) back into solution in the austenite. The treatment also homogenises dendritic weld metal structures, and relieves all remnant stresses from cold working. Annealing temperatures usually are above 1040°C, although some types may be annealed at closely controlled temperatures as low as 1010°C when fine grain size is important. Time at temperature is often kept short to hold surface scaling to a minimum or to control grain growth, which can lead to 'orange peel' in forming.

Quench annealing

Annealing of austenitic stainless steel is occasionally called quench annealing because the metal must be cooled rapidly, usually by water quenching, to prevent sensitisation (except for stabilised and extra-low carbon grades).

Stabilising anneal

A stabilising anneal is sometimes performed after conventional annealing for grades 321 and 347. Most of the carbon content is combined with titanium in grade 321 or with niobium in grade 347 when these are annealed in the usual manner. A further anneal at 870° to 900°C for 2 to 4 hrs followed by rapid cooling precipitates all possible carbon as a titanium or niobium carbide and prevents subsequent precipitation of chromium carbide. This special protective treatment is sometimes useful when service conditions are rigorously corrosive, especially when service also involves temperatures from about 400° to 870°C, and some specifications enable this treatment to be specified for the product.

Cleaning

Before annealing or other heat treating operations are performed on austenitic stainless steels, the surface must be cleaned to remove oil, grease and other carbonaceous residues. Such residues lead to carburisation during heat treating, which degrades corrosion resistance.

Process annealing

All martensitic and most ferritic stainless steels can be subcritical annealed (process annealed) by heating into the upper part of the ferrite temperature range, or full annealed by heating above the critical temperature into the austenite range, followed by slow cooling. Usual temperatures are 760° to 830°C for sub-critical annealing. When material has been previously heated above the critical temperature, such as in hot working, at least some martensite is present even in ferritic stainless steels such as grade 430. Relatively slow cooling at about 25°C/hr from full annealing temperature, or holding for one hour or more at subcritical annealing temperature, is required to produce the desired soft structure of ferrite and spheroidised carbides. However, parts that have undergone only cold working after full annealing can be sub-critically annealed satisfactorily in less than 30 minutes.

The ferritic types that retain predominantly single-phase structures throughout the working temperature range (grades 409, 442, 446 and 26Cr-1Mo) require only short recrystallisation annealing in the range 760° to 955°C.

Controlled atmospheres

Stainless steels are usually annealed in controlled atmospheres to prevent or at least reduce scaling. Treatment can be in salt bath, but the best option is "bright annealing" in a highly reducing atmosphere. Products such as flat rolled coil, tube and wire are regularly bright annealed by their producers, usually in an atmosphere of nitrogen and hydrogen. The result is a surface requiring no subsequent scale removal; the product is as bright after as before annealing. These products are often referred to as 'BA'.

Hardening

Martensitic stainless steels are hardened by austenitising, quenching and tempering much like low alloy steels. Austenitising temperatures normally are 980° to 1010°C, well above the critical temperature. As-quenched hardness increases with austenitising temperature to about 980°C and then decreases due to retention of austenite. For some grades the optimum austenitising temperature may depend on the subsequent tempering temperature.

Preheating before austenitising is recommended to prevent cracking in high-carbon types and in intricate sections of low-carbon types. Preheating at 790°C, and then heating to the austenitising temperature is the most common practice.

Cooling and quenching

Martensitic stainless steels have high hardenability because of their high alloy content. Air cooling from the austenitising temperature is usually adequate to produce full hardness, but oil quenching is sometimes used, particularly for larger sections. Parts should be tempered as soon as they have cooled to room temperature, particularly if oil quenching has been used, to avoid delayed cracking. Parts sometimes are frozen to approximately –75°C before tempering to transform retained austenite, particularly where dimensional stability is important, such as in gauge blocks made of grade 440°C.

Tempering at temperatures above 510°C should be followed by relatively rapid cooling to below 400°C to avoid '475°C' embrittlement.

Some precipitation-hardening stainless steels require more complicated heat treatments than standard martensitic types. For instance, a semi-austenitic precipitation-hardening type may require annealing, trigger annealing (to condition austenite for transformation on cooling to room temperature), sub-zero cooling (to complete the transformation of austenite) and ageing (to fully harden the alloy). On the other hand, martensitic precipitation-hardening types (such as grade 630) often require nothing more than a simple ageing treatment.

Stress relieving

Stress relieving at temperatures below 400°C is an acceptable practice but results in only modest stress relief. Stress relieving at 425° to 925°C significantly reduces residual stresses that otherwise might lead to stress corrosion cracking or dimensional instability in service. One hour at 870°C typically relieves about 85 per cent of the residual stresses. However, stress relieving in this temperature range can also precipitate grain boundary carbides, resulting in sensitisation that severely impairs corrosion resistance in many media. To avoid these effects, it is strongly recommended that a stabilised stainless steel (grade 321 or 347) or an extra-low-carbon type (304L or 316L) be used, particularly when lengthy stress relieving is required.

Full solution treatment (annealing), generally by heating to about 1080°C followed by rapid cooling, removes all residual stresses, but is not a practical treatment for most large or complex fabrications.

Low temperature stress relieving

When austenitic stainless steels have been cold worked to develop high strength, low temperature stress relieving will increase the proportional limit and yield strength (particularly compressive yield strength). This is a common practice for austenitic stainless steel spring wire. A two hour treatment at 345° to 400°C is normally used; temperatures up to 425°C may be used if resistance to intergranular corrosion is not required for the application. Higher temperatures will reduce strength and sensitise the metal, and generally are not used for stress relieving cold worked products.

Annealing after welding

Stainless steel weldments can be heated to temperatures below the usual annealing temperature to decrease high residual stresses when full annealing after welding is impossible. Most often, stress relieving is performed on weldments that are too large or intricate for full annealing or on dissimilar metal weldments consisting of austenitic stainless steel welded to low alloy steel.

Stress relieving of martensitic or ferritic stainless steel weldments will simultaneously temper weld and heat affected zones, and for most types will restore corrosion resistance to some degree. However, annealing temperatures are relatively low for these grades, and normal subcritical annealing is the heat treatment usually selected if the weldment is to be heat treated at all.

Surface hardening

Only limited surface hardening treatments are applicable to the stainless steels. In most instances hardening of carbon and low alloy steels is due to the martensitic transformation, in which the achievable hardness is related to the carbon content— as most martensitic stainless steels have carbon contents ranging from fairly low to extremely low, this hardening mechanism is of little use.

Nitriding

It is possible to surface harden austenitic stainless steels by nitriding. As in nitriding of other steels the hard layer is very hard and very thin; this makes the process of limited use as the underlying stainless steel core is relatively soft and unsupportive in heavily loaded applications. A further drawback is that the nitrided case has a significantly lower corrosion resistance than the original stainless steel.

A number of alternative, proprietary surface hardening processes for austenitic stainless steels have been developed but these have not as yet become commercially available.

Physical vapour deposition (PVD)

An interesting recent development is the PVD (Physical vapour deposition) process. This enables very thin but hard layers to be deposited on many materials, including stainless steels. The most commonly applied coating is Titanium Nitride 'TiN', which in addition to being very hard is also an aesthetically pleasing gold colour. Because of its appearance this coating has been applied, generally on No8 mirror polished surface, to produce gold mirror finished architectural panels.

Chapter 5
Heat Treatment of Steel

INTRODUCTION

Heat treating/treatment is a group of industrial and metalworking processes used to alter the physical, and sometimes chemical, properties of a material. The most common application is metallurgical. Heat treatments are also used in the manufacture of many other materials, such as glass. Heat treatment involves the use of heating or chilling, normally to extreme temperatures, to achieve a desired result such as hardening or softening of a material. Heat treatment techniques include annealing, case hardening, precipitation strengthening, tempering and quenching. It is noteworthy that while the term heat treatment applies only to processes where the heating and cooling are done for the specific purpose of altering properties intentionally, heating and cooling often occur incidentally during other manufacturing processes such as hot forming or welding.

Theoretically, steels are the alloys of iron and carbon in which the carbon content is between 0.008 to 2.0 per cent. Commercial steel always contain some amounts of other elements. If these elements are accidentally present without any intention, they are called impurities. However, if they are added purposely, they are called alloying elements. Sulphur and phosphorus are the most common impurities which come from the coke and are used in the manufacture of steel.

To overcome the undesirable effects of sulphur, manganese is always added in some amount to the steel. Many other elements are also present in certain amounts and hence commercial steels are rather complex alloys. Presence of these elements in small amounts do not appreciably change the heat treatment behaviour and microstructures of steels. Steels with other elements in small amounts are called plain carbon steels and their structures and properties can be discussed with the help of Fe-C (or Fe-Fe$_3$C) equilibrium diagram.

In certain cases, some of the elements are intentionally added to steels to increase some of the required properties. These steels are called alloy steels. The properties of alloy steels can also be discussed with the help of Fe-C (or Fe-Fe$_3$C) equilibrium diagram by keeping in mind the influence of these elements on the above diagram or by using a modified diagram.

Therefore, it is highly essential to study the Fe-C (or Fe-Fe$_3$C equilibrium or phase diagram in detail.

IRON–IRON CARBIDE EQUILIBRIUM DIAGRAM

This equilibrium diagram is shown in Fig. 5.1.

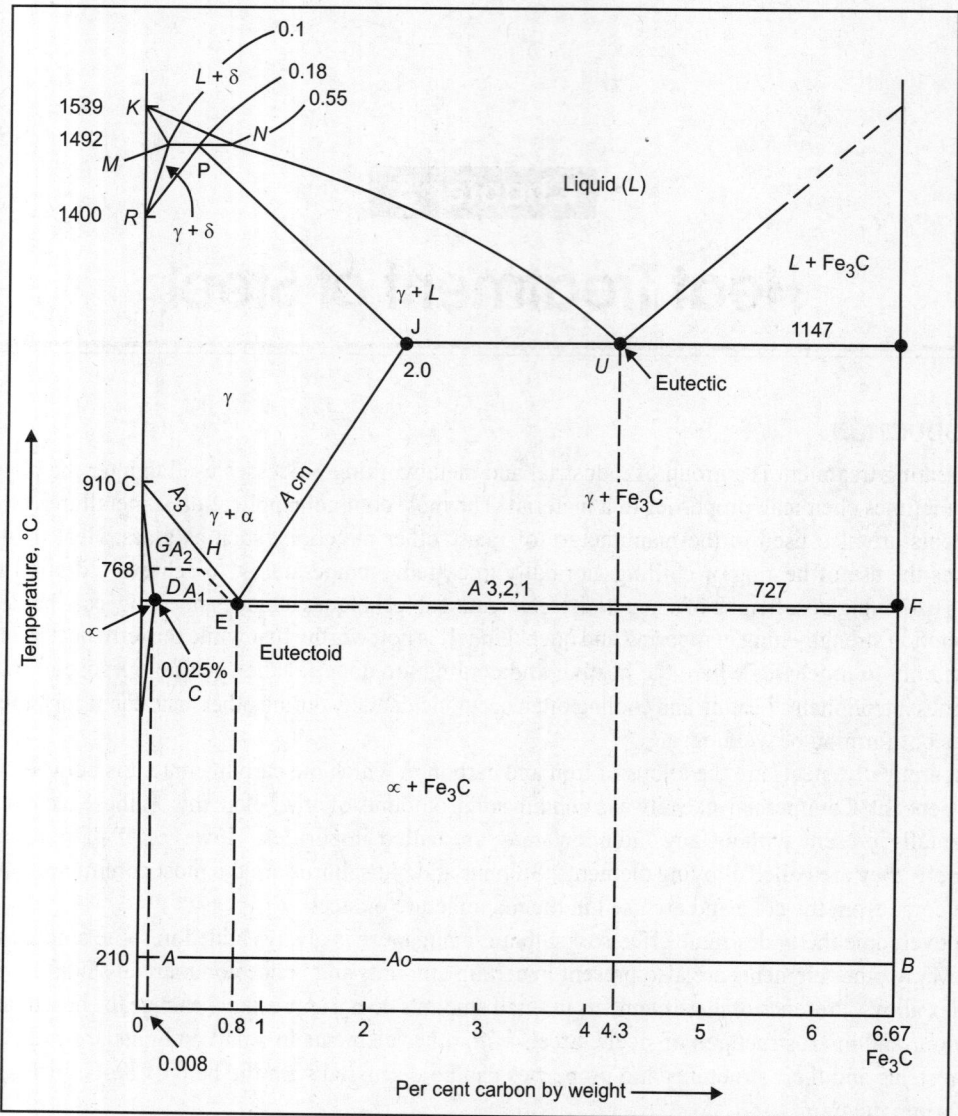

Fig. 5.1. Iron–Iron carbide equilibrium diagram.

Various Phases in Diagram

The various phases existing in the diagram are as below:
1. α (Ferrite): Ferrite is an interstitial solid solution of carbon in low temperature BCC α-iron. It is almost a pure iron and the name ferrite comes from the Latin word ferrum which means iron. The solubility of carbon in α-iron at room temperature is 0.008 per cent and increases with increasing temperature to about 0.025 per cent at 727°C. It is a relatively soft and ductile phase (hardness ≈ 80 BHN). It can be extensively cold worked without cracking. It is strongly

ferromagnetic upto 768°C and becomes paramagnetic at 768°C during heating. This temperature (768°C) at which ferrite becomes paramagnetic is called Curie temperature. The paramagnetic α which exists between 768°C and 910°C was denoted as β in old days.

2. γ (Austenite): Austenite is an interstitial solid solution of carbon in FCC γ-iron. The phase is called Austenite in honour of Sir Austin, who was one of the first metallographer to study its properties. It can dissolve upto 2.0 per cent carbon at 1147°C. The phase is stable only above 727°C. It is a soft, ductile, malleable and nonmagnetic (paramagnetic) phase. It can be extensively worked at the temperatures of its existence.

3. δ (δ-Ferrite): It is an interstitial solid solution of carbon in high temperature BCC δ-iron. It is similar to α-ferrite except its occurrence at high temperature.

4. Fe_3C (Cementite): It is an intermetallic compound of iron and carbon with a fixed carbon content of 6.67 per cent by weight. Cementite has a complex orthorhombic crystal structure with 12 iron atoms and 4 carbon atoms in a unit cell. It is extremely hard and brittle phase (hardness 900–1200 VPN). It is ferromagnetic upto 210°C and paramagnetic above this temperature. It is also called iron carbide or simply carbide in the discussion of Fe-C system.

The above diagram contains three different transformations which are described below:

Peritectic transformation

In general, peritectic transformation is denoted as:

$$S_1 + L \xrightarrow{\text{Constant temperature}} S_2$$

where, S_1 and S_2 are two different solids and L is liquid.

The peritectic region in the upper left hand corner of Fig. 5.1 is shown on an enlarged scale in Fig. 5.2. In Fe-C system, This transformation occurs at point P and is as below:

$$\underset{\text{(of 0.1\% C)}}{\delta} + \underset{\text{(of 0.55\% C)}}{L} \xrightarrow{1492°C} \underset{\text{(of 0.18\% C)}}{\gamma} \qquad \ldots (5.1)$$

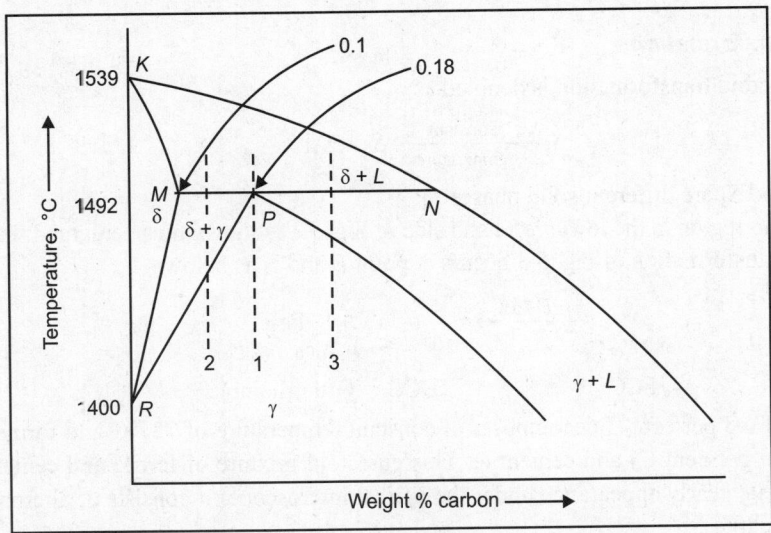

Fig. 5.2. Peritectic region of Fe-C phase diagram.

δ of 0.1 per cent C combines with liquid of 0.55 per cent C at 1492°C and forms γ of 0.18 per cent C. The amounts of δ and L can be found out by applying lever role:

$$\text{Amount of } \delta = \frac{0.55 - 0.18}{0.55 - 0.1} \times 100$$
$$= 82.2\%$$

$$\text{Amount of liquid} = \frac{0.18 - 0.1}{0.55 - 0.1} \times 100$$
$$= 17.8\%$$

For hypoperitectic steels (i.e. steels of carbon content less than 0.18 per cent), the transformation can be written as:

$$\delta + L \xrightarrow{1492°C} \delta + \gamma \qquad \ldots (5.2)$$

and for hyperperitectic steels (i.e. steels of carbon content more than 0.18 per cent), the transformation can be written as:

$$\delta + L \rightarrow \gamma + L \qquad \ldots (5.3)$$

Equations 5.2 and 5.3 are similar to peritectic transformation as shown by Eq. 5.1. Equation 5.2 indicates that for hypoperitectic steels, there is an excess of δ and Eq. 5.3 indicates that there is an excess of liquid for hyperperitectic steels before the start of transformation and hence some amount of these phases remain after the completion of transformation. This indicates that the peritectic transformation range is from 0.1 per cent C to 0.55 per cent C. All the steels containing carbon between 0.1 and 0.55 per cent exhibit peritectic transformation when cooled from the liquid state. Other steels (i.e. steels containing carbon from 0.008 to 0.1 per cent and 0.55 to 2.0 per cent) do not undergo peritectic transformation.

The above transformation occurs at a very high temperature where the steels, if heated, show burning and hence is of no use for the modification of properties of steels.

Eutectoid transformation

In general eutectoid transformation is denoted as:

$$S_1 \xrightarrow[\text{temperature}]{\text{Constant}} S_2 + S_3$$

where, S_1, S_2 and S_3 are different solid phases.

The eutectoid region in the lower left hand side of Fig. 5.1 is shown on an enlarged scale in Fig. 5.3. Eutectoid transformation in Fig. 5.3 occurs at point E and is as below:

$$\underset{\substack{\text{(of 0.8\% C)}\\ \text{FCC}}}{\gamma} \xrightarrow{727°C} \underset{\substack{\text{(of 0.025\% C)}\\ \text{BCC}}}{\alpha} + \underset{\substack{\text{(of 6.67\% C)}\\ \text{Orthorhombic}}}{Fe_3C} \qquad \ldots (5.4)$$

Austenite of 0.8 per cent C decomposes at constant temperature of 727°C and forms a mixture of ferrite (of 0.025 per cent C) and cementite. This eutectoid mixture of ferrite and cementite is called pearlite, due to its pearly appearance under the optical microscope. It consists of alternate lamillae of ferrite and cementite.

The amount of ferrite and cementite in pearlite at room temperature are as below:

Amount of ferrite $= \dfrac{6.67 - 0.8}{6.67 - 0.008}$

$= 88.1\%$

Amount of cementite $= \dfrac{0.8 - 0.008}{6.67 - 0.008}$

$= 11.9\%$

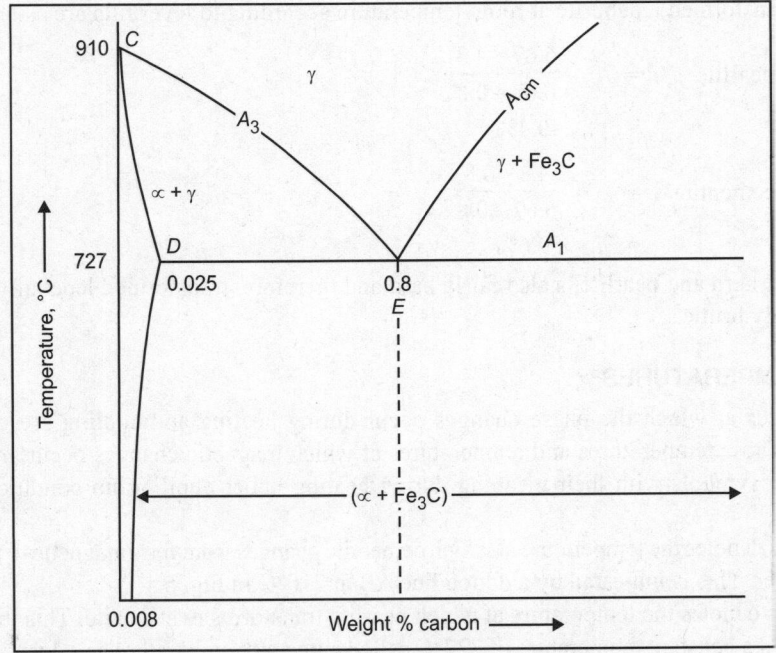

Fig. 5.3. Eutectoid region of Fe-C phase diagram.

This clearly reveals that the ferrite lamilla is 7.4 times (i.e. about 7 times) thicker than cementite lamilla. The properties of pearlite depend upon its interlamillar spacing. Smaller the spacing, higher are the mechanical properties. The interlamillar spacing depends on the cooling rate and within limit, the spacing becomes less and less with increasing cooling rates. The hardness of pearlite with the usual cooling rates is between 230 to 270 BHN. However, for all practical purposes, the value of hardness may be taken as 250 BHN. The interlamillar spacing of a pearlite is defined as the distance from the centre of a ferrite (or cementite) lamilla to the centre of the next adjacent ferrite (or cementite) lamilla.

Eutectic transformation

In general, eutectic transformation is denoted as:

$$L \xrightarrow[\text{temperature}]{\text{Constant}} S_1 + S_2$$

where, S_1 and S_2 are two different solids and L is liquid.

In Fe-C system, this reaction occurs at 1147°C and 4.3 per cent C and is as below:

$$\underset{\text{(of 4.3\% C)}}{L} \xrightarrow{1147°C} \underset{\text{(of 2.0\% C)}}{\gamma} + \underset{\text{(of 6.67\% C)}}{Fe_3C} \qquad \ldots (5.5)$$

Liquid of 4.3 per cent carbon transforms at constant temperature of 1147°C and gives an eutectic mixture of austenite (of 2.0 per cent C) and cementite. This eutectic mixture of austenite and cementite is called ledeburite. Austenite from the ledeburite is not stable at low temperatures and gets transformed to pearlite with slow rates of cooling at 727°C and hence at room temperature, structure consists of pearlite and cementite. This mixture is called transformed ledeburite. The amounts of pearlite and cementite in transformed ledeburite at room temperature according to lever rule are as follows:

$$\text{Amount of pearlite} = \frac{6.67 - 4.3}{6.67 - 0.8}$$
$$= 40.4\%$$

$$\text{Amount of cementite} = \frac{4.3 - 0.8}{6.67 - 0.8}$$
$$= 59.6\%$$

Cementite is hard and pearlite is also fairly hard and therefore, transformed ledeburite is also hard and subsequently brittle.

CRITICAL TEMPERATURES

The temperatures at which the phase changes occur during heating and cooling are called critical temperatures. These temperatures and temperatures at which magnetic changes occur are denoted by symbols. These symbols with their meaning during heating under equilibrium conditions are given below:

1. A_0: This denotes the temperature at which cementite changes from ferromagnetic to paramagnetic character. This is indicated by a dotted line AB at 210°C in Fig. 5.1.
2. A_1: This denotes the temperature at which pearlite transforms to austenite. This transformation occurs at a constant temperature of 727°C called eutectoid temperature and does not depend on the carbon content in the alloy. It is denoted by the line DEF in Fig. 5.1. This temperature is known as lower critical temperature.
3. A_2: This indicates the temperature at which ferromagnetic ferrite becomes paramagnetic. This is shown by a dotted line GH in Fig. 5.1 at 768°C (Curie temperature). The loss of ferromagnetism continues with the line HEF.
4. A_3: It is the temperature at which the last trace of free ferrite gets dissolved to from 100 per cent austenite. It represents the temperature of $(\alpha + \gamma)/\gamma$ phase boundary and is a function of carbon content. It decreases from 910°C at 0 per cent C to 727°C at 0.8 per cent C which is shown by a line CHE in Fig. 5.1. This temperature is known as upper critical temperature for ferrite.
   For steels containing about 0.5 to 0.8 per cent C disappearance of ferromagnetism (A_2) coincides with disappearance of ferrite (A_3), and hence the upper critical temperature in this region is frequently identified as $A_{3,2}$. In hypereutectoid steels, all A_1, A_2 and A_3 coincide with the eutectoid temperature and hence to the right of 0.8 per cent C, the lower critical temperature is often designated as $A_{3,2,1}$.

5. A_{cm}: It is the temperature at which last trace of free cementite gets dissolved to form 100 per cent austenite. It represents the temperature of $(\gamma + Fe_3C)/\gamma$ phase boundary and like A_3, is a function of carbon content. This temperature is shown by the line EJ in Fig. 5.1 and increases from 727° to 1147°C with increase in carbon from 0.8 to 2.0 per cent. It is also known as upper critical temperature for cementite. The A_{cm} line is considerably steeper than the A_3 line.

Critical phase transformation temperatures A_1, A_3 and A_{cm} are influenced by heating or cooling rates. During rapid heating, these temperatures are raised and during rapid cooling, they are lowered. For extremely slow cooling or heating rates, i.e. under equilibrium conditions, the critical temperatures are the same as shown by the equilibrium diagram. Under non-equilibrium conditions, the departure in critical temperatures from their equilibrium values will be more and more with increasing rates of heating or cooling. This change in temperature is due to thermal hysteresis and during heating, it is denoted by a suffix letter 'c' (c from the French word *chauffage*, means heating) and during cooling, by a letter 'r' (r from the French word, *refroidissement*, means cooling). Thus, for example, A_1 observed during heating becomes A_{c1} and during cooling becomes A_{r1}. For equilibrium cooling, letter 'e' is used. This method of notation is commonly used to explain the departures from equilibrium condition. However, such a change is not observed in A_0 and A_2 temperatures because of no hysteresis in magnetic transition.

SOLIDIFICATION AND MICROSTRUCTURES OF SLOWLY COOLED STEELS

The solidification starts at or just below the liquidus temperature (line KNU) with the separation of δ for steels of less than 0.55 per cent C and γ for steels of carbon between 0.55 and 2.0 per cent (Fig. 5.1). As the temperature decreases, more and more liquid solidifies and the solidification completes at the solidus temperature (line KMPJ). Below line RPJ, all the steels have austenitic structure. Further decrease in temperature results in solid-to-solid phase transformation at upper and lower critical temperatures. The changes in structures are described below separately for hypoeutectoid and hypereutectoid steels.

Microstructures of Hypoeutectoid Steels

These steels contain carbon from 0.008 to 0.8 per cent (less than the eutectoid carbon). For better illustration of changes in structures during cooling of steels from the austenitic region, the eutectoid region of Fe-C phase diagram is shown separately in Fig. 5.4. A typical steel from this group such as 0.2 per cent C is marked on the above diagram.

The structural changes for this steel are as below:
1. At point 1, α starts separating out at the grain boundaries of γ. As the temperature decreases, the amount of α increases. The composition of α varies along the line CD and that of γ along the line CE. This continues up to 2. The amounts of α and γ at any temperature between 1 and 2 can be found out by applying the lever rule. This α which has separated before the eutectoid transformation (i.e. point 2 temperature) is called primary or free or proeutectoid α (pro means before).
2. At 2, the existing γ transforms at constant temperature of 727°C to a lamillar mixture of ferrite and, cementite called pearlite by eutectoid transformation process.
3. Cooling from 2 to 3 does not result in significant change in the microstructure due to insignificant solubility of carbon in α and hence the same structure is observed at room temperature. The amounts of α and pearlite at room temperature according to the lever rule will be as below:

$$\text{Amount of } \alpha = \frac{0.8 - 0.2}{0.8 - 0.008} \approx 75\%$$

Amount of pearlite $= \dfrac{0.2 - 0.008}{0.8 - 0.008} \approx 25\%$

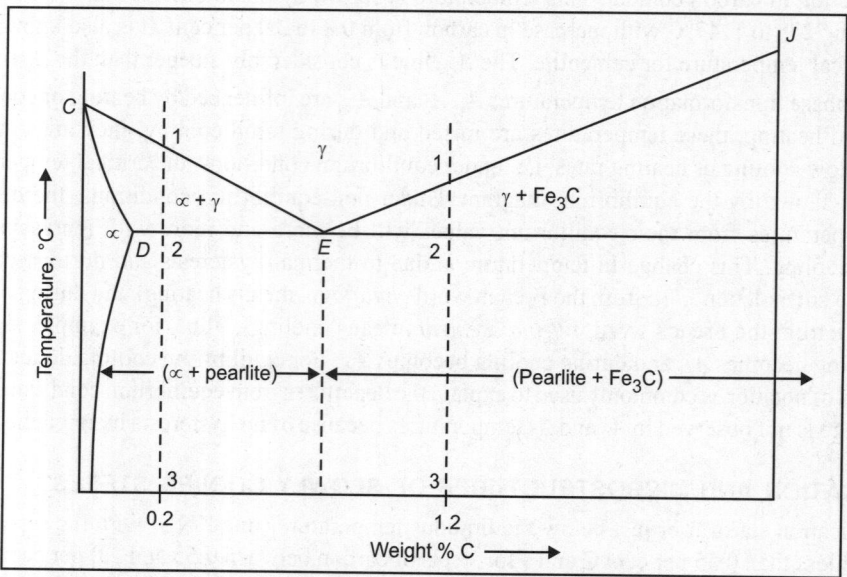

Fig. 5.4. Eutectoid transformation in Fe-C system.

For other steels, the sequence of structural changes are very much similar to the above; only the amounts of phases will be different for each steel. As the carbon increases, the amount of proeutectoid ferrite decreases and pearlite increases. For 0.8 per cent C, the amount of proeutectoid ferrite becomes 0 per cent and pearlite becomes 100 per cent. There is a linear variation in carbon content of the steel and the amount of pearlite or ferrite. For 0.008 per cent C, the amount of α is 100 per cent and for 0.8 per cent C, the amount of pearlite is 100 per cent. This means that every 0.1 per cent C approximately corresponds to 12.5 per cent pearlite. The variation of ferrite and pearlite with carbon is shown in Fig. 5.5.

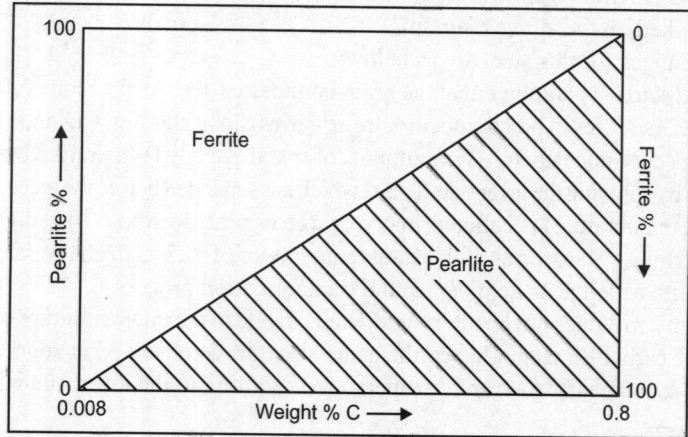

Fig. 5.5. The variation of pearlite and ferrite with carbon for hypoeutectoid steels.

Ferrite appears white and pearlite appears dark or lamillar under the microscope with most common etching reagents such as nital and picral used for steels and hence in most of the cases, they can be easily identified by microscopy.

Microstructures of Hypereutectoid Steels

These steels contain carbon from 0.8 to 2.0 per cent (more than the eutectoid carbon). A typical steel from this group such as 1.2 per cent C is marked in Fig. 5.4. The structural changes for the above steel are as below:

1. At point 1, Fe_3C starts separating out on the grain boundaries of austenite. As the temperature decreases, amount of Fe_3C increases and austenite decreases. The composition of austenite varies along line JE and the composition of Fe_3C does not change, since it is an intermetallic compound. This continues upto 2. The amounts of Fe_3C and austenite at 2 can be found out by applying the lever rule. This Fe_3C which has separated before the eutectoid transformation is called primary or free or proeutectoid Fe_3C.
2. At 2, the existing amount of austenite transforms at constant temperature of 727°C to pearlite.
3. Cooling from 2 to 3 does not result in significant change in microstructure and hence the same structure is observed at room temperature. The amounts of Fe_3C and pearlite according to the lever rule will be as below:

$$\text{Amount of } Fe_3C = \frac{1.2 - 0.8}{6.67 - 0.8} = 6.8\%$$

$$\text{Amount of pearlite} = \frac{6.67 - 1.2}{6.67 - 0.8} = 93.2\%$$

For any other steel from this group, the sequence of transformations are very much similar to the above; only the amounts of Fe_3C and pearlite will be different for the steel under consideration. As the carbon increases, the amount of Fe_3C increases and 'for a steel containing maximum amount of carbon (i.e. 2 per cent), the amount of Fe_3C will be:

$$\text{Maximum amount of } Fe_3C \text{ in steel} = \frac{2.0 - 0.8}{6.67 - 0.8}$$
$$= 20.4\%$$

Free cementite is 0 per cent for 0.8 per cent C steel and increases linearly with increasing carbon reaching to 20.4 per cent for 2.0 per cent carbon steel. This clearly indicates that every 0.1 per cent C corresponds to 1.7 per cent Fe_3C. The variation of Fe_3C and pearlite with carbon is shown in Fig. 5.6.

Cementite appears white and pearlite appears dark or lamillar under the microscope with the general etching reagents such as nital and picral and hence in many of the cases, they can be easily identified.

Even though, the maximum amount of free cementite that can appear in a steel is about 20 per cent, in most of the commercial steels it is less than 10 per cent because the carbon rarely exceeds 1.3/1.4 per cent. Therefore, it is quite possible that the microstructures of such slowly cooled hypereutectoid steels may appear similar to those of some of the slowly cooled hypoeutectoid steels which contain free ferrite less than 10 per cent (carbon content between 0.7 and 0.8 per cent).This is due to the fact that both the proeutectoid (free) ferrite and cementite appear white under the microscope with the usual etching reagents nital and picral. Under this situation, it is possible to distinguish the phases by using the following bases:

1. Relative hardness: Cementite is fairly hard and ferrite is soft. Therefore, a microhardness test can be used to identify the phases. Sometimes, it is also possible to identify the phases from the relief effect produced during polishing by observing the polished surface under the microscope. Cementite being hard will stand in relief above the plane of polish whereas ferrite being soft will go slightly below the plane of polish.
2. Special etchants: Most of the commonly used etchants for steels attack only at the grain boundaries and interfaces and do not attack and darken either the ferrite or the cementite appreciably. However, there are some etchants which preferentially attack either ferrite or cementite and allow a clear-cut distinction to be made between them. For example, boiling alkaline sodium picrate selectively darkens cementite and leaves ferrite white and hence it can be used to distinguish cementite from ferrite.
3. Shape of grains: Proeutectoid ferrite grains are typically thick and rather rounded, while proeutectoid cementite grains tend to be thin and sharply acicular.

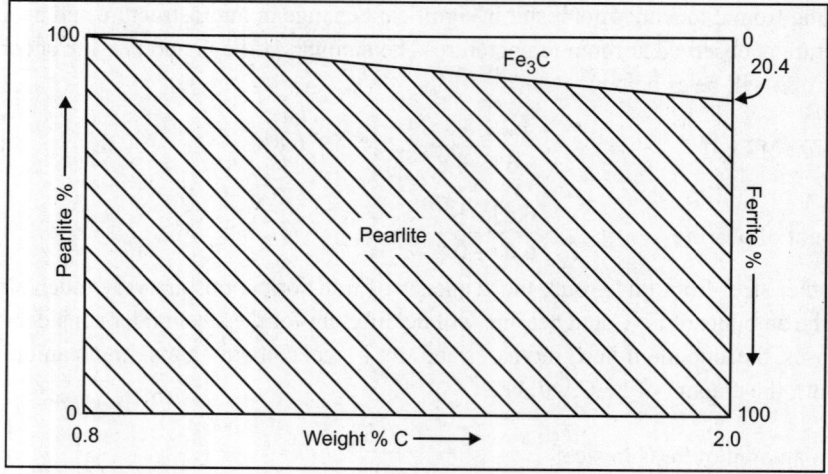

Fig. 5.6. The variation of pearlite and cementite with carbon for hypereutectoid steels.

The microstructures of hypereutectoid steels slowly cooled from the austenitic region will show a continuous network of cementite across the boundaries of pearlite regions. Cementite is a hard phase and hence it does not allow to move the dislocations from region to region via boundaries. Therefore, such a steel becomes more brittle and does not serve the purpose. This clearly indicates that slow cooling of hypereutectoid steels from austenitic region deteriorates the properties of steels. Also, no heat treatment process used in practice is aimed to obtain such structures and hence such structures are rare in commercial products.

If they are cooled with a moderate rate, proeutectoid cementite separates in the form of needles in austenite grains which later transform to pearlite. Such steels at room temperature show innumerable needles of cementite in pearlite. However, hypoeutectoid steels cooled under similar conditions do not show needles of ferrite. In such cases, identification of phases does not become a problem and the needle like appearance of proeutectoid phase becomes a typical character of hypereutectoid steels.

ESTIMATION OF CARBON FROM MICROSTRUCTURES

For plain carbon steels which are cooled slowly through the critical range, carbon content can be approximately determined from their microstructures. This is possible due to the fact that every 12.5 per cent proeutectoid ferrite in hypoeutectoid steels and 1.7 per cent proeutectoid cementite in hypereutectoid steels correspond to 0.1 per cent carbon. However, there are certain limits for estimation of carbon accurately by this method which are as below:

1. With slight fast cooling of steel from austenitic region, the amount of pearlite increases because of the departure of the eutectoid carbon from its equilibrium value. Due to this, in a given steel, the amount of proeutectoid phase decreases and pearlite increases changing the above mentioned ratios between the proeutectoid phase and carbon.
2. Alloying elements also affect the microstructure.
3. The phase distribution is in three dimensions and observation and estimation is usually done in two dimensions, i.e. on the plane of polish. This creates error in phase measurement.
4. For hypereutectoid steels the ratio of proeutectoid Fe_3C to carbon is very low as compared to the ratio of proeutectoid α to carbon in hypoeutectoid steels and hence for constant error in measurement of phase, the error in carbon estimation is more for hypereutectoid steels than for hypoeutectoid steels.
5. Normalising is a common heat treatment process used for steel components. The structure of normalised hypereutectoid steels contains large number of fine cementite needles which are difficult to measure by the usual quantitative microscopic techniques.

In most of the cases, the cooling rates of steels are not as slow as used in plotting of Fe-C equilibrium diagram and also due to the presence of some amount of other elements, carbon estimation from the structure is not accurate. The limits and errors are still more for hypereutectoid steels and therefore, this method should not be used for hypereutectoid steels. However, for hypoeutectoid steels, it gives fairly good results.

NON-EQUILIBRIUM COOLING OF STEELS

Due to non-equilibrium cooling, i.e. fast cooling of austenite through the critical range, microstructures produced are quite different from those produced by equilibrium cooling. This results in significant changes in properties of steels. Controlled departures from equilibrium conditions to obtain such different structures and thereby properties is the object of most of the common heat treatments of steels.

Eutectoid transformation of austenite to pearlite occurs by nucleation; and growth Temperature of transformation has a strong influence on the above mechanisms. Faster the cooling, lesser will be the eutectoid transformation temperature with shift of eutectoid carbon towards the composition of undercooled phase.

This means that the eutectoid carbon will shift to the lower values for hypoeutectoid steels and higher values for hypereutectoid steels. Due to this, in a given steels amount of proeutectoid phase decreases and pearlite increases, e.g. for a steel of 0.4 per cent C, the amount of pearlite may increase from its equilibrium value of 50 per cent to say 100 per cent with increasing cooling rates as shown by dotted lines in Fig. 5.7.

This also results in decrease of interlamillar spacing of pearlite, i.e. the pearlite becomes finer. This is due to the increase in nucleation rate because of decrease in transformation temperatures. Due to the above two simultaneous effects, mechanical properties sharply rise.

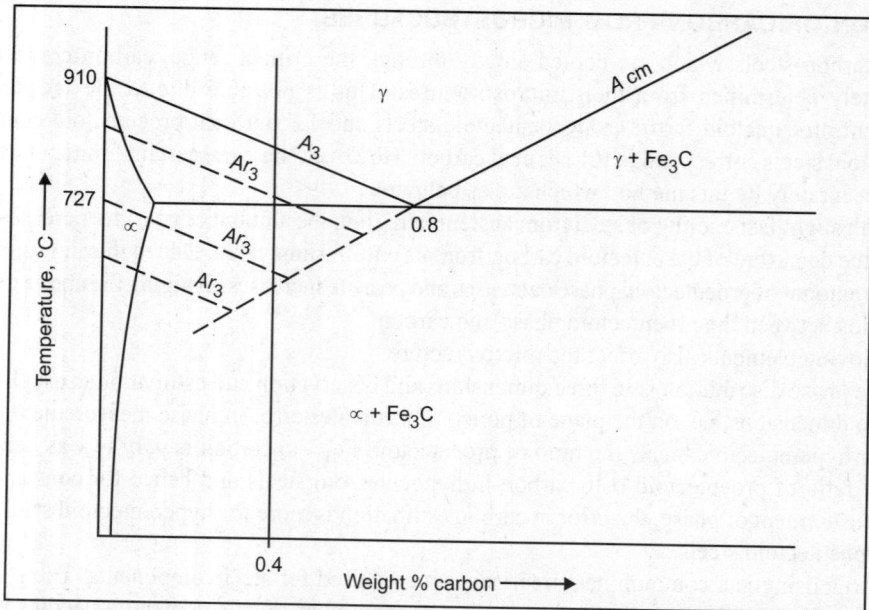

Fig. 5.7. Showing the displacement of eutectoid point due to undercooling of ferrite by increasing cooling rates.

It is clear from the above example that simply by adjusting the cooling rate through the critical range, the amount of pearlite in a given steel can be controlled so as to obtain the desired properties in the component. However, there is a certain limit to this because if the cooling rate exceeds a certain value called as critical cooling rate, austenite does not transform to pearlite but transforms to a phase called martensite. Moreover, a totally different type of transformation called Bainitic transformation will occur if austenite is cooled isothermally at some temperature below the lower critical temperature. Martensite and bainite have different properties from pearlite and more details about these transformations will be described at a later stage.

Iron–carbon equilibrium diagram indicates only the existence of equilibrium phases and martensite and bainite being non-equilibrium phases are not indicated by the above diagram.

WIDMANSTATTEN STRUCTURES

During cooling of steels from austenitic region, sometimes the proeutectoid phase separates not only along the grain boundaries but also in the grains along certain crystallographic planes and directions. During any transformation, the system tries to reduce its energy to the maximum level and hence the phase separation may occur at the interfaces having very similar atomic spacings. This means that the separating proeutectoid ferrite or cementite has a definite orientation relationship with the austenite phase. Because of this, the structure shows a typical geometric pattern under the microscope. Such structures are called Widmanstatten structures. Since the orientation of each grain of austenite is different, the character of Widmanstatten pattern is also different from grain to grain. Following factors govern the formation of Widmanstatten structures:

1. Composition of steel: This influences the amount of proeutectoid phase. Larger the departure from eutectoid point, the amount of proeutectoid phase will be higher and formation of

Widmanstatten structure is favoured. This is because, under identical conditions, the increased amount of proeutectoid phase will not be able to migrate to the grain boundaries and hence gets separated inside the grains.
2. Grain size of austenite: Larger the grain size, the proeutectoid phase has to diffuse to a higher distance to reach the grain boundaries. This promotes the separation of phase inside the grains unless the cooling rate is slow. Hence, with increased grain size, chances of formation of Widmanstatten structures are higher.
   The grain size of austenite depends on the temperature of austenitisation and the type of steel. Higher the temperature, more is the grain size and at the same temperature, alloy steels show less grain size than plain carbon steels.
3. Cooling rate: Faster the cooling, less will be the diffusion time and hence all the amount of proeutectoid phase will not be able to migrate to the grain boundaries and part of it gets precipitated inside the grains showing Widmanstatten structures.

Usually Widmanstatten structures are observed in steels with less than 0.6 per cent C and more than 1.0 per cent C when cooled from a high temperature in the austenitic region under non-equilibrium conditions with cooling rates not exceeding the critical cooling rate. They are very common in steel castings and weldings, and are sometimes observed in hot forged, rolled, or extruded components.

Hypoeutectoid steels with Widmanstatten structures are characterised by low toughness and ductility values. This is because the strong pearlite phase is isolated in ineffective patches by a weak ferrite along which the cracks can readily propagate. Therefore, Widmanstatten structures are not desirable in these steels. The deterioration in properties can be reduced by the addition of silicon which modifies the Widmanstatten structure into a feathery structure or such structures .can be eliminated by a suitable heat treatment which consists of heating the steel to just above A_3 temperature and slow cooling to below A_1 or to room temperature.

Hypereutectoid steels with Widmanstatten structures show large number of cementite needles in the matrix of pearlite and have slightly better properties as compared to those of slowly cooled steels. This is due to the fact that the dislocations can move via certain regions and avoid cementite phase. However, in slowly cooled steels, cementite completely envelopes the pearlite regions and almost stops the motion of dislocations. Due to this, these steels with Widmanstatten structures are not so brittle as the slowly cooled steels from austenitic region and hence are preferred typical Widmanstatten structures.

The morphology of structure affects the homogenisation time and at a given temperature in the austenitic region, the time required for complete homogenisation is less with Widmanstatten structures than with slow cooled structures. Appearance of Widmanstatten structures is a general phenomenon and such structures are observed not only in steels but also in many other alloys such as two phase brasses and aluminium bronzes. Here also a definite orientation relationship is observed between the separating phase and the matrix phase, e.g. in α-β brasses, when α separates from β, (111) plane of α is parallel to the (110) plane of β and [110] direction of α is parallel to the [111] direction of β.

This orientation relationship is shown as below:

$$(111)_\alpha \parallel (110)_\beta \text{ and } [110]_\alpha \parallel [111]_\beta$$

PROPERTY VARIATION WITH MICROSTRUCTURE

Mechanical properties are structure dependent or structure sensitive. They vary with the amounts of phases and the distribution of phases (morphology of structure). When influence of morphology is less, the property can be fairly accurately correlated with the amounts of phases, e.g. for a two phase material with α-β structure, the property on an average can be expressed as below:

Average property = (Amount of α × the property of α)
+ (Amount of β × the property of β)

Since the hardness of a steel is not much sensitive to the morphology of structure and the variation of proeutectoid ferrite or cementite is linear with the carbon content, it can be expressed as below:
1. For hypoeutectoid steels:
   Hardness (BHN) ≈ 80 × amount of α
   + 230 × amount of pearlite
2. For hypereutectoid steels:
   Hardness (VPN) ≈ 900 × amount of Fe_3C
   + 240 × amount of pearlite

Many of the properties like tensile strength, ductility and impact strength are sensitive to the morphology of structure. Therefore, unless the distribution of phases is known correctly, property prediction can not be done accurately.

The microstructural phases of hypoeutectoid steels are ferrite and pearlite. Since these steels show a continuous ferrite around the pearlite regions when cooled slowly from austenitic region and the ferrite has fairly good plasticity and strength, the following equations can be used to express their tensile strength (TS) with reasonable accuracy.

1. TS kg/mm^2 ≈ 28 × amount of α + 84 × amount of pearlite ... (5.6)

or

$$\approx 28\left(1 - \frac{\%C}{0.8}\right) + 84\frac{(\%C)}{0.8} \quad \ldots (5.7)$$

2. TS kg/mm^2 ≈ 0.36 × BHN ...(5.8)

This clearly indicates that with almost 0 per cent C, the tensile strength of steel is approximately 28 kg/mm^2 and with increase of every 0.1 per cent C, 'tensile strength rises by 7 kg/mm^2. These equations give fairly good result for plain carbon steels in annealed and normalised conditions. However, for hypereutectoid steels, cementite separates out as continuous network and since the phase is hard and brittle, the steel becomes brittle.

In these steels, morphology of structure strongly influences the mechanical properties except the hardness. Therefore, the above equations of TS cannot be used for hypereutectoid steels. The variation of properties with carbon is shown in Fig. 5.8. Tensile strength and ductility of hypereutectoid steels are highly sensitive to the morphology of structure and hence the variation of these properties with carbon is shown by dotted lines in the Fig. 5.8.

CLASSIFICATION AND APPLICATIONS OF STEELS

The steels are classified by various methods and each method is based on a definite criteria. The various criterions for the basis of classification are as follows:
1. Amount of carbon.
2. Amount of alloying elements and carbon.
3. Amount of deoxidation.
4. Grain coarsening characteristics.
5. Method of manufacture.

6. Depth of hardening.
7. Form and use.

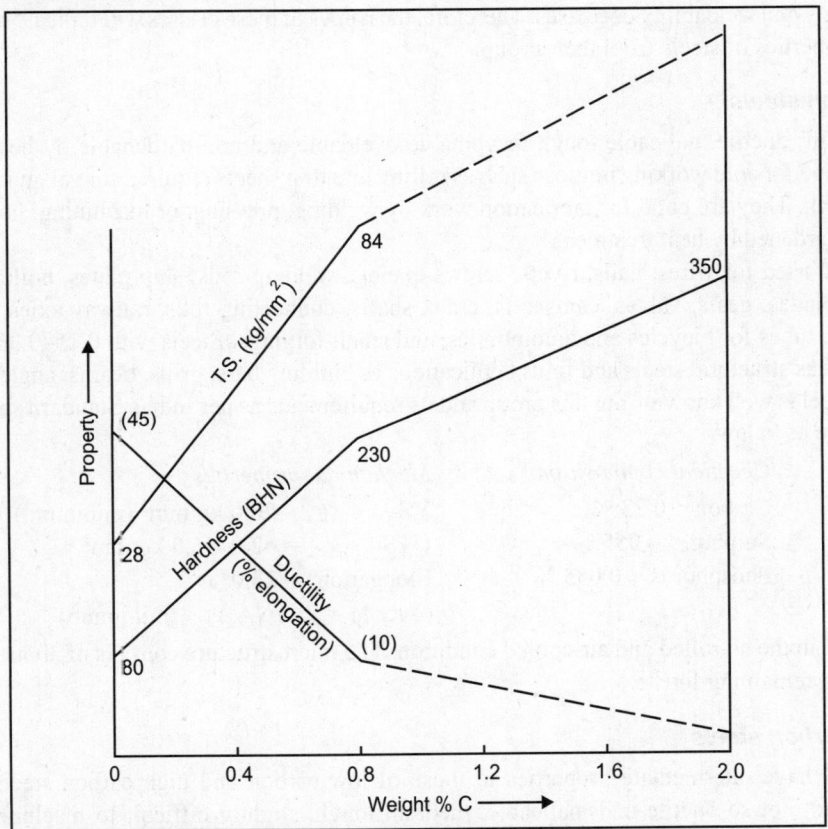

Fig. 5.8. Variation of properties with carbon in steels.

On the Basis of Carbon

Plain carbon steels are classified into three groups depending on the carbon content. These are:
1. Low carbon steels (0.008–0.30 per cent C).
2. Medium carbon steels (0.30–0.60 per cent C).
3. High carbon steels (0.60–2.00 per cent C).

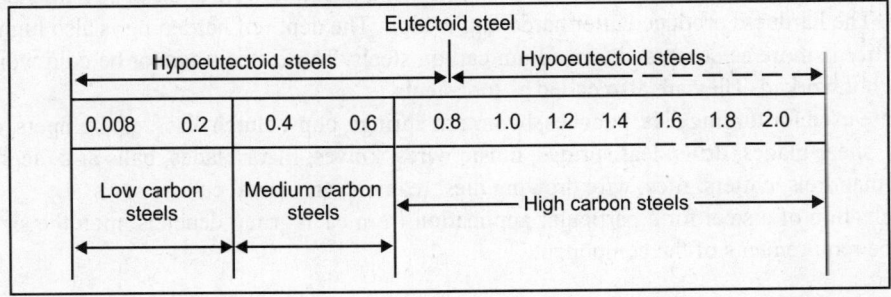

Carbon has a strong influence on the properties of steels. As the carbon, increases, hardness, TS fatigue resistance and hardenability increases; and ductility, malleability, formability, toughness, machinability and weldability decreases. Therefore, the names of these classes will indicate some general level of properties of steels from their group.

Low carbon steels

They are soft, ductile malleable tough machinable, weldable and non-hardenable by heat treatment. They are good for cold working purpose such as rolling into thin sheets required for galvanising, tinning or press work. They are good for fabrication work by welding, pressing, or machining; however, they cannot be hardened by heat treatment.

They are used for wires, nails, rivets, screws, panels, welding rods, ship plates, boiler plates and tubes, fan blades, gears, valves, camshafts, crank shafts, connecting rods, railway axles, fish plates, cross heads, tubes for bicycles and automobiles, and small forgings. Steels with 0.15–0.30 carbon are widely used as structural steels and finds applications as building bars, grills, beams, angles, channels, etc. Mild steel is well known from this group and its requirements as per Indian Standard specifications (IS-226) are as below:

Chemical composition
Carbon < 0.23 %
Sulphur < 0.055 %
Phosphorus < 0.055 %

Mechanical properties
YS = 26.0 kg/mm^2 (minimum)
UTS = 42.0–56.0 kg/mm^2
Elongation = 23.0%
(over lo = 5.65 $\sqrt{A_o}$) (minimum)

It is used in the as-rolled and air-cooled condition. The microstructure consists of about 25 per cent pearlite with remaining ferrite.

Medium carbon steels

These steels have intermediate properties to those of low carbon and high carbon steels. They are medium hard, not so ductile and malleable, medium tough, slightly difficult to machine, weld and harden. They require high cooling rates for hardening and the hardness produced after hardening is not so high. The depth of hardening is also less and hence they are of shallow hardening type. They are difficult to cold work and hence hot worked. They are also called as machinery steels.

They are used for bolts, axles, lock washers, large forging dies, springs, wires, wheel spokes, hammers, rods, turbine rotors, crank pins, cylinder liners, railway rails and railway tyres.

High carbon steels

They are hard, wear resistant, brittle, difficult to machine, difficult to weld and can be hardened by heat treatment. The hardness produced after hardening is high. The depth of hardening is also high, i.e. the hardenability is more as compared to medium carbon steels. These steels cannot be cold worked and hence are hot worked. They are also called as tool steels.

They are used for forging dies, punches, hammers, springs, clips, clutch discs, car bumpers, chiesels, vice jaws, shear blades, drills, leaf springs, music wires, knives, razor blades, balls and races for ball bearings, mandrels, cutters, files, wire drawing dies, reamers, and metal cutting saws.

The selection of a steel for a particular application from each group depends upon the size, shape and service requirements of the component.

On the Basis of Alloying Elements and Carbon

Alloying elements such as Ni, Cr, Mn, W, Mo, V, etc. are added to plain carbon steels in certain amounts to increase the desired properties. Such steels are classified on the basis of total alloy content in the following manner:
1. Low alloy steels.
2. High alloy steels.

Low alloy steels contain alloying elements less than 10 per cent and high alloy steels contain more than 10 per cent. Steels are also classified on the basis of alloying elements and carbon content as below:

Carbon content	Total content of alloying elements
Low (< 0.3%)	Low (<10%)
Medium (0.3–0.6%)	High (> 10%)
High (> 0.6%)	

These are: (i) low carbon low alloy, (ii) low carbon high alloy, (iii) medium carbon low alloy, (iv) medium carbon high alloy, (v) high carbon low alloy, and (vi) high carbon high alloy steels.

Each class has definite properties e.g. low carbon low alloy steels have good strength, low carbon high alloy steels have good corrosion resistance, and high carbon high alloy steels have excellent hardness and wear resistance at low and high temperatures.

On the Basis of Deoxidation

Depending on the deoxidation practice employed, steels are classified as below:
1. Rimmed steels.
2. Killed steels.
3. Semi-killed steels (balanced steels).

Rimmed steels

A molten steel contains large amount of dissolved oxygen and other gases. The solubility of gases is more in the liquid metal than in the solid metal and hence the dissolved oxygen along with other gases tries to go out as CO during solidification and a large part of it gets entrapped into the solidified ingot. The thin solidified layer of ingot, i.e. rim (skin) is of less carbon, more purity, free from blow holes and free from segregation of impurities. The entrapped gases form blow holes which compensate for the usual liquid to solid shrinkage reduce the pipe subsequently increasing the yield However, the ingot contains large number of blow holes and macrosegregation is also more [Fig. 5.9(a)]. These blow holes are eliminated during subsequent working operation. These steels cannot be continuously cast because the CO formed due to the reaction $2C + O_2 \rightarrow 2CO$ during solidification tries to come out and can puncture holes in the thin solidified layer (rim) through which the liquid metal may come out. These steels coarsen rapidly during heating in the austenitic region and hence are not much suitable for forging and carburising processes. Low carbon steels containing less than 0.15 per cent carbon are produced in sheet form in rimmed condition and are used for deep drawing and forming operations.

Killed steels

The dissolved oxygen from the melt is completely removed by the addition of strong deoxidising agents like Al, Si or Mn. The additions of silicon and manganese are done in the form of ferro-silicon and ferro-manganese master alloys.

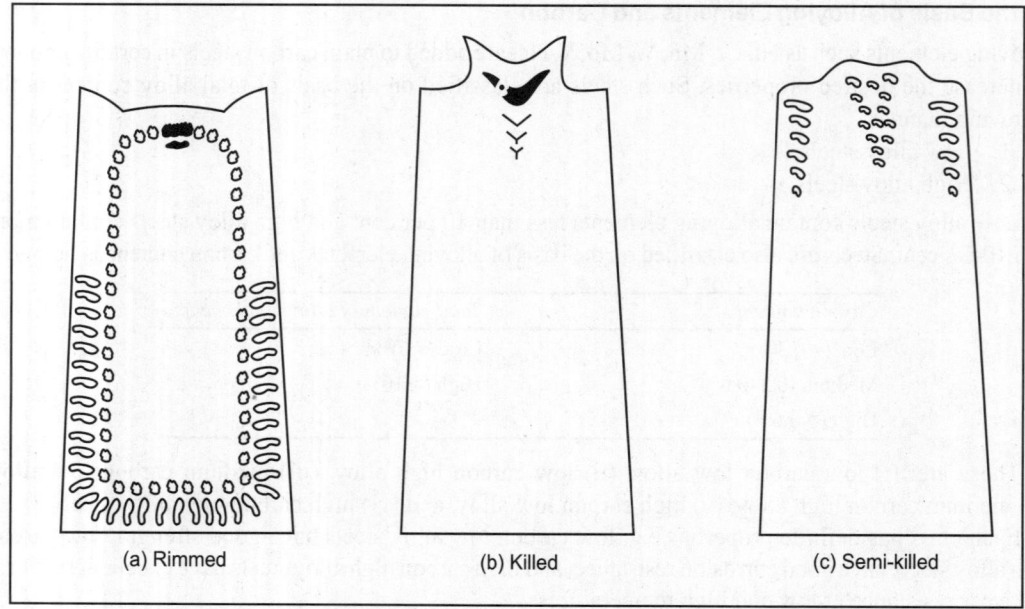

Fig. 5.9. Types of steel ingot.

These deoxidisers are added to the steel in the furnace or in the ladle prior to pouring into the mould. They rapidly combine with the dissolved oxygen from the melt and form respective oxides. Due to this, dissolved oxygen in the melt decreases but the content of inclusions (oxide particles) increases. The deoxidised steel shows more pipe because of absence of blow holes [Fig. 5.9(b)]. This pipe is removed before further processing of steel ingot and hence the yield decreases. These steels can be continuously cast without a problem in contrast to rimmed steels.

Aluminium deoxidised steels do not coarsen in the austenitic region upto about 950°C, but coarsen very fast beyond this temperature. However, silicon deoxidised steels show rapid coarsening with temperature above the upper critical temperature. Killed steel ingot has a sound, defect free, less segregated structure throughout the cross section and is used when the final product is to be made to exacting specifications, when subsequent mechanical working is limited, and when uniform properties throughout the section are required. Usually high carbon steels and alloy steels are produced in the killed condition. However, low carbon and medium carbon steels can also be produced in the killed condition, if cost permits. These steels are used, for components-which have to be forged, carburised, or heat treated.

Semi-killed steels

In these steels, part of the dissolved oxygen is removed by the addition of deoxidisers. The blow holes formed by the evolution of CO compensate for the part of the shrinkage and hence the pipe is less [Fig. 5.9(c)]. They show intermediate grain coarsening characteristics to those of rimmed and killed steels. Usually steels containing carbon between 0.15 and 0.25 per cent are produced in this condition and used for sheets, plates, structural shapes, etc.

On the Basis of Grain Coarsening Characteristics

During heating, 100 per cent austenite is formed at just above the upper critical temperature and the grains are of smallest size. AB the temperature increases above this, the grain size may increase. Depending on the grain coarsening characteristics, steels are classified into two types as:
1. Coarse grained steels.
2. Fine grained steels.

Coarse grained steels coarsen rapidly with temperature. However, fine grained steels do not coarsen much up to a definite temperature (Fig. 5.10), and this temperature is a characteristic of each steel. Above this temperature, they coarsen very fast and may reach a size greater than those of the coarse grained steels. Usually rimmed steels behave coarse grained and aluminium killed or alloy steels behave as fine grained steels. The oxide inclusions in killed steels and undissolved alloy carbides in alloy steels inhibit the grain boundary migration, reducing the grain coarsening. These steels maintain a relatively fine and uniform grain size even after holding for a long time at high temperatures. In the absence of such particles as in the rimmed steels, grain coarsening is rapid.

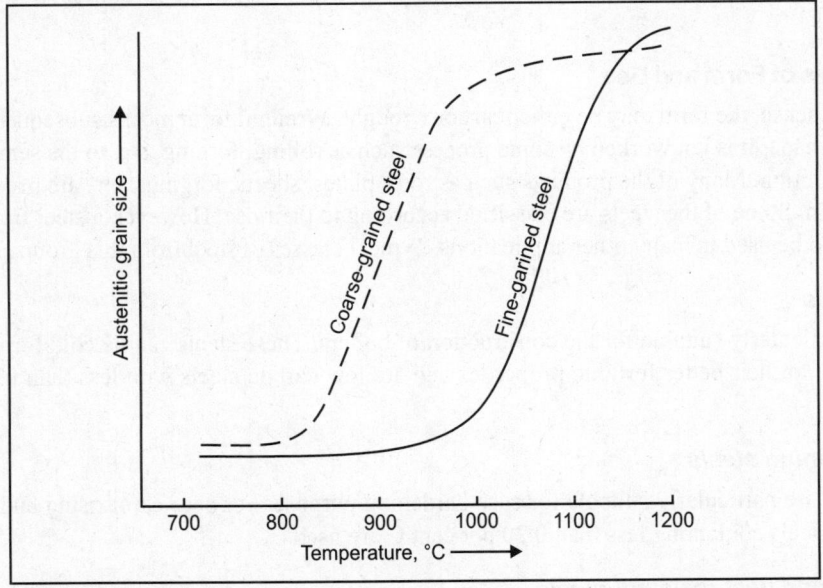

Fig. 5.10. Grain coarsening behaviour of steels.

On the Basis of Method of Manufacture

According to the method of manufacture, the steels are classified as:
1. Basic open hearth.
2. Electric furnace.
3. Basic oxygen process.
4. Acid open hearth.
5. Acid Bessemer.

This method of classification does not throw light on composition or mechanical properties of steels.

On the Basis of Depth of Hardening

The steels are classified as below:
1. Non-hardenable steels.
2. Shallow hardening steels.
3. Deep hardening steels.

The idea about the depth of hardening is obtained from the hardenability of a given steel and the hardenability is a function of carbon and alloying elements with all other factors constant. Non-hardenable steels contain less carbon and almost no alloying elements. Shallow hardening steels are medium carbon with or without alloying elements and are intermediate to those of non-hardening and deep hardening types. Deep hardening steels contain more carbon and alloying elements.

The selection of a particular steel is governed by its service requirements. Non-hardenable steels are suitable for fabrication by cold working and welding. They have applications similar to those of low carbon steels. Shallow hardening steels get hardened only at the surface and hence are sometimes used for gears, camshafts and such other applications. Deep hardening steels are used where depth of hardening required is more or thorough hardening is necessary and have applications similar to those of high carbon steels.

On the Basis of Form and Use

In the broad sense, the form may be either cast or wrought. Wrought form means subsequent to casting to a simple shape, it is hot worked by some process such as rolling, forging, etc. to the semifinished or finished condition. Many of the products such as rods, plates, sheets, forgings, etc. are produced in the wrought form. Some of the steels are classified according to their use. However, a steel from so-called class can also be used in many other applications. Typical classes of steel from this group are as below.

Boiler steels

They are particularly suitable for the construction of boilers. These steels can be cold formed without cracking due to their better forming properties and are low carbon steels with less than 0.25 per cent carbon.

Case hardening steels

These steels are particularly suitable for case hardening purpose. For case carburising and hardening, low carbon steels containing less than 0.20 per cent C are used.

Corrosion and heat resistant steels

They are alloy steels having high corrosion and oxidation resistance and used for corrosive and high temperature conditions, e.g. stainless steels and high chromium steels.

Deep drawing steels

These are suitable for deep drawing purpose due to their high formability and used for automobile bodies, stoves, refrigerators, etc. The carbon content of these steels is generally below 0.10 per cent.

Electrical steels

These steels have good electrical characteristics and are used for the manufacture of electrical equipments. They contain Si and the carbon is usually less than 0.05 per cent.

Free cutting (or machining) steels

These steels can be easily machined and are used for the manufacture of nuts, bolts, screws, etc. Elements like S, P, Se, Te and Pb increase machinability and hence, these steels contain one or more of the above elements.

Machinery steels

They are used for the manufacture of automotive and machinery parts and the carbon content is between 0.30 to 0.55 per cent. They belong to medium carbon category of steels.

Structural steels

These steels are used in the construction of ships, cars, buildings, bridges, etc. and contain carbon from 0.15 to 0.30 per cent.

Tool steels

They are used as tools for machining or cutting of metals and contain carbon above 0.6 per cent. They belong to high carbon category of steels.

TRANSFORMATION PRODUCTS OF AUSTENITE

Transformation of Austenite to Pearlite

Pearlite formation starts by the nucleation of cementite plate at the grain boundaries of homogeneous austenite and grow as platelets by edge-wise growth into the austenite matrix. During this growth, carbon from austenite matrix diffuses towards its flat faces as shown in Fig. 5.11.

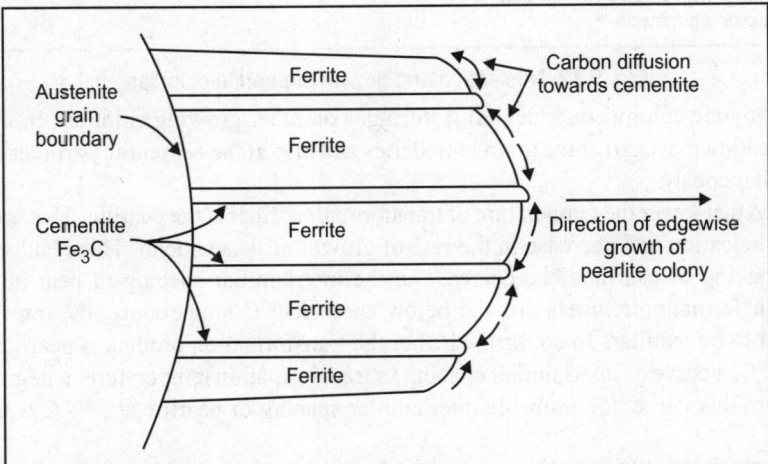

Fig. 5.11. Shows the growth of pearlite colony in austenite. The edgewise growth of a pearlite colony takes place by carbon diffusion in the austenite ahead, along directions indicated by arrows.

This reduces the carbon in the adjacent region of the growing cementite plate. When it reduces to a critical value, two ferrite plates, one on either side of the cementite plate, nucleate in these carbon deficient regions. These ferrite plates grow by rejecting carbon in excess of their solubility limit to the adjacent austenite. The rejected carbon then helps to nucleate of parallel cementite plates on both the sides. Repetition of this with sidewise nucleation of pairs of lamellae results in the creation of a colony of parallel cementite and ferrite platelets.

This first colony in turn nucleates other colonies and the process continues till a nodule containing many pearlite colonies is formed (Fig. 5.12).

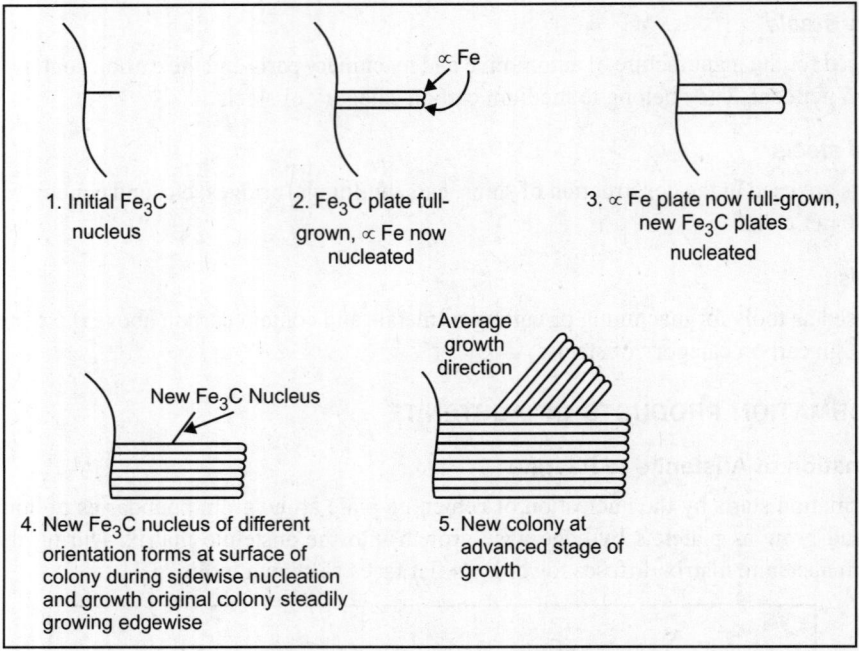

Fig. 5.12. Nucleation and growth of pearlite colonies.

Growth of anyone colony continues till it infringes on other growing colonies. In inhomogeneous austenite, nucleation may start at the grain boundaries and also at the cementite particles in the grains of austenite simultaneously.

It is observed that lower the temperature of transformation, finer is the pearlite. This is due to increase in the rate of nucleation and decrease in the rate of growth of these nuclei. This results in decrease in interlamillar spacing of pearlite. The decrease in the interlamillar spacing of pearlite is linear with decrease in transformation temperature and below about 550°C temperature, the transformed region does not appear to be lamillar. To confirm whether the transformation product is pearlite or something else below 550°C, a curve of interlamillar spacing vs transformation temperature in degrees Kelvin was plotted and from this curve, the probable interlamillar spacing of pearlite at 550°C was estimated by extrapolation.

This value of interlamillar spacing came out to less than the atomic dimensions. This is obviously impossible and hence the transformation product below 550°C is not pearlite. These studies were first done by a scientist Bain and hence the product is named as Bainite.

Transformation of Austenite to Bainite

The transformation product of austenite at below 550°C is not lamillar but is of different morphology and is called as Bainite. Bainite is an extremely fine mixture of ferrite and cementite and is formed by a different mechanism from that of pearlite. Bainitic transformation starts by the nucleation of ferrite, in contrast to the nucleation of cementite in pearlitic transformation (Fig. 5.13). Since the transformation occurs at low temperatures, nucleation rate is very high but the growth rate is very low due to relatively less mobility of carbon atoms at lower temperatures.

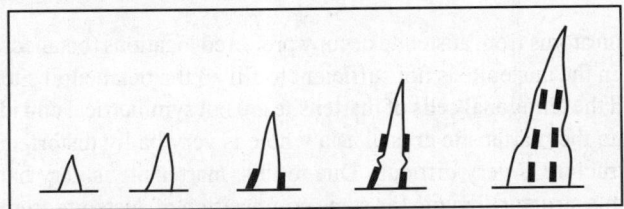

Fig. 5.13. Nucleation and growth of bainite colonies.

This results in a structure with very fine distribution of ferrite and cementite phases and is usually unresolvable by the optical microscopes. The bainite formed at higher temperatures is called as upper bainite and has a feathery appearance, whereas the bainite formed at lower temperatures is called as lower bainite and has an acicular (needle like) appearance. The distribution of carbides is finer in lower bainite than in upper bainite and hence lower bainite is harder, stronger and tougher than upper bainite. The hardness of bainite depends upon the carbon content in the steel and also on the temperature at which it is formed, but for a given steel, it is intermediate to that of pearlite and martensite. For eutectoid steel, the hardness of upper bainite is in the range of 40–50 Rc and that of lower bainite is between 50–60 Rc.

Transformation of Austenite to Martensite

The transformation product of austenite at low temperatures is totally different from that of pearlite or bainite and is called as martensite. At temperatures below the bainitic region, austenite very rapidly transforms to martensite by a shear mechanism involving no diffusion and the transformation proceeds at a speed close to the speed of sound.

$$\text{Austenite} \rightarrow \text{Martensite}$$
$$\text{(FCC)} \qquad \text{(BCT)}$$

Martensite is a supersaturated solid solution of carbon in BCC iron having BCT structure. The austenite to martensite transformation is diffusionless (i.e. time independent) and involves no change in composition. It depends only on temperature (i.e. athermal) and cannot be suppressed by rapid cooling. The basic mechanism is illustrated in Fig. 5.14.

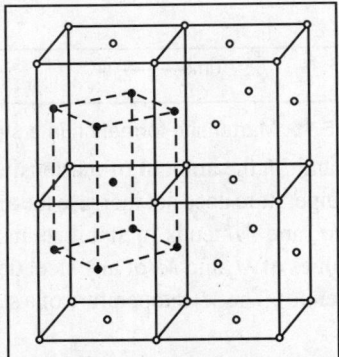

Fig. 5.14. The mechanism of formation of BCT martensite from FCC austenite by shear (Bain model).

A BCT unit cell is outlined within the adjacent FCC unit cells. During the shear transformation, the vertical axis (c) is contracted and horizontal axis (a and b) are extended slightly until the axis become equal, resulting in body centred a iron. However, the presence of carbon in austenite inhibits the complete alteration of the lattice, so that the axis do not become equal but retain a final axial ratio which depends upon carbon content.

The interstitial carbon atoms from austenite occupy preferred locations (octahedral sites) in martensite. The amount of carbon in the austenite is not sufficient to fill all the octahedral sites in every unit cell of martensite and hence all the tetragonal cells of martensite are not symmetrical and identical in dimensions to each other. Therefore, the martensite crystal as a whole is very badly distorted and slip propogation within this distorted structure is very difficult. Due to this, martensite is very hard, strong and brittle. Martensite is a metastable structure having the same composition of austenite from which it has formed. The properties of martensite depend on the carbon content in the steel, i.e. austenite.

During cooling from austenitic region, austenite starts transforming to martensite at some temperature. This temperature is denoted as M_s (martensite starts) temperature. As temperature decreases below M_s the amount of martensite progressively increases and at some temperature almost 99 per cent austenite transforms to martensite. This temperature is denoted as M_f (martensite finishes) temperature. Martensitic transformation does not go to completion and some small amount of austenite may still exist at below M_f temperature.

The austenite which has not transformed to martensite is called retained austenite or untransformed austenite. The amount of martensite formed between M_s and M_f is shown by dotted lines in Fig. 5.15.

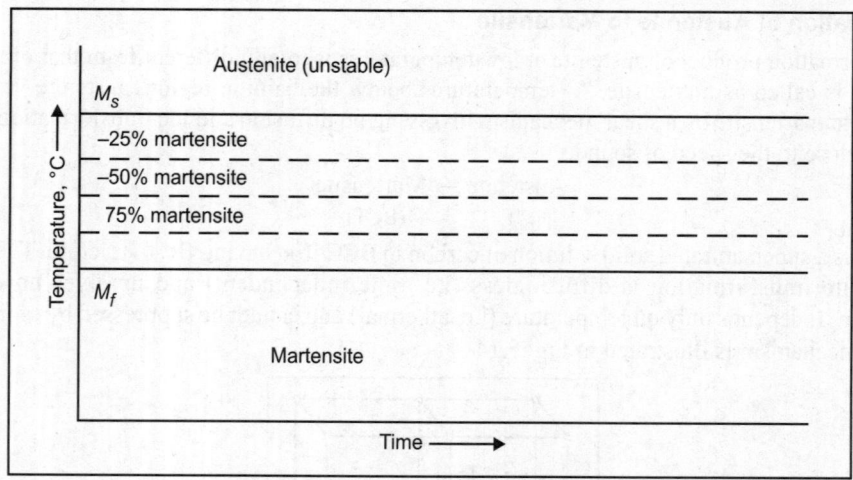

Fig. 5.15. Martensite formation in a steel.

At any temperature between M_s and M_f the amount of martensite characteristic of that temperature forms instantly, and holding at that temperature does not increase the amount of martensite. An appreciable delay at any temperature between M_s and M_f tends to stabilise austenite and the amount of retained austenite below M_f increases. The values of M_s and M_f of any steel depend upon the carbon and alloying elements present in the steel (i.e. austenite). The M_s temperature of a steel can be approximately calculated by the following equation:

$$M_s°C = 561 - 474\,(\%\,C) - 33\,(\%\,Mn) - 17\,(\%\,Ni) - 17\,(\%\,Cr) - 21\,(\%\,Mo) \quad \ldots (5.9)$$

The usual difference between M_s and M_f is in the range of 150° to 215°C. The variation of M_s and M_f with carbon in the austenite is shown in Fig. 5.16.

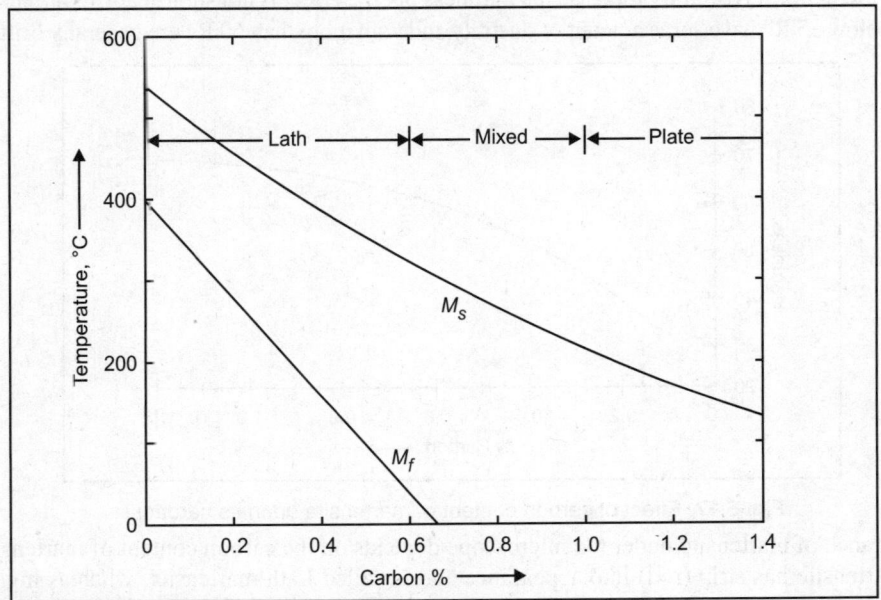

Fig. 5.16. The effect of carbon on the M_s and M_f temperatures and on the morphology of martensite in plain carbon steels.

At about 0.7 per cent carbon, M_f is very close to room temperature and for steels containing carbon above 0.7 per cent, M_f is actually below room temperature. Under this situation, if the steel is cooled only up to room temperature, all austenite will not transform to martensite but a part of it will remain untransformed. Such steels show retained austenite in their structure alongwith martensite at room temperature. The austenite is relatively soft and hence, its presence detracts from the hardness usually desired in a steel requiring full hardening. Since martensite occupies a greater volume than austenite, austenite to martensite transformation is accompanied by a volume increase of about 2 to 5 per cent depending on the carbon content and alloying elements in the austenite. With no alloying elements, volume increase is [4.64–0.53 (%C)]%. Due to this, the components are likely to distort or crack during martensitic transformation and particularly the tendency is more at the end of transformation. The tendency of cracking is reduced with the increase in amount of retained austenite. However, the retained austenite may get transformed to bainite or martensite under certain situations, resulting in volume changes of the components which may not be desirable for certain applications like precision gauges and measuring instruments. Therefore, the presence of retained austenite is not desirable for the above applications.

The hardness of martensite depends on the carbon content in the austenite as shown in Fig. 5.17. The extent to which a tetragonal unit cell of martensite departs from the cubic symmetry is a direct function of carbon content. Thus, a low carbon martensite is so little distorted by the presence of carbon that the axial ratio of its unit cell (c/a) is almost unity and such a low carbon martensite closely approaches ferrite in both structure and properties. With increasing carbon content, the axial ratio of martensite increases as an essentially linear function of % carbon, to a maximum value of 1.08 for high carbon steels. Due to this, the distortion in the lattice also increases, increasing the hardness of martensite as shown in Fig. 5.17. The hardness of martensite is solely dependent on the carbon in steel i.e. in austenite. (Alloying elements may slightly increase the hardness but the effect is not significant.) Martensites with hardness below 55 Rc have some amount of ductility and with more than 60 Rc are generally brittle.

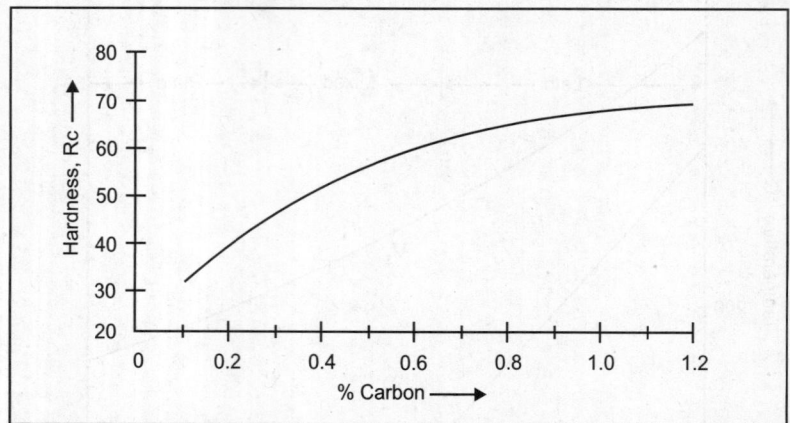

Fig. 5.17. Effect of carbon content of martensite upon its hardness.

Appearance of martensite under the microscope depends on the carbon content of martensite. Low carbon martensite has strip (rod) like appearance and is called Lath martensite, whereas high carbon martensite appears in needle form and is called as Plate martensite and with increasing carbon the appearance of martensite changes from strip like to more needle like shape. In high carbon martensites, the plates are arranged in a rig-zag fashion, partitioning the austenite grains into several smaller pockets. These strips or needles appear white with nital etching reagent.

ISOTHERMAL TRANSFORMATION DIAGRAM

Isothermal transformation diagrams (also known as time-temperature-transformation or TTT diagrams) are plots of temperature versus time (usually on a logarithmic scale). They are useful for understanding the transformations of an alloy steel that is cooled isothermally. Isothermal transformation diagrams are generated from percentage transformation vs logarithm of time measurements.

An isothermal transformation diagram is only valid for one specific composition of material, and only if the temperature is held constant during the transformation, and strictly with rapid cooling to that temperature. Though usually used to represent transformation kinetics for steels, they also can be used to describe the kinetics of crystallisation in ceramic materials. Time-temperature-precipitation diagrams and time-temperature-embrittlement diagrams have also been used to represent kinetic changes in steels.

Determination of TTT Diagram

For a given steel, TTT diagram can be experimentally determined as below:
1. Heat large number of steel pieces of a size suitable for metallography in the austenitic region. Throughout the experiment the austenitising temperature must be kept constant. During heating, oxidation and decarburisation should be avoided by suitable measures such as by the use of salt baths.
2. Soak these samples for sufficient time so as to obtain homogeneous austenite. The time of soaking should also be kept constant throughout the study.

3. Transfer all these samples quickly into a salt bath kept in another furnace at some constant temperature between A_1 and M_s.
4. Remove these samples one by one at fixed interval of time and quench them in brine or cold water. Due to this, the untransformed austenite is transformed to martensite.
5. Study these samples metallographically and find out the time of start of that particular transformation and the end of transformation.

    For example, if the study is done for eutectoid steel at say 600°C temperature, first few samples may show martensite (i.e. before quenching it was austenite) indicating that the transformation has not started; next few samples will show pearlite and martensite indicating that the pearlitic transformation is in progress; and after the pearlitic transformation is complete, rest of the samples will show only pearlite in, their microstructures. In the above example, we will have to note down the times of start and end of pearlitic transformation.

    Proeutectoid ferrite or cementite first separates out from austenite in hypoeutectoid or hypereutectoid steels and hence we have to note down the time of start of proeutectoid ferrite or cementite, time of start of pearlite, and time of end of pearlite transformation in the steels of off-eutectoid composition.
6. Similar studies are conducted at different temperatures and times of start and end of transformation are determined.
7. The obtained times at different isothermal transformation temperatures are plotted on temperature vs time graph and smooth curves are drawn through these points. For showing martensitic transformation two straight lines are drawn one at M_s and the other at M_f which indicate the start and finish of martensite transformation.

The resulting diagram is called as TTT diagram. The above diagram is also known as isothermal transformation (IT) diagram because it is plotted from the study of transformation products at constant temperatures. Because of its shape similar to letter C or S, it is also called as C or S curve.

Typical TTT diagrams of hypoeutectoid, eutectoid and hypereutectoid steels are shown in Fig. 5.18. The letters marked on the above curves have the following meaning:

1. F_s: Start of formation of proeutectoid ferrite.
2. C_s: Start of formation of proeutectoid cementite.
3. P_s: Start of pearlite formation.
4. P_f: Finish of pearlite formation.
5. B_s: Start of bainite formation.
6. B_f: Finish of bainite formation.

The transformation product between A_1 and the nose temperature is pearlite and the fineness of pearlite increases as the transformation temperature decreases, becoming unresolvably fine near the nose temperature.

The transformation product between the nose temperature and M_s is bainite. The morphology of bainite below the nose temperature is feathery and above M_s temperature is acicular. Martensitic transformation occurs between M_s and M_f as a linear function of temperature and below M_f the product is martensite. The hardness values of these products for eutectoid steel are marked on the TTT diagram. Pearlite is relatively soft, bainite is medium hard and martensite is hard. This clearly shows that as the transformation temperature decreases, hardness of a given steel increases. This helps in suitably adjusting the heat treatment cycle so as to obtain the desired properties in the components.

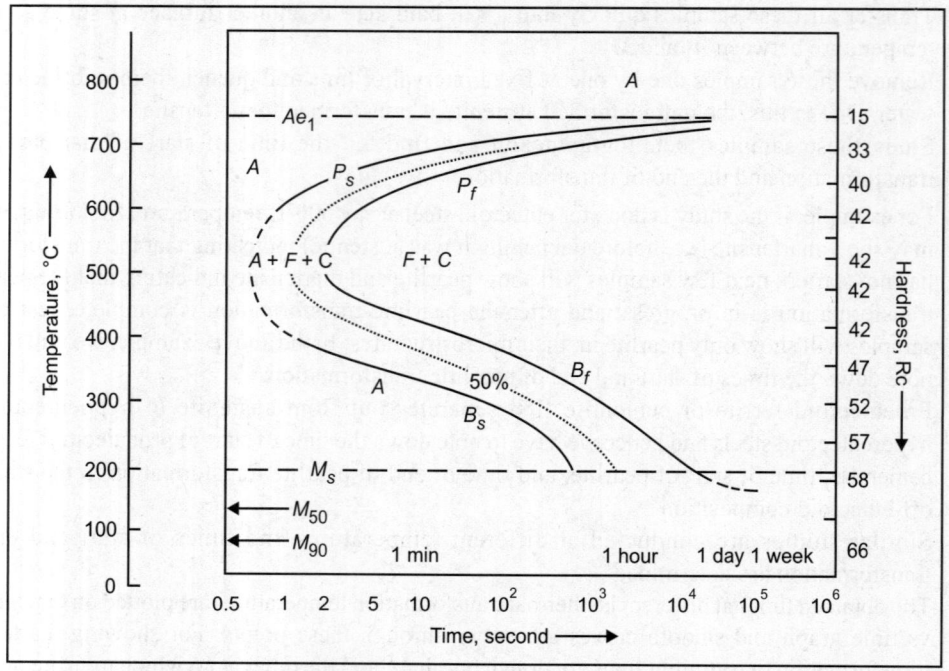

Fig. 5.18(b). TTT diagram of eutectoid steel.

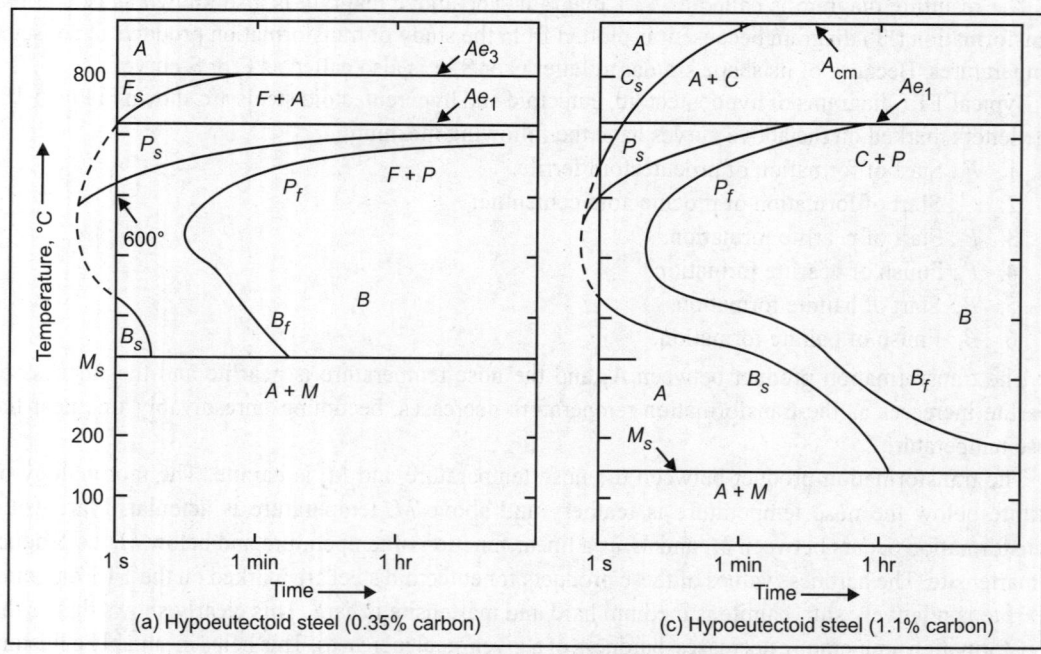

Fig. 5.18(a and c). Temperature–time transformation diagrams.

Carbon has the following effects on the TTT diagram:
1. The nose of S curves of hypoeutectoid and hypereutectoid steels are closer to the temperature axis as compared to the nose of eutectoid steel. This indicates that faster coolings are required for hypo and hyper eutectoid steels than eutectoid steels for martensitic transformation.
2. Carbon content has only a minor effect on the time required for the pearlitic reaction.
3. Dissolved carbon greatly retards the initiation and completion of the bainite reaction, displacing bainitic part of the curve strongly to the right side.
4. Dissolved carbon stabilises austenite and reduces M_s temperature.

CRITICAL COOLING RATE

The critical cooling rate is a rate which just bypasses the nose of the IT diagram (Fig. 5.19).

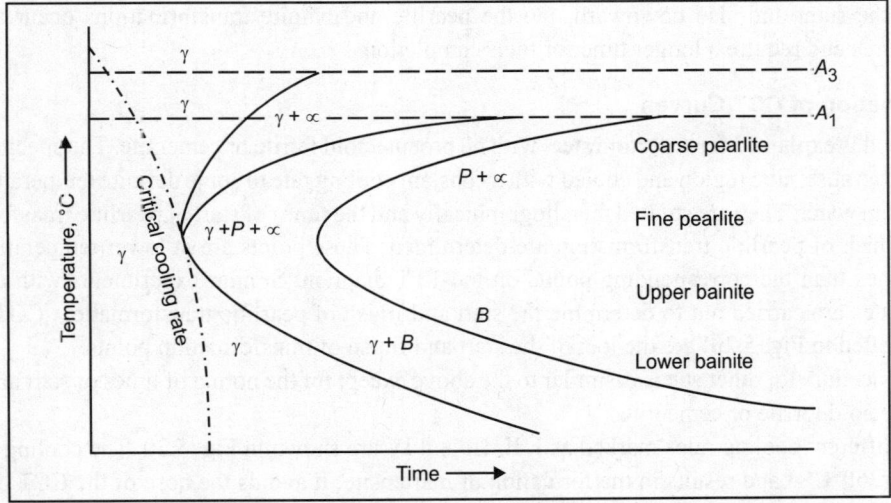

Fig. 5.19. Showing the critical cooling rate on TTT diagram.

It depends upon the shift of the nose of IT diagram to the right side. For hardening, steels from austenitic region must be cooled with such a rate that no transformation of austenite should occur upto M_s, i.e. the diffusion transformations should be stopped so that the austenite transforms to martensite by diffusionless transformation. The rate of cooling necessary to just suppress the diffusion transformation or to avoid the nose of IT diagram is called as the critical cooling rate. The critical cooling rate depends on many factors but the most important being the content of carbon and the alloying elements in steel. With higher carbon and/or alloying elements, critical cooling rate decreases. Most of the alloying elements (except cobalt) shift the IT diagram to the right side, i.e. retard transformation of austenite to pearlite or bainite decreasing the critical cooling rate. The shift of the nose of IT diagram to the right side gives an idea about the hardenability of steel. Thus, less the critical cooling rate, more is the hardenability. Alloying elements significantly reduce the critical cooling rate, permitting transformation of austenite to martensite at relatively low cooling rates. Thus, a steel with about 5 per cent Cr can be hardened by air cooling from austenitic region. A slower cooling rate reduces the danger of warping and cracking and becomes an advantage for hardening of complicated shaped components such as tools and dies compensating the cost of alloying elements.

Low carbon steels of plain type have very high critical cooling rate and hence rapid cooling is necessary to suppress the pearlitic or bainitic transformation. In some of the steels, it is not possible to achieve this even by water or brine quenching. Even if the critical cooling rate is exceeded by certain techniques, the martensite produced is not so hard because of less carbon in the steel. Since such steels are difficult to harden and cannot be effectively hardened, they are called as non-hardenable steels.

CONTINUOUS COOLING TRANSFORMATION (CCT) DIAGRAMS

TTT diagrams are valid only for isothermal transformations of austenite. They are not valid as the usual heat treating operations like full annealing, normalising and hardening, because in these processes steel is not cooled isothermally but cooled continuously.

When steel is cooled continuously from a high temperature to a low temperature, the TTT curve shifts to the right and also downward, i.e. the pearlite and bainite transformations occur at lower temperatures and require a longer time for their completion.

Determination of CCT Curves

The method is explained for eutectoid steel with no proeutectoid ferrite or cementite. The specimens are heated to the austenitic region and cooled with a constant cooling rate to some definite temperatures and quenched in water. They are studied metallographically and the times of start of pearlitic transformation and the finish of pearlitic transformation are determined. These points are at lower temperatures and longer times than the corresponding points on the TTT diagram. Similar experiments with different cooling rates are carried out to determine the start and finish of pearlitic transformation. CCT curves (shown dotted in Fig. 5.20) are the loci of the start and finish of transformation points.

The procedure for other steels is similar to the above except for the noting of times of start and finish of proeutectoid ferrite or cementite.

Four different cooling rates marked as I, II, III and IV are shown in Fig. 5.20. The cooling rate I is very fast (350°C/s) and results in the formation of martensite. It avoids the nose of the CCT diagram. The Cooling rate marked II (140°C/s) also results in the formation of martensite. It just touches the nose of the CCT diagram and is called as the critical cooling rate. It is the minimum cooling rate necessary to suppress the pearlitic transformation so as to obtain complete martensite. The cooling rate marked III (35°C/s) gives complete pearlite. The cooling rate marked IV (5°C/s) also gives complete pearlite. However, the pearlite formed with cooling rate IV is coarse than the pearlite formed with cooling rate III.

Bainite is not formed during continuous cooling because it is hidden below the nose of CCT diagram. Before the steel enters in the bainitic region, either pearlitic transformation is complete or starts and its formation and growth continues even when the steel passes through the B_s–B_f region.

HEAT TREATMENT OF STEEL

The heat treatment is a very broad term and includes any heating and cooling operation—or any sequence of two or more such operations-applied to any material in order to modify its internal structure or to alter its physical, mechanical or chemical properties. Usually it consists of heating the material to some specific temperature, holding at this temperature for a definite period and cooling to room temperature or below room temperature with a definite rate.

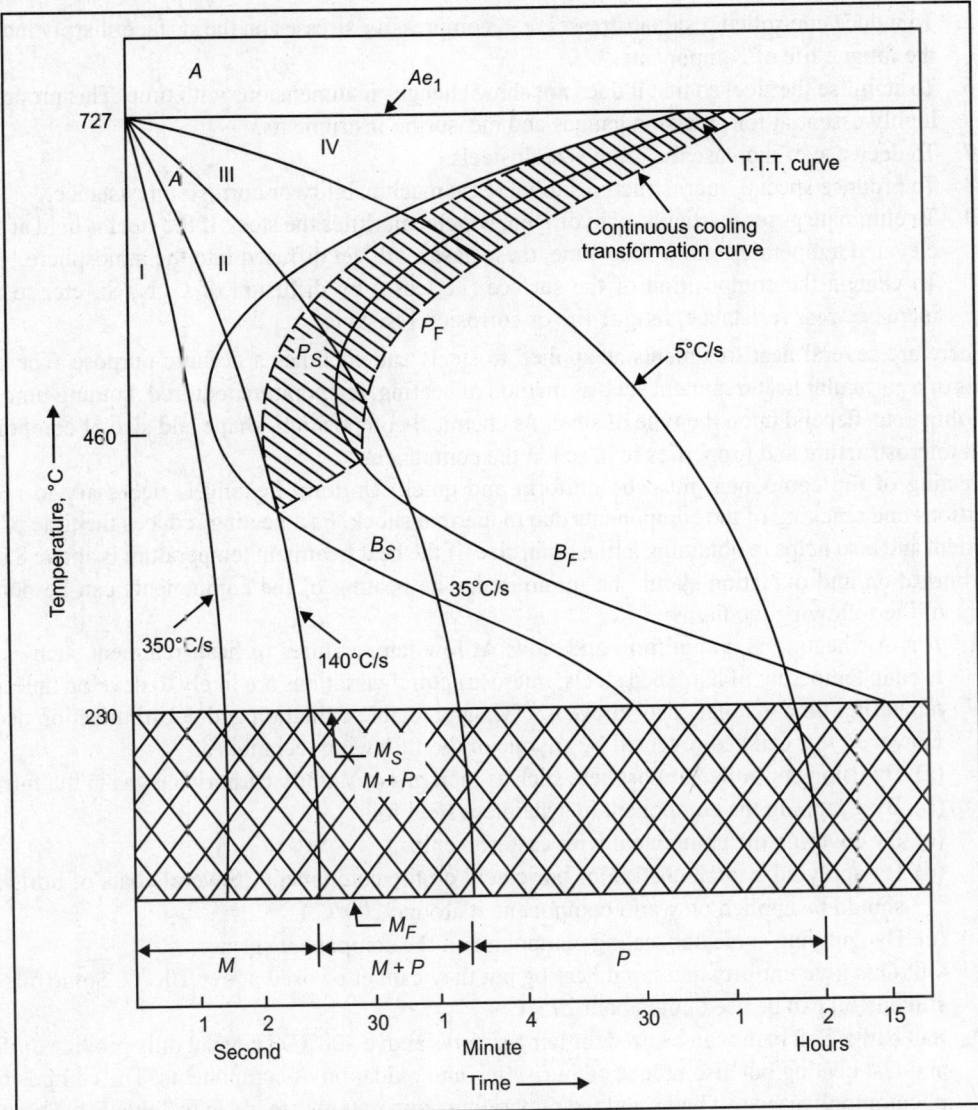

Fig. 5.20. Various cooling rates superimposed on time–temperature transformation (TTT) and continuous cooling transformation (CCT) curves of eutectoid steel.

The objects of various heat treatments commonly used for steels are one or more of the following:
1. To increase hardness, wear and abrasion resistance and cutting ability of steels.
2. To resoften the steel after it has been hardened by heat treatment or cold working.
3. To adjust its other mechanical, physical or chemical properties such as hardness, TS, ductility, electrical and magnetic properties, microstructure or corrosion resistance.
4. To reduce or eliminate internal residual stresses. Internal stresses lead to premature and brittle failures of the components. They also reduce corrosion resistance and hence are not desirable.

5. To induce controlled residual stresses, e.g. compressive stresses on the surface sharply increase the fatigue life of components.
6. To stabilise the steel so that it does not show changes in dimensions with time. This property is highly essential for precision gauges and measuring instruments.
7. To decrease or increase the grain size of steels.
8. To produce special microstructures to increase machinability or corrosion resistance.
9. To eliminate gases, particularly hydrogen, which embrittles the steel. If the steel is held at some elevated temperature for a short time, these gases will get diffused into the atmosphere.
10. To change the composition of the surface (i.e. case) by diffusion of C, N, Si, etc. so as to increase wear resistance, fatigue life or corrosion resistance.

There are several heat treatments as applied to steels and each has a definite purpose. The exact details of a particular heat treatment such as method of heating, temperature required, holding time, rate of cooling, etc. depend upon the type of steel, its chemical composition, shape and size of component, initial microstructure and properties required in the component.

Heating of the component must be uniform and quick. Uniform heating is necessary to reduce distortions and cracking of the components due to thermal shock. Fast heating reduces the time of heat treatment and also helps in obtaining a fine grain size. If the heat treatment temperature is above 850°C, decarburisation and oxidation should be minimised. The beating of the components can be done in anyone of the following mediums:

1. Air: Air heating is nonuniform and slow. At low temperatures of heat treatment such as that used in tempering of hardened steels, microstructural variations are likely to develop unless the tempering time is long. Also, above 850°C, appreciable oxidation and decarburisation occurs. However, this can be prevented by anyone of the following techniques.
    (a) By using controlled atmosphere such as inert gas or slightly carburising gas in the furnace.
    (b) By wrapping the component in a stainless steel foil.
    (c) By covering the component with cast iron chips.
    (d) By applying a thick coating of boric acid on the component. (Several coats of boric acid should be applied on warm component at around 200°C.)
    (e) By applying some antiscaling compound on the component surface.
2. Oil: Oils give uniform and rapid heating but they cannot be used above 200°C. Some oils like silicone oil can be used upto about 275°C.
3. Salt baths: Salt baths can be used for temperatures above 200°C. They not only provide uniform and fast heating but also reduce carburisation and oxidation of components. The compositions of commonly used salt baths and their operating temperatures are given in Table 5.1. These salt baths can also be used for obtaining uniform cooling rates in the components.

Table 5.1. Compositions and operating temperatures of salt baths used in heat treatments.

Sl. No.	Composition of salt bath	Melting point, °C	Range of application, °C
1	40–50 $NaNO_2$ 50–60 KNO_3	135	160–550
2	45–55 $NaNO_3$ 45–55 KNO_3	220	280–550

(Contd...)

Sl. No.	Composition of salt bath	Melting point, °C	Range of application, °C
3	45–55 NaCO$_3$ 45–55 KCl	450	550–900
4	10–15 NaCl 20–30 KCl 40–50 BaCl$_2$ 15–20 CaCl$_2$	400	500–800
5	70–96 BaCl$_2$ 4–30 NaO	600–800	700–1250

If the heat treatment temperature is more than 900°C, preheating of the component at some intermediate temperature is necessary to reduce distortions and cracking. During preheating of the components, decarburisation and oxidation are not much and hence there is no need of using any measures to reduce the above. Soaking of the components at the austenitising temperature is necessary to dissolve all the carbides into the austenite. The time of soaking depends on the size of component, type of steel (i.e. plain carbon or alloy steel) and initial microstructure of the component. For some of the alloy steels particularly containing large amounts of Cr, W, V, Mo, Ti, etc. the time of soaking is more because the complex alloy carbides do not dissolve fast in austenite due to their low diffusivity. If the initial microstructure is coarse and phase distribution is nonuniform, more time of soaking is necessary to dissolve these phases for obtaining homogeneous austenite. Time of soaking also depends on the size of component; larger the size, more is the time of soaking. About 20 minutes per cm thickness of the component is the approximate time required for this purpose. Unless the austenite is homogeneous in composition, the response to heat treatment will not be uniform. During heating at anyone temperature in the austenitic region, time necessary to form 99 per cent austenite is far less than the time required to form 100 per cent homogeneous austenite. The rate of austenitisation for 0.8 per cent carbon steel with initial microstructure of fine pearlite is shown in Fig. 5.21. It will be clear from Fig. 5.21 that the rate of austenite formation is more with temperature than with time. The residual carbides dissolve more slowly and hence the time of complete homogenisation is much more than for the formation of 99 per cent austenite.

COOLING MEDIA

Cooling can be done by using any one of the following mediums:
1. Brine (cold water + 5 to 10 per cent salt)—The salt may be sodium chloride, sodium hydroxide or calcium chloride.
2. Cold water.
3. Water + soluble oil.
4. Oil.
5. Fused salts.
6. Air.

They are arranged in order of decreasing cooling rates. Each medium provides a different cooling rate and hence depending upon the requirements, an appropriate quenching medium (quenchant) should be selected. Liquid cooling media remove the heat from the component through the following stages:
1. Vapour blanket stage: As soon as the component is quenched from a high temperature into the liquid medium, the liquid gets vaporised and forms a vapour blanket around the component. This vapour blanket does not allow to extract the heat and reduces the cooling rate.

2. **Vapour transport stage:** After sometime the vapour blanket breaks and the liquid comes in contact with the surface of hot component and hence, the cooling rate is highest during this stage.
3. **Liquid cooling stage:** This occurs when temperature of the component reaches the boiling point of quenching medium. During this stage, heat is removed by conduction and convection and hence cooling rate is the lowest.

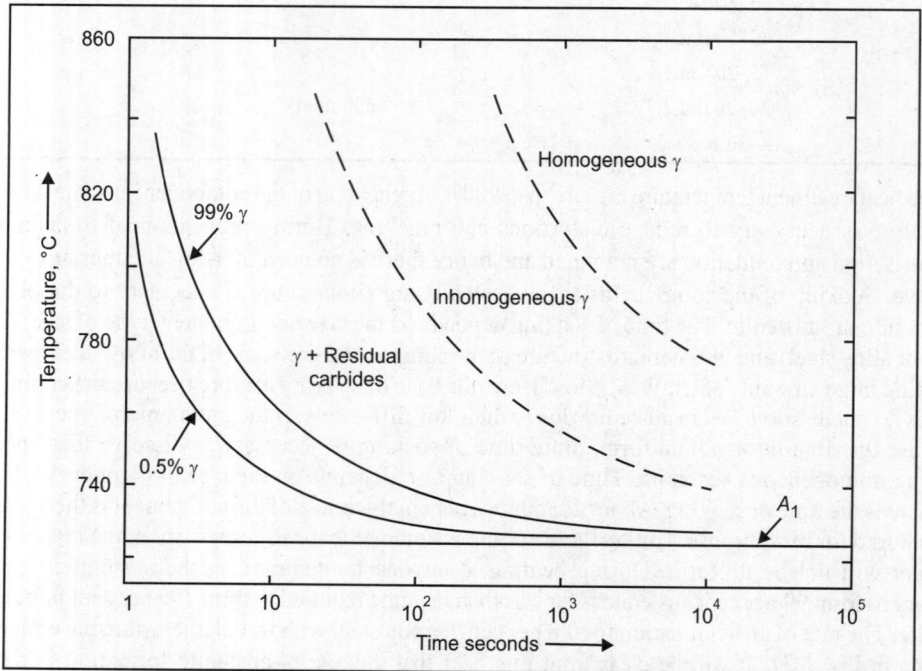

Fig. 5.21. The kinetics of austenite formation on heating above eutectoid temperature for 0.8 per cent carbon steel.

For hardening of steel components, it is necessary to cool them in some medium with a rate exceeding the critical cooling rate of that steel from austenitic region for the transformation of austenite to martensite. During quenching, the components does not crack as long as the structure is austenitic because austenite is soft, ductile and tough. However, there is a heavy tendency of cracking at lower temperatures when the austenite starts transforming to martensite and particularly it becomes severe at the end of transformation because martensite is hard and brittle phase. Therefore, the quenching medium should be such that it should extract heat rapidly at high temperatures and slowly at low temperatures. For such a requirement, liquid medium with sufficiently high boiling point will be most ideal. In this respect, hot water is not at all suitable because at high temperatures, it gives slow cooling rate due to the continuous formation of vapour blanket and at low temperatures, it gives high cooling rate due to almost direct contact of water because of delayed formation of vapour blanket. This leads to heavy distortions and cracking of components. Therefore, hot water should not be used for quenching of steel components. However, hot oil can be used for cooling rates lesser than that obtained by cold oil.

The vapour blanket that forms around the component acts as an insulator and slows down the cooling rate. This can result in incomplete or nonuniform hardening of the component. Therefore, it is essential to agitate the component or the liquid medium for quick breaking of the vapour blanket to increase the severity of quenching, i.e. to increase the cooling rate. Long components should be quenched vertically downwards and up and down motion should be given in the quenching medium. This way of quenching not only breaks up the vapour blanket, but also reduces unequal cooling rates reducing the bending of components during quenching.

Water and oil are the most common quenching mediums for hardening of steels. However, water gives a fast cooling rate at lower temperatures and oil gives a slow cooling rate at higher temperatures. This goes against the requirements of an ideal quenching medium for hardening purpose. The above drawbacks of water and oil are overcome by using a new quenching medium called Polymer Quenchant. This quenching medium provides a faster cooling rate in the high temperature range and a slow cooling rate in the low temperature range, thus satisfying the requirements of an ideal quenching medium. A polymer quenchant is a solution of high molecular weight organic compound in water.

A few well known organic compounds used as polymer quenchants are polyvinyl alcohol (PVA), poly-alkylene glycol (VCON), sodium poly acrylate (ACR) and poly-oxyalkylene glycols (GLY).

Polymer quenchants have distinct advantages over the usual quenchants and are as below:
1. They provide a wide range of cooling rates depending upon the type of polymer, concentration and temperature of the solution.
2. They reduce distortions and cracking of components.
3. They virtually eliminate smoke, fume and fire hazards in contrast to oil quenching because they are noninflammable.
4. They provide uniform cooling rate because of the deposition of polymer film, which results in uniform hardening of the component.
5. As compared to oils, polymer solutions result in reduced drag out and fluid losses.

AUSTENITIC AND FERRITIC GRAIN SIZE IN STEELS

Fine grained structures have better strength, ductility, toughness and some other properties and hence many times heat treatments are carried out to obtain fine grained structures. Also, most of the heat treatments carried out on steels alter the grain size and therefore it is necessary to control the grain size to achieve better properties. The effect of grain size on properties is given in Table 5.2. Grain size is reported for austenite as well as ferrite and whenever the grain size is mentioned, it always means the austenitic grain size, unless specifically mentioned as ferritic grain size. Austenitic grain size means it is the grain size of austenite that existed prior to its transformation to ferrite and cementite or martensite. Ferritic grain size is the grain size of ferrite produced by such a transformation. Austenite usually exists at high temperatures, but the nature and the distribution of the transformation products of austenite are dependent on its grain size and hence the properties of steels are strongly influenced by the prior austenitic grain size. In low carbon steels, the amount of ferrite is maximum and hence the properties of these steels are strongly influenced by ferritic grain size and are not much dependent on the austenitic grain size. However, fine austenitic grain size produces fine ferritic grain size and hence finer the austenite grain size, better are the mechanical properties.

GRAIN SIZE CONTROL

Since austenite appears above the lower critical temperature (A_1), it is necessary to heat the steel above A_1 to change and control the grain size. The grain size of austenite is minimum at just above A_1 temperature. However, these fine grains of austenite will be associated with either proeutectoid ferrite or cementite, except in steels of eutectoid composition. If the steel is heated to A_3 or A_{cm} (upper critical temperature), some growth of austenite grains occurs during heating. In most of the heat treatments of hypoeutectoid steels, complete austenitisation is desirable and hence this slight coarsening is tolerated in order to completely eliminate the ferrite. Due to this it is usually assumed that for hypoeutectoid steels, the finest grain size produced is at the A_3 temperature. However, this is not true for hypereutectoid steels because heating of these steels to above A_{cm} temperature leads to excessive coarsening of austenite and hence most of the heat treatments of these steels are carried out from just above A_1 temperature where the grain size of austenite is minimum.

Table 5.2. Effect of grain size on properties.

Property	Coarse grained structure	Fine grained structure
Yield strength	Less	More
Tensile strength	Less	More
Ductility	Less	More
Toughness	Less	More
Resilience	Less	More
Hardness	Less	More
Work hardening exponent (n)	Less	More
Strain rate sensitivity (SRS) of flow stress	Less	More
Fatigue resistance	Less	More
Creep resistance	More	Less
Corrosion resistance	More	Less
Machinability	More	Less
Surface finish	Less	More
Hardenability	More	Less
Retained austenite	More	Less
Tendency of formation of quench cracks	More	Less
Behaviour in carburising	Deep case	Shallow case

In order to produce complete austenitisation for hypoeutectoid steels and austenite plus cementite for hypereutectoid steels within a short time, it is necessary to heat the steel to above the critical temperature A_3 or A_1. Higher the temperature, more rapid is the phase transformation and shorter will be soaking time required to obtain the above condition. This increase in temperature leads to coarsening of austenite grains already existing in the structure. Therefore, a compromise is achieved between short soaking time, for economy and high production rate, and somewhat less austenitic grain size by selecting not too high or too low austenitising temperature such as 40° to 60°C above A_3 for hypoeutectoid steels and above A_1 for hypereutectoid steels.

The equilibrium grain size is usually not attained with the soaking periods usually employed in practice and hence the austenite grains continue to grow during subsequent cooling. However, their growth rate during cooling is less. Unless the cooling is extremely slow, no appreciable increase in size is observed during cooling. It is also very clear that the grains formed at any one austenitising temperature cannot be reduced in size during cooling by employing any cooling rate but only their further coarsening can be reduced by rapid cooling. Hence, it can be stated that in a steel, grain refinement occurs during heating within or through the critical temperature range, and it never occurs during cooling. Therefore, a coarse grained structure can only be refined by reheating the steel to just above A_3 temperature and cooling.

The grain size obtained at any given temperature depends on the type of steel. Rimmed steels show progressive increase in grain size with increase in austenitisation temperature and soaking time. However, killed steels, particularly killed with Al, Ti and V, are very resistant to grain coarsening and show fine and uniform grain size even after long soaking periods at relatively high temperatures. These killed steels show fine grain size upto a certain definite temperature which is a characteristic of each steel. When this temperature is exceeded, sudden grain growth starts and within a short time, the grain size increases to a level even higher than the grain size observed in rimmed steel of identical composition.

Working of austenite also reduces the grain size by recrystallisation process. Since temperature at which austenite exists is higher than the recrystallisation temperature, any working of austenite is simultaneously accompanied by recrystallisation resulting in refinement of grain structure. To avoid subsequent coarsening of austenite grains, working should be carried out to the lowest possible temperature limited by the deformation capability of steel, e.g. the working of low carbon steels can be continued up to 600°C, steels with 0.3 to 0.8 per cent carbon can be continued upto just above A_1 and the working of hypereutectoid steels should be stopped at just above A_{cm} temperature.

The ferritic grain size of hypoeutectoid steels depends on the following factors:
1. The austenitic grain size from which the ferrite is formed: Finer the austenitic grain size, finer is be the ferritic grain size.
2. Cooling rate employed: Higher the cooling rate, i.e. faster the cooling smaller is the ferritic grain size.

GRAIN SIZE MEASUREMENT

The grain size can be measured by the following methods:
1. Comparison method.
2. Heyn's intercept method.
3. Jefferies planimetric method.

Comparision Method

This method is applicable for equiaxed grains. Here the grain size of steel is reported by ASTM (American Society for Testing of Materials) grain size number. This number is found out by measuring the number of grains (N) per square inch at 100 × magnification and using the following relationship:

$$N = 2^{n-1} \qquad \ldots (5.10)$$

where, n = ASTM grain size number.

Fractional grain sizes (e.g. ASTM 1.5) are also sometimes reported, but this degree of precision is generally not required.

ASTM grain size numbers with corresponding average number of grains and average grain diameters are given in Table 5.3. Standard charts are prepared for the convenience of measurement of grain size (ASTM E 112–63 or IS 4748–1968 method). The grain structure is compared with the sizes given in the above charts at 100 × magnification and the matching number is reported. These charts are given in Figs 5.22 to 5.29.

Table 5.3. ASTM grain size numbers.

ASTM grain size number	Average number of grains per square inch at 100 ×	(Unmagnified) Average diameter of equivalent spherical grain in microns (1 micron = 10^{-3} mm)
1	1	287.0
2	2	203.0
3	4	144.0
4	8	101.0
5	16	71.8
6	32	50.7
7	64	35.9
8	128	25.4
9	256	18.0
10	512	12.7
11	1024	9.0
12	2048	6.4

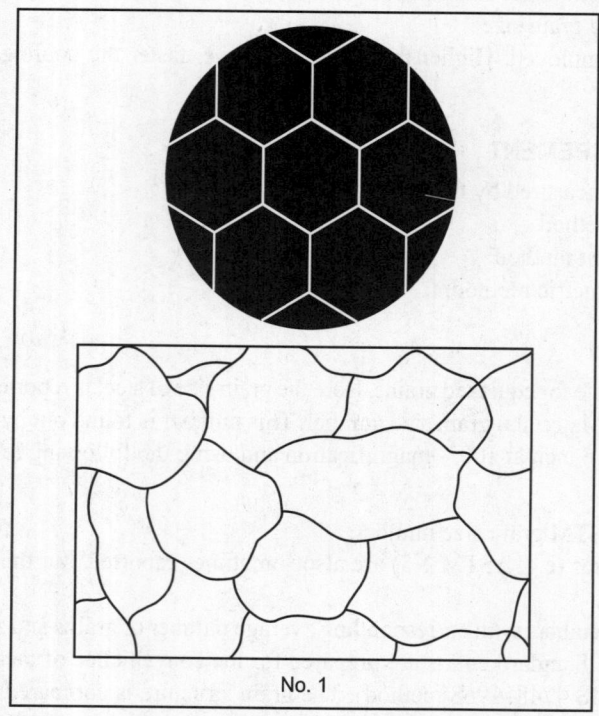

Fig. 5.22. Upper, idealised hexagonal network for mean grain size No.1, ASTM scale, 1 gr per sq. inch. Lower, ASTM standard grain size No.1, upto 1 1/2 gr per sq. inch at 100 ×.

Heat Treatment of Steel **121**

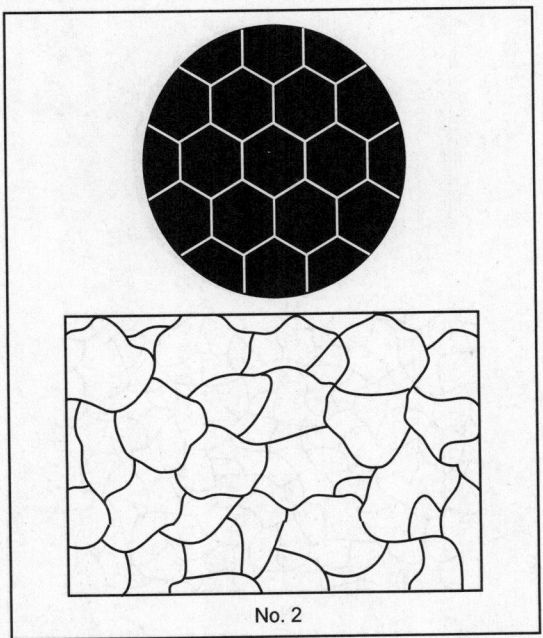

Fig. 5.23. Upper, idealised hexagonal network for mean grain size no. 2, ASTM scale, 2 gr per sq. inch. Lower, ASTM standard grain size No.2, 1½ gr per sq. inch at 100 ×.

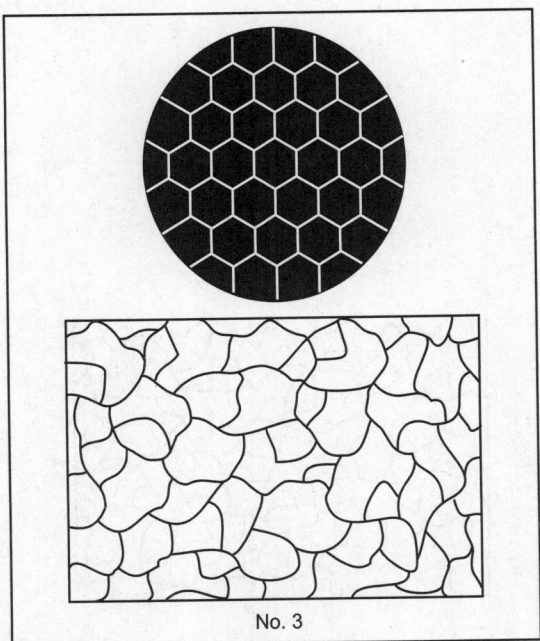

Fig. 5.24. Upper, idealised hexagonal network for mean grain size no. 3, ASTM scale, 4 gr per sq. inch. Lower, ASTM standard grain size no. 3, 3 to 6 gr per sq. inch at 100 ×.

122 Physical Metallurgy

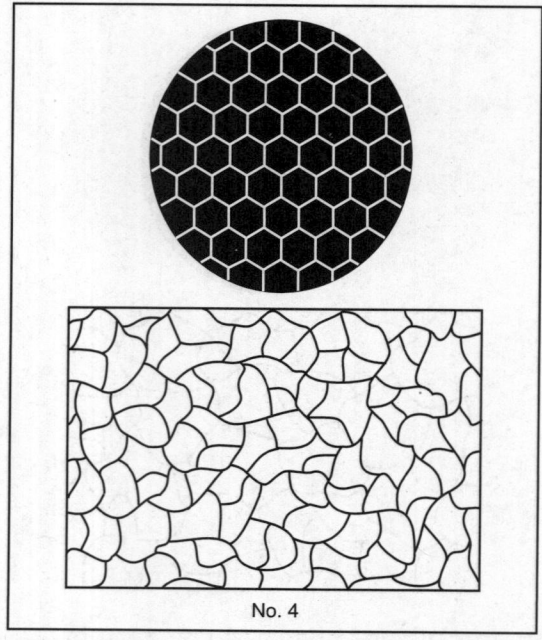

Fig. 5.25. Upper, idealised hexagonal network for mean grain size No.4, ASTM scale, 8 gr per sq. inch. Lower, ASTM standard grain size No.4, 6 to 12 gr per sq. inch at 100 ×.

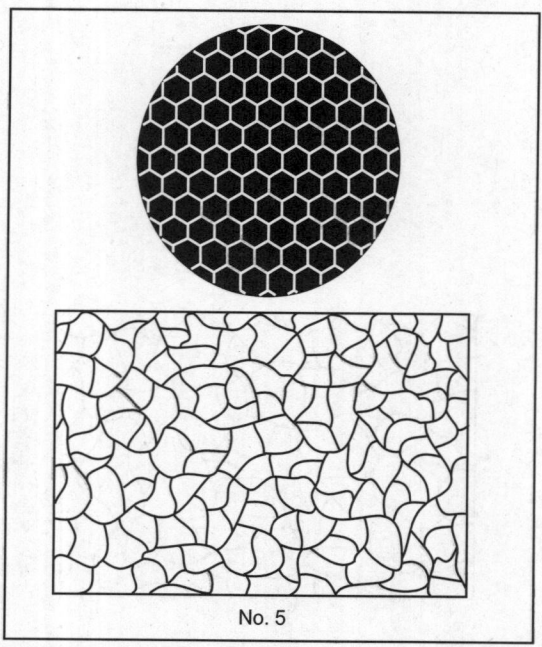

Fig. 5.26. Upper, idealised hexagonal network for mean grain size No.5, ASTM scale, 16 gr per sq. inch. Lower, ASTM standard grain size No.5, 12 to 24 gr per sq. inch at 100 ×.

Heat Treatment of Steel 123

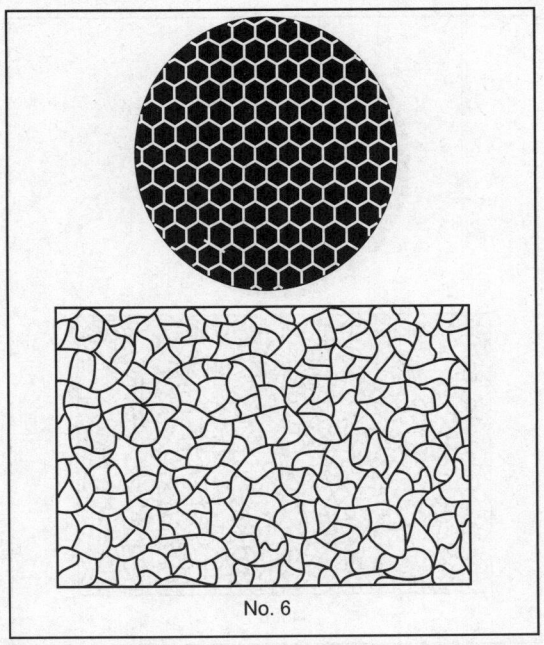

Fig. 5.27. Upper, idealised hexagonal network for mean grain size No.6, ASTM scale, 32 gr per sq. inch. Lower, ASTM standard grain size No.6, 24 to 48 gr per sq. inch at 100 ×.

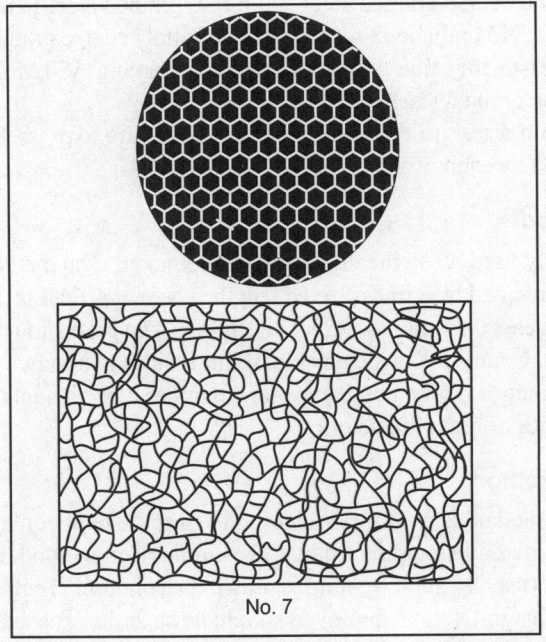

Fig. 5.28. Upper, idealised hexagonal network for mean grain size No.7, ASTM scale, 64 gr per sq. inch. Lower, ASTM standard grain size No.7, 48 to 96 gr per sq. inch at 100 ×.

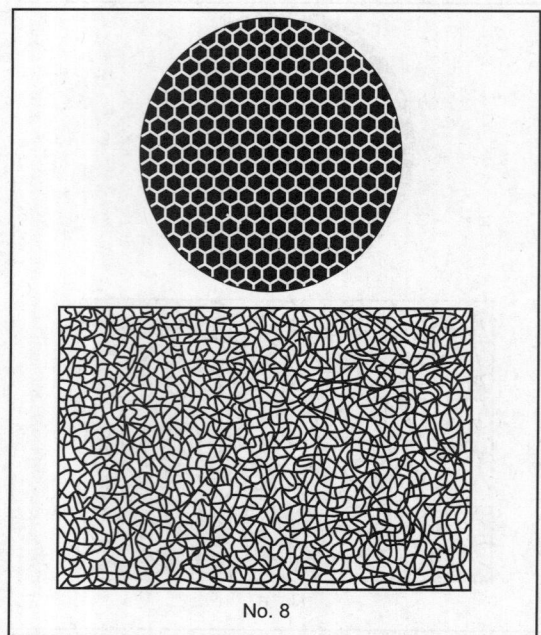

Fig. 5.29. Upper, idealised hexagonal network for mean grain size No.8, ASTM scale, 128 gr per sq. inch. Lower, ASTM standard grain size No.8, 96 to 192 gr per sq. inch at 100 ×.

A distinction between a coarse grained steel and a fine grained steel is not very clear. However, a grain size number below ASTM number 3 represents a definitely coarse grained steel and above ASTM number 6 represents a reasonably fine grained steel. Steels having ASTM grain size number greater than 8 are called ultra fine grained steels.

Sometimes mixed grain sizes are observed in steels. These are expressed by giving the estimated area percentages occupied by each of the ranges of sizes.

Heyn's Intercept Method

This method is particularly used when the grains are not equiaxed. The method consists of finding out the number of grains intercepted by a line of fixed length. The magnification employed should be such that the area covered is atleast 0.5 mm^2 on the actual sample. The grains touched by the end of the line are counted as half grains. Counts are made on at least three fields to assure a reasonable accuracy. The length of the line in millimetres divided by the average number of grains intercepted by that line gives the average intercept length or grain diameter.

Jefferies Planimetric Method

The Jefferies planimetric method is used for measuring the grain size of equiaxed grains, and in case of dispute the results of this method are preferred over the comparison method. In this method, a circle or a rectangle of known area (usually 5000 sq. mm) is drawn on a photomicrograph or on the ground glass of the metallograph. The magnification employed should be such that at least 50 grains should be seen in the above field. The total number of grains are counted in this area which is the sum of grains included in the above area plus half the grains intersected by the circumference or perimeter of the area.

From this the number of grains per square millimetre is determined by multiplying the total number of whole grains by the corresponding magnification factor (Jefferies' multiplier) 'f' given in Table 5.4.

Table 5.4. Relationship between magnification used and Jefferies multiplier 'f' for an Area of 5000 sq.mm.

Magnification used	f
1	0.0002
10	0.02
25	0.125
50	0.50
75	1.125
100	2.00
150	4.50
200	8.00
250	12.50
300	18.00
500	50.00
750	112.50
1000	200.00
1500	450.00
2000	800.00

CONVENTIONAL ANNEALING (FULL ANNEALING)

Purpose of full annealing is:
1. To relieve the internal stresses induced due to cold working, welding, etc. Internal stresses are not desirable because they lead to premature, sudden, and brittle failures of the components. They also decrease the corrosion resistance.
2. To reduce hardness (i.e. to make the metal soft) and to increase ductility.
3. To increase the uniformity of phase distribution and to make the material isotropic in respect of mechanical properties.
4. To refine the grain size.
5. To make the material homogeneous in respect of chemical composition.
6. To increase machinability.
7. To make the steel suitable for subsequent heat treatment like hardening.

Process of Annealing

The process consists of heating the steel to above A_3 temperature for hypoeutectoid steels and above A_1 temperature for hypereutectoid steels by 30°–50°C, holding at this temperature for a definite period and slow cooling to below A_1 or to room temperature usually in furnace. Due to slow cooling, eutectoid reaction occurs very nearly in accordance with conditions represented by the Fe–C phase diagram. To insure equalisation of temperature throughout the cross section of the component and complete austenitisation, a holding (soaking) period of at least 20 minutes per cm of the thickest section is necessary.

Hypereutectoid steels are always annealed from above A_1 temperature and never annealed from above A_{cm} temperature because of the following reasons:

1. If slowly cooled from above A_{cm} temperature, proeutectoid completely separates along the grain boundaries of austenite and completely envelopes the austenite grains which transform to pearlite at A_1 temperature. The microstructure of such a steel at room temperature shows a continuous network of cementitic areas all around the pearlite regions. Due to this the dislocations get blocked at cementite regions and are not able to move from one pearlite region to another (Fig. 5.30). This increases the brittleness of steel, departing from the aim of annealing.
2. A_{cm} temperature is high and therefore, heating to above A_{cm} results in more oxidation and decarburisation of steel.
3. Heavy grain coarsening of austenite occurs above A_{cm} temperature. This is because the last part of cementite dissolves at A_{cm} and grain boundary migration occurs without any hindrance above A_{cm} temperature. This leads to deterioration of mechanical properties because coarse grained structures are inferior to fine grained structures in respect of mechanical properties.

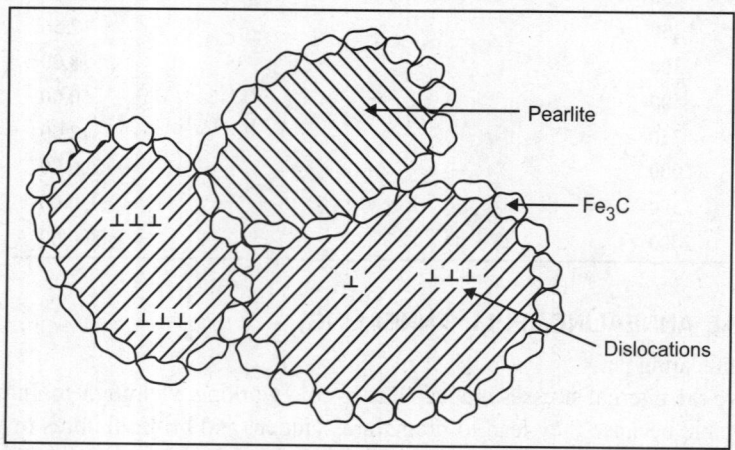

Fig. 5.30. Schematic illustration of blocking of dislocations by cementite regions.

TYPES OF ANNEALING

Bright Annealing

Annealing of steel components is carried out using some protective medium to prevent oxidation and surface discolouration. Such a type of annealing keeps the surface bright and hence is called bright annealing. The surface protection is obtained by the use of an inert gas such as argon or nitrogen or by using reducing atmospheres. A typical composition of a reducing gas is 15 per cent H_2, 10 per cent CO, 5 per cent CO_2, 1.5 per cent CH_4 and remainder N_2.

Box Annealing

Here annealing is carried out in a sealed container under conditions that minimise oxidation. The components are packed with cast iron chips, charcoal or clean sand and annealed in a way similar to full annealing. It is also called black annealing, close annealing or pot annealing.

Isothermal (Cycle) Annealing

In this process, the components are slightly fast cooled from the usual austenitising temperature of conventional annealing to a constant temperature just below A_1, held at this temperature for sufficient period for the completion of transformation and then cooled to room temperature in air.

Isothermal annealing has distinct advantages over conventional annealing which are as below:
1. It reduces the annealing time, especially for alloy steels which need very slow cooling to obtain the required reduction in hardness with the conventional annealing.
2. Because of equalisation of temperature, transformation occurs at the same time throughout the cross-section. This leads to more homogeneity in structure.
3. It shows improved machinability, improved surface finish after machining and less warping during subsequent hardening process.

Isothermal annealing is chiefly used for medium carbon, high carbon and some of the alloy steels to improve their machinability. The increase in machinability is due to the formation of spheroidised structure. Heat treatment cycles of full annealing, i.e. conventional annealing and isothermal annealing are shown in Fig. 5.31.

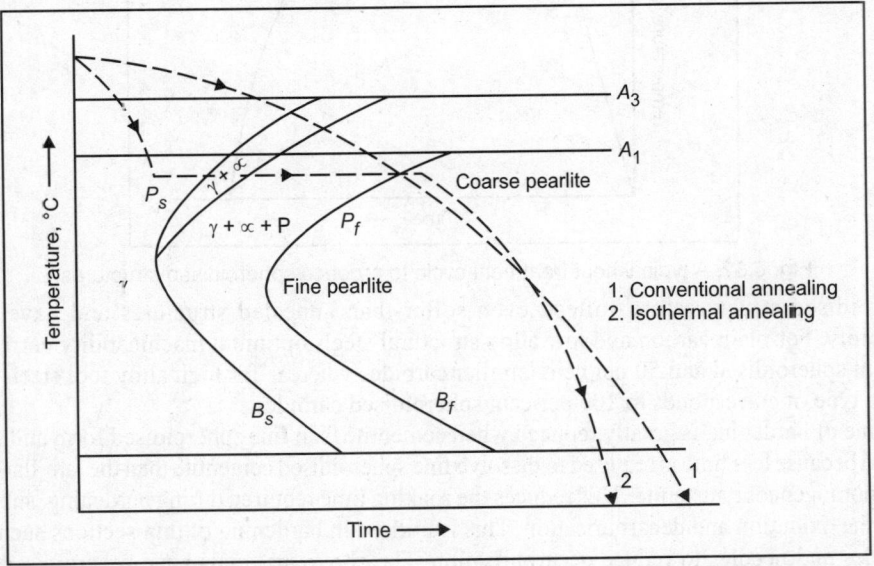

Fig. 5.31. Heat treatment cycles of full annealing and isothermal annealing.

Spheroidise Annealing

This heat treatment is given to high carbon and air hardening alloy steels to soften them and to increase machinability. The microstructure typical of this heat treatment shows globules (rounded particles) of cementite or carbides in the matrix of ferrite. Any heat treatment that produces a structure of the above type is called spheroidising or spheroidise annealing.

Following methods produce spheroidised structures:
1. Hardening and high temperature tempering: Due to tempering of hardened steels at 650°–700°C for a long time, cementite globules are formed in the matrix of ferrite from martensite.

   Martensite → Cementite (in globuler form) + Ferrite.

2. **Holding at just below A_1**: Due to holding for a long time at just below the lower critical temperature, cementite from pearlite globularises, The process is very slow and requires more time for obtaining spheroidised structures. It can be accelerated by prior cold working of steel. However, this may not be possible in many cases where the steel is brittle e.g. alloy steels and high carbon steels cannot be worked much in the annealed or normalised condition without cracking.
3. **Thermal cycling around A_1**: Due to thermal cycling in a narrow temperature interval around A_1, cementite lamillae from pearlite become spheroidal. During heating above A_1, cementite or carbides try to dissolve and during cooling they try to form. This repeated action spheroidises the carbide particles. A typical heat treatment cycle of this type is shown in Fig. 5.32.

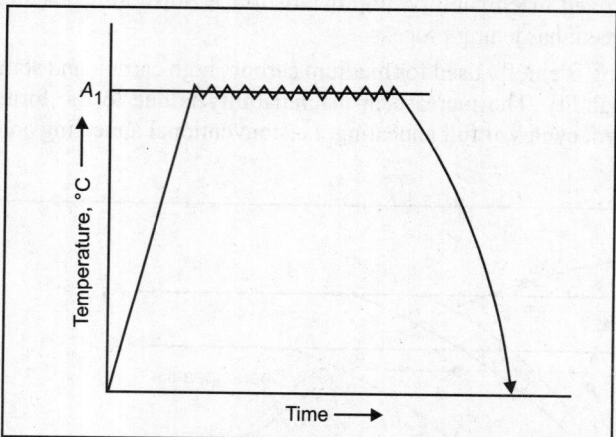

Fig. 5.32. A typical heat treatment cycle to produce spheroidised structures.

Spheroidised structures are softest, even softer than annealed structures and have excellent machinability. For plain carbon and low alloy structural steels optimum machinability corresponds to 50 per cent spheroidised and 50 per cent lamillar carbides whereas for high alloy tool steels of the air hardening type, it corresponds to 100 per cent spheroidised carbides.

The time of hardening is greatly reduced when cementite is in fine spheroidised form and uniformly distributed because less time is required to dissolve fine spheroidised cementite than the lamillar cementite to obtain homogeneous austenite. This reduces the soaking time required during hardening, subsequently reducing the oxidation and decarburisation. This is utilised in hardening of thin sections such as safety razor blades and needles to reduce decarburisation. The above materials have spheroidised structure prior to their hardening.

Subcritical Annealing

In these processes of annealing, the cold worked steel is heated to some temperature below the lower critical temperature and hence they are classified as subcritical annealing processes. They are used after cold working of steels to relieve the internal stresses or to reduce the hardness or to refine and modify the structure.

Stress-relief annealing

In this process, cold worked steel is heated to a temperature between 500° and 550°C, i.e. below its recrystallisation temperature ($\approx 600°C$), kept at this temperature for 1–2 hours and cooled to room temperature in air. Due to this, internal stresses are partly relieved without loss of strength and hardness, i.e. without change of microstructure. It reduces the risk of distortion in machining, and also increases corrosion resistance. Since only low carbon steels can be cold rolled/worked, the process is applicable to hypoeutectoid steels containing less than 0.4 per cent carbon.

Stress relief annealing is also carried out on components in which internal stresses are developed from other sources like rapid cooling and phase changes.

Recrystallisation annealing

This is done below A_1 temperature, i.e. at temperature between 625° and 675°C. The cold worked ferrite recrystallises and cementite tries to spheroidise during this annealing process. Not only internal stresses are eliminated but also the steel becomes soft and ductile. Refinement in grain size is also possible by control of degree of cold work prior to annealing or by control of annealing temperature and time.

Process annealing (intermediate annealing)

In this method, cold worked metal is heated to above its recrystallisation temperature. This is also accomplished by the formation of strain free equiaxed grains. This is given to metals to soften them during mechanical processing so as to continue the cold working process without cracking of metals. It may or may not involve full recrystallisation of the cold worked metal. In principle, process annealing and recrystallisation annealing are same and both the processes involve recrystallisation and formation of new stress free equiaxed grains from strained and distorted cold worked grains.

NORMALISING

Normalising is a type of heat treatment applicable to ferrous metals only. It differs from annealing in that the metal is heated to a higher temperature and then removed from the furnace for air cooling. The purpose of normalising is to remove the internal stresses induced by heat treating, welding, casting, forging, forming, or machining. Stress, if not controlled, leads to metal failure; therefore, before hardening steel, you should normalise it first to ensure the maximum desired results. Usually, low-carbon steels do not require normalising; however, if these steels are normalised, no harmful effects result. Castings are usually annealed, rather than normalised; however, some castings require the normalising treatment.

Note that the soaking time varies with the thickness of the metal. Normalised steels are harder and stronger than annealed steels. In the normalised condition, steel is much tougher than in any other structural condition. Parts subjected to impact and those that require maximum toughness with resistance to external stress are usually normalised. In normalising, the mass of metal has an influence on the cooling rate and on the resulting structure. Thin pieces cool faster and are harder after normalising than thick ones. In annealing (furnace cooling), the hardness of the two are about the same.

Process

The process consists, of heating to above the upper critical temperature (A_3) for hypoeutectoid steels and above A_{cm} (or between A_1 and above A_{cm}) for hypereutectoid steels by 30° to 50°C, holding long enough at this, temperature for homogeneous austenitisation and cooling to room temperature in still air.

Due to air cooling which is slightly fast as compared to furnace cooling employed in full annealing, normalised components show slightly different structure and properties than annealed components, which are shown in Table 5.5.

Table 5.5. Different structure and properties of normalised and annealed components.

Annealed	Normalised
Less hardness, TS and toughness.	Slightly more hardness, TS and toughness.
For plain carbon steels, microstructure shows pearlite almost in accordance with the Fe-C equilibrium diagram.	Microstructure shows more pearlite than observed in annealed components.
Pearlite is coarse and usually gets resolved by the optical microscope.	Pearlite is fine and usually appears unresolved with optical microscope.
Grain size distribution is more uniform.	Grain size distribution is slightly less uniform.
Internal stresses are least.	Internal stresses are slightly more.

The properties of normalised components are not much different from those of annealed components. However, normalising takes less time and is more convenient and economical than annealing and hence is a more common heat treatment in industry. Full annealing is specifically used for complex shapes where even air cooling may cause cracking or considerable warping of the components.

Hypereutectoid steels are usually normalised from above A_{cm} temperature. This is because due to air cooling from above A_{cm}, the proeutectoid Fe_3C separates in the form of needles in the grains of austenite which transforms to pearlite at A_1. Thus, the microstructure at room temperature shows innumerable needles of Fe_3C in the matrix of pearlite (Widmanstatten structure). Such structures are less brittle because the dislocations can move via certain regions avoiding these needles. However, slow cooled structures from the same temperature are more brittle.

These steels can also be normalised from above A_1 temperature. The microstructure of such steels show fine, quite rounded particles of proeutectoid Fe_3C and needles of Fe_3C in the matrix of pearlite. Such structures also have less brittleness.

HARDENING

Purpose: (i) to harden the steel to the maximum level by austenite to martensite transformation (due to increase in hardness, brittleness also increases), and (ii) to increase the wear resistance and cutting ability of steel. Steels can be hardened by the following methods.

Conventional Hardening

The conventional hardening process consists of heating the steel to above A_3 temperature for hypoeutectoid steels and above A_1 temperature for hypereutectoid steels by 50°C, austenitising for a sufficient time and cooling with a rate just exceeding the critical cooling rate of that steel to room temperature or below room temperature. Due to this, the usual diffusion transformations are stopped and the austenite transforms to martensite by a diffusionless process.

All the time, hypoeutectoid steels are hardened from above A_3 temperature. They are not hardened from temperatures between A_1 and A_3, because the phases which exist at this temperature are austenite and proeutectoid ferrite and only austenite gets transformed to martensite with no change in ferrite. Such steels show free ferrite in their microstructures and since ferrite is a soft phase, the hardness of hardened steel gets reduced.

On the other hand, hypereutectoid steels are always hardened from temperatures between A_1 and A_{cm} (i.e. from above A_1). At this temperature, austenitisation is not complete and some proeutectoid Fe_3C will exist along with austenite at the temperature of heating. Such steels after hardening show free Fe_3C

alongwith martensite in their microstructures. Since Fe_3C being a hard phase, the hardness of hardened-steels does not get reduced. Moreover, this free Fe_3C does not increase the brittleness of steels because usually it is fine, well distributed and partially spheroidised. Also, the grain size remains fine because the Fe_3C particles do not allow to coarsen the austenite. However, if these steels are hardened from above A_{cm} temperature, the following drawbacks are observed:

1. Since A_{cm} line is steep, higher temperatures are required to cross the A_{cm} line. Due to this and absence of Fe_3C above A_{cm} temperature, heavy grain coarsening occurs during austenitisation and results in coarse grained martensite which is extremely brittle.
2. Quenching from such a high temperature results in more distortions and may lead to cracking of the components.
3. Due to higher temperatures, oxidation and decarburisation is more.
4. The amount of retained austenite increases because of higher thermal stresses.

Due to these reasons, hypereutectoid steels are never hardened from above A_{cm} temperature. They are always hardened from above A_1 temperature which produces the desired hardening with almost elimination of the above drawbacks. Also, the free carbides present in the structure increase the wear resistance and cutting ability of these steels.

A proper quenching medium should be used such that the component gets cooled at a rate just exceeding the critical cooling rate of that steel. Faster cooling than the above also produces martensite but the tendency of warping and cracking is more and hence should be avoided. The critical cooling rate of a steel largely depends on the alloying elements and to a lesser extent on the carbon present in the steel. Alloy steels have less critical cooling rate and hence some of the alloy steels can be hardened by simply air cooling. High carbon steels have slightly more critical cooling rate and has to be hardened by oil quenching. Medium carbon steels have still higher critical cooling-rates and hence water or brine quenching is necessary for their hardening. Low carbon steels with very low carbon content such as less than 0.1 per cent carbon cannot be hardened by quenching because of their high critical cooling rate which is not possible to exceed even by brine quenching.

For high carbon steels containing more than 0.7 per cent carbon and some of the alloy steels, M_f is below room temperature. If these steels are cooled only upto room temperature all austenite will not transform to martensite but a part of it will appear as retained austenite. This retained austenite reduces the hardness of hardened steels. Therefore, in such cases, the steel is cooled below room temperature to eliminate part of the retained austenite by transforming it to martensite.

The heat treatment cycle for eutectoid steel is shown in Fig. 5.33. Hardening is invariably followed by tempering and hence tempering cycle is also shown alongwith hardening cycle in the Fig. 5.33.

Timed Quench (Interrupted Quench)

For plain carbon steels of low to medium carbon, critical cooling rates are high and therefore, very fast cooling from austenitising temperature is necessary to prevent the formation of pearlite or bainite at temperatures near the nose of the TTT diagram. However, once this region of rapid transformation has been passed, the transformation of austenite becomes slow. Therefore, it is possible to obtain a completely martensitic structure in a steel of low harden ability (i.e. of high critical cooling rate) by cooling it rapidly to a temperature below the nose of the IT diagram and then cooling it more slowly through the temperature range in which martensite is formed. Such a cycle of hardening employing two cooling rates, one fast and the other slow, is shown in Fig. 5.34 for a medium carbon steel.

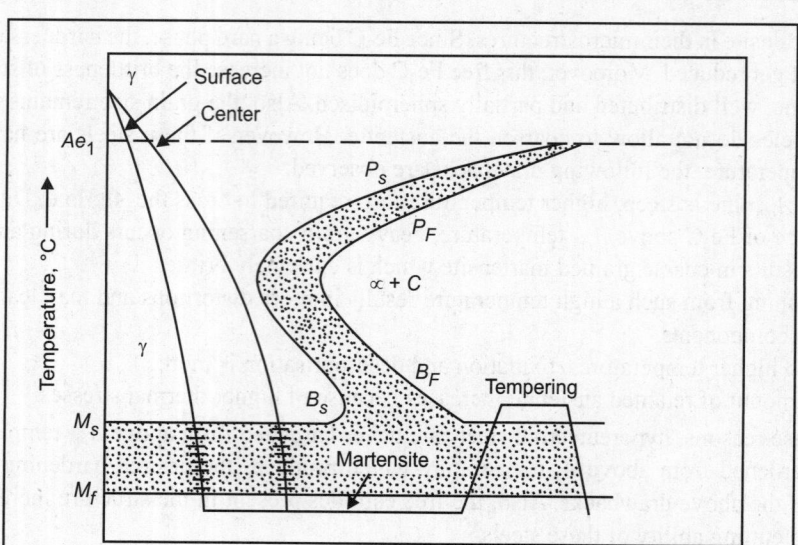

Fig. 5.33. Heat treatment cycle for conventional hardening process.

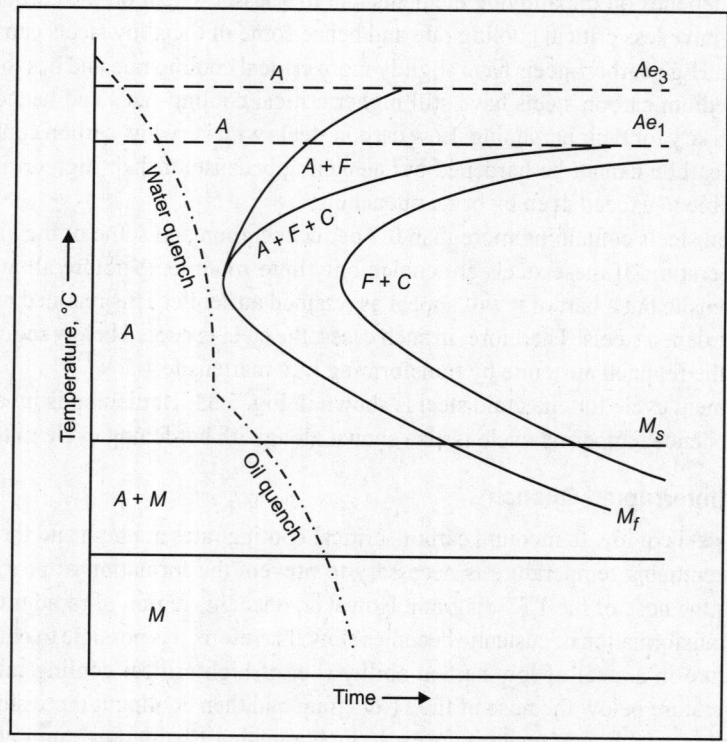

Fig. 5.34. Hardening cycle for the timed quench process.

Since the cooling rate between M_s and M_f is reduced, the cracking tendency also gets reduced and this becomes the chief advantage of the process. The process consists of heating the steel to the austenitisation temperature, quenching for a short period in cold water or brine to a temperature between the nose and M_s and then cooling in some other medium like oil to room temperature. Since the time of first quench is very small (0.1–0.3 sec.), it is very difficult to control the process to obtain consistent results.

For steels of slightly high hardenability (i.e. of slightly less critical cooling rate) like high carbon steels and low alloy steels, the initial; quench may be in oil with subsequent cooling in air. In such cases, the time of quench can be easily adjusted and the process becomes simpler to use.

Martempering (Marquenching)

In this process, the austenitised steel is cooled rapidly avoiding the nose of the IT diagram to a temperature between the nose and M_s, soaked at this temperature for a sufficient time for the equalisation of temperature but not long enough to permit the formation of banite and then cooled to room temperature in air or oil. The hardening cycle is shown in Fig. 5.35.

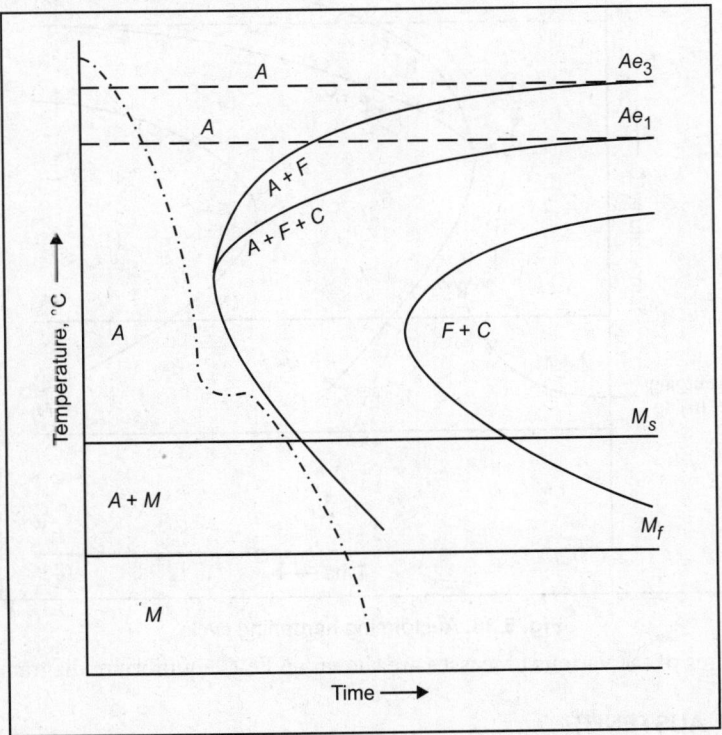

Fig. 5.35. Martempering hardening cycle.

Since the component has to be held for some time for equalisation of temperature, the process will be applicable to steels of slightly high hardenability such as high carbon steels and low alloy steels. The process produces martensitic structures with the following advantages:
1. It results in less distortions and warping, since the martensite formation occurs at the same time throughout the cross section of the component.
2. There is less possibility of quenching cracks appearing in the component.

This is a hardening process and therefore, the name martempering (an abbreviation for 'martensite tempering') is a misnomer for the treatment.

Ausforming

In this process, austenitised steel is cooled with a rate exceeding the critical cooling rate of that steel to a temperature between the nose and M_s, forged or rolled at this temperature and cooled to room temperature in oil. Due to the plastic deformation of austenite, the martensite formed is fine. Also this results is increased dislocation density in martensite and a finer distribution of carbides on tempering. Ausformed structures on tempering at low temperatures show better combination of TS and ductility. Steels with sufficient hardenability can only be ausformed. A typical ausforming cycle is shown in Fig. 5.36.

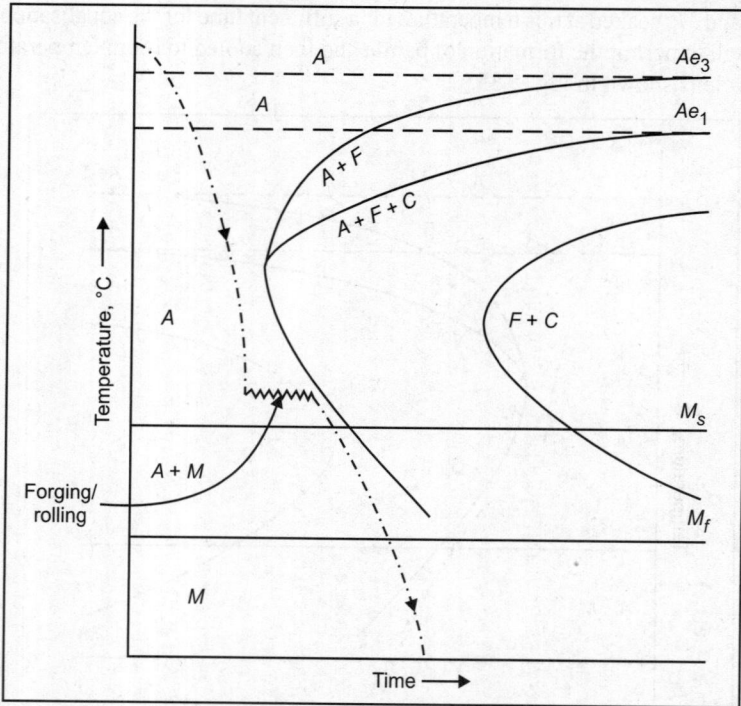

Fig. 5.36. Ausforming hardening cycle.

The temperatures of the various processes are shown on Fe-C equilibrium diagram in Fig. 5.37.

RETENTION OF AUSTENITE

Austenite to martensite transformation is temperature dependent and with decrease in temperature, some additional martensite forms characteristic of that temperature. However, the transformation never goes to completion, i.e. 100 per cent by cooling to any temperature.

The progress of martensitic transformation occurs as below:

    As the steel is cooled to some temperature below M_s, a certain amount of martensite forms in the austenite. Formation of martensite is accompanied by volume expansion which develops high compressive stresses in the austenite, opposing its further transformation to martensite, i.e. at any given temperature an apparent equilibrium is reached when a definite proportion of martensite has formed. When the steel is cooled to some lower temperature, both the phases will contract, but the volume contraction of martensite is greater than that of austenite. Due to this, the intensity of compressive stresses in austenite gets reduced and the equilibrium is upset Hence, some additional austenite transforms until the stress is again sufficient to develop equilibrium. Thus sequence of transformation continues and with each decrement of temperature an increment of austenite transforms to martensite till M_f temperature is reached. Below M_f, some small amount of austenite (less than 1 per cent) remains in the steel in a highly compressed condition without undergoing transformation to martensite and hence for all practical purposes, it is assumed that the transformation is complete at M_f, where the martensite is about 99 per cent.

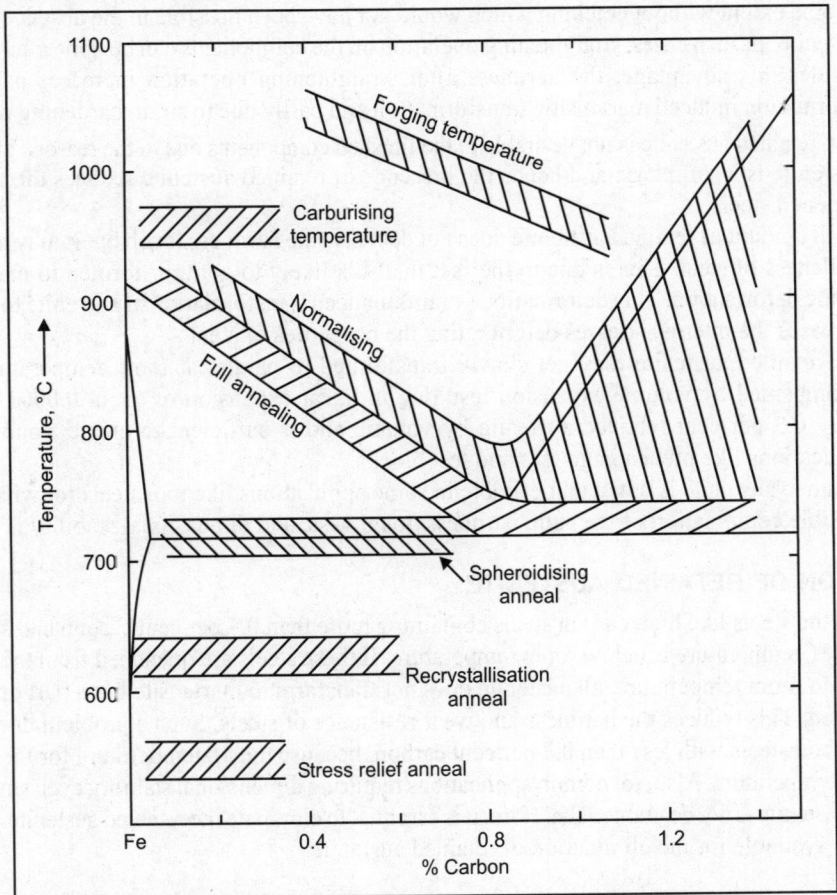

Fig. 5.37. The heating temperatures for various processes.

The amount of retained austenite varies from surface to centre in a hardened steel component. It is less at or near the surface and more in the centre. This is due to the fact that the surface cools first and there is a minimum of restraint on the expansion accompanying martensite formation at the surface. This reduces retained austenite at the surface. The centre is subjected to more restraint and hence shows more retained austenite.

The amount of retained austenite also depends on the quenching temperature. Higher the quenching temperature, more is the difference in temperature at the surface and centre of a component. The greater the temperature difference, higher will be the thermal stresses developed and higher will be the opposition for martensitic transformation resulting in higher proportion of retained austenite.

EFFECTS OF RETAINED AUSTENITE

The retained austenite in hardened steels has some advantages as below:
1. Austenite reduces the tendency of cracking during hardening and hence about 10 per cent retained austenite is desirable for this purpose.
2. If the amount of retained austenite is more such as 30–40 per cent, the steel can be cold worked to some extent without cracking which would not have been possible in the absence of retained austenite. In such cases, straightening operation on the components can be done after hardening. Besides this advantage, the hardness after straightening operation increases partly due to deformation induced martensitic transformation and partly due to strain hardening of austenite.

However, retained austenite is not desirable in the finished components due to the reasons given below:
1. Austenite is a soft phase and hence the presence of retained austenite reduces the hardness of hardened steels.
2. Small amount of retained austenite does not decrease the hardness much but it may increase the brittleness of steel. This is due to the fact that it is likely to get transformed to martensite by plastic deformation. This deformation (strain) induced transformation of austenite to martensite increases the internal stresses deteriorating the properties of steel.
3. The retained austenite may get slowly transformed to bainite at room temperature. This is accompanied by volume expansion resulting in linear expansion of about 0.0001 cm/cm for every 0.3 per cent retained austenite by volume and is sufficient to create trouble in some applications like precision gauges and test blocks.
4. Retained austenite is not at all desirable in some applications like tool steels for which the best possible combination of strength, hardness, toughness, and dimensional stability is essential.

ELIMINATION OF RETAINED AUSTENITE

For some of the steels like high carbon steels containing more than 0.7 per cent carbon and some of the alloy steels, M_f temperature is below room temperature. If these steels are quenched from the hardening temperature to room temperature, all austenite does not transform to martensite but a part of it remains untransformed. This reduces the hardness and wear resistance of steels. Such a problem does not arise for plain carbon steels with less than 0.7 per cent carbon, because the M_f temperature for these steels is above room temperature. Also, for certain applications requiring dimensional stability even small amount of retained austenite is not desirable. Therefore, it is essential to eliminate the retained austenite. Following methods are available for the elimination of retained austenite.

Cold Treatment (Subzero Treatment)

The steel components are cooled to a temperature below M_f by using a suitable medium from the following:

	Minimum temperature that can be obtained, °C
Ice + salt (sodium chloride)	23
Ice + calcium chloride	55

Acetone + dry ice (Frozen CO_2)	76
Liquid air	183
Liquid nitrogen	196
Liquid hydrogen	253
Liquid helium	269

Due to this, the retained austenite gets transformed to martensite. If the quenched steel is held at room temperature for some time before cooling, less austenite is transformed to martensite, i.e. the austenite gets stabilised.

Therefore, the subzero treatment should be done immediately after hardening. This treatment can be used to eliminate retained austenite from hardened components like tool and die steels. Some of the tool steels with almost negligible amount of retained austenite at room temperature have shown a sharp improvement in their performance due to their gradual cooling to around –200°C or below. This is likely to be due to the change in their stress distribution pattern.

Since there is some danger of cracking of hardened steel components when cooled to subzero temperatures, they are usually tempered at 150°–175°C before subjecting them to cold treatment.

Plastic Deformation

Plastic deformation of austenite can induce martensitic transformation. This phenomenon is called deformation (strain) induced martensitic transformation. If austenite is plastically deformed at a temperature somewhat above M_s, martensite formation starts. This temperature is denoted as M_d. M_d is the temperature at which deformation induced martensitic transformation starts. This method is applicable to steels containing large amounts of retained austenite like low and medium carbon high alloy steels in which the martensite formed is not so hard and brittle. This cannot be used for high carbon steels like tool steels because the martensite formed in these steels is hard and brittle and therefore, the extent of deformation possible in advance of fracture is not enough to transform a significant proportion of austenite to martensite.

TEMPERING

Tempering consists of heating the hardened steels to some temperature below A_1 and then cooling to room temperature. This eliminates retained austenite from the steel. The method is applicable to all steels with small as well as large amount of retained austenite. Since tempering involves many other effects, it is described below separately in detail.

Purpose

1. To relieve the internal stresses developed due to rapid cooling of steels during hardening process (i.e. austenite to martensite transformation) and due to volume changes occurring in the above transformation, to reduce brittleness.
   The high internal stresses produced due to hardening are likely to cause cracking of components if tempering operation is delayed. Therefore, tempering should be immediately done after hardening. Also, the components should not be ground before tempering because hardened and untempered components are extremely liable to stress cracking during grinding.
2. To reduce hardness, and to increase ductility and toughness. This is necessary to adjust the properties of the component according to the service requirements.
3. To eliminate retained austenite.

Process

The process consists of heating the hardened components to a temperature between 100° and 700°C [below A_1], holding at this temperature for specific period (1–2 hours), and cooling to room temperature, usually in air. After hardening heat treatment, steel contains martensite and retained austenite. In some of the steels like hypereutectoid steels and alloy steels, carbides are also present. Martensite and austenite are not stable phases and try to transform to more stable phases during heating. Depending on the transformation behaviour, tempering is classified in the following types:
1. Low temperature tempering (100°–200°C).
2. Medium temperature tempering (200°–500°C).
3. High temperature tempering [500°–700°C (below A_1)].

Low temperature tempering

During low temperature tempering, martensite decomposes and gives low carbon martensite (tempered martensite) and transition carbide called ε-carbide ($Fe_{2.4}C$).

$$\text{Martensite} \rightarrow \text{low carbon martensite} + \text{ε-carbide}$$

This decomposition is almost complete at 200°C. Due to the separation of ε-carbide, the structure etches rapidly and appears dark with the common etching reagents used for steels like nital and picral. Since the structure is unresolvably fine, it was identified as dark etching martensite in the old days. There is no appreciable change in the retained austenite.

Due to the above change in structure the hardness may slightly increase but the effect is insignificant for plain carbon steels. The brittleness of steel decreases due to sharp decrease in the internal stresses.

Medium temperature tempering

Due to heating in this temperature range, cementite is formed and a very fine distribution of cementite particles is observed in the matrix of ferrite as below:
1. The retained austenite may get transformed to bainite or decompose and form carbides and martensite. This transformation of austenite to martensite is due to increase in M_s temperature because of decrease in carbon content of austenite. This freshly formed martensite also decomposes.
2. The low carbon martensite and ε-carbide transform to ferrite and cementite. The particles of Fe_3C are very fine and cannot be resolved by optical microscopes.

These changes in microstructure result in decrease of hardness with increasing tempering temperature. The decrease in hardness is gradual upto 350°C and rapid thereafter, reaching to almost a minimum value at about 500°C. These changes are accompanied by simultaneous increase in toughness and ductility.

High temperature tempering

During this stage of tempering, cementite particles become coarse. Except this, there is no other change in the structure. When the particles are resolvable by optical microscope, they appear to be spheroidal in shape and the structure is called as spheroidite.

When the particles are sufficiently fine which hardly can be resolved, the structure is called as sorbite. Except these two, all other structures are called as tempered martensites.

Coarsening of particles results in a slight decrease in hardness and toughness. Since the coarsening rate is very less, the decrease in properties with time is also very less. Spheroidised structures can be machined with high speeds because of their excellent machinability. Some of the steels which are difficult to machine like high carbon steels and few of the alloy steels can be machined easily after spheroidising. The overall phase changes during hardening and tempering are shown in Fig. 5.38.

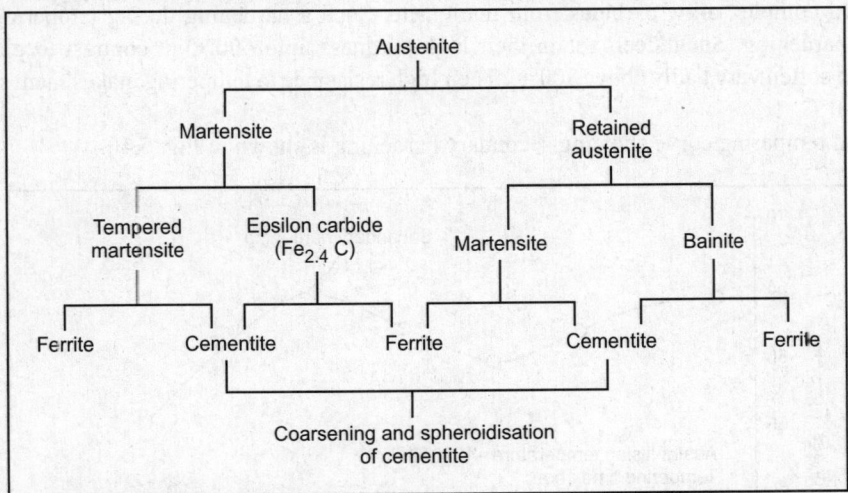

Fig. 5.38. Phase changes during hardening and tempering.

The variation of properties with tempering temperature are shown in Fig. 5.39.

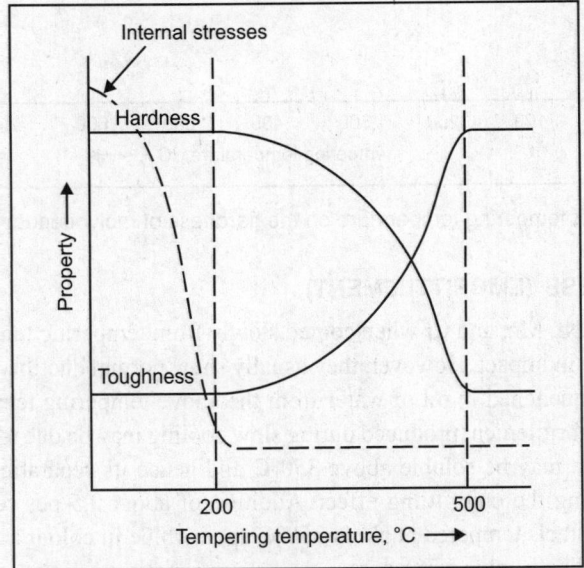

Fig. 5.39. Schematic representation of variation in properties with tempering temperature.

Auto tempering

Low carbon steels have a high M_s temperature and therefore, some tempering of martensite often occurs during its formation from M_s to M_f. This tempering is called auto tempering.

SECONDARY HARDENING

For alloy steels containing Cr, W, Mo, V, etc. hardness rises during tempering. This is due to the separation of very hard complex alloy carbides from martensite. Such a hardening during tempering is called secondary hardening. Such steels retain their high hardness upto 600°C in contrast to plain carbon steels which soften very badly above 300°C. Their high resistance to tempering makes them suitable for use upto 600°C.

A typical tempering curve showing secondary hardening is shown in Fig. 5.40.

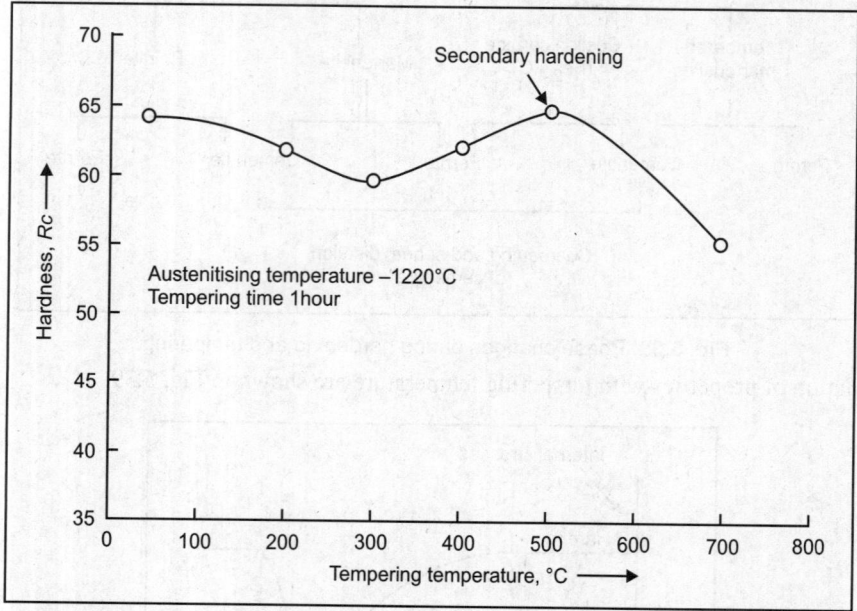

Fig. 5.40. Effect of tempering temperature on the hardness of molybdenum high speed steel.

TEMPER BRITTLENESS (EMBRITTLEMENT)

Alloy steels containing Ni, Mn, and Cr when cooled slowly from tempering temperature of about 350° or 550°C become brittle in impact. However, they usually show normal ductility in the standard tension test. If these steels are quenched in oil or water from the above tempering temperatures, they remain tough in impact. The embrittlement produced during slow cooling may be due to the separation of some brittle phase. This phase may be soluble above 350°C and hence its separation is suppressed during rapid cooling, eliminating the embrittling effect. Addition of about 0.5 per cent Mo also eliminates temper embrittlement. Steels tempered at about 350°C appear blue in colour and hence the brittleness observed at 350°C is called as blue brittleness.

QUENCH CRACKS

During quenching, surface of component cools rapidly and centre cools slowly; therefore, phases appearing at the surface and centre are likely, to be different. This results in non uniform volume changes. The overall effect of non uniform cooling and non uniform volume changes is to cause heavy distortions and cracking of the components. The cracking may result during quenching or sometimes after quenching, if tempering is delayed or in the early stages of tempering.

Quench cracks are liable to occur due to the following reasons:
1. Excessive amount of non metallic inclusions in steel.
2. Quenching from high temperature. Higher austenitising temperatures lead to grain coarsening of austenite resulting in coarse grained martensite which is more prone to cracking.
3. Improper selection of quenching medium. Quenching medium should just exceed the critical cooling rate. Use of mediums which give higher cooling rate than the one necessary may lead to cracking, e.g. if oil exceeds the critical cooling rate, use of water and brine may lead to cracking of the components.
4. Improper selection of the steel.
5. Improper design of key ways, holes, sharp changes in cross-section, mass distribution and non uniform sections.
6. Improper entry of the component into the quenching medium with respect to the shape of the component. This leads to nonuniform and eccentric cooling.
7. Time delays between hardening and tempering operations.

OTHER HEAT TREATMENTS

1. **Austempering:** Austempering consists of cooling the austenitised steel with a rate exceeding the critical cooling rate in a molten bath held at some constant temperature between the nose of TTT diagram and M_s temperature, i.e. in the bainitic region, holding at this temperature for a sufficient period for the completion of bainitic transformation and cooling to room temperature at any desired rate (Fig. 5.41).

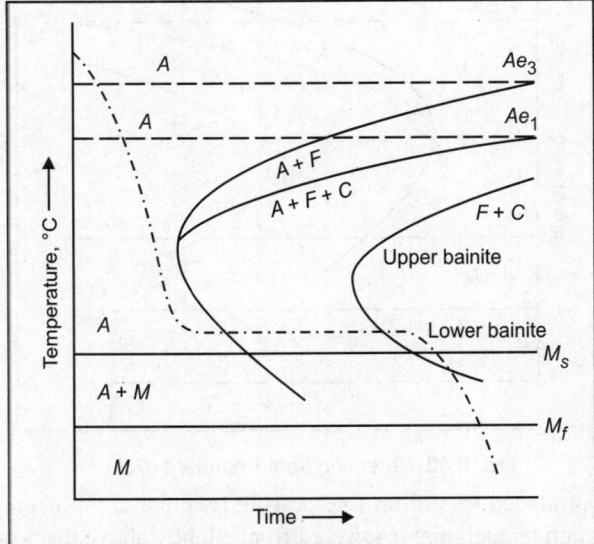

Fig. 5.41. Austempering cycle for a hypoeutectoid steel of reasonably high hardenability.

Depending on the temperature of transformation the product may be upper bainite or lower bainite. Properties of bainite are intermediate to those of martensite and pearlite and are very much similar to that of tempered martensite.

The most important advantage of austempering is that it produces structures and properties very much similar to tempered martensites without involving in martensitic transformation. Also, the dimensional stability of components is more due to the absence of retained austenite because the austenite to bainite transformation proceeds to 100 per cent in contrast to austenite to martensite transformation which never proceeds to 100 per cent. However, it has some definite disadvantages as compared to hardening and tempering process, which are as below:

1. The hardness produced is not so high as that produced by martensitic transformation. Also, wide range of property variation can be achieved by variation of tempering temperature which is not possible by this process.
2. Since the critical cooling rate has to be exceeded during cooling, the process is applicable only to slightly high hardenability steels.
3. The holding times are long and hence the process is expensive.

Patenting

The process is very much similar to austempering except in the range of temperature used for the isothermal transformation. It consists of quenching an austenitised steel in a molten bath maintained at some constant temperature slightly above or below the nose of TTT, diagram, holding at this temperature until the transformation is complete, and cooling to room temperature at any desired rate (Fig. 5.42).

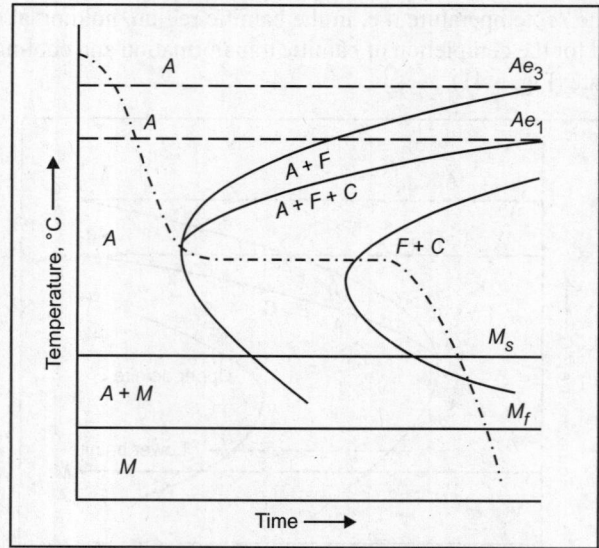

Fig. 5.42. Patenting heat treatment cycle.

The microstructures produced vary from fine pearlite (without any proeutectoid ferrite) to upper bainite as the transformation temperature is lowered from/slightly above the nose to below the nose of TTT diagram.

This process is chiefly used in wire drawing industry because the microstructures produced have good toughness to resist the severe stresses encountered during the wire drawing operation. With these structures the wire can be drawn to a reduction of area upto 90 per cent without intermediate heat treatment which is not possible with the annealed structures. It is chiefly used for plain carbon steels with carbon between 0.3 to 0.6 per cent and is equally applicable to alloy steels.

Isoforming

Austenite is worked, i.e. rolled or forged at the isothermal transformation temperature in the pearlitic region till the transformation of austenite to pearlite is complete. This results in refinement of structure with improvement in the fracture toughness. A typical heat treatment cycle is shown in Fig. 5.43.

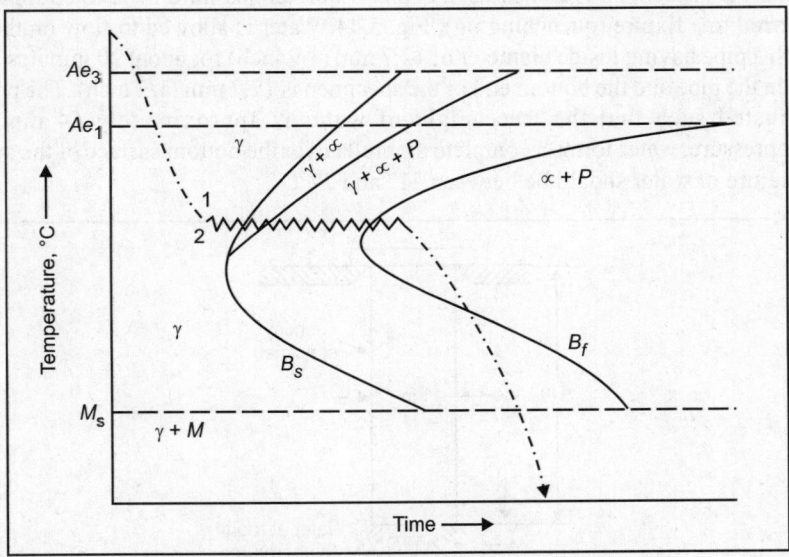

Fig. 5.43. Isoforming heat treatment cycle.

HARDENABILITY OF STEEL

Maximum Hardness

Maximum hardness in steels is obtained by producing a fully martensitic structure. This can be done by austenitising the steel and then quenching it. During the austenitising treatment all of the carbides dissolve and the ferrite transforms into austenite. Quenching this structure causes the austenite to transform via a shear mechanism into martensite. This transformation is so fast (Martensite needles grow at close to the speed of sound) that there is no time to the carbon to diffuse out of the martensite grains or to form carbide phases. The martensite, supersaturated with carbon, is very hard and also very brittle.

Carbon, being a very effective solid solution strengthening agent, essentially determines the hardness of the martensite. Cases where a lesser degree of hardening can be attributed to the presence of other alloying elements, but these elements tend to also make it more difficult to obtain a fully martensitic microstructure. So while maximum hardness in a given steel is dependent on our ability to produce a fully martensitic microstructure, the hardness of the martensite is largely determined by its carbon content.

Hardenability

Hardenability is the ease with which a steel piece can be hardened by martensitic transformation or it is the depth of hardening produced under the given conditions of cooling. It is evaluated by determining

144 Physical Metallurgy

the minimum cooling rate to transform an austenitised steel to a structure that is predominately or entirely martensitic, or by determining the thickness of the largest steel section that can be converted to such a structure under the given conditions of cooling.

Hardenability is most commonly measured by the Jominy End Quench Test. In this test, the specimen dimensions and test conditions are standardised and are as below:

The specimen is of cylindrical shape with 25.4 mm (1.0 inch) diameter and approximately 102 mm (4.0 inch) in length and has a machined shoulder (or a fitted detachable collar ring) at one end. This specimen is austenitised at a constant temperature for a fixed time and quickly transferred to a fixture (quenching jig), Fig. 5.44. Water is allowed to flow on the bottom end through a pipe having inside diameter of 12.7 mm (1/2 inch) for about 20 minutes. The distance between the pipe and the bottom end of the specimen is 12.7 mm (1/2 inch). The pressure should be adjusted such that the free height of water is approximately 64 mm (2.5 inch). At this pressure, water forms a complete umbrella over the bottom surface of the specimen. The temperature of water should be between 21° and 27°C.

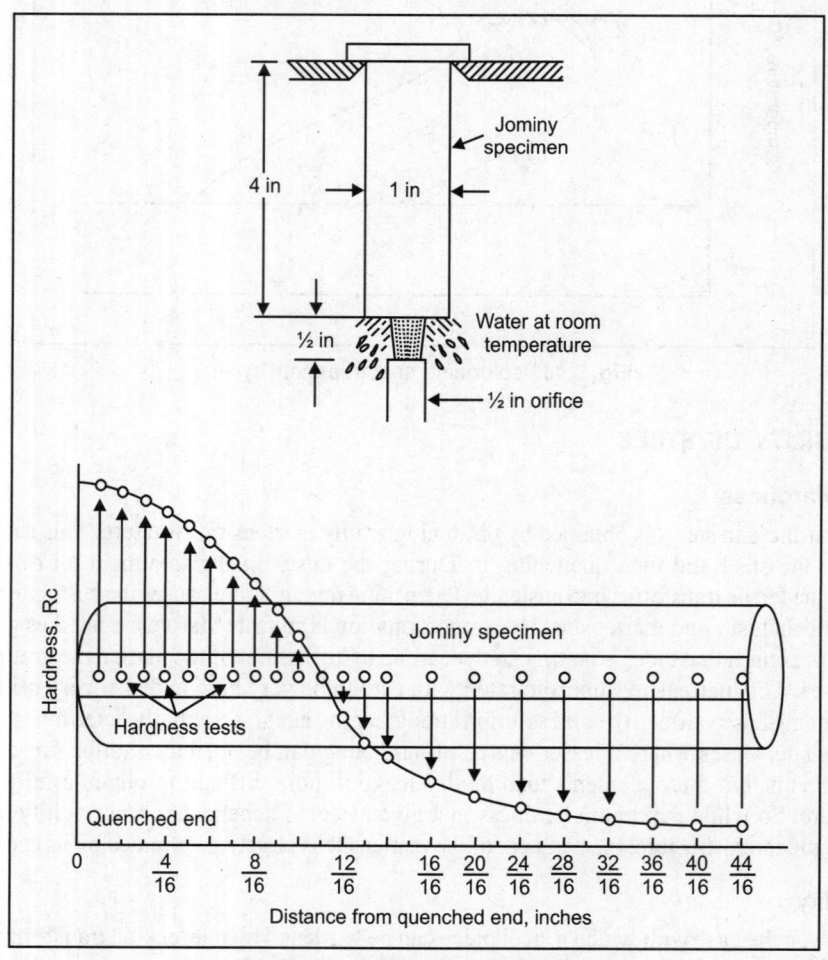

Fig. 5.44. Jominy end-quench test.

In order to form a fully martensitic structure the steel must be quenched at a rate that is equal to or greater than a critical cooling rate. If the quench is indeed fast enough and the part is thin then one can usually assume that this cooling rate can be achieved through the whole cross-section, producing a fully hardened part. However, this may not be the case for thick sections because the interior cools more slowly than the surface. But if one could modify this steel such that critical cooling rate is lower then thick pieces can be hardened throughout and even thicker pieces can be hardened to a considerable depth. This is of great practical importance not only in terms of our ability to produce a fully hardened part (which will also be fully brittle) but because subsequent tempering will be successful in producing the desired strength and ductility throughout the part. In addition, one could use less severe quenches to avoid problems with warping and cracking.

This ability of a steel to be hardened to a specified depth is called hardenability. In general, the hardenability of a steel is improved through alloying and all alloy additions except cobalt will improve the hardenability of a steel. Coarse grain size and homogeneity of the austenite also improve the hardenability. The reason this is so is not clear but is probably related to the retardation of nucleation and growth of the ferrite, carbide and bainite phases.

Jominy End-Quench

The most direct measure of the hardenability of a steel is the 'critical cooling rate'. Hardenability is also demonstrated in cases where large part fails to fully harden. One can measure this in terms of the depth of full hardening, the diameter of bar which will just harden to the center and the depth where the microstructure consists of 50 per cent martensite. A more convenient and very widely used method of measuring hardenability is the Jominy end-quench test. (Developed by Jominy and Boegehold in 1939, standardised in ASTM A255.) In this test a 1-inch diameter by 4-inches long bar is austenitised then quickly removed from the furnace and placed in a fixture where a jet of water of specified temperature and pressure impinges on one end of the specimen. Once cool, the specimen is removed, cleaned, a flat is ground along the length of the specimen and then is hardness tested every 0.0625 to 0.25 inches from the quenched end. The result is a plot of hardness versus distance from the quenched end. This curve is used to compare the hardenabilities of different steels.

Ideal Diameter

The ideal diameter D_I is another measure of the hardenability of steel. It is defined as the diameter of a bar which would contain 50 per cent martensite at its center following a quench in an ideal medium. Clearly, the larger the ideal diameter, the higher the hardenability of the steel. The ideal diameter of a plain carbon steel having a carbon content of 0.4 per cent (1040 steel) and whose ASTM grain size number is 7 is 0.215 inches. Naturally, varying the grain size or changing the concentration of alloying elements will change the ideal diameter. An empirical method of accounting for these effects utilises a series of multiplying factors:

$$D_I = D_{I,\,base} f_{Mn} f_{Si} f_S f_P f_{Cr} \ldots$$

where the base ideal diameter is a function of grain size and carbon content and the multiplying factors f_i are function of composition of element I. The ideal diameter for a 4340 steel (0.8 Cr, 1.75 Ni, 0.25 Mo) is over 6 inches.

The objective of this experiment is the measure the hardenability of several plain carbon and low alloy steels. The results will be used to explain the influence of alloy composition on the kinetics of martensite formation. They will also be compared to the calculated values of the ideal diameter.

Safety Considerations

This experiment involves heating several steel rods to as high as 875°C, quickly taking them out of the furnace and loading the hot specimens into a quenching fixture and then quenching the specimen. After this the specimens are ground flat along several sides and hardness tested along the length of the specimen. Extreme care should be exercised during the heat treating phase of the experiment as the temperatures are quite high and therefore pose severe burn hazards to personnel and fire hazards to the building. Grinding will be done by technicians in the machine shop so this will not be an issue during this experiment. Hardness testing, however, involves the use of a special fixture and a diamond brale indentor. One should be very careful when using this fixture and the brale indentor so that neither are damaged.

Chemical hazards

None. No chemicals are used and the specimens are 1-inch diameter rods made from conventional steels.

Physical hazards

1. The potential for very serious burns exists. Temperatures approaching 900°C are used during these experiments. At these temperatures one can easily be burned while loading and unloading specimens from the furnaces, even if the hot specimens and furnace are not touched. It will be important to wear heat resistant gloves and to use long tongs. One should also take care to prepare a clear area to work, have an emergency procedure in place in case hot specimens are dropped on the floor, etc. It would be a good idea to rehearse the procedures for handling hot specimens.
2. Hardness testing poses very little hazard if proper testing procedures are followed. Using the proper anvil and indentor and a clean specimen will minimise the chance of damaging the equipment or injuring personnel.

Biohazards

None.

Radiation hazards

None.

Protective equipment

1. Recommended: The use of safety glasses is recommended during the hardness testing phase of the experiment. The use of protective coverings for the floor and counter tops is also recommended.
2. Required: safety glasses, heat resistant gloves and long tongs for the heat treatment phases of the experiment.

Waste

Used specimens can be recycled as scrap steel.

Materials

The alloys used in this experiment are standard grades of the following steels: 1045, 4140, 4340 and 8620. Several have the same carbon content but have different concentrations of the other alloying elements. The specimens are standard Jominy specimens, 1 inch in diameter and 4 inches long with a flat washer pressed onto one end. (This washer can be removed after quenching.) On the end which has the washer a single letter which identifies the steel by composition has been stamped. During the austenitising treatment this stamp will probably be lost due to oxidation or carburisation. A more substantial marking should be used.

Procedure

Preliminary

Obtain a copy of ASTM A255 and read it. Consult the reference books and databases to find out what the ideal diameters for the steels being tested are. Calculate the ideal diameters and the Jominy curves for your steels. List the nominal compositions of each of the alloys. Mark, engrave or notch each specimen so that they can still be identified after having spent an hour or so in the furnace.

Prepare the Jominy quench tank

Set up the quench tank over a sink and connect a hose to the faucet. Place a specimen in the quench tank. Open the valve on the quench tank and, using the valve on the faucet, adjust the flow of water so that the height of the column of water is ½-inch above the bottom of the specimen. Close the valve on the quench tank but do not adjust the valve on the faucet.

Austenitising treatments

Preheat a furnace to 850°C and place the specimens in a container filled with graphite and place this in the furnace. Allow the specimens to soak at this temperature for one hour.

Prepare to quench the specimens

The purpose here is to prepare the work area for handling red-hot steel safely. Start by clearing a path between the furnace and the Jominy quench tank. Next, devise a plan for dealing with accidents such as dropping a hot specimen on the floor. Collect up gloves, tongs and safety equipment that will be used to move the specimens to the quench tank. Decide who will remove the specimen from the furnace and place it in the quenching fixture, who will assist in pushing the specimen through the hole in the quenching fixture (if necessary), who will turn on the water, who will monitor the time it took to start the quench, and who will execute the emergency procedures. Rehearse the procedure several times using a cold specimen.

Quench the specimens

Clear a path between the furnace and Jominy quench tank. Quickly but carefully remove a specimen from the furnace and place it in the quenching fixture and immediately turn on the water using the valve on the quench tank. Continue the quench until the specimen is cool enough to handle using bare hands. Remove the specimen from the fixture and engrave or paint an ID code on it.

Hardness test of the specimens

Clean the specimens and grind a flat surface 0.015 inches deep along four sides (90° apart) of the specimen. This will have to be done in the machine shop. Set up a Rockwell-type hardness tester for measuring hardness values on the C scale. Hardness test a couple of test blocks to make sure everything is working properly. Install the Jominy hardness testing fixture.

Take a hardness reading every 1/16 inch from the quenched end of the specimen. After the first ½ inch increase this interval to c inches and after the first full inch increase the interval to ¼ inches. Repeat this procedure for each of the flats on the specimen and then plot each of the four sets of results on a single graph.

Analysis

1. Compare the results (maximum hardness and the hardenability curves) with published data.
2. Compare the results with the calculated Jominy curves and ideal diameters.
3. Compare the maximum hardnesses obtained for the four alloys.
4. Compare the Jominy curves to the ideal diameters.
5. Discuss the differences in the hardenabilities of the four alloys. You can use depth to obtain a specified hardness value or the inflection point on the curves as your basis for comparison.
6. Discuss the results in terms of composition and the TTT curves.

Case Hardening

Case hardening or surface hardening is the process of hardening the surface of a metal, often a low carbon steel, by infusing elements into the material's surface, forming a thin layer of a harder alloy. Case hardening is usually done after the part in question has been formed into its final shape, but can also be done to increase the hardening element content of bars to be used in a pattern welding or similar process. The term face hardening is also used to describe this technique, when discussing modern armour.

Carbon itself is solid at case-hardening temperatures and so is immobile. Transport to the surface of the steel was as gaseous carbon monoxide, generated by the breakdown of the carburising compound and the oxygen packed into the sealed box. This takes place with pure carbon, but unworkably slowly. Although oxygen is required for this process it's recirculated through the CO cycle and so can be carried out inside a sealed box.

The sealing is necessary to stop the CO either leaking out, or being oxidised to CO_2 by excess outside air. Adding an easily decomposed carbonate 'energiser' such as barium carbonate breaks down to $BaO + CO_2$ and this encourages the reaction:

$$C \text{ (from the donor)} + CO_2 \leftrightarrow 2CO$$

increasing the overall abundance of CO and the activity of the carburising compound. It's 'common knowledge' that case-hardening was done with bone, but this is misleading. Although bone was used, the main carbon donor was hoof and horn. Bone contains some carbonates, but is mainly calcium phosphate (as hydroxylapatite). This doesn't have the beneficial effect on encouraging CO production and it can also supply phosphorus as an impurity into the steel alloy.

Both carbon and alloy steels are suitable for case-hardening; typically mild steels are used, with low carbon content, usually less than 0.3 per cent. These mild steels are not normally hardenable due to the low quantity of carbon, so the surface of the steel is chemically altered to increase the hardenability. Case hardened steel is formed by diffusing carbon (carburisation), nitrogen (nitriding) and/or boron (boriding) into the outer layer of the steel at high temperature, and then heat treating the surface layer to the desired hardness.

The term case hardening is derived from the practicalities of the carburisation process itself, which is essentially the same as the ancient process. The steel work piece is placed inside a case packed tight with a carbon-based case hardening compound. This is collectively known as a carburising pack. The pack is put inside a hot furnace for a variable length of time. Time and temperature determines how deep into the surface the hardening extends. However, the depth of hardening is ultimately limited by the inability of carbon to diffuse deeply into solid steel, and a typical depth of surface hardening with this method is up to 1.5 mm. Other techniques are also used in modern carburising, such as heating in a carbon-rich atmosphere. Small items may be case hardened by repeated heating with a torch and quenching in a carbon rich medium, such as the commercial products Kasenit/Casenite or 'Cherry Red'. Older formulations of these compounds contain potentially toxic cyanide compounds, such as ferrocyanide compounds, while the more recent types such as Cherry Red do not.

Processes

Flame and induction hardening

Flame or induction hardening are processes in which the surface of the steel is heated to high temperatures (by direct application of a flame, or by induction heating) then cooled rapidly, generally using water; this creates a 'case' of martensite on the surface. A carbon content of 0.4–0.6 wt% C is needed for this type of hardening.

Typical uses are for the shackle of a lock, where the outer layer is hardened to be file resistant, and mechanical gears, where hard gear mesh surfaces are needed to maintain a long service life while toughness is required to maintain durability and resistance to catastrophic failure.

Carburising

Carburising is a process used to case harden steel with a carbon content between 0.1 and 0.3 wt% C. In this process steel is introduced to a carbon rich environment and elevated temperatures for a certain amount of time, and then quenched so that the carbon is locked in the structure; one of the simpler procedures is repeatedly to heat a part with an acetylene torch set with a fuel-rich flame and quench it in a carbon-rich fluid such as oil.

Carburisation is a diffusion-controlled process, so the longer the steel is held in the carbon-rich environment the greater the carbon penetration will be and the higher the carbon content. The carburised section will have a carbon content high enough that it can be hardened again through flame or induction hardening.

It's possible to carburise only a portion of a part, either by protecting the rest by a process such as copper plating, or by applying a carburising medium to only a section of the part.

The carbon can come from a solid, liquid or gaseous source; if it comes from a solid source the process is called pack carburising. Packing low carbon steel parts with a carbonaceous material and heating for some time diffuses carbon into the outer layers. A heating period of a few hours might form a high-carbon layer about one millimetre thick.

Liquid carburising involves placing parts in a bath of a molten carbon-containing material, often a metal cyanide; gas carburising involves placing the parts in a furnace maintained with a methane-rich interior.

Nitriding

Nitriding heats the steel part to 482°–621°C (900°–1150°F) in an atmosphere of ammonia gas and dissociated ammonia. The time the part spends in this environment dictates the depth of the case. The hardness is achieved by the formation of nitrides. Nitride forming elements must be present for this method to work; these elements include chromium, molybdenum, and aluminium. The advantage of this process is it causes little distortion, so the part can be case hardened after being quenched, tempered and machined.

Advantages of nitriding

1. Nitriding is carried out at ~550°C and the increase in hardness produced is due to the formation of inherently hard alloy nitrides. It does not require a hardening treatment as is required for carburised components. Therefore, the distortions are minimum. It can be applied to finish machine parts requiring close dimensional tolerances such as precision gears, boring bars, forming rolls for paper and rubber, forming dies, camshafts crankshafts, bushings, cylinder liners, etc.
2. Nitride precipitation is accompanied by expansion and therefore, nitriding leaves the surface layers of steel parts in high residual compression. This effectively reduces the notch sensitivity and sharply increases the fatigue life of components. Also, they have better corrosion resistance than the carburised and hardened components.
3. Because of non metallic nature of nitrides, nitrided surfaces have less coefficient of friction. They also have exceptionally high resistance to galling and seizing even under poorly lubricated conditions. Due to this, nitrided surfaces have excellent bearing properties.
4. Nitrided cases have higher hardness (1000–1200 VPN) than the carburised and hardened cases (maximum 830 VPN equivalent to Rc 65). Not only this, but also they maintain high hardness upto about 600°C where, most of the hardened steels temper rapidly and become soft.

Disadvantages of nitriding

1. Since alloy steels containing appreciable amount of one or more of the alloying elements listed above (i.e. Al, Cr, Mo, V, W, Mn and Ti) are suitable for nitriding, such steels are costly. These steels are sold in the market under the trade name Nitralloy.
2. Nitrided cases are relatively thin, usually less than 0.5 mm. A case depth between 0.25 to 0.50 mm can be obtained in a period of 24 to 72 hours at the usual temperature (~550°C) of nitriding.
3. The presence of white layer on the surface is necessary for the nitriding reactions and a very thin white layer (0.02100.06 mm) remains on the component surfaces when nitriding is complete. This white layers has to be removed by precision grinding or lapping which is difficult and expensive. (Alternatively, the white layer can be reduced or eliminated by reducing the nitrogen concentration in the medium at the end of nitriding process or the white layer can be converted into dark layer by heating the nitrided steel in some neutral atmosphere such as molecular nitrogen or nonoxidising salt bath. Nitrogen from white layer diffuses into the neutral atmosphere or nonoxidising salt bath and the white layer gets eliminated. Due to heating, nitrogen diffusion occurs from the nitrided layer to the outside converting the white layer into the dark layer.)
4. No heat treatment can be done after nitriding. Therefore, the core properties should be adjusted before the components are nitrided. Tempered martensite structures show best properties after nitriding. The tempering should be done at a temperature of at least 40°C higher than the intended nitriding temperature, so that the properties of core does not get affected during nitriding treatment. The surface of steel must be free from decarburisation and residual stresses for obtaining best performance of the nitrided case.

Cyaniding

Cyaniding is a case hardening process that is fast and efficient; it is mainly used on low carbon steels. The part is heated to 871°–954°C (1600°–1750°F) in a bath of sodium cyanide and then is quenched and rinsed, in water or oil, to remove any residual cyanide.

This process produces a thin, hard shell [between 0.254–0.762 mm (0.010 and 0.030 inches)] that is harder than the one produced by carburising, and can be completed in 20 to 30 minutes compared to several hours so the parts have less opportunity to become distorted. It is typically used on small parts such as bolts, nuts, screws and small gears. The major drawback of cyaniding is that cyanide salts are poisonous.

Carbonitriding

Carbonitriding is similar to cyaniding except a gaseous atmosphere of ammonia and hydrocarbons is used instead of sodium cyanide. If the part is to be quenched then the part is heated to 775°–885°C (1427°–1625°F); if not then the part is heated to 649°–788°C (1200°–1450°F).

It has been observed that the nitrided cases containing more carbon show better behaviour in service which indicates that carbon helps in increasing the service life of nitrided cases. In this process both carbon and nitrogen are diffused into the surface of steel. The source of carbon and nitrogen may be fused salt bath or a gaseous medium containing CH_4, C_2H_6, etc. (carburising gases) with 5–10 per cent ammonia. The temperature of the process is between A_1 and A_3 of the steel (i.e. between 750°–850°C), but usually is slightly above A_1. The phases present in steel at this temperature are ferrite and austenite. Nitrogen diffuses in ferrite and carbon diffuses in austenite. If temperature is lower, nitrogen diffusion is promoted and the process becomes similar to nitriding and if temperature is higher, carbon diffusion is promoted and the process approaches to that of carburising. Nitrogen absorption at the surface of steel retards carbon diffusion so much that, within an hour or so, further increase in case depth becomes extremely slow. Therefore, the treatment times for carbonitriding are usually less than one hour and correspondingly the case depths are also smaller (0.075 to 0.25 mm). To transform the carburised areas into fine martensite, the carbonitrided steel is always quenched from the carbonitriding temperature in oil or water. Nitrogen and carbon diffusion increases the hardenability of surface steel and hence in many cases oil quenching is sufficient to produce martensite. The components are generally not ground or lapped after carbonitriding because of very small case depth.

Best results from carbonitriding are obtained when the steel is of an alloy type suitable for nitriding. However, it does produce a superficial file-hard skin on plain carbon steels of less than 0.5 per cent carbon and alloy steels that cannot be effectively nitrided.

Depending on the medium used in this process, the process is called liquid carbonitriding or gas carbonitriding.

Liquid carbonitriding is very much similar to liquid nitriding and is done in a similar salt both containing higher amount of sodium cyanide (20–30 per cent). This is also called cyaniding (or cyanide hardening) because of the use of cyanide salt both. Cyaniding and liquid carburising are also almost similar processes with the following differences:

1. The salt bath used in cyaniding does not contain alkaline earth salts. However, these salts are present in liquid carburising bath.
2. Cyaniding is performed in a bath containing a higher percentage of sodium cyanide.
3. The case produced by cyaniding is higher in nitrogen and lower in carbon content whereas reverse is the case for liquid carburising.
4. Cyanided case depths are less (usually less than 0.25 mm thickness) while liquid carburising permits thick cases.

Gas carbonitriding is almost similar to gas nitriding or gas carburising. The gas used is a mixture of carburising and nitriding gases. In this treatment, the carbonitriding medium contains no cyanide.

However, it produces a case equivalent to that of cyaniding and hence it is often known as dry cyaniding, gas cyaniding, nitrocarburising, and ni-carbing.

In the methods of surface hardening discussed so far, the composition of surface was altered to increase its hardness and wear resistance with or without subsequent heat treatment. There are few other methods like flame hardening and induction hardening in which the hardness and wear resistance of surface is increased without altering the composition of steel. They are based on locally heating the hardenable steel (or cast iron) to a temperature in the austenitic region for the formation of austenite and quenching in some appropriate medium to produce martensite.

Ferritic nitrocarburising

Ferritic nitrocarburising diffuses mostly nitrogen and some carbon into the case of a workpiece below the critical temperature, approximately 650°C (1202°F). Under the critical temperature the workpiece's microstructure does not convert to an austenitic phase, but stays in the ferritic phase, which is why it is called ferritic nitrocarburisation.

Applications

Parts that are subject to high pressures and sharp impacts are still commonly case hardened. Examples include firing pins and rifle bolt faces or engine camshafts. In these cases, the surfaces requiring the hardness may be hardened selectively, leaving the bulk of the part in its original tough state.

Firearms were a common item case hardened in the past, as they required precision machining best done on low carbon alloys, yet needed the hardness and wear resistance of a higher carbon alloy. Many modern replicas of older firearms, particularly single action revolvers, are still made with case hardened frames, or with case colouring, which simulates the mottled pattern left by traditional charcoal and bone case hardening. Another common application of case hardening is on screws, particularly self-drilling screws. In order for the screws to be able to drill, cut and tap into other materials like steel, the drill point and the forming threads must be harder than the material(s) that it is drilling into. However, if the whole screw is uniformly hard, it will become very brittle and it will break easily. This is overcome by ensuring that only the case is hardened and the core remains relatively soft. For screws and fasteners, case hardening is less complicated as it is achieved by heating and quenching in the form of heat treatment. For theft prevention, lock shackles and chains are often case hardened to resist cutting, whilst remaining less brittle inside to resist impacts. As case hardened components are difficult to machine, they are generally shaped before hardening.

INDUCTION HARDENING

This process also increases surface hardness by heating and quenching a thin surface layer of hardenable steel or cast iron component. Here heating is done within thin layer of surface metal by using high frequency induced currents. The component, is heated by means of an inductor coil (heating coil) which consists of one or several turns of water-cooled copper tube. High frequency alternating currents flowing through the inductor generate alternating magnetic field. This electromagnetic field induces eddy currents of the same frequency in the surface layers which rapidly heat the surface of the component. Within a short period of 2 to 5 minutes, the temperature of surface layer comes, to above the upper critical temperature of that steel. The high frequency induced currents chiefly flow through the surface layer—a phenomenon known as skin effect. The layer through which these currents flow is inversely proportional to the square root of frequency of induced currents and hence, the depth of hardened layer can be controlled by controlling the frequency of supply voltage. The usual range of frequency is from 1000 Hz to 1,00,000 Hz and the hardened depths obtained are from 0.5 to 6 mm. After the necessary temperature is attained, the component is quenched by water spray usually without removing from the inductor coil. Due to very fast heating and no holding time, the austenitic grain size is very fine which results in fine grained martensite. Induction hardening is commonly followed by low temperature tempering at 160° to 200°C. Frequently a self tempering occurs because usually the component does not cool completely and the heat from centre flows to the surface to cause the tempering. To obtain optimum core properties, the component is suitably heat treated prior to induction hardening.

Steels with carbon between 0.4 to 0.5 per cent are most suitable for induction hardening. However, case carburised components can also be hardened. Some of the examples are crankshafts, camshafts, axles, gears, rolls of rolling mills, boring bars, brake drums, over head travelling crane wheels, etc.

Some of the advantages of the process are as below:
1. Fast heating and no holding time leads to increase in production rates.
2. No scaling and decarburisation.
3. Less distortion because of heating of only surface.
4. Easy control over the depth of hardening by control of frequency of supply voltage and/or time of holding.

The process has few drawbacks as below:
1. Irregular shaped parts are not suitable for induction hardening.
2. Because of high cost of induction hardening unit, the process is not economical for small scale production.

Chapter 6

Heat Treatment of Tool Steel

INTRODUCTION

Tool steel refers to a variety of carbon and alloy steels that are particularly well-suited to be made into tools. Their suitability comes from their distinctive hardness, resistance to abrasion, their ability to hold a cutting edge, and/or their resistance to deformation at elevated temperatures (red-hardness). Tool steel is generally used in a heat-treated state.

With a carbon content between 0.7 per cent and 1.5 per cent, tool steels are manufactured under carefully controlled conditions to produce the required quality. The manganese content is often kept low to minimise the possibility of cracking during water quenching. However, proper heat treating of these steels is important for adequate performance, and there are many suppliers who provide tooling blanks intended for oil quenching.

Tool steels are made to a number of grades for different applications. Choice of grade depends on, among other things, whether a keen cutting edge is necessary, as in stamping dies, or whether the tool has to withstand impact loading and service conditions encountered with such hand tools as axes, pickaxes, and quarrying implements. In general, the edge temperature under expected use is an important determinant of both composition and required heat treatment. The higher carbon grades are typically used for such applications as stamping dies, metal cutting tools, etc. Tool steels are also used for special applications like injection moulding because the resistance to abrasion is an important criterion for a mould that will be used to produce hundreds of thousands of parts.

AISI-SAE GRADES

The AISI-SAE grades of tool steel is the most common scale used to identify various grades of tool steel. Individual alloys within a grade are given a number; for example: A2, O1, etc. (Table 6.1).

Water-Hardening Grades

W-grade tool steel gets its name from its defining property of having to be water quenched. W-grade steel is essentially high carbon plain-carbon steel. This type of tool steel is the most commonly used tool steel because of its low cost compared to other tool steels. They work well for small parts and applications where high temperatures are not encountered; above 150°C (302°F) it begins to soften to a noticeable degree. Hardenability is low so W-grade tool steels must be quenched in water. These steels can attain high hardness (above HRC 60) and are rather brittle compared to other tool steels.

The toughness of W-grade tool steels are increased by alloying with manganese, silicon and molybdenum. Up to 0.20 per cent of vanadium is used to retain fine grain sizes during heat treating.

Table 6.1. AISI-SAE tool steel grades.

Defining property	AISI-SAE grade	Significant characteristics
Water-hardening	W	
Cold-working	O	Oil-hardening
	A	Air-hardening; medium alloy
	D	High carbon; high chromium
Shock resisting	S	
High speed	T	Tungsten base
	M	Molybdenum base
Hot-working	H	H1–H19: chromium base
		H20–H39: tungsten base
		H40–H59: molybdenum base
Plastic mould	P	
Special purpose	L	Low alloy
	F	Carbon tungsten

Typical applications for various carbon compositions are:
1. 0.60–0.75 per cent carbon: machine parts, chisels, setscrews; properties include medium hardness with good toughness and shock resistance.
2. 0.76–0.90 per cent carbon: forging dies, hammers, and sledges.
3. 0.91–1.10 per cent carbon: general purpose tooling applications that require a good balance of wear resistance and toughness, such as drills, cutters, and shear blades.
4. 1.11–1.30 per cent carbon: small drills, lathe tools, razor blades, and other light-duty applications where extreme hardness is required without great toughness.

Air-Hardening Grades

The first air hardening grade tool steel was mushet steel, which was known as air-hardening steel at the time. A2 and D2 are currently the most commonly used air hardening grade.

1.2767: ISO 1.2767, also known as DIN X 45 NiCrMo 4, AISI 6F7, and BS EN 20 B, is an air hardening tool steel with a primary alloying element of nickel. It possesses good toughness, stable grains, and is highly polishable. It is primarily used for dies in plastic injection moulding application that involve high stresses. Other applications include blanking dies, forging dies, and industrial blades.

Cold-Working Grades

Grade-O refers to oil hardening tool steels, while grade-A refers to air hardening tool steels. These tool steels are used on larger parts or parts that require minimal distortion during hardening. The use of oil quenching and air hardening helps reducing distortion as opposed to higher stress caused by quicker water quenching. More alloying elements are used in these steels, as compared to water-hardening grades. These alloys increase the steels' hardenability, and thus require a less severe quenching process. These steels are also less likely to crack and are often used to make knife blades.

D-grade tool steels contain between 10 per cent and 18 per cent chromium. These steels retain their hardness up to a temperature of 425°C (797°F). Common applications for these grade of tool steel is forging dies, die-casting, die blocks and drawing dies. Due to high chromium content, certain D-grade tool steel grades are often considered stainless or semi-stainless tool steels.

Composition

Here are composition for some of the most common cold-working tools, quantities of minor ingredients may vary slightly with manufacturer:

O-1 contains 0.90 per cent carbon, 1.0–1.4 per cent manganese, 0.50 per cent chromium, 0.50 per cent nickel, and 0.50 per cent tungsten. It is a very good cold work steel and also makes very good knives. It can be hardened to about 57–61 HRC.

A-2 steel contains 1.0 per cent carbon, 5.0 per cent chromium, and 1.0 per cent molybdenum.

D-2 steel contains 1.5 per cent carbon and 11.0–13.0 per cent chromium; additionally it is composed of 0.45 per cent manganese, 0.030 per cent max phosphorus, 0.030 per cent max sulphur, 1.0 per cent vanadium, 0.7 per cent molybdenum, and 0.30 per cent silicon. D2 is very wear resistant but not as tough as lower alloyed steels. It is widely used for shear blades, planer blades and industrial cutting tools, sometimes used for knives.

Shock Resisting Grades

S-grade tool steel are designed to resist shock at both low and high temperatures. A low carbon content is required for the necessary toughness (approximately 0.5 per cent carbon). Carbide-forming alloys provide the necessary abrasion resistance, hardenability, and hot-working characteristics. This family of steels displays very high impact toughness and relatively low abrasion resistance, it can attain relatively high hardness (HRC 58/60). This type of steel is used in applications such as jackhammer bits.

High Speed Grades

T-grade and M-grade tool steels are used for cutting tools where strength and hardness must be retained at temperatures up to or exceeding 760°C (1400°F). M-grade tool steels were developed to reduce the amount of tungsten and chromium required.

T1 (also known as 18–4–1) is a common T-grade alloy. Its composition is 0.7 per cent carbon, 18 per cent tungsten, 4 per cent chromium, and 1 per cent vanadium. M2 is a common M-grade alloy.

Hot-Working Grades

H-grade tool steels were developed for strength and hardness during prolonged exposure to elevated temperatures. All of these tool steels use a substantial amount of carbide forming alloys. H1 to H19 are based on a chromium content of 5 per cent; H20 to H39 are based on a tungsten content of 9–18 per cent and a chromium content of 3–4 per cent; H40 to H59 are molybdenum based.

Special Purpose Grades

1. P-grade tool steel is short for plastic mould steels. They are designed to meet the requirements of zinc die casting and plastic injection moulding dies.
2. L-grade tool steel is short for low alloy special purpose tool steel. L6 is extremely tough.
3. F-grade tool steel is water hardened and substantially more wear resistant than W-grade tool steel.

Tool steel is normally delivered in the soft annealed condition. This is to make the material easy to machine with cutting tools and to give it a microstructure suitable for hardening.

The microstructure consists of a soft matrix in which carbides are embedded. In carbon steel, these carbides consist of iron carbide, while in the alloyed steel they are chromium (Cr), tungsten (W), molybdenum (Mo) or vanadium (V) carbides, depending on the composition of the steel. Carbides are compounds of carbon and these alloying elements and are characterised by very high hardness. A higher carbide content means higher resistance to wear.

In alloy steels, it is important that the carbides are evenly distributed. Other alloying elements are also used in tool steel, such as cobalt (Co) and nickel (Ni), but these do not form carbides. Cobalt is normally used to improve red hardness in high speed steels, nickel to improve through-hardening properties.

HARDENING AND TEMPERING

When a tool is hardened, many factors influence the result.

Theoretical Aspects

In soft annealed tool steel, most of the alloying elements are bound up with carbon in carbides. In addition to these there are the alloying elements cobalt and nickel, which do not form carbides but are instead dissolved in the matrix. When the steel is heated for hardening, the basic idea is to dissolve the carbides to such a degree that the matrix acquires an alloying content that gives the hardening effect— without becoming coarse grained and brittle. Note that the carbides are partially dissolved. This means that the matrix becomes alloyed with carbon and carbide-forming elements.

When the steel is heated to the hardening temperature (austenitizing temperature), the carbides are partially dissolved, and the matrix is also altered. It is transformed from ferrite to austenite. This means that the iron atoms change their position in the atomic lattice and make room for atoms of carbon and alloying elements. The carbon and alloying elements from the carbides are dissolved in the matrix.

If the steel is quenched sufficiently rapid in the hardening process, the carbon atoms do not have time to reposition themselves to allow the reforming of ferrite from austenite, i.e. as in annealing. Instead, they are fixed in positions where they really do not have enough room, and the result is high microstresses that can be defined as increased hardness. This hard structure is called martensite. Thus, martensite can be seen as a forced solution of carbon in ferrite (Fig. 6.1).

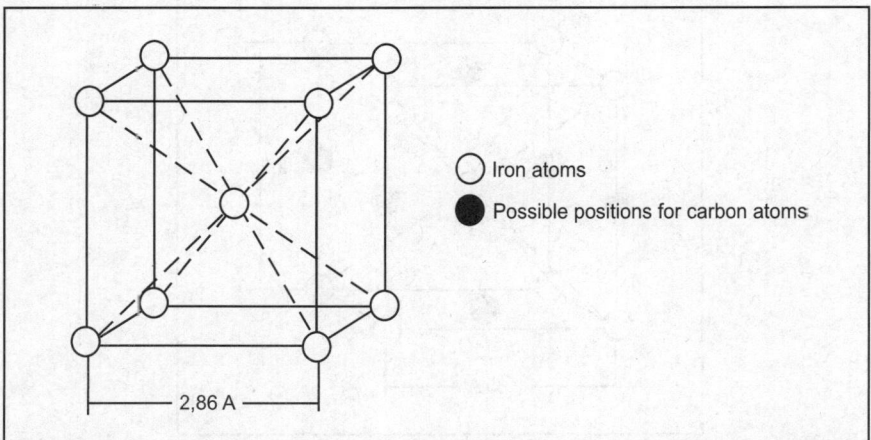

Fig. 6.1. Unit cell in a ferrite crystal body centred cubic (BCC).

When a steel is hardened, the matrix is not completely converted into martensite. Some austenite is always left and is called 'retained austenite'. The amount increases with increasing alloying content, higher hardening temperature and longer soaking times (Fig. 6.2).

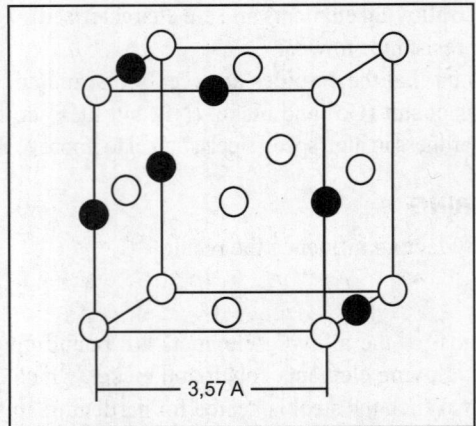

Fig. 6.2. Unit cell in an austenite crystal face centred cubic (FCC)

After quenching, the steel has a microstructure consisting of martensite, retained austenite and carbides. This structure contains inherent stresses that can easily cause cracking. But this can be prevented by reheating the steel to a certain temperature, reducing the stresses and transforming the retained austenite to an extent that depends upon the reheating temperature. This reheating after hardening is called tempering. Hardening of a tool steel should always be followed immediately by tempering.

It should be noted that tempering at low temperatures only affects the martensite, while tempering at high temperature also affects the retained austenite. After one tempering at high temperature, the microstructure consists of tempered martensite, newlyformed martensite, some retained austenite and carbides (Fig. 6.3).

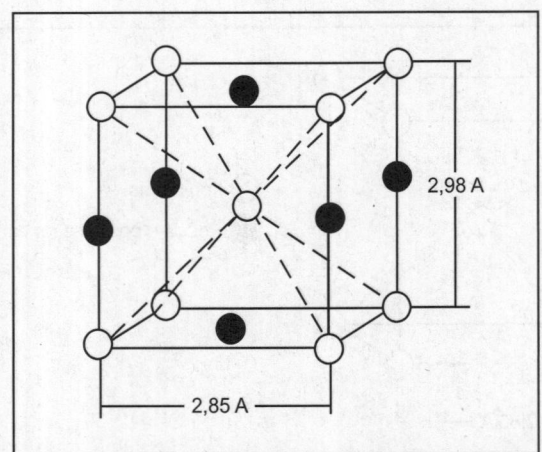

Fig. 6.3. Unit cell in a martensite crystal.

Precipitated secondary (newly formed) carbides and newly formed martensite can increase hardness during hightemperature tempering. Typical of this is the so-called secondary hardening of, e.g. high speed steel and high alloyed tool steels (Fig. 6.4).

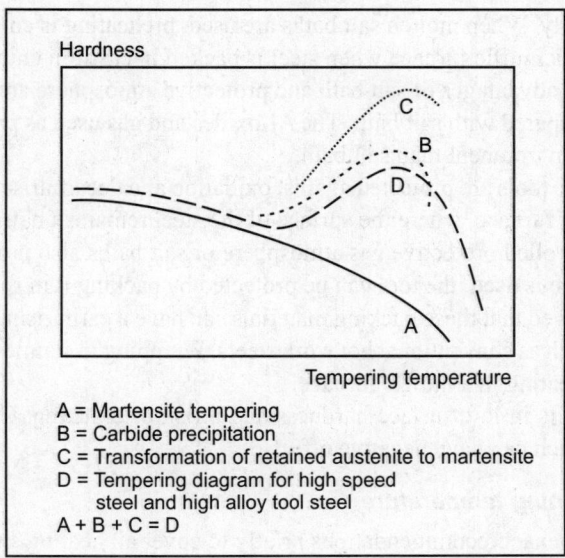

Fig. 6.4. The diagram shows the influence of different parameters on the secondary hardening.

Tool steel should always be double-tempered. The second tempering takes care of the newly formed martensite formed after the first tempering. Three tempers are recommended for high speed steel with a high carbon content.

How Hardening and Tempering is Done in Practice

Distortion due to hardening must be taken into consideration when a tool is rough-machined. Rough machining causes local heating and mechanical working of the steel, which gives rise to inherent stresses. This is not serious on a symmetrical part of simple design, but can be significant in asymmetrical machining, for example of one half of a die casting die. Here, stress relieving is always recommended.

Stress relieving

This treatment is done after rough machining and entails heating to 550°–650°C (1020°–1200°F). The material should be heated until it has achieved uniform temperature all the way through and then cooled slowly, for example in a furnace.

The idea behind stress relieving is that the yield strength of the material at the elevated temperature is so low that the material cannot resist the inherent stresses. The yield strength is exceeded and these stresses are released, resulting in a greater or lesser degree of distortion.

Correct work sequence is: rough machining, stress relieving and semifinish machining

The excuse that stress relieving takes too much time is hardly valid. Rectifying a part during semifinish machining of an annealed material is with few exceptions cheaper than making dimensional adjustments during finish machining of a hardened tool.

Heating to hardening temperature

The fundamental rule for heating to hardening temperature is that it should take place slowly. This minimises distortion. In vacuum furnaces and furnaces with controlled protective gas atmosphere, the heat is increased gradually. When molten salt baths are used, preheating is employed, whereas heating is automatically slow in a muffle furnace when steel is packed in castiron chips.

In a fluidised bed the advantages of salt bath and protective atmosphere are combined. Heating and cooling rates can be compared with salt bath. The Al-oxides and gas used as protective atmosphere are less detrimental to the environment than salt bath.

It is important that the tools are protected against oxidation and decarburisation. The best protection is provided by a vacuum furnace, where the surface of the steel remains unaffected.

Furnaces with a controlled protective gas atmosphere or salt baths also provide good protection. If an electric muffle furnace is used, the tool can be protected by packing it in spent charcoal or cast iron chips. It should be observed that these packing materials can have a carburising effect if the steels have a low carbon content, such as conventional hot work steels. Wrapping in stainless steel foil also provides good protection when heating in a muffle furnace.

Decarburisation results in low surface hardness and a risk of cracking. Carburisation results in a harder surface layer, which can have negative effects.

Holding time at hardening temperature

It is not possible to state exact recommendations briefly to cover all heating situations. Factors such as furnace type, furnace rating, temperature level, the weight of the charge in relation to the size of the furnace, etc. must be taken into consideration in each case.

We can, however, give one recommendation that is valid in virtually all situations:

> When the steel has reached hardening temperature through its entire thickness, hold at this temperature for 30 minutes. An exception to this rule is for thin parts heated in salt baths at high temperature, or high speed steel. Here the entire period of immersion is often only a few minutes.

Quenching

The choice between a fast and slow quenching rate is usually a compromise; to get the best microstructure and tool performance, the quenching rate should be rapid; to minimise distortion, a slow quenching rate is recommended.

Slow quenching results in less temperature difference between the surface and core of a part, and sections of different thickness will have a more uniform cooling rate.

This is of great importance when quenching through the martensite range, below the M_S temperature. Martensite formation leads to an increase in volume and stresses in the material. This is also the reason why quenching should be interrupted before room temperature has been reached, normally at 50°–70°C (120°–160°F).

However, if the quenching rate is too slow, especially with heavier cross-sections, undersirable transformations in the microstructure can take place, risking a poor tool performance.

Water is used as a quenching medium for unalloyed steels. 8–10 per cent sodium chloride (salt) or soda should be added to the water in order to achieve optimum cooling efficiency. Water hardening can often cause problems in the form of distortion and quench cracks.

Oil hardening is safer, but hardening in air or martempering is best of all. Oil should be used for low alloyed steels. The oil should be of good quality, and preferably of the rapid quenching type. It should be kept clean and must be changed after a certain period of use. Hardening oils should have a temperature of 50°–70°C (140°–160°F) to give the best cooling efficiency. Lower temperatures mean higher viscosity, i.e. the oil is thicker (Fig. 6.5).

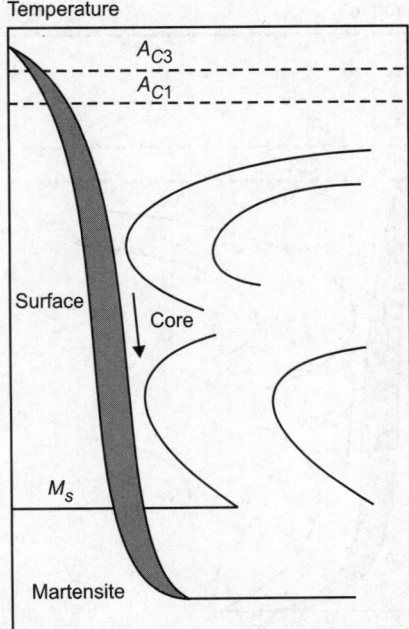

Fig. 6.5. The quenching process as expressed in a TTT graph.

Hardening in oil is not the safest way to quench steel, in view of the risks of distortion and hardening cracks. These risks can be reduced by means of martempering. In this process, the material is quenched in two steps. First it is cooled from hardening temperature in a salt bath whose temperature is just above the M_S temperature. It is kept there until the temperature has equalised between the surface and the core, after which the tool can be allowed to cool freely in air down through the martensite transformation range.

When martempering oil hardening steels, it should also be kept in mind that the material transforms relatively rapid and should not be kept too long at the martempering bath temperature. This can lead to excessive bainite transformation and the risk of low hardness.

High alloy steels can be hardened in oil, a martempering bath or air. The advantages and disadvantages of the different methods can be discussed.

Oil gives a good finish and high hardness, but it also maximises the risk of excessive distortion or cracking. In the case of thick parts, quenching in oil is often the only way to achieve maximum hardness.

Martempering in salt bath produces a good finish, high hardness and less risk of excessive distortion or cracking. For certain types of steel, the temperature of the salt bath is normally kept at about 500°C (930°F). This temperature ensures a relatively mild thermal shock, but a sufficient cooling rate to avoid phase transformations.

Full martensite transformation has, in many cases, time to occur when the steel is cooled in air from the martempering bath temperature. However, if the dimensions are big, it is often necessary to use a forced quenching rate depending of the hardenability of the steel.

Air quenching entails the least risk of excessive distortion. A tendency towards lower hardness is noticeable at greater thicknesses. One disadvantage is a poorer finish. Some oxidation takes place when the material comes into contact with air and cools slowly from the high hardening temperatures (Fig. 6.6).

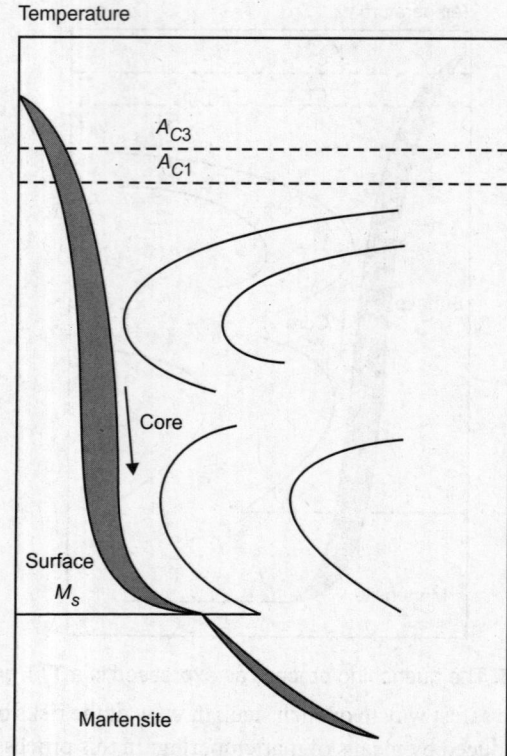

Fig. 6.6. Martempering.

The choice of quenching medium must be made from job to job, but a general recommendation could perhaps be made as shown in Fig. 6.7.

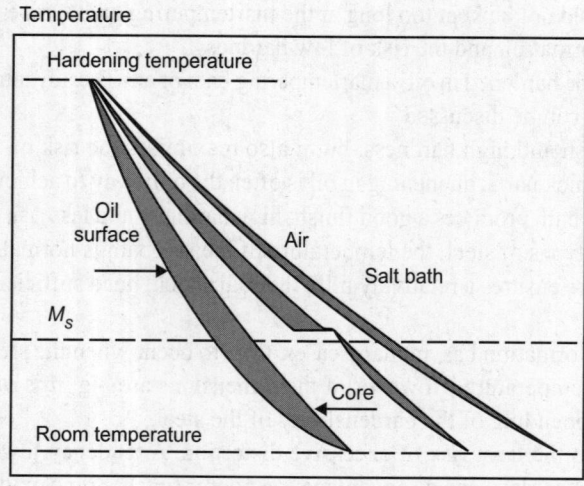

Fig. 6.7. Cooling rates for various media.

A martempering bath is the safest in most cases. Air is used when dimensional stability is crucial. Oil should be avoided and used only when it is necessary to achieve satisfactory hardness in heavy sections. Three well-known quenching methods have been mentioned here. Some new concepts have been introduced with modern types of furnaces, and the technique of quenching at a controlled rate in a protective gas atmosphere or in a vacuum furnace when gas is becoming increasingly widespread. The cooling rate is roughly the same as in air for protective gas atmosphere, but the problem of oxidised surfaces is eliminated.

Modern vacuum furnaces have the possibility to use overpressure during quenching which increases the quenching speed. The surfaces are completely clean after a vacuum hardening.

With these techniques, as with quenching in air, the risks of excessively slow cooling must be borne in mind, even for vacuum furnaces if no overpressure is used. The effect is that surface hardness is normally lower than expected. Hardness in the centre of heavy sections is even lower.

This effect can be critical with high speed steel and hot work steel, where a centre section can be cooled so slowly that carbide precipitation takes place on the way down. Here, the matrix becomes depleted of carbon and carbide forming alloying elements. The result is reduced hardness and strength of the core.

Tempering

The material should be tempered immediately after quenching. Quenching should be stopped at a temperature of 50°–70°C (120°–160°F) and tempering should be done at once. If this is not possible, the material must be kept warm, e.g. in a special 'hot cabinet', awaiting tempering.

The choice of tempering temperature is often determined by experience. However, certain guidelines can be drawn and the following factors can be taken into consideration:

1. Hardness.
2. Toughness.
3. Dimension change.

If maximum hardness is desired, temper at about 200°C (390°F), but never lower than 180°C (360°F). High speed steel is normally tempered at about 20°C (36°F) above the peak of the secondary hardening temperature.

If a lower hardness is desired, this means a higher tempering temperature. Reduced hardness does not always mean increased toughness. Avoid tempering within temperature ranges that reduce toughness. If dimensional stability is also an important consideration, the choice of tempering temperature must often be a compromise. If possible, however, priority should be given to toughness.

How many tempers are required?

Two tempers are recommended for tool steel and three are considered necessary for high speed steel with a high carbon content, e.g. over 1 per cent. Two tempers are always recommended. If the basic rule in quenching is followed—to interrupt at 50°–70°C (120°–160°F)—then a certain amount of austenite remains untransformed when the material is to be tempered. When the material cools after tempering, most of the austenite is transformed to martensite. It is untempered. A second tempering gives the material optimum toughness at the hardness in question.

The same line of reasoning can be applied with regard to retained austenite in high speed steel. In this case, however, the retained austenite is highly alloyed and slow transforming. During tempering, some diffusion takes place in the austenite, secondary carbides are precipitated, the austenite becomes lower alloyed and is more easily transformed to martensite when it cools after tempering. Here, several temperings can be beneficial in driving the transformation of the retained austenite further to martensite.

Holding times in connection with tempering

Here also, one should avoid all complicated formulae and rules of thumb, and adopt the following recommendation. After the tool is heated through, hold the material for at least 2 hrs at full temperature each time.

DIMENSIONAL AND SHAPE STABILITY

Distortion During the Hardening and Tempering of Tool Steel

When a piece of tool steel is hardened and tempered, some warpage or distortion normally occurs. This distortion is usually greater at high temperature.

This is well-known, and it is normal practice to leave some machining allowance on the tool prior to hardening. This makes it possible to adjust the tool to the correct dimensions after hardening and tempering by grinding, for example.

How does distortion take place?

The cause is stresses in the material. These stresses can be divided into:
 1. Machining stresses.
 2. Thermal stresses.
 3. Transformation stresses.

Machining stresses

This type of stress is generated during machining operations such as turning, milling and grinding. (For example, such stresses are formed to a greater extent during cold forming operations such as blanking, bending and drawing.) If stresses have built up in a part, they will be released during heating. Heating reduces strength, releasing stresses through local distortion. This can lead to overall distortion (Fig. 6.8).

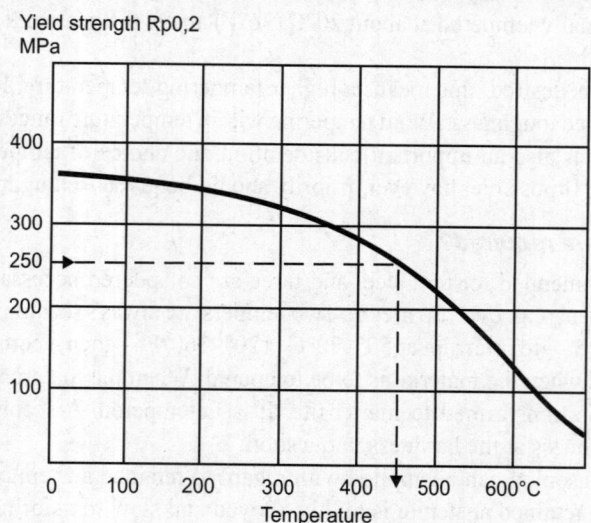

Fig. 6.8. Effect of temperature on the yield strength of Uddeholm Orvar 2 microdised, soft annealed.

In order to reduce this distortion while heating during the hardening process, a stress relieving operation can be carried out prior to the hardening operation. It is recommended that the material be stress relieved after rough machining. Any distorsion can then be adjusted during semifinish machining prior to the hardening operation.

Thermal stresses

These stresses are created when a piece is heated. They increase if heating takes place rapidly or unevenly. The volume of the steel is increased by heating. Uneven heating can result in local variations in volume growth, leading to stresses and distortion.

As an alternative with large or complex parts, heating can be done in preheating stages in order to equalise the temperature in the component (Fig. 6.9).

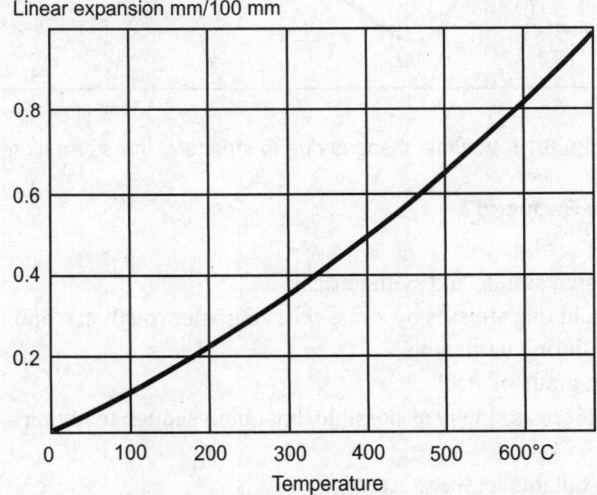

Fig. 6.9. Effect of temperature on the linear expansion of Uddeholm Orvar 2 microdised, soft annealed.

An attempt should always be made to heat slowly enough so that the temperature remains virtually equal throughout the piece.

What has been said regarding heating also applies to quenching. Very powerful stresses arise during quenching. As a general rule, the slower that quenching can be done, the less distortion will occur due to thermal stresses.

It is important that the quenching medium is applied as uniformly as possible. This is especially valid when forced air or protective gas atmosphere (as in vacuum furnaces) is used. Otherwise temperature differences in the tool can lead to significant distortion.

Transformation stresses

This type of stress arises when the microstructure of the steel is transformed. This is because the three microstructures in question — ferrite, austenite and martensite — have different densities, i.e. volumes.

The greatest effect is caused by transformation from austenite to martensite. This causes a volume increase. Excessively rapid and uneven quenching can also cause local martensite formation and thereby volume increases locally in a piece and give rise to stresses in this section. These stresses can lead to distortion and, in some cases, quenching cracks (Fig. 6.10).

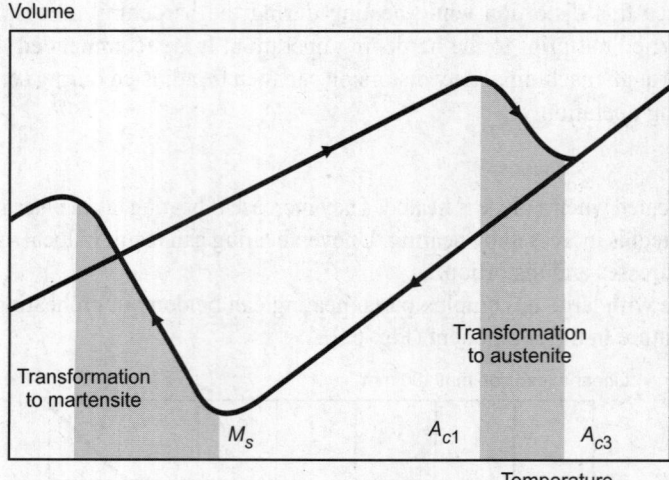

Fig. 6.10. Volume changes due to structural transformation.

How can Distortion be Reduced?

Distortion can be minimised by:
1. Keeping the design simple and symmetrical.
2. Eliminating machining stresses by stress relieving after rough machining.
3. Heating slowly during hardening.
4. Using a suitable grade of steel
5. Quenching the piece as slowly as possible, but quick enough to obtain a correct microstructure in the steel
6. Tempering at a suitable temperature.

Subzero Treatment

Tools requiring maximum dimensional stability in service can be subzero treated as follows:

Immediately after quenching, the tool should be subzero treated to −70° to −80°C (−95° to −110°F), soaking time 1–3 hrs, followed by tempering.

The subzero treatment leads to a reduction of retained austenite content. This, in turn, will result in a hardness increase of 1–2 HRC in comparison to not subzero treated tools if low temperature tempering is used. For high temperature tempered tools there will be little or no hardness increase and when referencing the normal tempering curves, a 25° to 50°C (45° to 90°F) lower tempering temperature should be chosen to achieve the required hardness.

Tools that are high temperature tempered, even without a subzero treatment, will normally have a low retained austenite content and in most cases, a sufficient dimensional stability. However, for high demands on dimensional stability in service it is also recommended to use a subzero treatment in combination with high temperature tempering.

For the highest requirements on dimensional stability, subzero treatment in liquid nitrogen is recommended after quenching and after each tempering.

SURFACE TREATMENT

Nitriding

The purpose of nitriding is to increase the surface hardness of the steel and improve its wear properties. This treatment takes place in a medium (gas or salt) which gives off nitrogen. During nitriding, nitrogen diffuses into the steel and forms hard, wear resistant nitrides. This results in an intermetallic surface layer with good wearing and frictional properties.

Nitriding is done in gas at about 510°C (950°F) and in salt or gas at about 570°C (1060°F) or as ion nitriding, normally at around 500°C (930°F). The process therefore requires steels that are resistant to tempering in order not to reduce the core strength.

Examples of applications

1. Nitriding is used in some cases on prehardened plastic moulds in order to prevent indentation and defects on the parting faces. It should be noted, however, that a nitrided surface cannot be machined with cutting tools and can only be ground with difficulty. A nitrided surface will cause problems in weld repairing as well. Nitriding can also have a stress relieving effect. Heavily machined parts may, therefore, undergo some distortion during nitriding due to the release of residual stresses from machining and in such a case, a stress relieving between rough and finish machining is recommended.
2. The life of forging dies can be increased by nitriding. It must be noted, though, that the treatment can give rise to higher susceptibility to cracking in sharp corners. Furthermore, the edge of the flash land must be given a rounded profile.
3. Extrusion dies of Uddeholm Orvar 2 Microdised can be nitrided to advantage — especially in the case of aluminium alloys. Exceptions can be profiles with sharp corners and thin sections of the dies.

Nitrocarburising

A widely known method is nitriding in a salt bath. The temperature is normally 570°C (1060°F). Due to aeration the cyanate content of the bath can be better controlled and the nitriding effect is very good. A nitrocarburising effect can also be achieved in gas atmosphere at 570°C (1060°F). The results after these methods are comparable.

The total nitriding time must be varied for different tool types and sizes. In the case of large sizes, the heating time to the specified nitriding temperature can be considerably longer than in the case of small tools.

Ion Nitriding

This is a new nitriding technology. The method can be summarised as follows:

The part to be nitrided is placed in a process chamber filled with gas, mainly nitrogen. The part forms the cathode and the shell of the chamber the anode in an electric circuit. When the circuit is closed, the gas is ionised and the part is subjected to ion bombardment. The gas serves both as heating and nitriding medium.

The advantages of ion nitriding include a low process temperature and a hard, tough surface layer. The depth of diffusion is of the same order as with gas nitriding.

Case Hardening

In this method, the steel is heated in a medium that gives off carbon (gas, salt or dry carburising compound). The carbon diffuses into the surface of the material and after hardening this gives a surface layer with enhanced hardness and wear resistance. This method is used for structural steel, but is not generally recommended for alloy tool steels.

Hard Chromium Plating

Hard chromium plating can improve the wear resistance and corrosion resistance of a tool. Hard chromium plating is done electrolytically. The thickness of the plating is normally between 0.001 and 0.1 mm (0.00004–0.004 inch). It can be difficult to obtain a uniform surface layer, especially on complex tools, since projecting corners and edges may receive a thicker deposit than large flat surfaces or the holes. If the chromium layer is damaged, the exposed steel may corrode rapidly.

Another advantage of the chromium layer is that it greatly reduces the coefficient of friction on the surface. During the chromium plating process, hydrogen absorption can cause a brittle surface layer. This nuisance can be eliminated by tempering immediately after plating at 180°C (360°F) for 4 hours.

Surface Coating

Surface coating of tool steel is becoming more common. Not only for cold work applications, but also for plastic moulds and hot work dies.

The hard coating normally consists of titanium nitride and/or titanium carbide. The very high hardness and low friction gives a very wear resistant surface, minimising the risk for adhesion and sticking.

To be able to use these properties in an optimal way one has to choose a tool steel of high quality or a powder metallurgy manufactured steel as substrate.

TESTING MECHANICAL PROPERTIES OF TOOL STEEL

When the steel is hardened and tempered, its strength is affected, so let us take a closer look at how these properties are measured.

Hardness Testing

Hardness testing is the most popular way to check the results of hardening. Hardness is usually the property that is specified when a tool is hardened.

It is easy to test hardness. The material is not destroyed and the apparatus is relatively inexpensive. The most common methods are Rockwell C (HRC), Vickers (HV) and Brinell (HBW). We shouldn't entirely forget the old expression 'file-hard'. In order to check whether hardness is satisfactory, for example above 60 HRC, a file of good quality can provide a good indication.

Rockwell (HRC)

In Rockwell hardness testing, a conical diamond is first pressed with a force F_0, and then with a force $F_0 + F_1$ against a specimen of the material whose hardness is to be determined. After unloading to F_0, the increase (e) of the depth of the impression caused by F_1 is determined. The depth of penetration (e) is converted into a hardness number (HRC) which is read directly from a scale on the tester dial or read-out (Fig. 6.11).

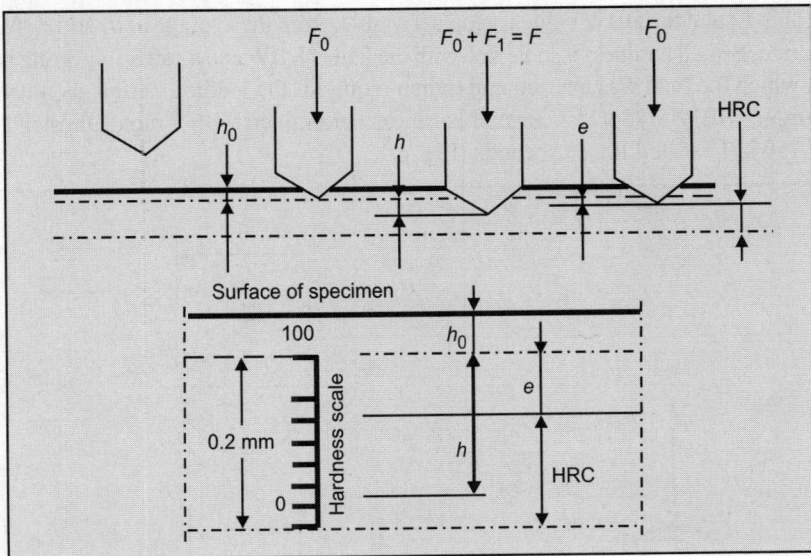

Fig. 6.11. Principle of Rockwell hardness testing.

Vickers (HV)

In Vickers hardness testing a pyramidshaped diamond with a square base and a peak angle of 136° is pressed under a load F against the material whose hardness is to be determined. After unloading, the diagonals d_1 and d_2 of the impression are measured and the hardness number (HV) is read off a table.

When the test results are reported, Vickers hardness is indicated with the letters HV and a suffix indicating the mass that exerted the load and (when required) the loading period, as illustrated by the following example: HV 30/20 = Vickers hardness determined with a load of 30 kgf exerted for 20 seconds (Fig. 6.12).

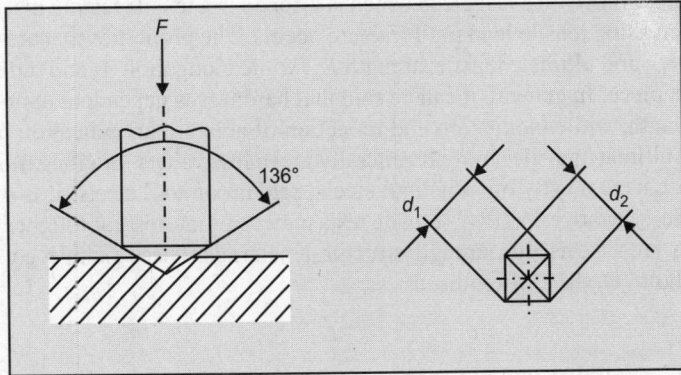

Fig. 6.12. Principle of Vickers hardness testing.

Brinell (HBW)

In Brinell hardness testing, a Tungsten (W) ball is pressed against the material whose hardness is to be determined. After unloading, two measurements of the diameter of the impression are taken at 90° to each other (d_1 and d_2) and the HBW value is read off a table, from the average of d_1 and d_2. When the test results are reported, Brinell hardness is indicated with the letters HBW and a suffix indicating ball diameter, the mass with which the load was exerted and (when required) the loading period, as illustrated by the following example: HBW 5/750/15 = Brinell hardness determined with 5 mm Tungsten (W) ball and under load of 750 kgf exerted for 15 seconds (Fig. 6.13).

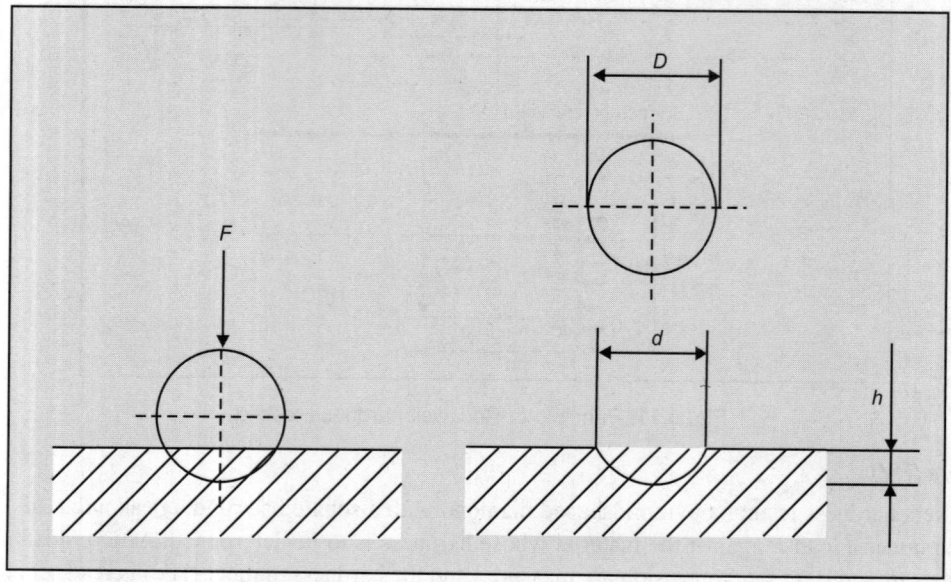

Fig. 6.13. Principle of Brinell hardness testing.

Tensile Strength

Tensile strength is determined on a test piece which is gripped in a tensile testing machine and subjected to a successively increasing tensile load until fracture occurs. The properties that are normally recorded are yield strength $Rp_{0,2}$ and ultimate tensile strength R_m, while elongation A_5 and reduction of area Z are measured on the test piece. In general, it can be said that hardness is dependent upon yield strength and ultimate tensile strength, while elongation and reduction of area are an indication of toughness. High values for yield and ultimate tensile strength generally mean low values for elongation and reduction of area. Tensile tests are used mostly on structural steels, seldom on tool steels. It is difficult to perform tensile tests at hardnesses above 55 HRC. Tensile tests may be of interest for tougher types of tool steel, especially when they are used as high strength structural materials. These include, e.g. Uddeholm Impax Supreme and Uddeholm Orvar 2 Microdised.

Impact Testing

A certain quantity of energy is required to produce a fracture in a material. This quantity of energy can be used as a measure of the toughness of the material, a higher absorption of energy indicating better toughness. The most common and simplest method of determining toughness is impact testing. A rigid pendulum is allowed to fall from a known height and to strike a test specimen at the lowest point of its swing. The angle through which the pendulum travels after breaking the specimen is measured, and the amount of energy that was absorbed in breaking the specimen can be calculated.

Several variants of impact testing are in use. The various methods differ in the shape of the specimens. These are usually provided with a V- or U-shaped notch, the test methods being then known as Charpy V and Charpy U respectively.

For the most part, tool steel has a rather low toughness by reason of its high strength. Materials of low toughness are notch sensitive, for which reason smooth, un-notched specimens are often used in the impact testing of tool steels. The results of the tests are commonly stated in joules, or alternatively in kgm (strictly speaking kgfm), although J/cm^2 or kgm/cm^2 is sometimes used instead, specially in Charpy U testing.

There are several other variants of impact testing which are used outside Sweden, e.g. DVM, Mesanger and — especially in English speaking countries — Izod.

SOME WORDS OF ADVICE TO TOOL DESIGNERS

Choice of Steel
Choose air-hardening steels for complex tools.

Design
Avoid:
1. Sharp corners.
2. Notch effects.
3. Large differences in section thicknesses.

These are often causes of quench cracks, especially if the material is cooled down too far or allowed to stand untempered.

Heat Treatment
Choose suitable hardnesses for the application concerned. Be particularly careful to avoid temperature ranges that can reduce toughness after tempering.

Keep the risk of distortion in mind and follow recommendations concerning machining allowances. It is a good idea to specify stress relieving on the drawings.

Chapter 7
Corrosion Technology of Metals

INTRODUCTION

The basic cause of corrosion is the instability of metal in its refined form. The process of corrosion is the tendency of a metal to revert to its natural state. What dictates the level of corrosion is the combination of the material type and the environment it is exposed to. All environments are corrosive in some manner. Understanding the environment helps to determine what factors contribute to corrosion activity and what the appropriate control methods could be. Corrosion environments can be placed into four major categories: liquid, underground, atmospheric and high temperature. In most industrial applications, the process system is exposed to many, if not all of these environments.

A material that is inert in one environment may not be in another. It is for this reason that material selection is important to ensure that adequate performance characteristics, especially life span, are obtained. Cost and availability dictate the materials that are used in industrial processes. This trade-off is what causes most corrosion problems. With the exception of some forms of high-temperature corrosion, all forms of corrosion occur through the action of the electrochemical cell. This cell contains what is known as an oxidation/reduction reaction. In this reaction, an exchange of electrons (due to a difference in potential) occurs, where an anode is the site of oxidation and a cathode is the site of reduction. The electrons given off at the anode travel through the metal to the cathode, where they are consumed in a reduction reaction. Corrosion is often classified as wet or dry.

Wet corrosion occurs when a liquid phase is present and dry corrosion occurs in the absence of a liquid phase or above the dew point of the environment. In most cases, the combination of the metals found in equipment and structures, combined with the wide range of possible environments, will result in more than one form of corrosion within a system. Corrosion is the deterioration of materials by chemical interaction with their environment.

The term corrosion is sometimes also applied to the degradation of plastics, concrete and wood, but generally refers to metals. The most widely used metal is iron (usually as steel) and the following discussion is mainly related to its corrosion.

CONSEQUENCES OF CORROSION

The consequences of corrosion are many and varied and the effects of these on the safe, reliable and efficient operation of equipment or structures are often more serious than the simple loss of a mass of metal. Failures of various kinds and the need for expensive replacements may occur even though the amount of metal destroyed is quite small.

Some of the major harmful effects of corrosion can be summarised as follows:
1. Reduction of metal thickness leading to loss of mechanical strength and structural failure or breakdown. When the metal is lost in localised zones so as to give a crack-like structure, very considerable weakening may result from quite a small amount of metal loss.
2. Hazards or injuries to people arising from structural failure or breakdown (e.g. bridges, cars, aircraft).
3. Loss of time in availability of profile-making industrial equipment.
4. Reduced value of goods due to deterioration of appearance.
5. Contamination of fluids in vessels and pipes (e.g. beer goes cloudy when small quantities of heavy metals are released by corrosion).
6. Perforation of vessels and pipes allowing escape of their contents and possible harm to the surroundings. For example a leaky domestic radiator can cause expensive damage to carpets and decorations, while corrosive sea water may enter the boilers of a power station if the condenser tubes perforate.
7. Loss of technically important surface properties of a metallic component. These could include frictional and bearing properties, ease of fluid flow over a pipe surface, electrical conductivity of contacts, surface reflectivity or heat transfer across a surface.
8. Mechanical damage to valves, pumps, etc. or blockage of pipes by solid corrosion products.
9. Added complexity and expense of equipment which needs to be designed to withstand a certain amount of corrosion, and to allow corroded components to be conveniently replaced.

CHEMISTRY OF CORROSION

Common structural metals are obtained from their ores or naturally-occurring compounds by the expenditure of large amounts of energy. These metals can therefore be regarded as being in a metastable state and will tend to lose their energy by reverting to compounds more or less similar to their original states. Since most metallic compounds, and especially corrosion products, have little mechanical strength a severely corroded piece of metal is quite useless for its original purpose.

Virtually all corrosion reactions are electrochemical in nature, at anodic sites on the surface the iron goes into solution as ferrous ions, this constituting the anodic reaction. As iron atoms undergo oxidation to ions they release electrons whose negative charge would quickly build up in the metal and prevent further anodic reaction, or corrosion. Thus this dissolution will only continue if the electrons released can pass to a site on the metal surface where a cathodic reaction is possible. At a cathodic site the electrons react with some reducible component of the electrolyte and are themselves removed from the metal. The rates of the anodic and cathodic reactions must be equivalent according to Faraday's Laws, being determined by the total flow of electrons from anodes to cathodes which is called the 'corrosion current', I_{cor}. Since the corrosion current must also flow through the electrolyte by ionic conduction the conductivity of the electrolyte will influence the way in which corrosion cells operate. The corroding piece of metal is described as a 'mixed electrode' since simultaneous anodic and cathodic reactions are proceeding on its surface. The mixed electrode is a complete electrochemical cell on one metal surface.

The most common and important electrochemical reactions in the corrosion of iron are thus

Anodic reaction (corrosion)
$$Fe \rightarrow Fe^{2+} + 2e \qquad \ldots (7.1)$$
Cathodic reactions (simplified)
$$2H^+ + 2e \rightarrow H_2 \qquad \ldots (7.2a)$$

or
$$H_2O + \tfrac{1}{2}O_2 + 2e \rightarrow 2OH^- \qquad \ldots (7.2b)$$

Recaction 7.2(a) is most common in acids and in the pH range 6.5–8.5 the most important reaction is oxygen reduction 7.2(b). In this latter case corrosion is usually accompanied by the formation of solid corrosion debris from the reaction between the anodic and cathodic products.

$$Fe^{2+} + 2OH^- \rightarrow Fe(OH)_2 \text{, iron (II) hydroxide}$$

Pure iron (II) hydroxide is white but the material initially produced by corrosion is normally a greenish colour due to partial oxidation in air.

$$2Fe(OH)_2 + H_2O + O_2 \rightarrow 2Fe(OH)_3 \text{, hydrated iron (III) oxide}$$

Further hydration and oxidation reactions can occur and the reddish rust that eventually forms is a complex mixture whose exact constitution will depend on other trace elements which are present. Because the rust is precipitated as a result of secondary reactions it is porous and absorbent and tends to act as a sort of harmful poultice which encourages further corrosion. For other metals or different environments different types of anodic and cathodic reactions may occur. If solid corrosion products are produced directly on the surface as the first result of anodic oxidation these may provide a highly protective surface film which retards further corrosion, the surface is then said to be 'passive'. An example of such a process would be the production of an oxide film on iron in water, a reaction which is encouraged by oxidising conditions or elevated temperatures.

$$2Fe + 3H_2O \rightarrow Fe_2O_3 + 6H^+ + 6e$$

FACTORS THAT CONTROL THE CORROSION RATE

Certain factors can tend to accelerate the action of a corrosion cell. These include:

1. *Establishment of well-defined locations on the surface for the anodic and cathodic reactions*: This concentrates the damage on small areas where it may have more serious effects, this being described as 'local cell action'. Such effects can occur when metals of differing electrochemical properties are placed in contact, giving a 'galvanic couple'. Galvanic effects may be predicted by means of a study of the Galvanic Series which is a list of metals and alloys placed in order of their potentials in the corrosive environment, such as sea water. Metals having a more positive (noble) potential will tend to extract electrons from a metal which is in a more negative (base) position in the series and hence accelerate its corrosion when in contact with it. The Galvanic Series should not be confused with the Electrochemical Series, which lists the potentials only of pure metals in equilibrium with standard solutions of their ions. Galvanic effects can occur on metallic surfaces which contain more than one phase, so that 'local cells' are set up on the heterogeneous surface. Localised corrosion cells can also be set up on surfaces where the metal is in a varying condition of stress, where rust, dirt or crevices cause differential access of air, where temperature variations occur, or where fluid flow is not uniform.
2. *Stimulation of the anodic or cathodic reaction*: Aggressive ions such as chloride tend to prevent the formation of protective oxide films on the metal surface and thus increase corrosion. Sodium chloride is encountered in marine conditions and is spread on roads in winter for de-icing.

Quite small concentrations of sulphur dioxide released into the atmosphere by the combustion of fuels can dissolve in the invisibly thin surface film of moisture which is usually present on metallic surfaces when the relative humidity is over 60–70 per cent. The acidic electrolyte that is formed under these conditions seems to be capable of stimulating both the anodic and the cathodic reactions.

In practical terms it is not usually possible to eliminate completely all corrosion damage to metals used for the construction of industrial plant. The rate at which attack is of prime importance is usually expressed in one of two ways:
1. Weight loss per unit area per unit time, usually mdd (milligrams per square decimetre per day).
2. A rate of penetration, i.e. the thickness of metal lost. This may be expressed in American units, mpy (mils per year, a mil being a thousandth of an inch) or in metric units, mmpy (millimetres per year).

Taking as an example the corrosion of heat exchanger tubes in industrial cooling water a typical corrosion rate in untreated water would be 40–50 mpy (210–260 mdd); the use of a corrosion inhibitor could reduce this to less than 5 mpy (26 mdd). The mild steel tubing used in heat exchangers is a maximum of 200 thousandths of an inch thick, thus with corrosion rates of 40–50 mpy in untreated water, severe problems might be expected within four or five years. If suitable water treatment with corrosion inhibitors is used a life of at least twenty years might be expected. This, of course, is ignoring the fact that at some time before the metal corrodes away the tubing may have thinned to a point where its required mechanical strength is not attained. When designing equipment for a certain service life engineers often add a 'corrosion allowance' to the metal thickness, permitting a certain amount of thinning before serious weakening occurs. In a cooling water system the factors influencing the rate of attack are:
1. The condition of the metal surface:
    (a) Corrosion debris and other deposits: Corrosion under the deposits, with a possibility of pitting (severe attack in small spots).
2. The nature of the environment:
    (a) pH: In the range of 4-10 corrosion rate is fairly independent of pH, but it increases rapidly when the pH falls below 4.
    (b) Oxygen content: Increase in oxygen concentration usually gives an increase in corrosion rate.
    (c) Flow rate: Increased water flow increased oxygen access to the surface and removes protective surface films, so usually increases corrosion, but can sometimes improve access for corrosion inhibiting reactants.
    (d) Water type: Very important, in general low corrosion rates are found with scale-forming (hard) waters. Aggressive ions which accelerate corrosion are Cl^-, SO_4^{2-} but quite complex interactions may occur between the various dissolved species in natural waters.

CORROSION PREVENTION

By retarding either the anodic or cathodic reactions the rate of corrosion can be reduced. This can be achieved in several ways:

Conditioning the Metal

This can be subdivided into two main groups.

Coating the metal

Coating the metal, in order to interpose a corrosion resistant coating between metal and environment. The coating may consist of:
1. Another metal, e.g. zinc or tin coatings on steel.

2. A protective coating derived from the metal itself, e.g. aluminium oxide on 'anodised' aluminium.
3. Organic coatings, such as resins, plastics, paints, enamel, oils and greases.

The action of protective coatings is often more complex than simply providing a barrier between metal and environment. Paints may contain a corrosion inhibitor: zinc coating in iron or steel confers cathodic protection.

Alloying the metal

Alloying the metal to produce a more corrosion resistant alloy, e.g. stainless steel, in which ordinary steel is alloyed with chromium and nickel. Stainless steel is protected by an invisibly thin, naturally formed film of chromium sesquioxide Cr_2O_3.

Conditioning the Corrosive Environment

Removal of oxygen

By the removal of oxygen from water systems in the pH range 6.5–8.5 one of the components required for corrosion would be absent. The removal of oxygen could be achieved by the use of strong reducing agents, e.g. sulphite.

However, for open evaporative cooling systems this approach to corrosion prevention is not practical since fresh oxygen from the atmosphere will have continual access.

Corrosion inhibitors

A corrosion inhibitor is a chemical additive, which, when added to a corrosive aqueous environment, reduces the rate of metal wastage. It can function in one of the following ways:

1. Anodic inhibitors: As the name implies an anodic inhibitor interferes with the anodic process.

$$Fe \rightarrow Fe^{++} + 2e^- \qquad \ldots (7.3)$$

   If an anodic inhibitor is not present at a concentration level sufficient to block off all the anodic sites, localised attack such as pitting corrosion can become a serious problem due to the oxidising nature of the inhibitor which raises the metal potential and encourages the anodic reaction (Eq. 7.3). Anodic inhibitors are thus classified as 'dangerous inhibitors'. Other examples of anodic inhibitors include orthophosphate, nitrite, ferricyanide and silicates.

2. Cathodic inhibitors: The major cathodic reaction in cooling systems is the reduction of oxygen.

$$\tfrac{1}{2}O_2 + H_2O + 2e \rightarrow 2OH^- \qquad \ldots (7.4)$$

   There are other cathodic reactions and additives that suppress these reactions called cathodic inhibitors. They function by reducing the available area for the cathodic reaction. This is often achieved by precipitating an insoluble species onto the cathodic sites. Zinc ions are used as cathodic inhibitors because of the precipitation of $Zn(OH)_2$ at cathodic sites as a consequence of the localised high pH [See reaction 7.2(b)]. Cathodic inhibitors are classed as safe because they do not cause localised corrosion.

3. Adsorption type corrosion inhibitors: Many organic inhibitors work by an adsorption mechanism. The resultant film of chemisorbed inhibitor is then responsible for protection either by physically blocking the surface from the corrosion environment or by retarding the electrochemical processes. The main functional groups capable of forming chemisorbed bonds with metal surfaces are amino (–NH_2), carboxyl (–COOH), and phosphonate (–PO_3H_2) although other functional groups or atoms can form co-ordinate bonds with metal surfaces.

4. Mixed inhibitors: Because of the danger of pitting when using anodic inhibitors alone, it became common practice to incorporate a cathodic inhibitor into formulated performance was obtained by a combination of inhibitors than from the sum of the individual performances. This observation is generally referred to a 'synergism' and demonstrates the synergistic action which exists between zinc and chromate ions.

Electrochemical Control

Since corrosion is an electrochemical process its progress may be studied by measuring the changes which occur in metal potential with time or with applied electrical currents. Conversely, the rate of corrosion reactions may be controlled by passing anodic or cathodic currents into the metal. If, for example, electrons are passed into the metal and reach the metal/electrolyte interface (a cathodic current) the anodic reaction will be stifled while the cathodic reaction rate increases. This process is called cathodic protection and can only be applied if there is a suitable conducting medium such as earth or water through which a current can flow to the metal to be protected In most soils or natural waters corrosion of steel is prevented if the potential of the metal surface is lowered by 300 or 400 mV. Cathodic protection may be achieved by using a DC power supply (impressed current) or by obtaining electrons from the anodic dissolution of a metal low in the galvanic series such as aluminium, zinc or magnesium (sacrificial anodes). Similar protection is obtained when steel is coated with a layer of zinc. Even at scratches or cut edges where some bare metal is exposed the zinc is able to pass protective current through the thin layer of surface moisture.

In certain chemical environments it is sometimes possible to achieve anodic protection, passing a current which takes electrons out of the metal and raises its potential. Initially this stimulates anodic corrosion, but in favourable circumstances this will be followed by the formation of a protective oxidised passive surface film.

DRY CORROSION

Dry corrosion or oxidation occurs when oxygen in the air reacts with metal without the presence of a liquid. Typically, dry corrosion is not as detrimental as wet corrosion, but it is very sensitive to temperature. If you hold a piece of clean iron in a flame, you will soon see the formation of an oxide layer. Most engineering metals have a slow oxidation rate in the atmosphere at ambient temperature (Fig. 7.1).

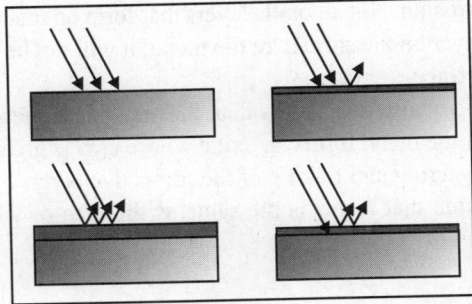

Fig. 7.1. Dry corrosion vary from metal to metal.

The differences in the rate of dry corrosion vary from metal to metal as a result of the mechanisms involved. In dry corrosion the oxygen has to be able to make contact with the metal surface. Initially this is not a problem, but as soon as corrosion starts to occur the oxide layer, that forms on the metal surface, will limit the amount of oxygen that can further react with the metal.

Formation of an Oxide Layer

The different in oxidation rates depends on the conductivity of the oxides because the ions have to move through the oxide layer. Oxidation occurs much more rapidly as temperature increases because the mobility of ions within the oxide layer increases (Fig. 7.2).

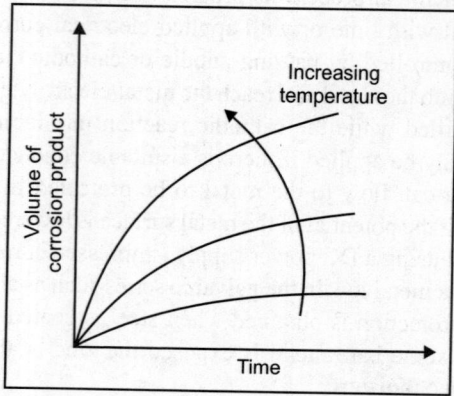

Fig. 7.2. Formation of oxide layer.

In some cases, dry corrosion is actually encouraged. The formation of an oxide layer on the surface of a metal will, in some instances, lead to a reduction in the rate of corrosion. When a metal oxidises and forms an outer layer, this layer can remain on the surface of the metal and limit further corrosion by inhibiting the ability of oxygen or other corrodents to reach the metal surface. This is known as passivation.

Passivation

Passivation of a metal surface through the formation of an oxide layer is found in many common metals and alloys. Aluminium naturally forms a protective oxide layer (or scale) which slows down further oxidation and corrosion. Stainless steel has chromium added to it, which forms a very protective oxide layer that prevents further corrosion. Not all oxide layers that form on metals are protective. If the oxide does not form a continuous layer on the surface of the metal, it will not be able to reduce the amount of oxygen reaching the metal surface.

If the metal forms an oxide whose area is less than the area of the metal then the surface will show gaps in the protective layer. If the metal forms an oxide whose area is greater than the area of the metal then the surface will show blistering and flaking of the protective layer.

Only if the area of the oxide that forms is the same as the area of the metal will the oxide layer protect the metal from further corrosion.

Anodising

Aluminium is often anodised, which means it has an oxide layer artificially induced to protect it from further corrosion. Apart from giving increased corrosion resistance, the strong protective film or passivating layer also increases the hardness of the component and allows it to be dyed different colours.

To anodise a piece of aluminium, the surface must be very clean and smooth. If the surface is not clean then the presence of contaminants such as oils and grease will result in the formation of an incomplete oxide layer. If the surface is not smooth rough patches may cause cracks in the oxide layer. To anodise aluminium, you will need:

1. A container or beaker.
2. Moderate strength sulphuric acid or chromic acid.
3. A clean piece of aluminium that you wish to use as the anode.
4. A lead or stainless steel cathode.
5. A piece of wire as a connection between the aluminium and the cathode.
6. A power supply.

Dry Corrosion Reactions

The basic reaction involved in dry corrosion is:

$$M \Rightarrow M^{n+} + n \times e^{-1}$$

where, M is a metal element.

The metal loses electrons to form an ion and some free electrons. The ionic metal can then react with oxygen to form a metal oxide. In dry corrosion, the oxygen comes from the air, in wet corrosion, the oxygen is supplied by aerated water.

PILLING-BEDWORTH RATIO

The Pilling-Bedworth ratio (P-B ratio), in corrosion of metals, is the ratio of the volume of the elementary cell of a metal oxide to the volume of the elementary cell of the corresponding metal (from which the oxide is created). On the basis of the P-B ratio, it can be judged if the metal is likely to passivate in dry air by creation of a protective oxide layer. The P-B ratio is defined as:

$$R_{PB} = \frac{V_{oxide}}{V_{metal}} = \frac{M_{oxide} \cdot \rho_{oxide}}{n \cdot M_{metal} \cdot \rho_{oxide}}$$

where,

R_{PB} = the Pilling-Bedworth ratio.
M = The atomic or molecular mass.
n = Number of atoms of metal per one molecule of the oxide.
ρ = Density.
V = The molar volume.

N.B. Pilling and R.E. Bedworth suggested in 1923 that metals can be classed into two categories: those that form protective oxides, and those that cannot. They ascribed the protectiveness of the oxide to the volume the oxide takes in comparison to the volume of the metal used to produce this oxide in a corrosion process in dry air. The oxide layer would be unprotective if the ratio is less than unity because the film that forms on the metal surface is porous and/or cracked. Conversely, the metals with the ratio higher than 1 tend to be protective because they form an effective barrier that prevents the gas from further oxidising the metal.

Application

On the basis of measurements, the following connection can be shown:

1. RPB < 1: the oxide coating is broken, no protective effect (for example magnesium).

2. RPB > 2: the oxide coating chips off, no protective effect (example iron).
3. RPB = 1–2: the oxide coating is passivating (examples aluminium, titanium, chromium-containing steels).

However, the exceptions to the above P-B ratio rules are numerous. Many of the exceptions can be attributed to the mechanism of the oxide growth: the underlying assumption in the P-B ratio is that oxygen needs to diffuse through the oxide layer to the metal surface; in reality, it is often the metal ion that diffuses to the air-oxide interface.

FORMATION AND GROWTH OF FILMS

The formation and growth of films occur by three successive stages as below:
1. Adsorption: When a completely clean (oxide-free) surface of metal is exposed to the gaseous environment such as air which contains oxygen, an instantaneous adsorption of gas occurs at the metal surface. This is due to the existence of secondary attraction forces between the residual valency of the metal atoms at the surface and the oxygen molecules. All the gases are adsorbed by metals and hence the process of adsorption is not selective, and has a purely physical character.
2. Chemisorption: The oxygen molecules at the surface gradually enter into chemical combination with the surface metal atoms by electron transfer or electron sharing mechanism. This is known as chemisorption. For chemisorption, the oxygen (or gas) must dissociate into atoms or ions or the metal must dissociate into ions. The dissociation may occur due to high chemical affinity of the gas for the metal or due to high temperature.
3. Growth of film: Once the surface of a metal is covered with a monolayer of oxide, the growth of film continues perpendicular to the metal surface. The mechanisms of growth of film for nonporous and porous films are as below.

Growth of Nonporous Films

Here growth of film occurs by movement of ions and electrons through the oxide film. This is enhanced by the presence of crystal defects such as vacancies present in the film. The contact between the environment and metal surface is maintained by diffusion of metal ions and/or oxygen (or gas) ions by the processes as shown below:
1. Inward diffusion of oxygen ions and outward diffusion of electrons [Fig. 7.3(a)].
2. Outward diffusion of metal ions and electrons [Fig. 7.3(b)].
3. Combination of (1) and (2), i.e. simultaneous inward diffusion of oxygen ions and outward diffusion of metal ions and electrons [Fig. 7.3(c)].

It is clear from the mechanisms (1), (2) and (3) that the rate of growth of film will depend on the diffusivity of oxygen ions and metal ions through the oxide film and also on the electronic conductivity of the oxide. Any difference in the diffusivities of these ions will arrest the rate of growth of film.

Growth of Porous Films

Here the oxygen molecules penetrate through the pores of the oxide film and keep a direct contact with the surface of metal [Fig. 7.2(d)]. Under this situation, the chemical reaction at the metal surface proceeds at a constant rate.

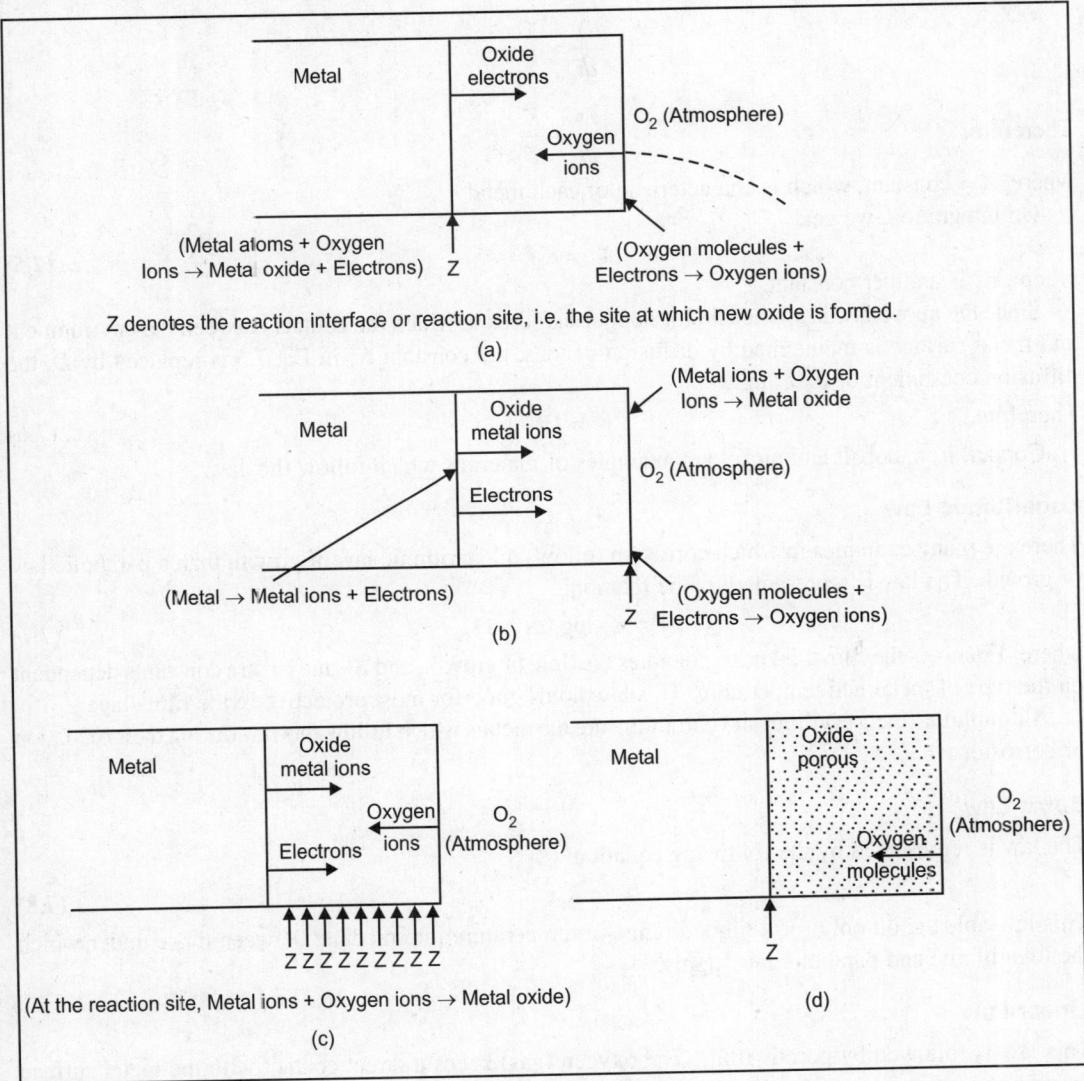

Fig. 7.3. Mechanisms of film growth.

GROWTH LAWS

The growth of film can occur by certain rules. These rules are called growth laws. Nonporous films can grow by parabolic, logarithmic and cubic laws; whereas porous films follow a linear law during their growth.

Parabolic Law

The rate of oxidation or corrosion or increase in the thickness of film with time (t) is inversely proportional to the thickness of film (Y), i.e.

$$\frac{dY}{dt} \propto \frac{1}{Y}$$

Therefore,
$$\frac{dY}{dt} = \frac{K}{Y}$$

where, K = constant, which is characteristic of each metal.

On integration, we get:
$$Y^2 = K_1 t \qquad \ldots (7.5)$$

where, K_1 is another constant.

Since the above law is applicable for nonporous films in which the contact between the environment and metal surface is maintained by diffusion of ions, the constant K_1 in Eq. 7.5 is replaced by D, the diffusion coefficient of the film.

Therefore,
$$Y^2 = Dt \qquad \ldots (7.6)$$

Copper, iron, cobalt and nickel are examples of materials which follow this law.

Logarithmic Law

There are many examples in which corrosion follows a logarithmic law of growth than a parabolic law of growth. The law is represented by the relation:
$$Y = K_2 \log(at + 1) \qquad \ldots (7.7)$$

where, Y denotes the film thickness, t denotes the time of growth, and K_2 and 'a' are constants dependent on the type of metal and temperature. This law holds good for most protective oxide films/layers.

Aluminium, zinc, beryllium and chromium are the metals which follow this law during their oxidation or corrosion.

Cubic Law

The law is represented by the following equation:
$$Y^3 = K_3 t \qquad \ldots (7.8)$$

This law holds good only for a limited range of temperature intermediate between those under which the logarithmic and parabolic laws apply.

Linear Law

This law is followed by porous films. The oxygen (gas) keeps a direct contact with the metal surface through the pores in the film. Here the corrosion proceeds by a direct chemical attack and not by an electrochemical reaction as is for nonporous films. The rate of oxidation is controlled by the passage of oxygen inwards or metal outwards through a continuous pseudomorphic layer next to the metal surface. This layer maintains a constant thickness.

The outer layer next to the pseudomorphic layer is broken up by cracks, so that it is permeable to the passage of oxygen. Under such conditions, the rate of oxidation at a given temperature remains constant. The law can be represented by the equation:
$$\frac{dY}{dt} = K_4$$

i.e.
$$Y = K_4 t \qquad \ldots (7.9)$$

where, K_4 is a constant characteristic of each metal. This law is applicable for alkali and alkaline earth metals which give porous films, e.g. calcium, barium, strontium, magnesium, etc.

The above four laws are schematically shown in Fig. 7.4. It can be seen from this figure that the metals which follow logarithmic or cubic law of growth are most suitable for high temperature service. This is because the thickness of the film formed in a given time is smallest when the law followed by the film is either logarithmic or cubic.

Thus aluminium and chromium are highly resistant to oxidation at elevated temperatures, even at the temperatures close to their melting points. Their alloys also have high oxidation resistance at elevated temperatures.

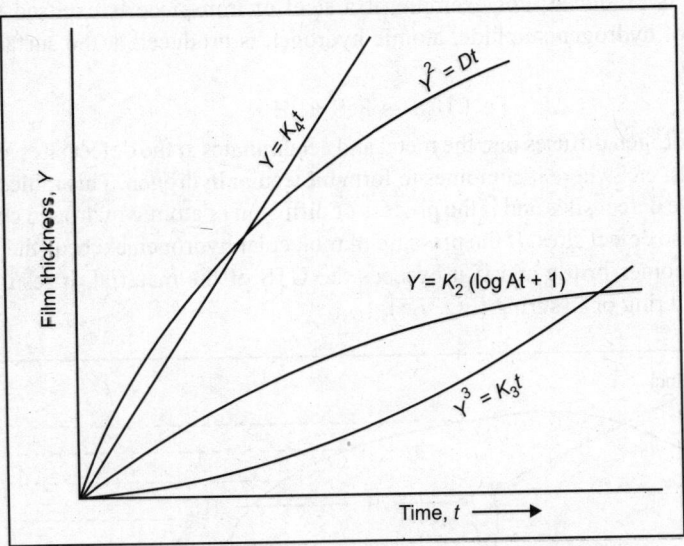

Fig. 7.4. Schematic graphical representation of growth laws.

EFFECT OF TEMPERATURE

For nonporous films, growth of film occurs by diffusion of ions and hence the variation of corrosion rate or oxidation rate with temperature is governed by the Arrhenius equation:

$$K = A\, e^{-E/RT} \qquad \ldots (7.10)$$

where, K is the rate of corrosion (oxidation), or rate of reaction leading to the formation of corrosion products, A is the frequency factor, E is the activation energy, R is the gas constant, and T is the absolute temperature.

The Arrhenius equation can be verified by determining the values of K at different temperatures and plotting $\log K$ versus $1/T$. This plot will be a straight line if the growth of oxide film follows anyone particular law.

However, when the growth law changes with temperature, the plot will not be a straight line. Example of this type is titanium which shows a transition from logarithmic to parabolic law at about 360°C and from parabolic law to linear law at about 800°C. Also at a given temperature, the growth law may change with time of oxidation.

ACTION OF HYDROGEN

The action of hydrogen on metals is of two types as given below.

Hydrogen Embrittlement

Hydrogen embrittlement occurs at low temperatures. Due to the diffusion of hydrogen into the metal, the metal becomes brittle leading to the failure of component. The embrittlement of component due to the diffusion of atomic hydrogen formed by chemical or electrochemical action on the surface of the component at ordinary temperatures is called hydrogen embrittlement.

In certain environments, due to the action of environment with the metal at the surface, atomic or nascent hydrogen is produced. For example, if a steel or iron piece is exposed to the action of an aqueous solution of hydrogen sulphide, atomic hydrogen is produced at the surface according to the following reaction:

$$Fe + H_2S \rightarrow FeS + 2H$$

This atomic hydrogen diffuses into the metal and accumulates at the defect sites such as dislocations, cracks, pores, voids, etc. where it combines to form molecular hydrogen. This molecular hydrogen gets trapped at the above defect sites and if the process of diffusion of atomic hydrogen continues, a pressure is developed in these defect sites. If the pressure of molecular hydrogen exceeds the YS of the material, the component becomes brittle and if it exceeds the UTS of the material, it results in failure of the component by blistering or fissuring (Fig. 7.5).

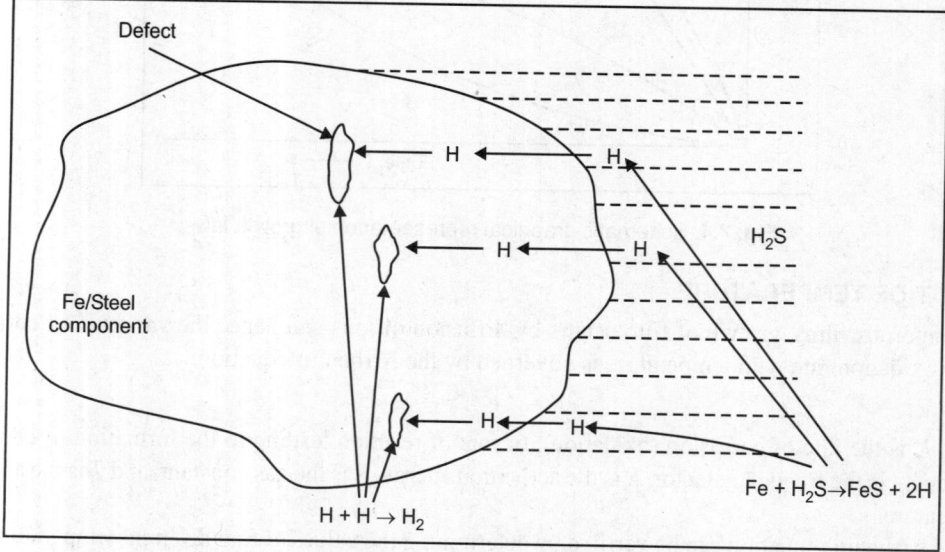

Fig. 7.5. Hydrogen embrittlement.

The embrittlement may also result due to the formation of metal hydrides at the defect boundaries. Formation of metal hydrides reduces strength and increases brittleness of the region around the defect or ahead of the crack tip.

Hydrogen embrittlement is also likely to occur when the component corrodes by hydrogen evolution mechanism with high hydrogen over potential. Hydrogen evolution occurs in two steps. In the first step electrons combine with hydrogen ions and form hydrogen atoms (i.e. $H^+ + e \rightarrow H$). These atoms get adsorbed at the metal surface. In the second step, the adsorbed atoms combine with each other and form molecules (i.e. $H + H \rightarrow H_2$) and this molecular hydrogen evolves at the cathode. The reaction $H + H \rightarrow H_2\uparrow$ is slow and requires an activation potential to keep it going at the rate required by the magnitude of the current flowing 'through the component (or the magnitude at which the anode corrodes). The extra potential necessary for the above is called hydrogen overvoltage or hydrogen overpotential. The metal surfaces for which hydrogen overpotential is more, the atomic hydrogen adsorbed at the surface may diffuse into the metal and can cause hydrogen embrittlement of the component.

Hydrogen Attack

Hydrogen attack also occurs by the diffusion of hydrogen atoms into the metal surface but usually at high temperatures. Due to high temperature, molecular hydrogen may dissociate into atomic hydrogen. The atomic hydrogen is highly reactive at high temperatures. While diffusing into the component, it combines with carbon, sulphur, oxygen, or nitrogen which are usually present in small amounts in metals. This results in the formation of methane, hydrogen sulphide, water vapour or ammonia gas. The high pressure of these gases causes failure of the component. Particularly for steels, the reaction between hydrogen and carbon from the steel results in the formation of high pressure methane which causes inter granular cracking, fissuring or blistering. This leads to decarburisation and considerably reduces the strength of steel and causes brittleness.

WET CORROSION

Wet corrosion is the most common form of corrosion. It will occur if an 'electrochemical cell' is produced. An electrochemical cell consists of an anode, a cathode, a connection, and an electrolyte. The anode is the metal that corrodes. It undergoes oxidation and therefore loses electrons.

The cathode can be a metal or any other conducting material. It undergoes reduction and therefore gains electrons. The reaction that occurs at the cathode is not necessarily related to the material that it is made from. The connection is necessary for the electrons to travel between the anode and cathode and can be either physical direct contact or some form of wire. An electrolyte must also be present to allow for migration of ions between the cathode and anode and participate in the formation of corrosion products. Wet corrosion therefore involves an oxidation reaction at the anode and a reduction reaction at the cathode.

Description of a Wet Corrosion Process

The main features of corrosion of a divalent metal M in an aqueous solution containing oxygen are presented schematically in Fig. 7.6. The corrosion process consists of an anodic and a cathodic reaction. In the anodic reaction (oxidation) the metal is dissolved and transferred to the solution as ions M^{2+}. The cathodic reaction in the example is reduction of oxygen. It is seen that the process makes an electrical circuit without any accumulation of charges. The electrons released by the anodic reaction are conducted through the metal to the cathodic area where they are consumed in the cathodic reaction. A necessary condition for such a corrosion process is that the environment is a conducting liquid (an electrolyte) that is in contact with the metal. The electrical circuit is closed by ion conduction through the electrolyte. In accordance with the conditions this dissolution process is called wet corrosion, and the mechanism is typically electrochemical.

In the example in Fig. 7.6 the metal ions M^{2+} are conducted towards OH^- ions, and together they form a metal hydroxide that may be deposited on the metal surface. If, for instance, the metal is zinc and the liquid is water containing O_2 but not CO_2, the pattern in the figure is followed: Zn^{2+} ions join OH^- and form $Zn(OH)_2$. When CO_2 is dissolved in the liquid a zinc carbonate is deposited. Corrosion of substances like iron and copper follow similar patterns with modifications: divalent iron oxide, $Fe(OH)_2$, is not stable, thus with access of oxygen and water it oxidises to a trivalent hydrated iron oxide, $Fe_2O_3 \cdot nH_2O$, or an iron hydroxide, $Fe(OH)_3$, which also may be expressed as $FeOOH + H_2O$. FeOOH is the ordinary red (or brown) rust. If the access of oxygen is strongly limited, Fe_3O_4 is formed instead of the trivalent corrosion products. Fe_3O_4 is black (without water) or green (with water). Divalent copper hydroxide, $Cu(OH)_2$, is not stable either and tends to be dehydrated to CuO.

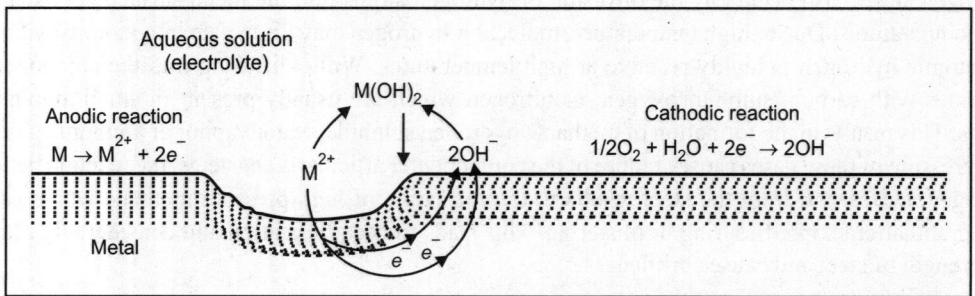

Fig. 7.6. Wet corrosion of a divalent metal *M* in an electrolyte containing oxygen.

Reduction of oxygen is the dominating cathodic reaction in natural environments like seawater, fresh water, soil and the atmosphere. However, under certain conditions there are also other important cathodic reactions: the hydrogen reaction $2H^+ + 2e^- \rightarrow H_2$, reduction of carbonic acid (H_2CO_3) (in oil and gas production), reduction of metal ions, etc.

Figure 7.6 illustrates an electrochemical cell, and the driving force for the electrochemical process (the corrosion) is the cell voltage, or in other words the potential difference between the anode and the cathode.

Crucial Mechanisms Determining Corrosion Rates

It is seen that the corrosion process in Fig. 7.6 depends on the availability of oxygen. When corrosion products, such as hydroxides, are deposited on a metal surface, they may cause a reduction in the oxygen supply because the oxygen has to diffuse through the deposits, which may form a more or less continuous layer on the metal surface. Since the rate of metal dissolution is equal to the rate of oxygen reduction (Fig. 7.6), a limited supply and limited reduction rate of oxygen will also reduce the corrosion rate. In this case it is said that the corrosion is under cathodic control. This is a very widespread mechanism for corrosion limitation by nature. If the corrosion products are removed from the metal surface by mechanisms such as the corrosion medium flowing at high velocity and corresponding strong fluid dynamical forces, the corrosion rate may be greatly increased.

In certain cases, the corrosion products form a dense and continuous surface film of oxide closely related to the crystallographic structure of the metal. Films of this type prevent the conduction of metal ions from the metal–oxide interface to the oxide–liquid interface to a great extent so that the corrosion rates may be very low (anodic control). This phenomenon is called passivation and is typical for materials like stainless steel and aluminium in many natural environments. Ordinary structural steels are also passivated in alkaline water. Passivation is promoted by ample access of oxygen on the material surface, which is obtained by high oxygen concentration in the liquid and by efficient transport of oxygen as a result of strong convection (high flow rates). Conversely, passivation may be hindered or a passive film may be broken down—by the lack of oxygen. This often happens underneath deposits and in narrow crevices that obstruct the oxygen supply.

Aggressive species like chlorides are other major causes of the local breakdown of passive films that occurs in crevice corrosion, pitting and other forms of corrosion. When more and less noble materials are placed in contact, the more noble material offers an extra area for the cathodic reaction. Therefore the total rate of the cathodic reaction is increased, and this is balanced with an increased anodic reaction, i.e. increased dissolution of the less noble material. If the more noble material (the cathodic material) has a large surface area and the less noble metal (the anodic metal) has a relatively small area, a large cathodic reaction must be balanced by a correspondingly large anodic reaction concentrated in a small area. The intensity of the anodic reaction, i.e. the corrosion rate (material loss per area unit and time unit) becomes high. Thus, the area ratio between the cathodic and the anodic materials is very important and should be kept as low as possible. It should be mentioned that in a galvanic corrosion process, the more noble material is more or less protected. This is an example of cathodic protection, by which the less noble material acts as a sacrificial anode.

Corrosion Prevention Measures

Corrosion prevention aims at removing or reducing the effect of one or more of the conditions leading to corrosion using the following measures:
1. Selecting a material that does not corrode in the actual environment.
2. Changing the environment, e.g. removing the oxygen or adding anticorrosion chemicals (inhibitors).
3. Using a design that will avoid corrosion, e.g. preventing the collection of water so that the metal surface can be kept dry.
4. Changing the potential, most often by making the metal more negative and thus counteracting the natural tendency of the positive metal ions to be transferred from the metal to the environment.
5. Applying coatings on the metal surface, usually in order to make a barrier between the metal and the corrosive environment.

Expressions and Measures of Corrosion Rates

There are three main methods that are used to express the corrosion rate:
1. Thickness reduction of the material per unit time.
2. Weight loss per unit area and unit time.
3. Corrosion current density.

Thickness reduction per unit time is the measure of most practical significance and interest. In the metric system this measure is usually expressed in mm/year. In some literature one can still find the unit mils per year (mpy) = 1/1000 inches per year, possibly also inches per year (ipy). Weight loss per unit area and unit time was commonly used in earlier times, mainly because weight loss was usually the directly determined quantity in corrosion testing. Here the test specimens were weighed before and after the exposure to the corrosion medium. On this basis one could calculate the thickness reduction as weight loss per unit area/density.

From Fig. 7.6 it can be understood that corrosion rate also can be expressed by corrosion current density. The dissolution rate (the corrosion rate) is the amount of metal ions removed from the metal per unit area and unit time. This transport of ions can be expressed as the electric current I_a per area unit, i.e. anodic current density i_a = corrosion current density i_{corr}.

If it is preferred to express the local corrosion current density in the anodic area in Fig. 7.6, one has $i_{corr} = i_a = I_a/A_a$, where, A_a is the anodic area. However, usually the average corrosion current density over the whole surface area A is given, i.e. $i_{corr} = i_a = I_a/A$. The most suitable measure to employ for calculating the corrosion rate depends on which form of corrosion one is dealing with.

Corrosion current density is a particularly suitable measure of corrosion rate when treating corrosion theory and in connection with electrochemical corrosion testing. Current density is also directly applicable for cathodic and anodic protection. In corrosion testing the unit µA/cm² is most often used. When dealing with cathodic protection the units mA/m² and A/m² are used for the cathode (structure to be protected) and the anode, respectively.

The relationship between thickness reduction per time unit ds/dt (on each corroding side of the specimen/component) and the corrosion current density i_{corr} is determined from Faraday's equations:

$$\frac{ds}{dt} = \frac{i_{corr} M}{zF\rho} \text{ cm/s} \qquad \ldots (7.11a)$$

or

$$\frac{\Delta s}{\Delta t} = 3268 \frac{i_{corr} M}{z\rho} \text{ mm/year} \qquad \ldots (7.11b)$$

where, i_{corr} is given in A/cm^2;
- z = Number of electrons in the reaction equation for the anodic reaction (dissolution reaction) (per atom of the dissolving metal).
- M = The mol mass of the metal (g/mol atoms) (the numerical value of M is the atomic weight of the metal).
- F = Faraday's constant = 96,485 coulombs/mole electrons = 96,485 C/mol $e^- \approx$ 96,500 As/mol e^-.
- ρ = The density of the metal (g/cm³).

Table 7.1 shows the conversion factors between the units of corrosion rates that are most frequently used in the literature.

Table 7.1. Corrosion rate conversion factors.

Material/reaction	Corrosion current density µA/cm²	Weight loss per unit area and unit time mdd*	Average attack depth increment per unit time	
			mm/year	mpy**
Fe → Fe²⁺ + 2e⁻	1	2.51	1.16 × 10⁻²	0.46
Cu → Cu²⁺ + 2e⁻	1	2.84	1.17 × 10⁻²	0.46
Zn → Zn²⁺ + 2e⁻	1	2.93	1.5 × 10⁻²	0.59
Ni → Ni²⁺ + 2e⁻	1	2.63	1.08 × 10⁻²	0.43
Al → Al³⁺ + 3e⁻	1	0.81	1.09 × 10⁻²	0.43
Mg → Mg²⁺ + 2e⁻	1	1.09	2.2 × 10⁻²	0.89

*mdd = mg per dm² per day.
**mpy = mils per year (1/1000 inches per year).

Note that, for most of the listed materials, a corrosion current density of 1 µA/cm² corresponds to a thickness reduction of roughly 0.01 mm/year. As an example of practical corrosion rates it can be mentioned that structural steels in seawater normally corrode by 0.1–0.15 mm/year ≈ 10–15 µA/cm² on average. The corrosion rate can be a few times higher locally.

Basic Properties that Determine if Corrosion is Possible and How Fast Material can Corrode

The corrosion process in Fig. 7.6 is an example of a so-called spontaneous electrochemical cell reaction. The driving force of the reaction is a reversible cell voltage. The cell voltage can be expressed as the difference between the potentials of the two electrodes (anode and cathode). Reversible cell voltage and the corresponding reversible potentials of the electrodes are determined by thermodynamic properties. These properties, mainly provide a possibility to determine the spontaneous direction which a given reaction tends to have. Applied to corrosion, the thermodynamics can tell us if corrosion is theoretically possible or not under given conditions.

The driving voltage of the cell reaction must cope with various types of resistance: (i) resistance against charge transfer between a metal and the adjacent electrolyte at the anode and cathode, respectively, (ii) resistance due to limited access of reactants or limited removal of reaction products at the electrodes, (iii) ohmic resistance in the liquid and possibly in the metal between the anode and the cathode. The driving voltage and the sum of the resistances will together determine how fast the reactions will proceed, i.e. how fast a given material will corrode.

Resistances against the reactions and the resulting reaction rates are described and explained under electrode kinetics. In other words by using kinetic relationships we can determine how fast a material will corrode under certain conditions. Thermodynamics and electrode kinetics make up the two main parts of corrosion theory. These are the key to understanding and explaining the majority of practical corrosion problems. It is normal to apply this corrosion theory in modern corrosion testing, and it provides a more rational basis for corrosion prevention and monitoring.

Electrochemical Theory of Wet Corrosion: Fundamentals

As with dry corrosion wet corrosion reactions are only possible if the free energy of the products of reaction is lower than the free energy of the reactants. This is the case however for the reaction of nearly all metals with water and oxygen to give metal hydroxides:

$$M + H_2O(l) \rightarrow M(OH)_2(s) \quad \quad \text{... (7.12)}$$

for example:
1. For Mg: $\Delta G = 597$ kJ/mol.
2. And for Cu: $\Delta G = 120$ kJ/mol.

In addition, and unfortunately, the rate of wet corrosion may often be very high compared with dry corrosion on the same metal at the same temperature. There are two underlying reasons for this:
1. The dipolar water molecule stabilises the free (dissociated) metal ions in solution.
2. The metallic structure and water in contact with it can both conduct electric current.

This enables reaction 7.12 above to proceed through the coupling of two primary corrosion reactions:

$$A: M \rightarrow M^{2+} + 2e^- \quad \quad \text{... (7.13)}$$

(Anode reaction: destroys metal, releases electrons, oxidation)

$$C: 2e^- + H_2O + \tfrac{1}{2}O_2 \rightarrow 2OH^- \quad \quad \text{... (7.14)}$$

(Cathode reaction: consumes electrons; electron sink reaction: reduction).

Electrons liberated in the anode reaction A flow to the site of the cathode reaction C through the conducting metal. The movement of dissociated ions carries an equal ionic current in the water. The distances over which these currents flow can vary from microns to many metres.

All wet corrosion processes can be analysed in terms of anodic and cathodic reactions. The anodic process is the direct cause of damage to metallic structures but both an anodic and a cathodic process must occur for a corrosion cell to be formed.

The corrosion of metals by reaction with air and water to form metal hydroxides as shown above is a very important wet corrosion process, especially in the construction industries. There are other corrosion reactions resulting from, for example, other cathode reactions (electron-consuming).

$$2e^- + 2H^+ \rightarrow H_2 \qquad \ldots (7.15)$$
$$2e^- + 2M^{2+} \rightarrow M \qquad \ldots (7.16)$$

or other anode reactions (electron releasing).

$$M + H_2O \rightarrow MO + 2H^+ 2e^- \qquad \ldots (7.17)$$

When a metal M is placed in pure water, some ions will immediately pass into solution:

$$M \rightarrow M^{2+} + 2e^- \qquad \ldots (7.18)$$

The build-up of negative charge on the metal and the build-up of metal ions in solution makes possible a back-reaction:

$$M \leftarrow M^{2+} + 2e^- \qquad \ldots (7.19)$$

and ultimately an equilibrium is established:

$$M \rightleftarrows M^{2+} + 2e^- \qquad \ldots (7.20)$$

At this stage, a steady potential difference now exists between metal and solution. The magnitude of this potential difference depends on the metal and composition of the solution. It is not possible to measure this potential difference for a single metal, but the potential difference (emf) between two metals dipping into a solution can be measured. Under well-defined conditions, this enables a single potential E_m (relative to a common reference) to be assigned to every metal.

Electrochemical series

The single electrode potential E_m developed by a material M acting as an electrode depends on the constitution of the material and the composition of the solution with which it is in contact. The electrochemical series lists electrodes according to the standard single potential $E_m^\ominus$ developed in contact with a 1 mol/l solution of the ion produced by the electrode reaction, at equilibrium (that is, no current flowing), at 25°C. On this scale, the hydrogen electrode $H_2 \rightleftarrows 2H^+ + 2e^-$, H_2 pressure 1 atm) is given the arbitrary value zero. The recommended sign convention (Stockholm) is such that the more noble metals show increasingly positive potentials (e.g. $Cu^{2+}|Cu\ E = +0.34$ V, not 0.34 V). Some older texts (especially American) use the opposite sign convention. Note that single potentials can be assigned to electrode reactions other than $M^{n+}|M$, including familiar cathode reactions.

Nernst equation

Nernst equation describes how E_m varies with concentration of metal ions for the electrode $M^{n+}|M$.

$$E_m = E_m^\ominus + \frac{b}{n}\log c \qquad \ldots (7.21)$$

where, $b = 0.059$ V at 25°C.

For the electrode $O_2 | 4OH^-$

$$E_{O_2} = E^\ominus_{O_2} + \frac{b}{4}\log\frac{p_{O_2}}{c^4_{OH^-}} \qquad \text{...(7.22)}$$

Practical use of reference electrodes

The hydrogen electrode is not a practical reference electrode for field use. The copper/copper sulphate electrode is perhaps the most widely used. In sea water, the even simpler zinc electrode is often employed.

Polarisation

In active corrosion cells, a net corrosion current flows at each electrode surface. At the anode, the electrode reaction is no longer in equilibrium (Fig. 7.7). The rate of the forward reaction exceeds the rate of the back reaction: $i_f > i_b$.

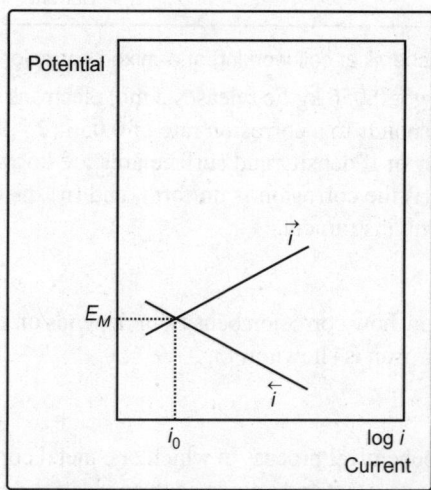

Fig. 7.7. Ideal polarisation curve for a metal surface in contact with water.

This net anodic current requires a shift of the electrode potential to a more positive value. This favours the forward reaction and disfavours the back reaction. A second surface acting as a cathode is cathodically polarised, as shown in Fig. 7.8.

$$X^{n-} \rightleftarrows X + ne^- \qquad \text{...(7.23)}$$

Here for example X may stand for $2H_2O + O_2$, with $n = 4$, and $X^{n-} \equiv 4OH^-$.
Potential–current (E–log i) diagrams are known as polarisation diagrams or Tafel plots.

Simple calculations of corrosion rates

The measured current and the corrosion rate are simply and directly related because 1 mol electrons has a total charge of 96500 C (coulombs). But 1 A s = 1 C (A current in amperes). Therefore, for example in the case of ferrous metals for which:

$$Fe \rightarrow Fe^{2+} + 2e^- \qquad \text{...(7.24)}$$

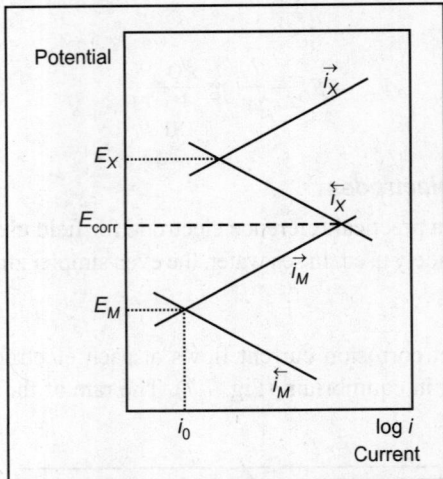

Fig. 7.8. Electrochemical cell working at a mixed corrosion potential E_{corr}.

The corrosion of 1 mol Fe = 56 g = 0.056 kg Fe releases 2 mol electrons = 2×96500 C electric charge; therefore a current of 1 A corresponds to a corrosion rate of $0.056/(2 \times 96500)$ kg/s iron.

More useful units are g/year; or if density and surface area are known mm/y depth of penetration. Assumptions in the treatment: (i) the corrosion is uniform, and (ii) the entire current of the corrosion cell passes through the measuring instrument.

Pourbaix diagram of iron

These widely used diagrams show how corrosion behaviour depends on electrical potential E and pH. A simplified Pourbaix diagram for iron is shown in Fig. 7.9.

GALVANIC CORROSION

Galvanic corrosion is an electrochemical process in which one metal corrodes preferentially to another when both metals are in electrical contact and immersed in an electrolyte. The same galvanic reaction is exploited in primary batteries to generate a voltage. Dissimilar metals and alloys have different electrode potentials and when two or more come into contact in an electrolyte a galvanic couple is set up. A galvanic couple can also be set up on a single metal or alloy due the metal surface not being homogeneous or if the electrolyte varies in composition, forming a concentration cell.

The electrolyte provides a means for ion migration whereby metallic ions can move from the anode to the cathode. This leads to the anodic metal corroding more quickly than it otherwise would; the corrosion of the cathodic metal is retarded even to the point of stopping. The presence of electrolyte and a conducting path between the metals may cause corrosion where otherwise neither metal alone would have corroded.

In some cases, this reaction is intentionally encouraged. For example, low-cost household batteries typically contain carbon–zinc cells. As part of a closed circuit (the electron pathway), the zinc within the cell will corrode preferentially (the ion pathway). Another example is the cathodic protection of buried or submerged structures. In this example, sacrificial anodes work as part of a galvanic couple, promoting corrosion of the anode, rather than the protected subject metal.

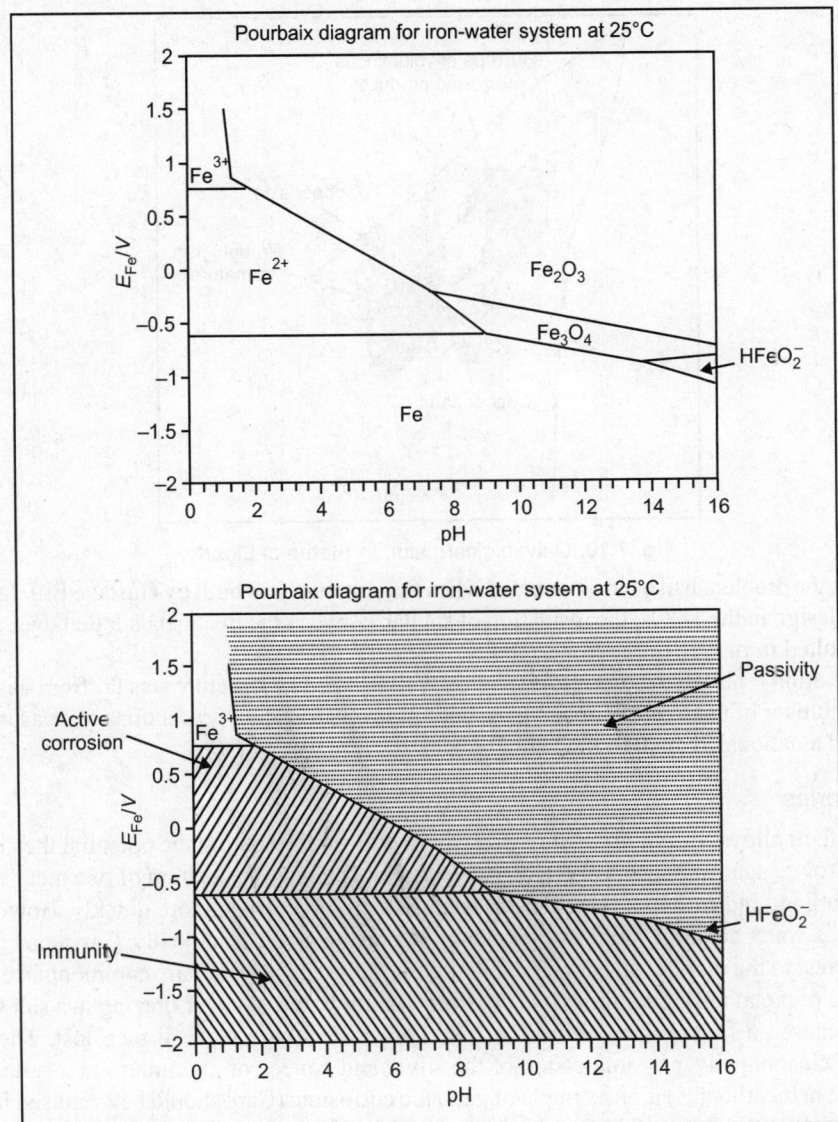

Fig. 7.9. Pourbaix diagram for iron, showing regions of active corrosion, passivity and immunity.

Examples: A common example of galvanic corrosion is the rusting of corrugated iron sheet, which becomes widespread when the protective zinc coating is broken and the underlying steel is attacked. The zinc is attacked preferentially because it is less noble, but when consumed, rusting will occur in earnest. With a tin can, the opposite is true because the tin is more noble than the underlying steel, so when the coating is broken, the steel is attacked preferentially.

A rather more spectacular example occurred in the Statue of Liberty when regular maintenance in the 1980s showed that galvanic corrosion had taken place between the outer copper skin and the wrought iron support structure (Fig. 7.10).

194 Physical Metallurgy

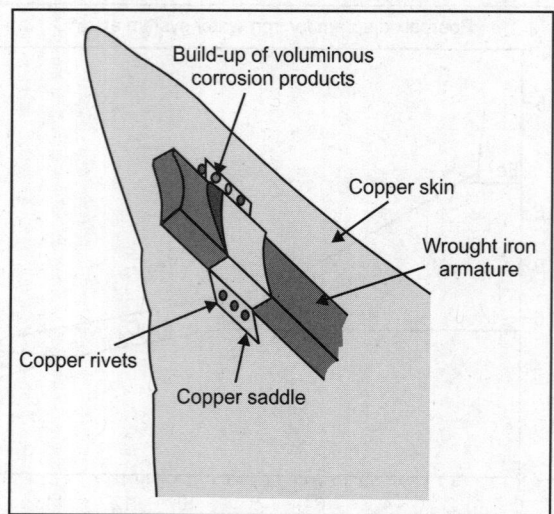

Fig. 7.10. Galvanic corrosion in Statue of Liberty.

Although the problem had been anticipated when the structure was built by Gustave Eiffel to Frédéric Bartholdi's design in the 1880s, the insulation of shellac between the two metals failed over a period of time and resulted in rusting of the iron supports.

The renovation replaced the original insulation with PTFE. The structure was far from unsafe owing to the large number of unaffected connections, but it was regarded as a precautionary measure for what is considered a national symbol of the United States.

Galvanic Series

Metals (and their alloys) can be arranged in a galvanic series representing the potential they develop in a given electrolyte against a standard reference electrode. The relative position of two metals on such a series gives a good indication of which metal is more likely to corrode more quickly. However, other factors such as water aeration and flow rate can influence the process markedly. Galvanic corrosion is of major interest to the marine industry. Galvanic series tables for seawater are commonplace due to the extensive use of metal in shipbuilding. It is possible that corrosion of silver brazing in a salt water pipe might have caused a failure that lead to the *USS Thresher* sinking with all men lost. The common technique of cleaning silver by immersion of the silver and a piece of aluminium in a salt water bath (usually sodium bicarbonate) is an example of galvanic corrosion. (Care should be exercised for reasons such as this will strip silver oxide from the silver which may be there for decoration. Use on plated silver is inadvisable as this may introduce unwanted galvanic corrosion with the base metal.)

Preventing Galvanic Corrosion

There are several ways of reducing and preventing this form of corrosion.
1. One way is to electrically insulate the two metals from each other. Unless they are in electrical contact, there can be no galvanic couple set up. This can be done using plastic or another insulator to separate steel water pipes from copper-based fittings or by using a coat of grease to separate aluminium and steel parts. Use of absorbent washers that may retain fluid is often counterproductive. Piping can be isolated with a spool of pipe made of plastic materials or

made of metal material internally coated or lined. It is important that the spool has a minimum length of approx. 500 mm to be effective.
2. Another way is to keep the metals dry and/or shielded from ionic compounds (salts, acids, bases), for example by painting or encasing the protected metal in plastic or epoxy, and allowing them to dry.
3. Coating the two materials or if it is not possible to coat both, the coating shall be applied to the more noble, the material with higher potential. This is necessary because if the coating is applied only on the more active material, in case of damage of the coating there will be a large cathode area and a very small anode area, and for the area effect the corrosion rate will be very high.
4. It is also possible to choose metals that have similar potentials. The more closely matched the individual potentials, the lesser the potential difference and hence the lesser the galvanic current. Using the same metal for all construction is the most precise way of matching potentials.

Electroplating or other plating can also help. This tends to use more noble metals that resist corrosion better. Chrome, nickel, silver and gold can all be used.

Cathodic protection uses one or more sacrificial anodes made of a metal which is more active than the protected metal. Metals commonly used for sacrificial anodes include zinc, magnesium, and aluminium. This is commonplace in water heaters. Failure to regularly replace sacrificial anodes in water heaters severely diminishes the lifetime of the tank. Water softeners tend to degrade these sacrificial anodes and tanks more quickly.

Finally, an electrical power supply may be connected to oppose the corrosive galvanic current.

For example, consider a system is composed of 316 SS (a 300 series stainless steel; it is a very noble alloy meaning it is quite resistant to corrosion and has a high potential) and a mild steel (a very active metal with lower potential). The mild steel will corrode in the presence of an electrolyte such as salt water. If a sacrificial anode is used (such as a zinc alloy, aluminium alloy, or magnesium), these anodes will corrode, protecting the other metals.

This is a common practice in the marine industry to protect ship equipment. Boats and vessels that are in salt water use either zinc alloy or aluminium alloy. If boats are only in fresh water, a magnesium alloy is used. Magnesium has one of the highest galvanic potentials of any metal. If it is used in a salt water application on a steel or aluminium hull boat, hydrogen bubbles will form under the paint, causing blistering and peeling.

Metal boats connected to a mains shore line will normally have to have the hull connected to earth for safety reasons. However the end of that earth connection is likely to be a copper rod buried within the marina, resulting in a steel-copper 'battery' of about 0.5 V. For such cases the use of a galvanic isolator is essential—typically 2 diodes in series, preventing any current flow while the applied voltage is less than 1.4V (i.e. 0.7V per diode), but allowing a full flow in case of an earth fault. It has been noted that there will still be a very minor leak through the diodes which may result in slightly faster corrosion than normal.

Factors that influence galvanic corrosion

1. Using a protective coating between dissimilar metals will prevent the reaction of the two metals.
2. Relative size of anode and cathode—This is known as the 'area effect'—as it is the anode that corrodes more quickly, the larger the anode in relation to the cathode, the lesser the corrosion. Conversely, a small anode and a large cathode will see the anode readily damaged. Painting and plating can alter the exposed areas.

3. Aeration of seawater—Poorly aerated water can affect stainless steels, moving them more towards the anodic end of a galvanic scale.
4. Degree of electrical contact—The greater the electrical contact, the easier for a galvanic current to flow.
5. Electrical resistivity of electrolyte—Higher resistivity of the electrolyte will decrease the current, slowing corrosion.
6. Range of individual potential difference—It is possible that different metals could overlap in their range of individual potential differences. This means that either of the metals could act as the anode or cathode depending upon the other conditions that affect the individual potentials.
7. Covering by bio-organisms—Slimes that build up on metals can affect the areas exposed as well as limiting flow rate, aeration, and altering pH.
8. Oxides—Some metals may be covered by a thin layer of oxide that is less reactive than the bare metal. Cleaning the metal can strip this oxide and thus increase reactivity.
9. Humidity—Can affect the electrolytic resistance and transport ions.
10. Temperature—Temperature can affect the rate resistance of metals to other chemicals. For example, higher temperatures tend to make steels less resistant to chlorides.
11. Type of electrolyte—Exposing one piece of metal to two different electrolytes (either different chemicals or concentrations) can cause a galvanic current to flow within the metal.

Lasagna Cell

A 'lasagna cell' or 'lasagna battery' is accidentally produced when salty food such as lasagna is stored in a steel baking pan and is covered with aluminium foil. After a few hours the foil develops small holes where it touches the lasagna, and the food surface becomes covered with small spots composed of corroded aluminium.

This metal corrosion occurs because whenever two metal sheets composed of differing metals are placed into contact with an electrolyte, the two metals act as electrodes, and an electrolytic cell or battery is formed. In this case, the two terminals of the battery are connected together. Because the aluminium foil touches the steel, this battery is shorted out, a significant electric current appears, and rapid chemical reactions take place on the surfaces of the metal in contact with the electrolyte. In a steel/salt/aluminium battery, the aluminium is higher on the electrochemical series, so the solid aluminium turns into dissolved ions and the metal experiences galvanic corrosion.

Galvanic Compatibility

Often when design requires that dissimilar metals come in contact, the galvanic compatibility is managed by finishes and plating. The finishing and plating selected facilitate the dissimilar materials being in contact and protect the base materials from corrosion.

Polarisation

In galvanic corrosion, when corrosion proceeds, i.e. when current flows, certain irreversible effects may occur at near the anode and cathode surfaces in the electrolyte. The changes occurring adjacent to the anode and cathode surfaces in the electrolyte make the potential of the anode to increase and that of the cathode to decrease, i.e. the position of anodic metal shifts towards cathodic end and that of cathodic metal shifts towards anodic end of the electrochemical or galvanic series. Due to this, the potential difference between the electrodes gradually decreases, decreasing the current flowing through the cell, i.e. decreasing the corrosion of anodic metal. This is known as polarisation. The potential change is always in such a way that it opposes the flow of corrosion current.

Causes of polarisation

Changes in ionic concentration

As the reaction at the electrodes proceeds, the ionic concentration near the electrode surfaces becomes different from that in the electrolyte away from the electrodes. For example, concentration of zinc ions increases and at near the cathode, concentration of copper ions decreases. Due to this, the electrode potential of zinc increases and that of copper decreases. The polarisation resulting from the changes in the concentration of ions near the electrode surfaces is called concentration polarisation. Concentration, polarisation is because of slow diffusion of ions in the electrolyte. It is greatly affected by the velocity of the solution, temperature of solution, and diffusivity of ions near the electrode surfaces. Concentration polarisation decreases with increase in anyone or all the above factors.

Hydrogen over potential or over voltage

The over potential of hydrogen is the difference between the potential of the electrode at which hydrogen gas is actually evolved and the theoretical value of the potential at which hydrogen gas is in equilibrium with the hydrogen ions.

Usually metal dissolution at anode is fast and hydrogen evolution at cathode (in acidic environments) is slow. First hydrogen atoms are formed and next they combine and form molecules which evolve at cathode. The process of formation of molecular hydrogen from atomic hydrogen is slow and requires an activation potential to keep it going at the same rate at which the anodic metal dissolves in the solution. This extra potential is called as hydrogen over voltage.

All metals above hydrogen in the electrochemical series should displace hydrogen from its ions in an acid solution of pH = 0. However, it is observed that some metals like lead, tin and cadmium do not displace hydrogen from dilute HCl solutions, i.e. they are not corroded by these acids, provided that there is no air present in these acids. This is due to the high value of hydrogen overpotential which makes these metals more noble than hydrogen. The value of hydrogen overpotential depends on physical characteristics of a metal, the nature of solution in contact, and the current density.

Passivity of the films

Under the service conditions, certain protective films may be formed on both the anode and cathode surfaces. These films inhibit further corrosion by separating the metals from the electrolyte. They also increase resistance of the cell and may decrease the diffusion rates. The overall result of this is the increase in polarisation at the anode and cathode.

Some of the metals and alloys become highly corrosion resistant in the presence of such films. Stainless steels (Fe-Cr alloys), nickel and nickel alloys, aluminium and aluminium alloys, and titanium and titanium alloys show high passivity in oxidising environments due to the formation of a thin film of oxide on their surfaces.

Due to polarisation, the electrode potentials (Ec and Ea) does not remain constant, but vary with the flow of corrosion current (or current density). The plot of variation of potentials of polarised anode and cathode with corrosion current or corrosion current density is called a polarisation curve. Figure 7.11 shows a typical polarisation curve for currents which are not too high or which do not vary radically with time. This diagram is known as Evan's polarisation diagram.

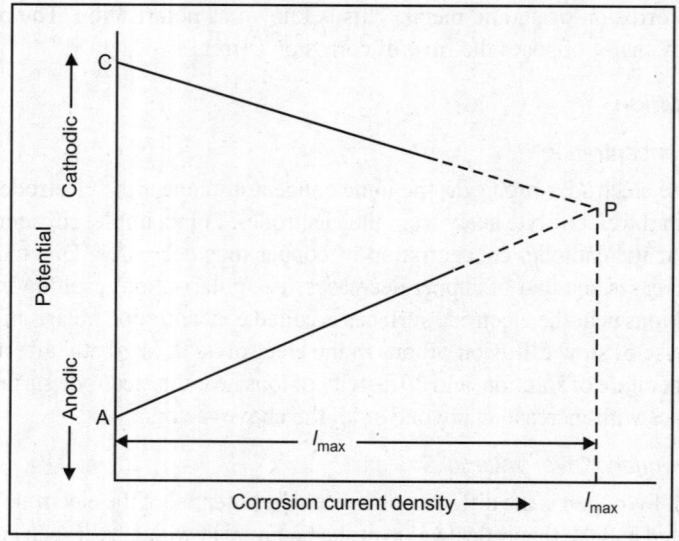

Fig. 7.11. Polarisation curves (mixed control).

Assuming polarisation curves to be straight lines, we get:

$$Ec = E°c - Pc\, I \qquad ...(7.25)$$

and

$$Ea = E°a - Pa\, I \qquad ...(7.26)$$

where, Ec and Ea are the polarised cathode and anode potentials, $E°c$ and $E°a$ are the cathode and anode potentials at zero current (i.e. open circuit potentials), Pc and Pa are the polarisation factors of the cathode and anode, and I is the current flowing through the cell.

In Fig. 7.11, points A and C are the open circuit potentials of anode ,and cathode, curves CP and AP are the cathode and anode polarisation curves and I_{max} is the maximum amount of current that can flow under the polarised conditions. The polarisation factors Pc and Pa are the slopes of the lines CP and AP.

It can be seen from the Fig. 7.11 that the magnitude of corrosion current will depend on the slope of the polarisation curves (i.e. Pc and Pa). If only anode undergoes polarisation without polarisation at the cathode, the rate of corrosion will be controlled by the degree of polarisation at the anode and the system is said to be under anodic control (Fig. 7.12). With increase in the anodic polarisation, the curve becomes steeper (curve API) so that the maximum current becomes I_1, which is less than I_{max}; and hence corrosion also becomes less. If the cathode alone undergoes polarisation without polarisation at anode, the system is said to be under cathodic control (Fig.7.13). If both the electrodes undergo polarisation, the system is said to be under mixed control as shown in Fig. 7.11.

It is very clear from the theory of polarisation that corrosion cannot be completely stopped by polarisation (i.e. corrosion current cannot be brought to zero) because for the maintenance of polarisation of the electrodes same current is necessary in the circuit.

CONCENTRATION CELL CORROSION

Concentration cell corrosion occurs when two or more areas of a metal surface are in contact with different concentrations of the same solution. There are three general types of concentration cell corrosion:
   1. Metal ion concentration cells.

2. Oxygen concentration cells.
3. Active-passive cells.

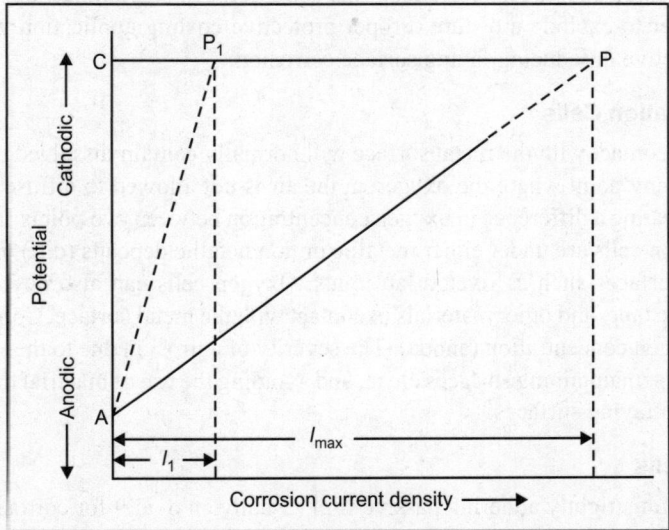

Fig. 7.12. Polarisation curve (anodic control).

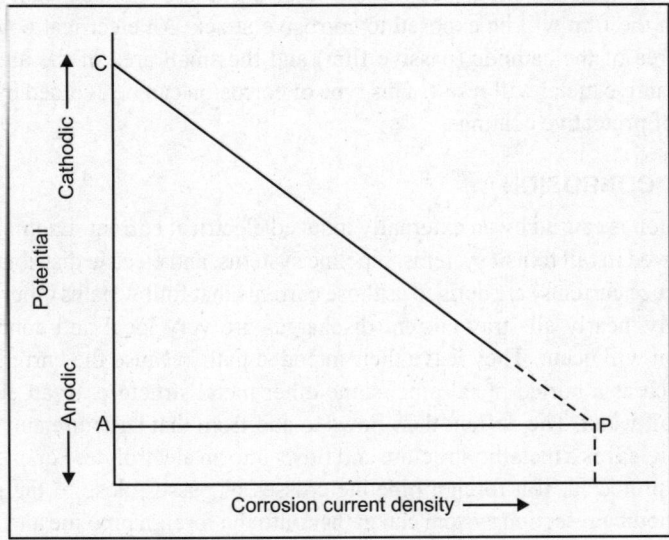

Fig. 7.13. Polarisation curve (cathodic control)

Metal Ion Concentration Cells

In the presence of water, a high concentration of metal ions will exist under faying surfaces and a low concentration of metal ions will exist adjacent to the crevice created by the faying surfaces. An electrical potential will exist between the two points. The area of the metal in contact with the low concentration of metal ions will be cathodic and will be protected, and the area of metal in contact with the high metal ion concentration will be anodic and corroded. This condition can be eliminated by sealing the faying surfaces in a manner to exclude moisture. Proper protective coating application with inorganic zinc primers is also effective in reducing faying surface corrosion.

Oxygen Concentration Cells

A water solution in contact with the metal surface will normally contain dissolved oxygen. An oxygen cell can develop at any point where the oxygen in the air is not allowed to diffuse uniformly into the solution, thereby creating a difference in oxygen concentration between two points. Typical locations of oxygen concentration cells are under either metallic or nonmetallic deposits (dirt) on the metal surface and under faying surfaces such as riveted lap joints. Oxygen cells can also develop under gaskets, wood, rubber, plastic tape, and other materials in contact with the metal surface. Corrosion will occur at the area of low-oxygen concentration (anode). The severity of corrosion due to these conditions can be minimised by sealing, maintaining surfaces clean, and avoiding the use of material that permits wicking of moisture between faying surfaces.

Active-Passive Cells

Metals that depend on a tightly adhering passive film (usually an oxide) for corrosion protection, e.g. austenitic corrosion-resistant steel, can be corroded by active-passive cells. The corrosive action usually starts as an oxygen concentration cell, e.g. salt deposits on the metal surface in the presence of water containing oxygen can create the oxygen cell. If the passive film is broken beneath the salt deposit, the active metal beneath the film will be exposed to corrosive attack. An electrical potential will develop between the large area of the cathode (passive film) and the small area of the anode (active metal). Rapid pitting of the active metal will result. This type of corrosion can be avoided by frequent cleaning and by application of protective coatings.

STRAY-CURRENT CORROSION

Stray-current corrosion is caused by an externally induced electrical current. Examples of this situation are commonly observed in rail transit systems, pipeline systems, and electric distribution systems. Stray currents (or interference currents) are defined as those currents that follow paths other than their intended circuit. Unfortunately, nearly all stray current discharges are very local and concentrated, ensuring accelerated corrosion will occur. They leave their intended path because the current finds a path with lower resistance, such as a buried metal pipe, some other metal structure, or an electrolyte with low resistance such as salt water. The current then flows to and from that structure and causes accelerated corrosion whenever it leaves a metallic structure and flows into an electrolyte. For example, in a pipeline that is cathodically protected, if a foreign pipeline crosses or passes close to the protected pipeline, current from the cathodic protection system can gather onto the foreign pipeline and then be discharged from the foreign line when it crosses or comes close to the protected pipeline. This is particularly true in higher resistivity soil. Accelerated corrosion occurs on the foreign line at the point of current discharge. The location of the discharge can be detected because the pipe-to-soil potential is very low at that point. Likewise in an oil or gas field, where the flowline system or the well casings from several wells are being protected using a centrally located rectifier and ground bed, the path of lowest resistance is usually to the nearest well, down the well casing until a low-resistant formation containing salt water is encountered. The current then travels through the saltwater formation to the other more remote wells in the field where it travels up the well casing to the flowline and then returns to the rectifier. Accelerated corrosion occurs on the well casings of the close wells where current is discharged from the casing to the formation.

This corrosion is extremely difficult to detect and is very expensive to correct. It can cause a blowout in the well to occur because of the corroded casing and can result in a fire or spill. Insulating flanges can cause corrosion from stray currents. Usually the insulating flange is separating pipes that have different ownership or different levels of cathodic protection. If current collects on the pipeline downstream of the protected pipeline, this current may flow back to the insulated flange, discharge into the earth on one side of the flange, and flow to the other side of the flange that is connected to the protected pipeline. Corrosion occurs where the current discharges from the unprotected, downstream pipeline.

Detection of Stray Currents

Detection of stray currents which may be causing corrosion is somewhat involved and involves technical operations for which field staff are usually not equipped. Their presence may be suspected when large direct-current installations are in the vicinity of the structure experiencing corrosion and especially when very rapid corrosion occurs. The services of a corrosion specialist should then be requested.

Stray Currents in Transit Systems

Stray current corrosion problems continue to affect several North American cities where the transit systems are typically installed in high-density urban areas. Obviously such urban areas are associated with underground cables and piping (water and gas) systems, that can also be highly susceptible to this form of corrosion damage.

The major characteristics of a solidly grounded system are direct metallic connection of the AC rectifier negative buses to the earthing mats at the substations and the absence of insulation on the running rails. Such a design allows stray current to flow totally unrestricted between the rectifier negative bus and any available underground metallic path. Consequently, stray-current corrosion occurs frequently on the transit rails, rail fasteners, tunnels, bridges and other transit structures.

The only advantage of a solidly grounded system is that the negative return voltage is at the same voltage as the earth ground, which eliminates the hazard of having electric potentials develop between station platforms and the earth ground. Electric potentials can vary from zero to 150 volts and can represent a hazard for passengers.

Ungrounded systems represent the other extreme of traction power system design. An ungrounded system has no direct metallic connection between earth and the rectifier bus at the substations. Rail fastener insulation is also important so that high, rail-to-earth resistances are maintained. In theory, stray currents from an ungrounded system should be low as long as rail shorts are not allowed to develop along the line.

Practically, however, because of the thousands of fasteners in parallel on the system, an earth ground does exist. In addition, special trackwork is often difficult to isolate completely, and represents areas where grounding can occur. The one disadvantage of an ungrounded system is that sufficiently high electric potentials can develop between platforms and earth ground.

Diode-grounded systems represent a compromise between a solidly grounded and ungrounded system. They are often used to eliminate the problems of stray-current corrosion from a solidly grounded system, but also to keep electric potentials to a safe level. Diode-grounded systems contain a direct metallic connection of the rectifier bus to the earthing mats at substations, but through a diode circuit. The diode circuit allows current to flow from the earthing mat to the negative bus when a certain threshold voltage is reached. The threshold can be as low as 10 volts or as high as 50 volts depending on the conditions at the substation. In this way, electric potentials are dissipated and not allowed to build up to unsafe levels. Stray-current corrosion can still occur on diode-grounded systems, especially on the rails and rail fasteners where low rail-to-earth resistances are seen. In addition, because of the diode-ground circuit path, the return rails periodically discharge current when a threshold voltage is exceeded. It has been observed that a rail designed for 35 years life on a diode-grounded transit system had to be replaced in seven years due to stray-current corrosion and rail cracks.

Nature of Stray Currents

Stray current problems stem from the fundamental design of electrified rail transit systems, whereby current is returned to substations via the running rails. The ground surrounding the rails can be viewed as a parallel conductor to the rails. The magnitude of stray current flow in the ground conductor will increase as its resistivity decreases. Any metallic structure buried in ground of this nature will tend to 'attract' stray current, as it represents a very low resistance current path. The highest rate of metal dissolution occurs where the current leaves the structure and undesirable overprotection effects can occur at the points of current pick-up.

The stray currents tend to be very dynamic in nature, with the magnitude of stray current varying with usage of the transit system and relative position and degree of acceleration of the electrified vehicles. Fundamentally, the following factors all have an effect on the severity of stray currents: magnitude of propulsion current, substation spacing, substation grounding method, resistance of the running rails, usage and location of cross bonds and isolated joints, track-to-earth resistance and the voltage of the traction power system.

At a particular location on an affected structure, the presence of stray currents can be identified when fluctuating pipe-to-soil potentials are recorded with time. The older DC transit systems generally produce the worst stray current problems due to the following factors:

1. Relatively high electrical resistance of the running rails (smaller rail cross sections, bolted connections, deterioration of connections over time, etc.).
2. Poor isolation from earth of the running rails (intentional grounded negative bus, intimate earth contact, moisture absorbing wood ties, etc.).
3. Widely spaced substations leading to a higher voltage drop in the rails.

In modern system designs stray current problems are ameliorated with two fundamental measures:
1. Decreasing the electrical resistance of the rail return circuit.
2. Increasing the electrical resistance between the rails and ground.

The first measure makes current return through the ground less likely. Steps taken in this direction include the use of heavier rail sections, continuously welded rails, improved rail bonding and reduced spacing between substations. It is desirable to combine substations with passenger stations. At passenger stations current flow is highest due to acceleration of trains. This combination ensures that these peak currents have a very short return path. The rail to soil resistance can be increased by using insulators placed between the rails and concrete or wooden ties and by using insulated rail fasteners. Stray current concerns are particularly relevant when older rail systems are integrated with newer designs. The higher current demand of modern, high-speed vehicles poses increased stray current risks in the older sections.

UNIFORM CORROSION

Uniform corrosion is characterised by corrosive attack proceeding evenly over the entire surface area, or a large fraction of the total area. General thinning takes place until failure. On the basis of tonnage wasted, this is the most important form of corrosion. However, uniform corrosion is relatively easily measured and predicted, making disastrous failures relatively rare. In many cases, it is objectionable only from an appearance standpoint. As corrosion occurs uniformly over the entire surface of the metal component, it can be practically controlled by cathodic protection, use of coatings or paints, or simply by specifying a corrosion allowance. In other cases uniform corrosion adds colour and appeal to a surface. Two classics in this respect are the patina created by naturally tarnishing copper roofs and the rust hues produced on weathering steels. The breakdown of protective coating systems on structures often leads to this form of corrosion. Dulling of a bright or polished surface, etching by acid cleaners, or oxidation (discolouration) of steel are examples of surface corrosion. Corrosion resistant alloys and stainless steels can become tarnished or oxidised in corrosive environments. Surface corrosion can indicate a breakdown in the protective coating system, however, and should be examined closely for more advanced attack. If surface corrosion is permitted to continue, the surface may become rough and surface corrosion can lead to more serious types of corrosion.

PITTING CORROSION

Pitting corrosion, or pitting, is a form of extremely localised corrosion that leads to the creation of small holes in the metal. The driving power for pitting corrosion is the depassivation of a small area, which becomes anodic while an unknown but potentially vast area becomes cathodic, leading to very localised galvanic corrosion. The corrosion penetrates the mass of the metal, with limited diffusion of ions. The mechanism of pitting corrosion is probably the same as crevice corrosion.

Mechanism

It is supposed by some that gravitation causes downward-oriented concentration gradient of the dissolved ions in the hole caused by the corrosion, as the concentrated solution is denser. This however is unlikely. The more conventional explanation is that the acidity inside the pit is maintained by the spatial separation of the cathodic and anodic half-reactions, which creates a potential gradient and electromigration of aggressive anions into the pit (Fig. 7.14).

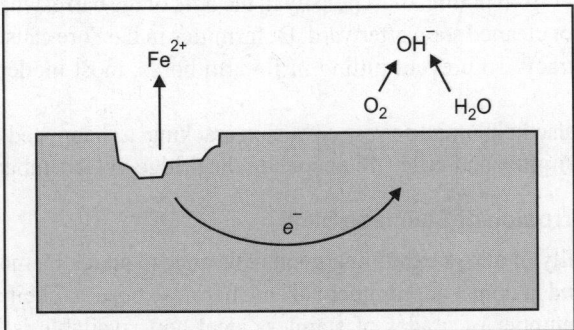

Fig. 7.14. Diagram showing a mechanism of localised corrosion developing on metal in a solution containing oxygen.

This kind of corrosion is extremely insidious, as it causes little loss of material with small effect on its surface, while it damages the deep structures of the metal. The pits on the surface are often obscured by corrosion products. Pitting can be initiated by a small surface defect, being a scratch or a local change in composition, or a damage to protective coating. Polished surfaces display higher resistance to pitting.

Susceptible Alloys

Alloys most susceptible to pitting corrosion are usually the ones where corrosion resistance is caused by a passivation layer: stainless steels, nickel alloys, aluminium alloys. Metals that are susceptible to uniform corrosion in turn do not tend to suffer from pitting. Thus, a regular carbon steel will corrode uniformly in sea water, while stainless steel will pit. Additions of about 2 per cent of molybdenum increases pitting resistance of stainless steels.

Environment

The presence of chlorides, e.g. in sea water, significantly aggravates the conditions for formation and growth of the pits through an autocatalytic process. The pits becomes loaded with positive metal ions through anodic dissociation. The Cl^- ions become concentrated in the pits for charge neutrality and encourage the reaction of positive metal ions with water to form a hydroxide corrosion product and H^+ ions. Now, the pits are weakly acidic, which accelerates the process.

Besides chlorides, other anions implicated in pitting include thiosulphates ($S_2O_3^{2-}$), fluorides and iodides. Stagnant water conditions favour pitting. Thiosulphates are particularly aggressive species and are formed by partial oxidation of pyrite, or partial reduction of sulphate. Thiosulphates are a concern for corrosion in many industries: sulphide ores processing, oil wells and pipelines transporting soured oils, kraft paper production plants, photographic industry, methionine and lysine factories.

Corrosion inhibitors, when present in sufficient amount, will provide protection against pitting. However, too low level of them can aggravate pitting by forming local anodes.

Examples

A single pit in a critical point can cause a great deal of damage. One example is the explosion in Guadalajara, Mexico on April 22, 1992, when gasoline fumes accumulated in sewers destroyed kilometers of streets. The vapours originated from a leak of gasoline through a single hole formed by corrosion between a steel gasoline pipe and a zinc-plated water pipe.

Firearms can also suffer from pitting, most notably in the bore of the barrel when corrosive ammunition is used and the barrel is not cleaned soon afterward. Deformities in the bore caused by pitting can greatly reduce the firearms accuracy. To prevent pitting in firearm bores, most modern firearms have a bore lined with chromium.

Pitting corrosion can also help initiate stress corrosion cracking, as happened when a single eyebar on the Silver Bridge, West Virginia and killed 46 people on the bridge in December, 1967.

Pitting and Crevice Corrosion of Stainless Steel

Stainless Steels are a family of alloys exhibiting good resistance to attack by many of the environments encountered in industry and in domestic, commercial and marine exposure. Their resistance is not perfect, however, and the large number of grades of stainless steel now available is largely because of this challenge of finding cost-effective resistance to these various environments.

The corrosion resistance of stainless steels to some environments can be described by corrosion resistance tables, as the corrosion which does occur is a fairly uniform metal thinning over time. This is termed 'General corrosion'. 'Localised corrosion' by contrast results in attack at certain specific sites while other parts of the metal may remain totally unaffected.

Studies of corrosion failures of stainless steel have indicated that pitting and crevice corrosion types are major problems, and together account for perhaps 25 per cent of all corrosion failures.

What is crevice corrosion?

Crevice Corrosion can be thought of as a special case of pitting corrosion, but one where the initial 'pit' is provided by an external feature; examples of these features are sharp re-entrant corners, overlapping metal surfaces, nonmetallic gaskets or incomplete weld penetration. To function as a corrosion site a crevice has to be of sufficient width to permit entry of the corrodent, but sufficiently narrow to ensure that the corrodent remains stagnant. Accordingly crevice corrosion usually occurs in gaps a few micrometres wide, and is not found in grooves or slots in which circulation of the corrodent is possible.

Environmental factors

The severity of the environment is very largely dependent upon two factors—the chloride (Cl^-) content and the temperature—and the resistance of a particular steel to pitting and crevice corrosion is usually described in terms of what %Cl^- (or ppm Cl^-) and °C it can resist. It should be noted that the most common grade of stainless steel, Type 304, may be considered susceptible to pitting corrosion in sea water (2 per cent or 20,000 ppm chloride) above about 10°C, and even in low chloride content water may be susceptible at only slightly elevated temperatures. A safe chloride level for warm ambient temperatures is generally about 150 ppm (150 mg/l). Grade 316 is more resistant and is commonly used in ambient sea water, but can be attacked in crevices or if the temperature increases even slightly.

The velocity of the liquid is also significant; a stagnant solution is more likely to result in pitting and crevice attack, particularly if there are particles to settle out of the liquid. Note that there may also be a problem from stress corrosion cracking if austenitic stainless steels are used in chloride containing water at temperatures over about 60°C.

All stainless steels grades can be considered susceptible, but their resistances vary widely. Their resistance to attack is largely a measure of their content of chromium, molybdenum and nitrogen. Another factor of importance is the presence of certain metallurgical phases (in particular the grades 303, 416 and 430F containing inclusions of manganese sulphide) have very low resistances, and ferrite may be harmful in austenitic grades in severe environments. A clean and smooth surface finish improves the resistance to attack. Contamination by mild steel or other 'free iron' greatly accelerates attack initiation.

Measurement of resistance to attack

Laboratory tests have been developed to measure the resistance of metals to both pitting and crevice corrosion. This testing has two main aims—firstly to enable ranking of each alloy in order of resistance, and secondly as a quality control measure, to ensure that particular batches of steel have been produced not just with correct composition, but also have been properly rolled and heat treated.

The most commonly used test is that in ASTM G48, which measures resistance to a solution of 6 per cent ferric chloride, at a temperature appropriate for the alloy, shown in the graph above. If an artificial crevice is added to the sample the test measures crevice corrosion resistance rather than pitting resistance. The temperature which is just high enough to cause failure of this test is termed the critical pitting temperature (CPT) or the critical crevice temperature (CCT). Alternative laboratory tests can be carried out using electrochemical cells with a variety of test solutions. The results obtained in laboratory tests are approximate only, as factors such as surface finish, water velocity, water contaminants and metallurgical condition of the steel are all important.

Pitting resistance equivalent number (PRE)

From experience it has been found that an estimate of resistance to pitting can be made by calculation from the composition as the pitting resistance equivalent number:

$$PRE = \% Cr + 3.3 \times \%Mo + 16 \times \%N$$

Various multipliers (up to 30) for nitrogen have been used in this equation; with the higher values often used for the austenitic stainless steel grades; in any case the effect of nitrogen is very important, hence the requirement by many suppliers (including Atlas) that the highly resistant grade 2205 have a minimum nitrogen content of 0.14 per cent. This also explains the trend in extremely high pitting resistant alloys for even higher nitrogen levels. The super duplex grade UR52N+ (UNS S32520/S32550) typically contains 0.2 per cent nitrogen, while the super austenitic grade 4565S (UNS S34565) typically contains 0.45 per cent nitrogen.

Effect of welding

The welding process results in metallurgical changes in both fusion zone and heat affected zone. In most alloy systems some degradation in pitting and crevice corrosion resistance occurs in welding, but these effects can be minimised if proper materials and practices are used. Proper materials usually involves over-alloyed consumables and practices includes proper heat inputs. It is important that correct information be sought from suppliers. Again looking at the extremely high pitting resistant alloys it has been found that the high molybdenum alloys are particularly susceptible to fusion zone micro-segregation, leading to lowered pitting resistance. Alloys such as 4565S which achieve their pitting resistance by high nitrogen rather than very high molybdenum levels have been found to be less affected by weld segregation.

Measures to reduce pitting and crevice corrosion

1. Control the environment to low chloride content and low temperature if possible.
2. Fully understand the environment.
3. Use alloys sufficiently high in chromium, molybdenum and/or nitrogen to ensure resistance.
4. Prepare surfaces to best possible finish. Mirror-finish resists pitting best.
5. Remove all contaminants, especially free-iron, by passivation.
6. Design and fabricate to avoid crevices.
7. Design and fabricate to avoid trapped and pooled liquids.
8. Weld with correct consumables and practices and inspect to check for inadvertent crevices.
9. Pickle to remove all weld scale.

STRESS CORROSION CRACKING

Stress corrosion cracking (SCC) is the unexpected sudden failure of normally ductile metals subjected to a tensile stress in a corrosive environment, especially at elevated temperature in the case of metals. SCC is highly chemically specific in that certain alloys are likely to undergo SCC only when exposed to a small number of chemical environments. The chemical environment that causes SCC for a given alloy is often one which is only mildly corrosive to the metal otherwise. Hence, metal parts with severe SCC can appear bright and shiny, while being filled with microscopic cracks. This factor makes it common for SCC to go undetected prior to failure. SCC often progresses rapidly, and is more common among alloys than pure metals. The specific environment is of crucial importance, and only very small concentrations of certain highly active chemicals are needed to produce catastrophic cracking, often leading to devastating and unexpected failure.

The stresses can be the result of the crevice loads due to stress concentration, or can be caused by the type of assembly or residual stresses from fabrication (e.g. cold working); the residual stresses can be relieved by annealing.

Metals Attacked

Certain austenitic stainless steels and aluminium alloys crack in the presence of chlorides, mild steel cracks in the presence of alkali (boiler cracking) and nitrates, copper alloys crack in ammoniacal solutions (season cracking). This limits the usefulness of austenitic stainless steel for containing water with higher than few ppm content of chlorides at temperatures above 50°C. Worse still, high-tensile structural steels crack in an unexpectedly brittle manner in a whole variety of aqueous environments, especially containing chlorides. With the possible exception of the latter, which is a special example of hydrogen cracking, all the others display the phenomenon of subcritical crack growth, i.e. small surface flaws propagate (usually smoothly) under conditions where fracture mechanics predicts that failure should not occur. That is, in the presence of a corrodent, cracks develop and propagate well below K_{Ic}. In fact, the subcritical value of the stress intensity, designated as K_{Iscc}, may be less than 1 per cent of K_{Ic}, as shown in Table 7.2.

Table 7.2. The subcritical value of the stress intensity.

Alloy	K_{Ic} $MN/m^{3/2}$	SCC environment	K_{Iscc} $MN/m^{3/2}$
13Cr steel	60	3% NaCl	12
18Cr-8Ni	200	42% $MgCl_2$	10
Cu-30Zn	200	NH_4OH, pH7	1
Al-3Mg-7Zn	25	Aqueous halides	5
Ti-6Al-1V	60	0.6M KCl	20

Polymers Attacked

A similar process occurs in polymers, when products are exposed to aggressive chemicals such as acids and alkalis. As with metals, attack is confined to specific polymers and particular chemicals. Thus polycarbonate is sensitive to attack by alkalis, but not by acids. On the other hand, polyesters are readily degraded by acids, and SCC is a likely failure mechanism. Polymers are also susceptible to environmental stress cracking where attacking agents do not necessarily degrade the materials chemically. Nylon is sensitive to degradation by acids, a process known as hydrolysis, and nylon mouldings will crack when attacked by strong acids. For example, the fracture surface of a fuel connector showed the progressive growth of the crack from acid attack (Ch) to the final cusp (C) of polymer.

In this case the failure was caused by hydrolysis of the polymer by contact with sulphuric acid leaking from a car battery. Cracks can be formed in many different elastomers by ozone attack, another form of SCC in polymers. Tiny traces of the gas in the air will attack double bonds in rubber chains, with natural rubber, styrene-butadiene rubber and NBR being most sensitive to degradation. Ozone cracks form in products under tension, but the critical strain is very small. The cracks are always oriented at right angles to the strain axis, so will form around the circumference in a rubber tube bent over. Such cracks are very dangerous when they occur in fuel pipes because the cracks will grow from the outside exposed surfaces into the bore of the pipe, so fuel leakage and fire may follow.

The problem of ozone cracking can be prevented by adding anti-ozonants to the rubber before vulcanisation. Ozone cracks were commonly seen in automobile tyre sidewalls, but are now seen rarely thanks to the use of these additives. On the other hand, the problem does recur in unprotected products such as rubber tubing and seals.

Crack Growth

The subcritical nature of propagation may be attributed to the chemical energy released as the crack propagates. That is,

Elastic energy released + Chemical energy = Surface energy + Deformation energy

The crack initiates at K_{Iscc} and thereafter propagates at a rate governed by the slowest process, which most of the time is the rate at which corrosive ions can diffuse to the crack tip. As the crack advances so K rises (because crack length appears in the calculation of stress intensity). Finally it reaches K_{Ic}, whereupon fast fracture ensues and the component fails. One of the practical difficulties with SCC is its unexpected nature. Stainless steels, for example, are employed because under most conditions they are 'passive', i.e. effectively inert. Very often one finds a single crack has propagated while the rest of the metal surface stays apparently unaffected. The crack propagates perpendicular to the applied stress.

Prevention

SCC is the result of a combination of three factors—a susceptible material, exposure to a corrosive environment, and tensile stresses above a threshold. If you eliminate any one of these factors SCC initiation becomes impossible. The conventional approach to controlling the problem has been to develop new alloys that are more resistant to SCC. This is a costly proposition and can require a massive time investment to achieve only marginal success.

Surface enhancement techniques such as needle peening and cavitation peening are also being used to impede SCC by inducing compressive residual stresses into the surface material. However, the depth of compression achieved is typically shallow and SCC can still occur. These operations also cause a considerable amount of cold working that can exceed 50 per cent. High levels of cold work further increase the risk of SCC initiation and produce a thermally unstable residual stress state. Retaining residual compression at high temperatures is particularly significant in nuclear applications like boiling water reactors or pressurised water reactor systems. SCC can also be prevented by using Ultrasonic Impact Treatment technique with depth of compression significantly deeper than with needle peening.

SEASON CRACKING

Season cracking is a form of stress-corrosion cracking of brass cartridge cases originally reported from British forces in India. During the monsoon season, military activity was temporarily reduced, and ammunition was stored in stables until the dry weather returned. Many brass cartridges were subsequently found to be cracked, especially where the case was crimped to the bullet. It was not until 1921 that the phenomenon was explained by Moor, Beckinsale and Mallinson: ammonia from horse urine, combined with the residual stress in the cold-drawn metal of the cartridges, was responsible for the cracking.

Season cracking is characterised by deep brittle cracks which penetrate into affected components. If the cracks reach a critical size, the component can suddenly fracture, sometimes with disastrous results. However, if the concentration of ammonia is very high, then attack is much more severe, and attack over all exposed surfaces occurs. The problem was solved by annealing the brass cases after forming so as to relieve the residual stresses.

Ammonia

Attack takes the form of reaction between ammonia and copper to form the cuprammonium ion, formula $[Cu(NH_3)_4]$, a chemical complex which is water-soluble, and hence washed from the growing cracks. So the problem of cracking can also occur in copper and any other copper alloy, such as bronze. The tendency of copper to react with ammonia was exploited in making rayon, and the deep blue colour of the aqueous solution of copper oxide in ammonia is known as Schweizer's reagent.

Materials

Although the problem was first found in brass, any alloy containing copper will be susceptible to the problem. It includes copper itself (as used in pipe for example), bronzes and other alloys with a significant copper content.

CAUSTIC EMBRITTLEMENT

Caustic embrittlement is the phenomenon in which the material of a boiler becomes brittle due to the accumulation of caustic substances.

Cause

As water evaporates in the boiler, the concentration of sodium carbonate increases in the boiler. Sodium carbonate is used in softening of water by lime soda process, due to this some sodium carbonate may be left behind in the water. As the concentration of sodium carbonate increases, it undergoes hydrolysis to form sodium hydroxide.

$$Na_2CO_3 + H_2O \rightarrow 2NaOH + CO_2$$

The presence of sodium hydroxide makes the water alkaline. This alkaline water enters minute cracks present in the inner walls of the boiler by capillary action. Inside the cracks, the water evaporates and amount of hydroxide keeps on increasing progressively. This sodium hydroxide attacks the surrounding material and the dissolves the iron of the boiler as sodium ferrate. This causes embrittlement of boiler parts like rivets, bends and joints, which are under stress.

Prevention

This can be prevented by using sodium phosphate instead of sodium carbonate as softening reagents. Adding tannin or lignin to boiler water, which block the hairline cracks and prevent infiltration of NaOH into these areas. Adding Na_2SO_4 to boiler water, which also blocks hairline cracks.

CORROSION FATIGUE

Corrosion fatigue is a special case of stress corrosion caused by the combined effects of cyclic stress and corrosion. No metal is immune from some reduction of its resistance to cyclic stressing if the metal is in a corrosive environment. Damage from corrosion fatigue is greater than the sum of the damage from both cyclic stresses and corrosion. Control of corrosion fatigue can be accomplished by either lowering the cyclic stresses or by corrosion control. The 'beach marks' on the propeller shown below mark the progression of fatigue on this surface.

EROSION-CORROSION

Erosion-corrosion is most prevalent in soft alloys (i.e. copper, aluminium and lead alloys). Alloys which form a surface film in a corrosive environment commonly show a limiting velocity above which corrosion rapidly accelerates. With the exception of cavitation, flow induced corrosion problems are generally termed erosion-corrosion, encompassing flow enhanced dissolution and impingement attack. The fluid can be aqueous or gaseous, single or multiphase. There are several mechanisms described by the conjoint action of flow and corrosion that result in flow-influenced corrosion.

Erosion-corrosion is associated with a flow-induced mechanical removal of the protective surface film that results in a subsequent corrosion rate increase via either electrochemical or chemical processes. It is often accepted that a critical fluid velocity must be exceeded for a given material. The mechanical damage by the impacting fluid imposes disruptive shear stresses or pressure variations on the material surface and/or the protective surface film. Erosion-corrosion may be enhanced by particles (solids or gas bubbles) and impacted by metaphase flows. The morphology of surfaces affected by erosion-corrosion may be in the form of shallow pits or horseshoes or other local phenomena related to the flow direction.

Mass Transport Control

Mass transport controlled corrosion implies that the rate of corrosion is dependent on the convective mass transfer processes at the metal/fluid interface. When steel is exposed to oxygenated water, the initial corrosion rate will be closely related to the convective flux of dissolved oxygen towards the surface, and later by the oxygen diffusion through the iron oxide layer. Corrosion by mass transport will often be streamlined and smooth.

Phase Transport Control

Phase transport controlled corrosion suggests that the wetting of the metal surface by a corrosive phase is flow dependent. This may occur because one liquid phase separates from another or because a second phase forms from a liquid. An example of the second mechanism is the formation of discrete bubbles or a vapour phase from boiler water in horizontal or inclined tubes in high heat-flux areas under low flow conditions. The corroded sites will frequently display rough, irregular surfaces and be coated with or contain thick, porous corrosion deposits.

Cavitation

Cavitation sometimes is considered a special case of erosion-corrosion and is caused by the formation and collapse of vapour bubbles in a liquid near a metal surface. Cavitation removes protective surface scales by the implosion of gas bubbles in a fluid. Calculations have shown that the implosions produce shock waves with pressures approaching 415 MPa. The subsequent corrosion attack is the result of hydro-mechanical effects from liquids in regions of low pressure where flow velocity changes, disruptions, or alterations in flow direction have occurred. Cavitation damage often appears as a collection of closely spaced, sharp-edged pits or craters on the surface. In offshore well systems, the process industry in which components come into contact with sand-bearing liquids, this is an important problem. Materials selection plays an important role in minimising erosion corrosion damage. Caution is in order when predicting erosion corrosion behaviour on the basis of hardness. High hardness in a material does not necessarily guarantee a high degree of resistance to erosion corrosion. Design features are also particularly important. It is generally desirable to reduce the fluid velocity and promote laminar flow; increased pipe diameters are useful in this context. Rough surfaces are generally undesirable. Designs creating turbulence, flow restrictions and obstructions are undesirable. Abrupt changes in flow direction should be avoided. Tank inlet pipes should be directed away from the tank walls, towards the center. Welded and flanged pipe sections should always be carefully aligned. Impingement plates of baffles designed to bear the brunt of the damage should be easily replaceable.

The thickness of vulnerable areas should be increased. Replaceable ferrules, with a tapered end, can be inserted into the inlet side of heat exchanger tubes, to prevent damage to the actual tubes. Several environmental modifications can be implemented to minimise the risk of erosion corrosion. Abrasive particles in fluids can be removed by filtration or settling, while water traps can be used in steam and compressed air systems to decrease the risk of impingement by droplets. De-aeration and corrosion inhibitors are additional measures that can be taken. Cathodic protection and the application of protective coatings may also reduce the rate of attack.

INTERGRANULAR CORROSION

Intergranular corrosion (IGC), also known as intergranular attack (IGA), is a form of corrosion where the boundaries of crystallites of the material are more susceptible to corrosion than their insides. This situation can happen in otherwise corrosion-resistant alloys, when the grain boundaries are depleted of the corrosion-inhibiting compound by some mechanism. In nickel alloys and austenitic stainless steels, where chromium is added for corrosion resistance, the mechanism involved is formation of chromium carbide at the grain boundaries, forming chromium-depleted zones (this process is called sensitisation). Around 12 per cent chromium is minimally required to ensure passivation, mechanism by which a thin invisible layer forms at the surface of stainless steels. This layer protects the metal from corrosive environments and it is, thus, stainless.

These zones also act as local galvanic couples, causing local galvanic corrosion. This condition happens when the material is heated to temperature around 700°C for too long time, and often happens during welding or an improper heat treatment. When zones of such material form due to welding, the resulting corrosion is termed weld decay. Stainless steels can be stabilised against this behaviour by addition of titanium, niobium, or tantalum, which form titanium carbide, niobium carbide and tantalum carbide preferentially to chromium carbide, by lowering the content of carbon in the steel and in case of welding also in the filler metal under 0.02 per cent or by heating the entire part above 1000°C and quenching it in water, leading to dissolution of the chromium carbide in the grains and then preventing its precipitation. Another possibility is to keep the welded parts thin enough to not hold elevated temperature for time sufficiently long to cause chromium carbide precipitation.

Other related kind of intergranular corrosion is termed knifeline attack (KLA). Knifeline attack impacts steels stabilised by niobium, such as 347 stainless steel. Titanium, niobium, and their carbides dissolve in steel at very high temperatures. At some cooling regimes, niobium carbide does not precipitate, and the steel then behaves like unstabilised steel, forming chromium carbide instead. This affects only a thin zone several millimeters wide in the very vicinity of the weld, making it difficult to spot and increasing the corrosion speed. Structures made of such steels have to be heated in a whole to about 1950°F, when the chromium carbide dissolves and niobium carbide forms. The cooling rate after this treatment is not important, as the carbon that would otherwise pose risk of formation of chromium carbide is already sequestered as niobium carbide. Aluminium based alloys may be sensitive to intergranular corrosion if there are layers of materials acting as anodes between the aluminium-rich crystals. High strength aluminium alloys, especially when extruded or otherwise subjected to high degree of working, can undergo exfoliation corrosion, where the corrosion products build up between the flat, elongated grains and separate them, resulting in lifting or leafing effect and often propagating from edges of the material through its entire structure. Intergranular corrosion is a concern especially for alloys with high content of copper.

Other kinds of alloys can undergo exfoliation as well; the sensitivity of cupronickel increases together with its nickel content. A broader term for this class of corrosion is lamellar corrosion. Alloys of iron are susceptible to lamellar corrosion, as the volume of iron oxides is about seven times higher than the volume of original metal, leading to formation of internal tensile stresses tearing the material apart. Similar effect leads to formation of lamellae in stainless steels, due to the difference of thermal expansion of the oxides and the metal. Copper based alloys become sensitive when depletion of copper content in the grain boundaries occurs.

Anisotropic alloys, where extrusion or heavy working leads to formation of long, flat grains, are especially prone to intergranular corrosion. Intergranular corrosion induced by environmental stresses is termed stress corrosion cracking. Intergranular corrosion can be detected by ultrasonic and eddy current methods.

SELECTIVE CORROSION

This process, also called 'dealloying' or 'selective leaching', involves the selective dissolution of one of the elements in a single phase alloy or one of the phases in a multiphase alloy. The most well known example is the dezincification of brass (e.g. 70Cu–30Zn). In this case, the brass takes on a red coppery tinge as the zinc is removed. It also becomes porous and very brittle, without modification to the overall dimensions of the part

This problem can be overcome by choosing an alloy that is less prone, such as a copper-rich cupronickel. Brasses with lower zinc contents or containing elements such as tin (1 per cent) and/or small quantities of arsenic, antimony, or phosphorus have much greater resistance.

Numerous other alloys are susceptible to selective corrosion in certain conditions. For example, denickelisation can occur in Cu-Ni alloys, and dealuminisation in aluminium bronzes, while the graphitisation phenomenon in grey cast irons is due to slow dissolution of the ferrite matrix.

CORROSION/SELECTION OF MATERIALS

Corrosion is the largest single cause of plant and equipment breakdown in the process industries. For most applications it is possible to select materials of construction that are completely resistant to attack by the process fluids, but the cost of such an approach is often prohibitive. In practice it is usual to select materials that corrode slowly at a known rate and to make an allowance for this in specifying the material thickness. However, a significant proportion of corrosion failures occur due to some form of localised corrosion, which results in failure in a much shorter time than would be expected from uniform wastage. Additionally, it is important to take into account that external atmospheric corrosion leads to many instances of loss of containment and tends to be a greater problem than internal corrosion. All these aspects of corrosive behaviour need to be addressed both at plant design time and during the life of the plant.

General Principles

The operator should demonstrate that procedures are in place to ensure that corrosion and the selection of the correct materials of construction are considered at the process design stage. Additionally the operator should demonstrate that it has appropriate inspection and maintenance programs in place in order to prevent corrosion causing loss of containment from its process operations. In doing so the following should be considered.

Process fluid corrosion

Corrosion in metallic components occurs when pure metals and their alloys form stable compounds with the process fluid by chemical reaction or electrochemical processes resulting in surface wastage. Appreciable corrosion can be permitted for tanks and piping if anticipated and allowed for in design thickness, but essentially no corrosion can be permitted in fine mesh wire screens, orifice plates and other items in which small changes in dimensions are critical.

Rates of corrosion can be heavily affected by temperature changes and whilst a material of construction may be suitable at one temperature it may not be appropriate for use at a higher temperature with the same process fluid.

The corrosion of nonmetallic materials is essentially a physiochemical process that manifests itself as swelling, cracking or softening of the material of construction. In many instances nonmetallic materials will prove to be attractive from an economic and performance view.

The use of various substances as additives to process streams to inhibit corrosion has found widespread use and is generally most economically attractive in recirculation systems, however it has also been found to be attractive in some once through systems such as those encountered in the petroleum industry. Typical inhibitors used to prevent corrosion of iron or steel in aqueous solutions are chromates, phosphates, and silicates. In acid solutions organic sulphides and amides are effective.

Localised corrosion

There are many forms of localised corrosion than can lead to early failure of equipment. The prevention of corrosion should be addressed at the mechanical design stage and proper design to minimise local corrosion should include free and complete drainage, minimising crevices, no dead spots in pipework and ease of cleaning and inspection. Some of the more common types of local corrosion are briefly discussed in this section. Pitting often occurs where certain impurities such as chlorides are present in process streams and cooling waters.

This is an extreme form of localised corrosion. Once initiated pits are usually self-accelerating and can result in rapid failures. Many metals suffer from stress corrosion cracking under certain conditions. In piping the most frequent failures from stress corrosion cracking occur with austenitic stainless steels in contact with solutions containing chloride. Even trace quantities of chlorides can cause problems at temperatures above 60°C.

Crevice corrosion may occur where liquid is trapped between close fitting metal surfaces, or between a metal surface and a nonmetallic material such as a gasket. Attention to detail at the design and fabrication stage should be given to areas such as jointing to prevent crevice corrosion.

Localised erosion can occur where equipment orientation causes fluid velocities to accelerate such as at bends. Some chemicals can be handled in carbon steel piping because they form protective coatings of ferric compounds in pipework. Careful design to ensure the coating is not eroded if necessary.

External corrosion

Exterior surface corrosion or rusting of pipework occurs by the formation of iron oxides. Painting to an appropriate specification will significantly extend the period to the onset of corrosion but the durability of the paint finish is largely dependent on the quality of the surface preparation. Improperly installed insulation can provide ideal conditions for corrosion and should be weather proofed or otherwise protected from moisture and spills to avoid contact of the wet material on equipment surfaces. Application of an impervious coating such as bitumen to the exterior of the pipework is beneficial in some circumstances.

Cathodic protection is an electrochemical method of corrosion control that has found widespread application in the protection of carbon steel underground structures such as pipelines and tanks from soil corrosion. The process equipment metal surface is made the cathode in an electrolytic circuit to prevent metal wastage.

Anodic protection is less commonly used and relies on an external potential control system to maintain the metal in a passive condition. This form of corrosion protection has found practical application in the sulphuric acid manufacturing industry.

Materials selection

Corrosion rates are expressed in terms of inches per year of surface wastage and are used to provide a corrosion allowance in the design thickness of equipment such as vessels and pipework. Operators will often use data based on historical experience from plant operations to aid them in determining appropriate corrosion allowances. Alternatively corrosion charts are widely available that give corrosion rates for many combinations of materials of construction and process fluids and normally a range of values will be provided for various process temperatures.

In some instances, particularly where there is a mixture of chemicals present, appropriate data may not exist and corrosion tests may be necessary in order to determine the suitability of equipment. Operators should be able to demonstrate the use of corrosion allowances in equipment specification and design. The sources of data used should be traceable.

Whilst carbon and stainless steels are commonly used materials of construction, increasing use is being made of nonmetallic and lined or plastic process equipment. The selection of the material of construction should taken into account worst case process conditions that may occur under foreseeable upset conditions and should be applied to all components including valves, pipe fittings, instruments and gauges. Both composition (e.g. chlorides, moisture) and temperature deviations can have a significant direct effect on the rate of corrosion. The operator should demonstrate that procedures are in place to ensure that potential deviations in process conditions such as fluid temperature, pressure and composition are identified by competent persons and assessed in relation to the selection of materials of construction for pipework systems.

A wide range of plastics are available for use as materials of construction and can be used in areas such as handling inorganic salt solutions where metals are unsuitable. The use of plastic linings is widespread in equipment such as tanks, pipes, and drums. However, their use is limited to moderate temperatures and they are generally unsuitable for use in abrasive duties. Some of the more commonly used plastics are PVC, PTFE and polypropylene. Special glasses can be bonded to steel, providing an impervious liner. Glass or 'epoxy' lined equipment is widely used in severely corrosive acid duties. The glass lining can be easily damaged and careful attention is required. The thin paint like coatings are unlikely to give full protection due to defects and the most dependable barrier linings are those that are built up in multiple layers to a depth in the region of 3 mm.

Performance tests

Normally testing is carried out in order to determine the suitability of a material of construction for handling a process fluid. However, testing can be used for different purposes. Typically this might be to justify a modified inspection frequency of equipment on an existing plant.

There are a variety of test methods available. Commonly test specimens consisting of small strips or 'coupons' of the material of interest are exposed to the process fluid. The weight loss of the test specimen over a time period is measured in order to determine the corrosion rate. Testing can be carried out on the plant, in the laboratory, or on a pilot plan depending on the situation.

Where laboratory testing is carried out using standard test methods there are difficulties in interpreting results and translating them into plant performance. Care is required to ensure that the test fluid is exactly the same as on the process plant. Discrepancies in test conditions such as trace impurities, dissolved gases, velocity, and turbulence can lead to erroneous results.

Maintenance requirements

Process equipment handling hazardous materials should be inspected at regular frequencies, both internally and externally. Localised corrosion can be unpredictable and fabrication defects such as poor welds can be present. Linings can deform or be damaged. Typically the glass lining on a jacketed reactor can suffer thermal shock or a static discharge may occur through the lining. The frequency of inspection can be amended once an inspection history has been built up and the condition of a piece of equipment can be reasonably predicted. The operator should demonstrate that it has inspection and maintenance programs in place for hazardous process equipment including lagged systems. Where equipment is lined electrical continuity tests for lining defects should be carried out where appropriate. Cathodic and anodic protection systems should be regularly checked to ensure continued protection.

Control of operating conditions

Where control of corrosion is dependent on the concentration of contaminants or moisture the operator should demonstrate that procedures and the necessary controls are in place to maintain a safe operating condition. Similarly where inhibitors are added or systems such as cathodic protection are used the operator should demonstrate that these systems are inspected and adequately maintained to ensure continued protection of the process.

Chapter 8

Cast Iron

INTRODUCTION

Cast iron usually refers to grey iron, but also identifies a large group of ferrous alloys, which solidify with a eutectic. The colour of a fractured surface can be used to identify an alloy. White cast iron is named after its white surface when fractured, due to its carbide impurities which allow cracks to pass straight through. Grey cast iron is named after its grey fractured surface, which occurs because the graphitic flakes deflect a passing crack and initiate countless new cracks as the material breaks.

Carbon (C) and silicon (Si) are the main alloying elements, with the amount ranging from 2.1 to 4 wt% and 1 to 3 wt%, respectively. While this technically makes these base alloys ternary Fe-C-Si alloys, the principle of cast iron solidification is understood from the binary iron-carbon phase diagram. Since the compositions of most cast irons are around the eutectic point of the iron-carbon system, the melting temperatures closely correlate, usually ranging from 1150° to 1200°C (2102° to 2192°F), which is about 300°C (572°F) lower than the melting point of pure iron.

Cast iron tends to be brittle, except for malleable cast irons. With its relatively low melting point, good fluidity, castability, excellent machinability, resistance to deformation and wear resistance, cast irons have become an engineering material with a wide range of applications and are used in pipes, machines and automotive industry parts, such as cylinder heads (declining usage), cylinder blocks and gearbox cases (declining usage). It is resistant to destruction and weakening by oxidisation (rust).

PRODUCTION OF CAST IRON

Cast iron is made by re-melting pig iron, often along with substantial quantities of scrap iron and scrap steel and taking various steps to remove undesirable contaminants such as phosphorus and sulphur. Depending on the application, carbon and silicon content are reduced to the desired levels, which may be anywhere from 2 to 3.5 per cent and 1 to 3 per cent respectively. Other elements are then added to the melt before the final form is produced by casting.

Iron is sometimes melted in a special type of blast furnace known as a cupola, but more often melted in electric induction furnaces. After melting is complete, the molten iron is poured into a holding furnace or ladle.

FACTORS INFLUENCING MICROSTRUCTURE

Microstructure (and also properties) of cast irons are influenced by the following factors.

Amount of Total Carbon

Carbon is a graphitiser. With increasing carbon, the tendency of graphitisation, i.e. formation of graphite by the decomposition of cementite ($Fe_3C \to 3Fe + C$) becomes more and hence leads to the formation of grey cast iron. With higher carbon and slower cooling, the matrix may become ferrite. At a moderate cooling rate and with less amount of carbon, the cast iron may solidify without graphitisation giving all carbon in the combined form and is identified as white cast iron.

Amount of Silicon

Silicon is a strong graphitiser and promotes graphitisation, i.e. decomposition of cementite to iron and graphite and hence its amount is controlled to control the amount of graphitisation. The amount of silicon varies from 0.5 to 3.0 per cent in various commercial cast irons. With lower amount of silicon, the cast iron solidifies as white and with higher amount, it solidifies as grey at a moderate cooling rate.

The effect of alloying elements other than silicon on graphitisation is described in terms of the silicon equivalent by Eq. 8.1.

$$\text{Si equivalent} = \% \text{ Si} + 3 (\% \text{ C}) + \% \text{ P} + 0.3 (\% \text{ Ni})$$
$$+ 0.3 (\% \text{ Cu}) + 0.5 (\% \text{ Al}) - 0.25 (\% \text{ Mn}) \qquad \ldots(8.1)$$
$$- 0.35 (\% \text{ Mo}) - 1.2 (\% \text{ Cr})$$

Non-carbide forming elements Cu, Ni, and Al have positive factors, i.e. they promote the graphitisation whereas carbide forming elements Mo, Cr and Mo have negative factors which limit the graphitisation.

Amount of Phosphorus

Phosphorus is also a strong graphitiser like silicon and its content varies from 0.1 to 0.3 per cent. Most of the phosphorus combines with iron and forms iron phosphide (Fe_3P). This iron phosphide separates out as eutectic mixture with cementite and austenitic. This ternary eutectic of iron phosphide, cementite, and austenitic is called steadite. Steadite has a freezing temperature of about 980°C and is the last to solidify and therefore occupies interdendritic regions. A relatively small percentage of phosphorus produces large volume of steadite and hence with higher amount of phosphorus, the steadite areas may merge to form a continuous network around the primary dendrites of austenitie. Steadite is brittle and therefore, it reduces toughness and increases the brittleness of cast irons. Due to this, the amount of phosphorus must be carefully controlled to obtain optimum mechanical properties. However, phosphorus increases the fluidity of cast irons and makes them, easy to cast into thin and complex sections.

Increasing silicon and phosphorus have almost similar effect as increasing the carbon on the microstructures of cast irons. Their effect in terms of carbon is considered and equivalent carbon is found out as below:

$$\text{Equivalent carbon} = \text{Total carbon} + 1/3 (\text{Silicon} + \text{Phosphorus})$$
$$\text{i.e. E.C} = \text{T.C} + 1/3 (\text{Si} + \text{P}) \qquad \ldots (8.2)$$

For a given cast iron, equivalent carbon may be used for predicting the amount of graphitisation (or graphitisation tendency) similar to that without silicon and phosphorus containing the same amount of total carbon by using $Fe-Fe_3C$ equilibrium diagram. Carbon equivalent value can also be used to predict whether the alloy will solidify as hypoeutectic, eutectic, or hypereutectic. It also predicts the chilling tendency of a given section at constant pouring temperature, cooling rate and alloying elements.

Amount of Sulphur

Sulphur combines with iron and forms iron sulphide (FeS) which is a hard and brittle compound. Due to its low melting point, it appears at interdendritic regions in a solidified casting and increases the brittleness of casting. Addition of manganese reduces the detrimental effect of sulphur. Sulphur has greater affinity for manganese than for iron and hence, in the presence of manganese, the reaction product is manganese sulphide (MnS) instead of iron sulphide (FeS). MnS appears as small and widely distributed inclusions of rounded or polyhedral shape. Unless MnS is present in large amount, it has little effect on the properties of cast iron. The usual sulphur content of any cast iron is between 0.06 to 0.12 per cent.

Also, sulphur, in the form of FeS promotes the formation of iron carbide without participating in its formation. It has a strong effect as carbide stabiliser and about 0.01 per cent sulphur is sufficient to neutralise the graphitising influence of 0.15 per cent silicon. However, when sulphur is present as, MnS, it has almost no influence on carbide or graphite formation.

Amount of Manganese

The most important effect of manganese is to reduce the brittleness likely to be introduced due to the formation of iron sulphide. It takes care of sulphur by forming manganese sulphide. Any excess amount of manganese present after combining with all sulphur and forming MnS serves as an useful alloying element. The usual amount of manganese in any commercial cast iron varies between 0.5 to 1.0 per cent (5 to 8 time the amount of sulphur).

In addition to the above elements, cast irons may contain alloying elements such as nickel, chromium, molybdenum, magnesium, copper, aluminium, boron, etc. which are added to obtain the desired properties and structure.

Cooling Rate

Cooling rate has a pronounced effect on the microstructure of cast irons. Rapid cooling suppresses the graphitisation (i.e. decomposition of Fe_3C to $Fe + C$) and results in white structure. Slow cooling favours the graphitisation of Fe_3C any may result in grey structure. This results in different structures in thin and thick sections of a casting or in a large casting in which the cooling rate varies from surface to centre.

Presence of relative amounts of various elements in cast irons greatly influence their microstructure for the given conditions of casting. The extent of graphitisation or chill depth depends on the amount of graphitising elements, particularly silicon, present in the cast iron alongwith its equivalent carbon, i.e. relative amounts of silicon and carbon determine whether a cast iron will contain cementite, graphite, or both as shown in Fig. 8.1.

In region I, cementite is stable and the structure is that of white cast iron. In region II, there is sufficient silicon to cause graphitisation of all the cementite except the eutectoid cementite (i.e. the cementite in pearlite). This results in grey cast iron with pearlitic matrix. In region III, the large amount of silicon promotes the decomposition of all the cementite and results in the formation of ferrite and graphite, giving a grey cast iron with ferrite matrix. In region II_a, the structures are typical of mottled cast iron and II_b the matrix is pearlitic-ferritic.

The properties of cast irons not only depend on the amount of graphite and type of matrix but also depend on the shape, size, and distribution of graphite present in the cast irons. Graphite is very soft and weak material and therefore, graphite occupied spaces behave almost similar to empty spaces like notches.

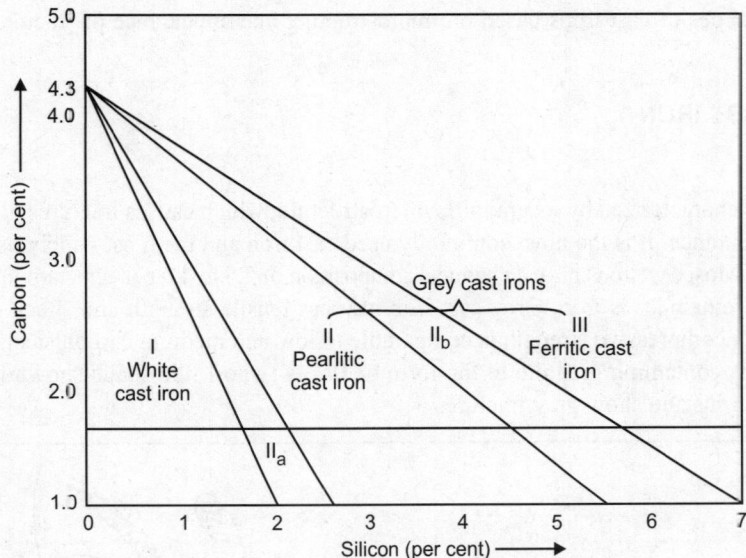

Fig. 8.1. Showing the relation between structures of carbon and silicon content of cast iron.

The amount of graphite can be controlled by controlling the total carbon and the amount of graphitising elements, particularly silicon; shape, size and distribution of graphite can be controlled by addition of certain alloying elements, and the matrix can be controlled by controlling the cooling rate or by a suitable heat treatment. Due to this, it is easy to control the properties of cast irons over a wider limit and because of low cost, they become an attractive engineering material for large number of general purpose applications. The overall factors influencing the mechanical properties of a cast iron are shown in Fig 8.2.

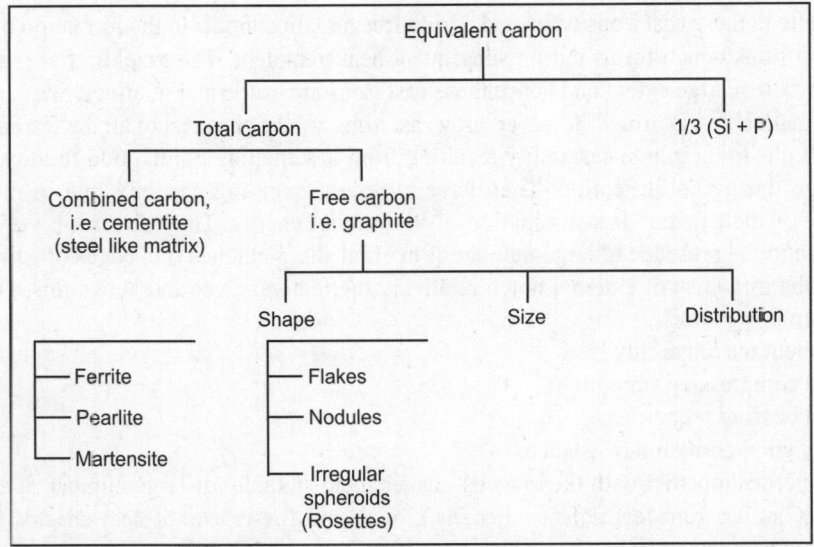

Fig. 8.2. The overall factors influencing the mechanical properties of a cast iron.

The various types of cast irons based on microstructure and appearance of fracture are described below in detail.

TYPES OF CAST IRON

Grey Cast Iron

Grey cast iron is characterized by its graphitic microstructure, which causes fractures of the material to have a grey appearance. It is the most commonly used cast iron and the most widely use cast material based on weight. Most cast irons have a chemical composition of 2.5 to 4.0 per cent carbon, 1 to 3 per cent silicon, and the remainder is iron. Grey cast iron has less tensile strength and shock resistance than steel, however its compressive strength is comparable to low and medium carbon steel.

The cast irons containing graphite in the form of flakes (whorl like shape-shown in Fig. 8.3) are called grey cast irons and show grey fracture.

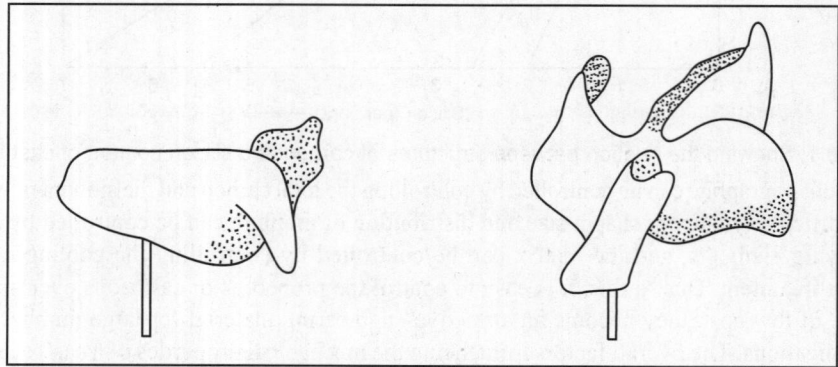

Fig. 8.3. Space models of flake graphite.

The graphite in these cast irons is formed during freezing, in contrast to the formation of graphite in malleable cast irons which forms during subsequent heat treatment. The graphite flakes interrupt the steel like matrix to a large extent and hence these cast irons are brittle and relatively weak in tension as compared to malleable cast irons. However, grey cast irons are the cheapest of all the ferrous alloys and easiest to cast due to their high castability resulting from low melting point, good fluidity of melt and low shrinkage during solidification. They have excellent damping capacity due to more internal discontinuities which favour fast dissipation of vibrational energy. They also have very low notch sensitivity due to the presence of large number of internal sharp notches (i.e. edges of graphite flakes) which make the influence of external notch relatively ineffective. Over and above this, they have the following useful properties:
1. Excellent machinability.
2. Good compressive strength.
3. Good bearing properties.
4. Fairly good corrosion resistance.

These properties together with the low cost makes them suitable for large number of applications. However, they suffer from few defects such, as growth and fire-cracks or heat checks. Growth, i.e. permanent expansion occurs when heated to about 400°C. This result in loss of strength with increased brittleness. Fire-cracks or heat checks occur in the form of cracks due to repeated local heating and cooling to a temperature of the order of 550°C and due to high thermal gradients between the surface and the interior, it leads to failure of the component. These drawbacks may be reduced by the addition of certain alloying elements like chromium, molybdenum and nickel and grain refiners to the grey cast irons.

The composition of the alloy is adjusted in such a way that all the proeutectic (from hypereutectic alloys) and eutectic cementite decomposes as soon as it forms and eutectoid cementite does not decompose. This is done by controlling carbon and silicon in the alloy. If the amount of these two elements is more, eutectoid cementite may also decompose with the normal cooling rates as encountered in sand moulds. This leads to ferritic matrix and the cast iron becomes soft and extremely weak thereby becoming unsuitable for engineering applications. Therefore, a control over the composition must be exercised in such a way that all the proeutectic and eutectic cementite must decompose—obviously this leads to the decomposition of all proeutectoid cementite and no eutectoid cementite should decompose. This is necessary to obtain pearlitic matrix in the grey cast irons. The matrix can also be controlled by controlling the cooling rate through the eutectoid transformation region. These cast irons have the following composition range:

C	3.2 to 3.7 per cent.
Si	2.0 to 3.5 per cent.
S	0.06 to 0.1 per cent.
P	0.1 to 0.2 per cent.
Mn	0.5 to 1.0 per cent.

Their properties depend on composition, and size and distribution of graphite flakes but are roughly in the following range.

T.S	15 to 40 kg/mm
Hardness	150 to 300 BHN
Elongation	Less than 1 per cent

Grey cast irons are widely used for machine bases, engine frames, drainage pipes, elevator and industrial furnace counter weights, pump housings, cylinders and pistons of I.C. engines, flow wheels, etc. Graphite produced due to graphitisation may have different shapes, sizes and distribution depending upon the cooling conditions, composition and presence of certain elements. Different sizes and distribution of graphite flakes leads to different mechanical properties of these cast irons. Depending upon the above variables, cast irons have been classified into different types and grades as follows.

Types of Grey Cast Iron

Depending up on the distribution of graphite flakes, American Foundrymen's Association (AFA) and American Society for Testing Materials (ASTM) jointly have classified the grey cast irons into five types such as type A to type E (Fig. 8.4).

Since graphite is very soft and weak, interdendritic segregation of graphite is not desirable because the cast iron becomes excessively brittle. Therefore, both the type D and E are not desirable and the more regular pattern of type E graphite is still more undesirable than type D. This type of distribution is observed when the alloy solidifies as hypoeutectic alloy with coarse primary dendrites of austenite.

Type C shows superimposed flake sizes and is mixture of few extremetly large and quite straight graphite flakes with large number of much finer flakes. Due to the large amount of graphite and long flakes (superimposed one over the other), this type is also not desirable. This is observed when the alloy solidifies as hypereutectic alloy.

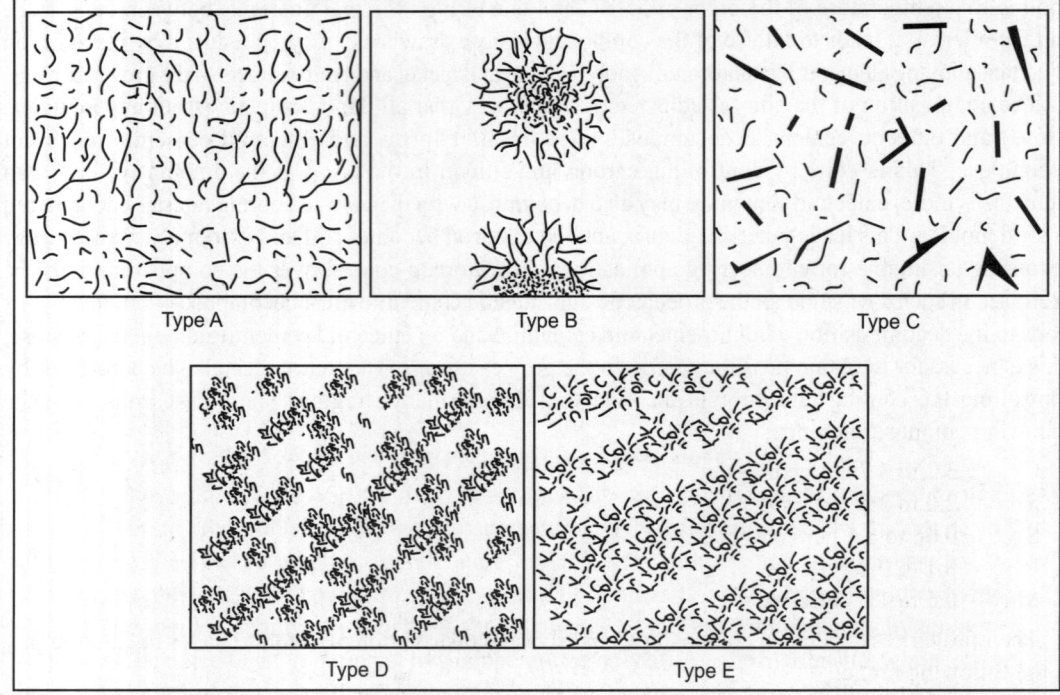

Fig. 8.4. Graphite flake types in grey cast iron: Type A, uniform distribution, random orientation; Type B, rosett groupings, random orientation; Type C, superimposed flakes of various sizes, random orientation; Type D, interdendritic flakes, ramdom orientation; Type E, interdendritic flakes, preferred orientation.

Type B graphite is observed in the mottled region lies between the white and grey. This type of graphite distribution also increases the brittleness and hence is undesirable.

Type A graphite is most desirable because of uniform distribution and random orientation of graphite flakes, since they do not seriously interrupt the continuity of the pearlitic matrix. This type of distribution is observed when the alloy solidifies as an eutectic alloy.

The various undesirable types of graphite flake distributions can be avoided as below:

Type C graphite can be prevented by avoiding the hypereutectic compositions, i.e. by reducing the carbon content of cast iron by the addition of steel scrap.

Type B can be avoided by using compositions high enough in carbon and silicon so that the cast iron does not solidify as mottled at the cooling rates encountered during its freezing.

Type D and E can avoided by using slow cooling rates during freezing. This results in complete divorcement giving A-type of distribution with slightly coarse graphite flakes. This can also be achieved by reducing the austenite dendrite size by the addition of certain grain refiners or inoculants which result in fine graphite flakes.

Once type A distribution is obtained, the properties of grey cast iron depend on the length of graphite flakes. Short graphite flakes create less interruptions in the continuity of steel like matrix and hence give better mechanical properties. Graphite flake sizes are described in terms of flake size number according to the Table 8.1 established jointly by AFA and ASTM.

Table 8.1. Designation of graphite flake sizes.

A.F.A. – A.S.T.M. Flake–size number	Length of longest flake at 100×
1	4 inches or more
2	2 to 4 inches
3	1 to 2 inches
4	1/2 to 1 inch
5	1/4 to 1/2 inch
6	1/8 to 1/4 inch
7	1/16 to 1/8 inch
8	1/16 inch or less

Standard charts have been prepared showing the pictures of these flake sizes at 100 × to facilitate the measurement of flake size number by comparison method (ASTM–A 247 method). These charts are shown in Fig. 8.5.

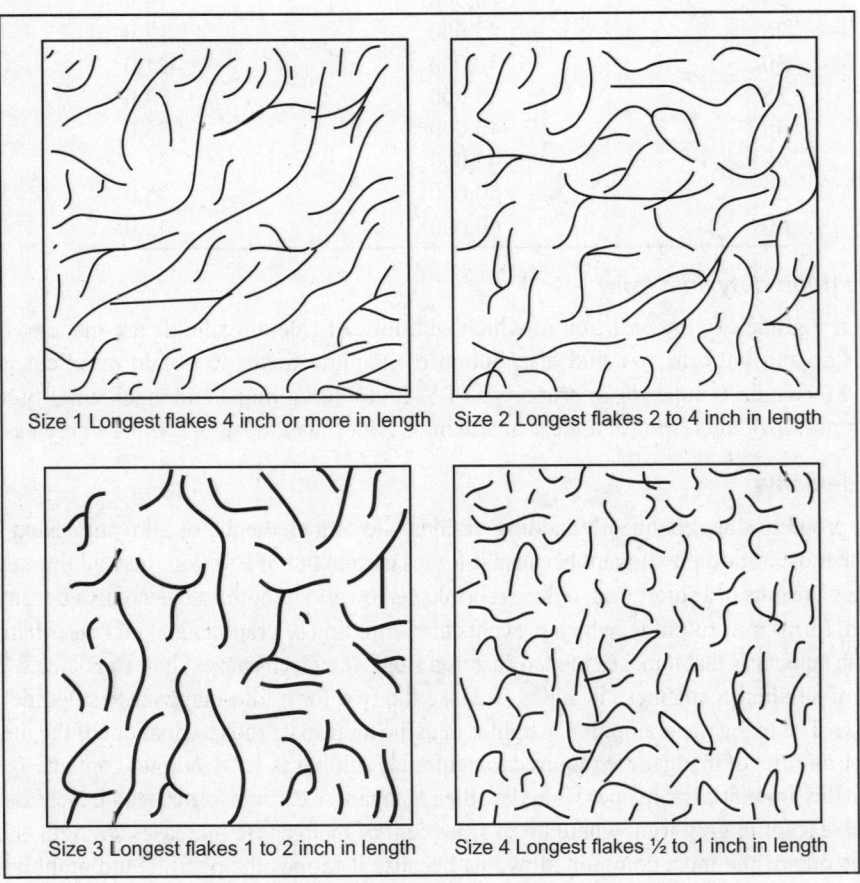

Fig. 8.5. Graphite flake sizes in grey cast iron.

The best method of reducing the size and improving the distribution of graphite flakes is by the addition of a small amount of material called as inoculant. Materials which have been successfully used as inoculants are calcium silicide, silicon carbide, metallic calcium, aluminium, titanium, zirconium or combination of these. The inoculating agent might be increasing the nucleation rate giving a fine grain size of austenite or it must be momentarily displacing the eutectic point to the left, i.e. towards low carbon side so that a hypoeutectic cast iron will solidify as an eutectic cast iron, eliminating the primary austenite crystals.

Grades of grey cast iron

Due to the wide range of compositions used to obtain grey cast irons and since the properties of these irons are dependent not only on the matrix structure but also on the length, distribution and orientation of graphite flakes, they are graded according to the tensile strength as below:

Grade	T.S. (minute) lb/in^2 (as per ASTM-AFS)	T.S. (minute in kg/mm^2)
20	20,000	14.0
25	25,000	17.0
30	30,000	21.0
35	35,000	24.0
40	40,000	28.0
45	45,000	31.0
50	50,000	35.0
60	60,000	42.0

Meehanite (high duty cast iron)

Meehanite is a grade of grey cast iron in which additions of calcium silicide are made to the melt to produce a fine and uniform size and distribution of graphite flakes to obtain excellent mechanical properties. Meehanite is superior in properties (T.S.-25 to 40 kg/mm^2) and machinability to ordinary grey cast irons. Also, the response to heat treatment is better than those of ordinary grey cast irons.

Alloying Elements

Cast iron's properties are changed by adding various alloying elements, or alloyants. Next to carbon, silicon is the most important alloyant because it forces carbon out of solution. Instead the carbon forms graphite which results in a softer iron, reduces shrinkage, lowers strength, and decreases density. Sulphur, when added, forms iron sulphide, which prevents the formation of graphite and increases hardness. The problem with sulphur is that it makes molten cast iron sluggish, which causes short run defects. To counter the effects of sulphur, manganese is added because the two form into manganese sulphide instead of iron sulphide. The manganese sulphide is lighter than the melt so it tends to float out of the melt and into the slag. The amount of manganese required to neutralise sulphur is 1.7 × sulphur content +0.3 per cent. If more than this amount of manganese is added, then manganese carbide forms, which increases hardness and chilling, except in grey iron, where up to 1 per cent of manganese increases strength and density.

Nickel is one of the most common alloyants because it refines the pearlite and graphite structure, improves toughness, and evens out hardness differences between section thicknesses. Chromium is added in small amounts to the ladle to reduce free graphite, produce chill, and because it is a powerful carbide stabiliser; nickel is often added in conjunction. A small amount of tin can be added as a substitute for 0.5 per cent chromium. Copper is added in the ladle or in the furnace, on the order of 0.5 to 2.5 per cent, to decrease chill, refine graphite, and increase fluidity. Molybdenum is added on the order of 0.3 to 1 per cent to increase chill and refine the graphite and pearlite structure; it is often added in conjunction with nickel, copper, and chromium to form high strength irons. Titanium is added as a degasser and deoxidiser, but it also increases fluidity 0.15 to 0.5 per cent vanadium are added to cast iron to stabilise cementite, increase hardness, and increase resistance to wear and heat. 0.1 to 0.3 per cent zirconium helps to form graphite, deoxidise, and increase fluidity.

In malleable iron melts, bismuth is added, on the scale of 0.002 to 0.01 per cent, to increase how much silicon can be added. In white iron, boron is added to aid in the production of malleable iron; it also reduces the coarsening effect of bismuth.

White Cast Iron

With a lower silicon content and faster cooling, the carbon in white cast iron precipitates out of the melt as the metastable phase cementite, Fe_3C, rather than graphite. The cementite which precipitates from the melt forms as relatively large particles, usually in a eutectic mixture, where the other phase is austenite (which on cooling might transform to martensite). These eutectic carbides are much too large to provide precipitation hardening (as in some steels, where cementite precipitates might inhibit plastic deformation by impeding the movement of dislocations through the ferrite matrix). Rather, they increase the bulk hardness of the cast iron simply by virtue of their own very high hardness and their substantial volume fraction, such that the bulk hardness can be approximated by a rule of mixtures. In any case, they offer hardness at the expense of toughness. Since carbide makes up a large fraction of the material, white cast iron could reasonably be classified as a cermet. White iron is too brittle for use in many structural components, but with good hardness and abrasion resistance and relatively low cost, it finds use in such applications as the wear surfaces (impeller and volute) of slurry pumps, shell liners and lifter bars in ball mills and autogenous grinding mills, balls and rings in coal pulverisers, and the teeth of a backhoe's digging bucket (although cast medium-carbon martensitic steel is more common for this application).

It is difficult to cool thick castings fast enough to solidify the melt as white cast iron all the way through. However, rapid cooling can be used to solidify a shell of white cast iron, after which the remainder cools more slowly to form a core of grey cast iron. The resulting casting, called a chilled casting, has the benefits of a hard surface and a somewhat tougher interior.

High-chromium white iron alloys allow massive castings (for example, a 10-ton impeller) to be sand cast, i.e. a high cooling rate is not required, as well as providing impressive abrasion resistance.

In these cast irons, all the carbon is present in the form of combined carbon, i.e. cementite and there is no free carbon, i.e. graphite. The appearance of a fractured surface is white because of absence of graphite and hence the name is 'white cast iron'. Since there is no graphitisation, the solidification of a white cast iron and the resulting microstructural changes can be exactly indicated by the $Fe-Fe_3C$ equilibrium diagram.

The graphitisation is supressed by controlling the chemical composition and cooling rate. Lower silicon content, lower carbon content and rapid cooling results in the prevention of decomposition of cementite.

Cooling of a Hypoeutetic Cast Iron with 3 per cent Carbon

The above cast iron is indicated at 3 per cent carbon on Fe–Fe$_3$C equilibrium diagram in Fig. 8.6 and cooling from the molten state is explained below:
1. From 1 to 2, the alloy is in the liquid state and there is no change in the state of the alloy.
2. Just below 2, austenite starts separating out from the liquid and further cooling will increase the amount of austenite. This continues upto 3. This primary or proeutectic austenite is in the dendritic form since it is separating out from the liquid state. The amount of austenite according to lever rule at just above 3 will be:

$$\text{Amount of austenite (of 2.0\% carbon)} = \frac{4.3 - 3.0}{4.3 - 2.0} = 56.5\%$$

 The remaining 43.5 per cent of the alloy still exists in the liquid state with 4.3 per cent carbon. The microstructure is shown in Fig. 8.7 (a).
3. At 3, the above liquid of eutectic composition solidifies at constant temperature (1147°C) and forms an eutectic mixture of austenite and cementite called ledeburite as indicated below:

$$\underset{\text{(of 4.3 \% C)}}{\text{Liquid}} \xrightarrow{1147°C} \underset{\text{(of 2.0 \% C)}}{\gamma} + \underset{\text{(of 6.67 \% C)}}{Fe_3C}$$

 Since ledeburite is formed at high temperature, its structure is coarse. The microstructure is shown in Fig. 8.7 (b).
4. From 3 to 4, almost there is no change in the morphology of the existing structure. However, due to the decrease in solubility of carbon in austenite, it — both primary and eutectic austenite-rejects Fe$_3$C to the adjacent eutectic cementitic areas. Due to this, the amount of Fe$_3$C increases. The Fe$_3$C which separates out from point 3 to 4 is called proeutectoid cementite.
5. At 4, all the austenite-primary as well as eutectic-transforms isothermally to an eutectoid mixture of ferrite and cementite, i.e. pearlite.

$$\underset{\text{(of 0.8 \% C)}}{\gamma} \xrightarrow{727°C} \underset{\text{(of 0.025 \% C)}}{\alpha} + \underset{\text{(of 6.67 \% C)}}{Fe_3C}$$

 The microstructure is shown in Fig. 8.4 (c).
6. From 4 to 5, there is almost no change in microstructure except slight increase in the amount of Fe$_3$C due to the decrease in solubility of carbon in ferrite from 0.025 per cent to 0.008 per cent.

At room temperature the microstructure consists of dendritic areas of transformed austenite, i.e. pearlite in a matrix of transformed ledeburite (Fe$_3$C + pearlite).

Cooling of an Eutectic Cast Iron

This alloy solidifies at eutectic temperature (i.e. 1147°C) by an eutectic transformation process and gives a mixture of austenite and cementite, i.e. ledeburite with no proeutectic phase. Further cooling from eutectic to eutectoid temperature (i.e. 1147° to 727°C) only increases the amount of Fe$_3$C without change of morphology of structure due to the separation of poroeutectoid Fe$_3$C from eutectic austenite because of decrease in solubility of carbon in austenite. At eutectoid temperature (i.e. 727°C), the austenite transforms to pearlite. Cooling from 727°C to room temperature slightly increases the amount of cementite due to decrease in solubility of carbon in ferrite.

At room temperature, the microstructure consists of cementite and pearlite called transformed ledeburite.

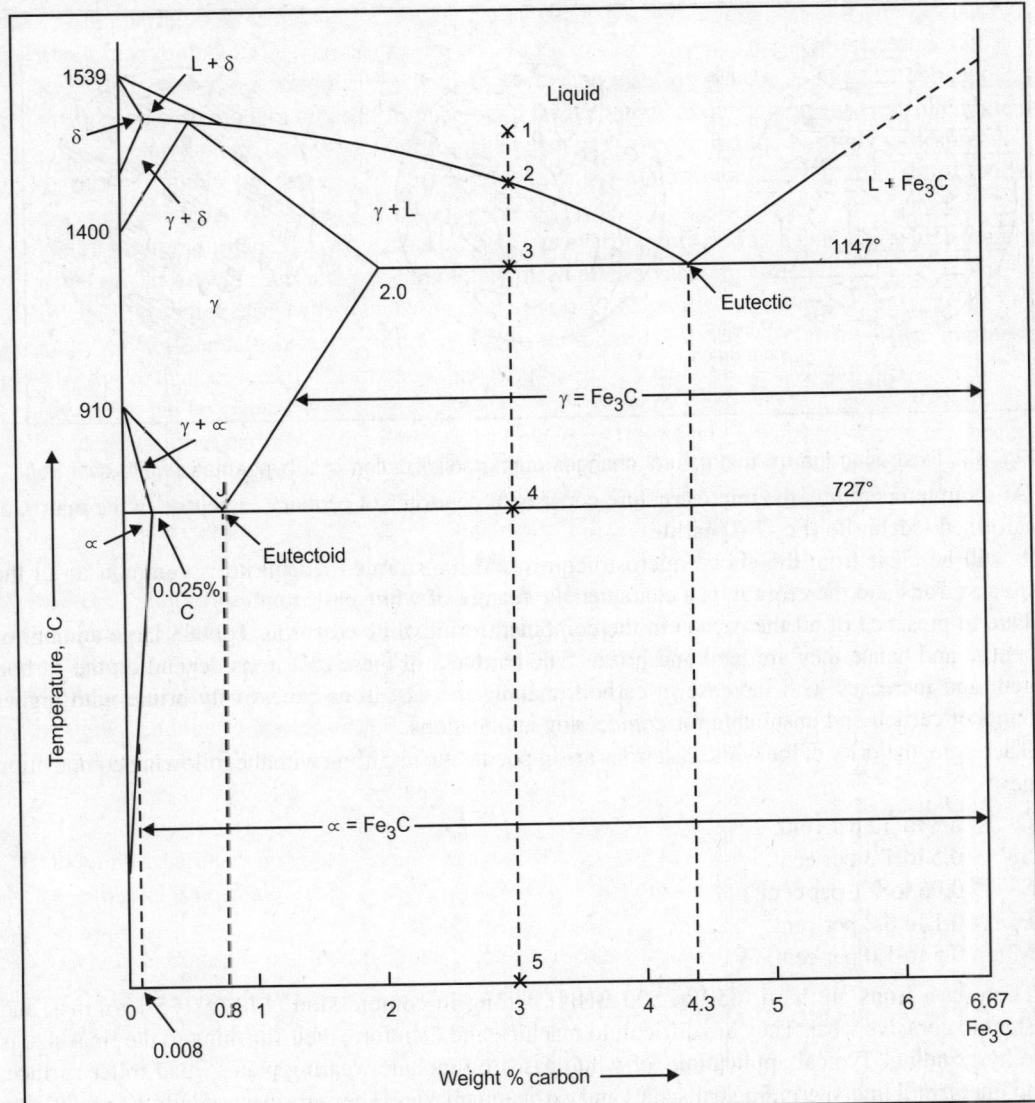

Fig. 8.6. Fe–Fe$_3$C equilibrium diagram used to explain the cooling of 3.0 per cent carbon alloy.

Cooling of a Hypereutectic White Cast Iron

The microstructural changes during cooling of this cast iron are almost similar to that explained for a hypoeutectic cast iron except the proeutectic phase separating our from liquid being cementite instead of austenite. During freezing, primary cementite separates out first from the liquid in the dendritic from upto eutectic temperature and at the eutectic temperature, the remaining liquid solidifies as eutectic mixture of cementite and austenite. Rest of the changes are similar to that explained for a hypoeutectic white cast iron.

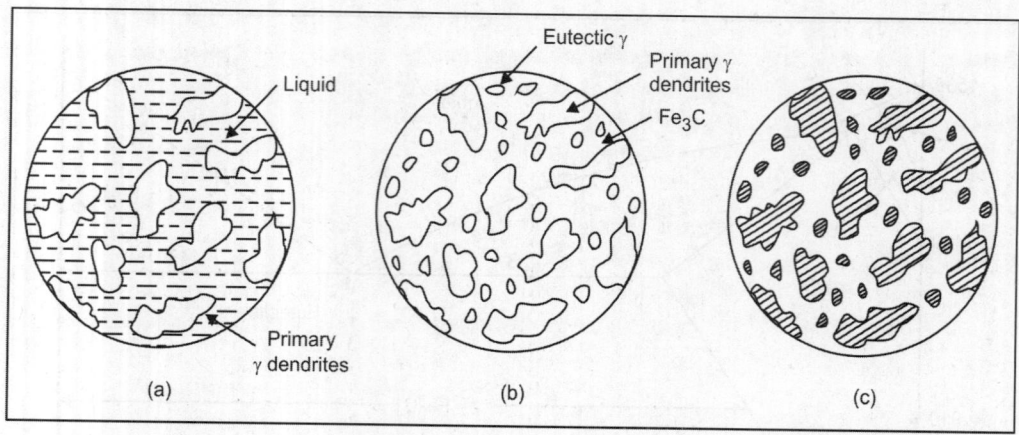

Fig. 8.7. Illustrating the microstructural changes during solidification of a hypoeutetic white cast iron.

At room temperature, the microstructure consists of dendrites of primary cementite in the matrix of transformed ledeburite (Fe_3C + pearlite).

It will be clear from the above microstructures that transformed ledeburite is common in all the white cast irons and therefore it, is a characteristic feature of white cast irons.

Due to presence of all the carbon in the combined form, white cast irons contain large amount of cementite and hence they are hard and brittle. The hardness of these cast irons depend on the carbon content and increases with increase in carbon, making the cast irons excessively brittle with higher amounts of carbon and unsuitable for engineering applications.

Therefore, majority of the white cast irons are hypoeutectic in carbon with the following composition range:

C	2.3 to 30 per cent.
Si	0.5 to 1.3 per cent.
S	0.06 to 0.1 per cent.
P	0.1 to 0.2 per cent.
Mn	0.5 to 1.0 per cent.

These cast irons are hard (350 to 500 BHN), strong in compression (140 to 175 kg/mm^2), and resistant to abrasive wear. They are difficult to machine and therefore, their finishing to the final size is done by grinding. Typical applications of white cast iron include wearing plates, road roller surface, pump liners, mill liners, grinding balls, dies and extrusion nozzles. They are also used for the production of malleable castings. They are not employed for structural parts because of their excessive brittleness.

Malleable Cast Iron

Malleable iron starts as a white iron casting that is then heat treated at about 900°C (1650°F). Graphite separates out much more slowly in this case, so that surface tension has time to form it into spheroidal particles rather than flakes. Due to their lower aspect ratio, spheroids are relatively short and far from one another, and have a lower cross section vis-a-vis a propagating crack or phonon. They also have blunt boundaries, as opposed to flakes, which alleviates the stress concentration problems faced by grey cast iron. In general, the properties of malleable cast iron are more like mild steel. There is a limit to how large a part can be cast in malleable iron, since it is made from white cast iron.

These cast irons are produced from white cast iron castings by a malleablising heat treatment (malleablising anneal). The heat treatment consists of heating the white castings slowly (to avoid cracking) to a temperature between eutectoid and eutectic temperatures, usually at around 900°C (800°–950°C) and holding at this temperature for a long time (24 hours to several days) followed by cooling to room temperature. The above heat treatment cycle is shown in Fig. 8.8.

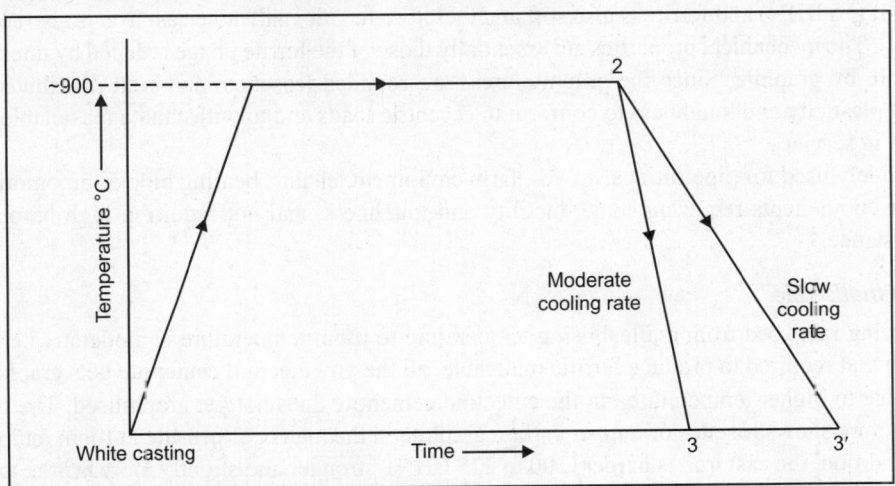

Fig. 8.8. Malleablising heat treatment cycle.

Due to heating to 900°C (i.e. at point 1), the structure of cast iron consists of austenite and cementite. Cementite being a metastable phase, decomposes to austenite and graphite (i.e. temper carbon graphite) with a long holding time.

The above graphitisation of cementite gives rise to rough, ragged irregular nodules or spheroids called as rosettes of temper carbon graphite. Therefore, at point 2 the structure consists of rosettes of temper carbon graphite in a matrix of austenite. Cooling to room temperature with moderate cooling rate results in the transformation of austenite to pearlite at eutectoid temperature and therefore at 3, the microstructure shows rosettes of temper carbon graphite in the matrix of pearlite.

However, if the cooling rate is slow (or if the silicon in the white casting is more), the cementite from pearlite may also decompose giving ferrite and graphite and the structure at room temperature, i.e. at 3′ may show rosettes of temper carbon graphite in the matrix of ferrite. For intermediate conditions, the matrix may be pearlite and ferrite.

These rosettes disrupt the steel like matrix (pearlite or ferrite) much less as compared to the flake graphite of grey cast irons and therefore they greatly diminish the internal notch effects. Due to this, these cast irons show some ductility, toughness and are bendable in contrast to grey cast irons which are brittle. Hence, they are called as malleable cast irons. In the ordinary sense, they are not malleable because they can not be rolled, forged, or extruded to an appreciable degree. Their properties vary with the matrix and are as below:

T.S.   25 to 70 kg/mm^2
Elongation 6 to 18 per cent
Hardness   80 to 275 BHN

Types of Malleable Cast Iron

Depending on the microstructure or appearance of fracture malleable cast irons are classified as below:

Ferritic malleable

The matrix is ferritic due to slow cooling from malleablising temperature to room temperature. Graphite is very soft (~5 BHN) and ferrite is also soft and therefore ferritic malleable cast iron is also soft (80 to 100 BHN). The mechanical properties are essentially those of the ferrite phage reduced by interruptions in structure by graphite. Since the graphite areas are rounded (rosettes) and well distributed, it has sufficient plasticity and toughness to conform to eccentric loads and to withstand a reasonable amount of impact in service.

It is widely used for pipe fittings, valves, farm equipment, chains, bearing blocks, automotive parts and other components requiring some ductility and toughness, and not requiring high hardness and wear resistance.

Pearlitic malleable

If the cooling rate used from malleablising temperature to room temperature is moderate, i.e. slightly more than that required to produce ferritic malleable, all the proeutectoid cementite gets graphitised as it forms due to higher temperature but the eutectoid cementite does not get graphitised. The resulting microstructure shows rosettes of temper carbon graphite in the matrix of pearlite at room temperature. In this condition, the cast iron is harder (200 to 275 BHN), stronger and slightly more brittle, and some what more difficult to machine than the ferritic (or ferritic-pearlitic) malleable cast iron.

If the cooling rate is increased, the matrix may result in martensite instead of pearlite and the cast iron becomes hard and brittle and its toughness—which is the major advantage of malleable cast iron—is lost. Therefore, cooling rates higher than needed to form a completely pearlitic matrix are never purposely used in the production of malleable cast irons. Some of the applications of pearlitic malleable cast iron are camshafts, crankshafts, axles, gears, links and ordnance parts. They are also used for electrical applications such as switch gear parts, fittings for high and low voltage transmission and distribution systems, and for railway electrification systems.

Pearlitic-ferritic malleable

This is produced due to intermediate cooling rate between those to produce ferritic malleable and pearlitic malleable cast irons.

The cooling rate used from malleablising temperature to room temperature is slow enough to graphitise all the proeutectoid cementite and a part of the eutectoid cementite. Since carbon itself is a graphitiser, the cementite from pearlite adjacent to the existing rosettes of temper carbon graphite decomposes rapidly without graphitising cementite away from these rosettes. Therefore, the microstructure at room temperature shows rosettes of temper carbon graphite surrounded by an envelope of ferrite. The matrix is usually coarse pearlite or slightly spheroidised due to slow cooling. They are intermediate in properties to those of ferritic and pearlitic malleable cast irons.

Black heart malleable

This cast iron shows dark grey appearance in the central region or core. This is due to decarburisation at the surface. This decarburised ferritic layer has no temper carbon and hence appears bright whereas the presence of graphite (which is black in colour) makes the core or centre to appear dark grey. Because of its unusual fracture, the cast iron is identified as black heart malleable. It is simply a ferritic (or pearlitic) malleable cast iron in which a decarburised layer of observable thickness has been formed.

White heart malleable

This cast iron shows white fracture from centre to surface. It is a cast iron completely free from temper carbon graphite with ferritic skin or case. If the graphite from a malleable cast iron is completely removed by decarburisation, it becomes a white heart malleable cast iron. The structure no more appears like a cast iron but is similar to steel. The chemical composition of the alloy, particularly carbon and silicon contents, play an important role in production, heat treatment and final properties of these cast irons. In the manufacture of malleable cast irons, it is desirable that the amount of graphitising elements should be as high as possible to minimise the malleablising period required for complete graphitisation. However, if the amount of graphitising elements are more, the melt will not solidify as white but may solidify as mottled or grey and hence a proper balance of carbon and silicon contents must be maintained to optimise the production of malleable castings. The mechanical properties are superior when the carbon content is less because of less amount of graphite formed (1 per cent free carbon by weight corresponds to about 4 per cent graphite by volume). However, reduction in carbon content raises the liquidus temperature and hence requires higher pouring temperatures which increases the general casting troubles.

Ductile Cast Iron

A more recent development is nodular or ductile cast iron. Tiny amounts of magnesium or cerium added to these alloys slow down the growth of graphite precipitates by bonding to the edges of the graphite planes. Along with careful control of other elements and timing, this allows the carbon to separate as spheroidal particles as the material solidifies. The properties are similar to malleable iron, but parts can be cast with larger sections. These cast irons contain graphite in the form of nodules or spheroids. Due to this, the interruption in the steel like matrix is less as compared to the interruptions produced by flake graphite of grey cast irons. This increases the tensile strength, ducitility and toughness. They are also called as spheroidal graphite cast irons (SGCI) or ductile cast irons.

They are produced from grey cast irons by the addition of small quality of certain elements called as nodulising elements such as magnesium, cerium, calcium, barium, lithium or zirconicum. The most common addition to grey cast iron for the production of nodular castings is magnesium. The addition of Mg (0.06 to 0.08 per cent) is done to the grey cast iron melt usually in the ladle just prior to pouring into the moulds. Any delay in pouring results in the distortion of nodular shape of graphite and reduction in properties of these cast irons. The effect of nodulising elements is purely temporary and is lost due to long holing time. Remelting of nodular cast iron produces grey cast iron, unless fresh nodulising addition is done. All the nodulising elements including Mg have low density and are highly chemically reactive. If they are added in the pure from, they simply float to the top of the bath and burn or decompose at the surface. Therefore, they are usually added in the form of master alloys.

Also, these elements have strong affinity for sulphur and they scavenge sulphur form the molten bath as an initial step in producing nodular graphite. The additions are expensive and hence for effective utilisation of these elements, the original grey iron melt must contain less amount of sulphur (< 0.03 per cent). The sulphur (and also phosphorus) is reduced by treating the melt with soda ash (sodium carbonate).

When nodulising element is added to the molten bath and stirred, large amount of gas is evolved and also gets dissolved in the melt. This dissolved gas gives rise to large number of blow holes in the solidified casting. Also, the contraction of nodular cast iron during freezing is considerably greater than that of ordinary grey cast iron. Due to this, careful design of the mould is necessary to avoid shrinkage cavities in the solidified casting. Inspite of these difficulties, nodular cast irons are popular due to their high tensile strength, ductility and toughness. They combine the advantages of cast irons and steels. They do not suffer from the defects of grey cast irons such as growth and fire-cracks when used at elevated temperatures. The mechanism by which graphite nodules are formed is not known with certainty. It is postulated that the addition of nodulising elements may be affecting the surface tension favouring the nodule formation. The matrix of a nodular cast iron can be controlled by controlling composition, i.e. carbon and silicon or alloying elements or by cooling rate. The range of properties of the cast irons is given below:

TS	38 to 80 kg/mm.
Elongation	6 to 20 per cent.
Hardness	100 to 300 BHN.

It is widely used for crankshafts, gears, punch dies, sheet metal dies, metal working rolls, furnace doors, pipes, pistons, cylinder blocks and heads and bearing blocks.

MOTTLED CAST IRONS

These cast irons shown free cementite as well as graphite flakes in their microstructure. For certain compositions, particularly in terms of carbon and silicon content, such structures are observed under the existing conditions of cooling. For a given composition, faster cooling gives white structure and slow cooling result in grey structure. For intermediate cooling rates, mottled structure is observed. Hence, mottled structure is also observed in certain region between the surface and centre of a chilled casting.

Mottled structures do not have good properties and should be avoided This is done by increasing the carbon and silicon contents in sufficient amount so that the melt solidifies as grey instead of mottled under the existing conditions of cooling.

CHILLED CAST IRONS

This type of cast iron shows white structure at surface and grey structure in the centre. Due to this, the good properties of white cast iron (hardness and were resistance) and grey cast iron (machinability, damping capacity and low notch sensitivity) can be coupled together in a chilled casting.

The composition of melt is adjusted in such a manner that rapid cooling gives white structure and usual cooling gives grey structure. Generally carbon content varies between 3.3 to 3.5 per cent with silicon between 2.0 to 2.5 per cent. Surface is cooled fast by using metal or graphite chillers or chill plates. The depth of chill, i.e. the thickness of white layer can be controlled by controlling the carbon and silicon contents and by other alloying additions which are either carbide formers or graphitisers. Increase in the amount of carbon, silicon, and graphitisers decreases the chill depth, whereas decreases in carbon, silicon, and increase in carbide formers increases the chill depth.

Chilled cast irons are used for railways-freight-car wheels, crushing rolls, grinding balls, road rollers, hammers, dies and such other applications. 'Chill test' is used to obtain the idea about the depth of chill in chilled castings. Chill depth is evaluated by solidifying the cast iron melt in a suitable shaped mould such as wedge or step bar which gives variable cooling rate during solidification. A test sample of melt from cupola or ladle is poured into a sand mould of the above shape. High rates of cooling prevent graphitisation and give white iron whereas low rates of cooling give grey iron. The test sample is fractured and the chill depth, i.e. the zone which appears white is estimated by observing the fracture surface. These change in structure at different places reflect in hardness values which are illustrated in Fig. 8.9 for a step bar casting.

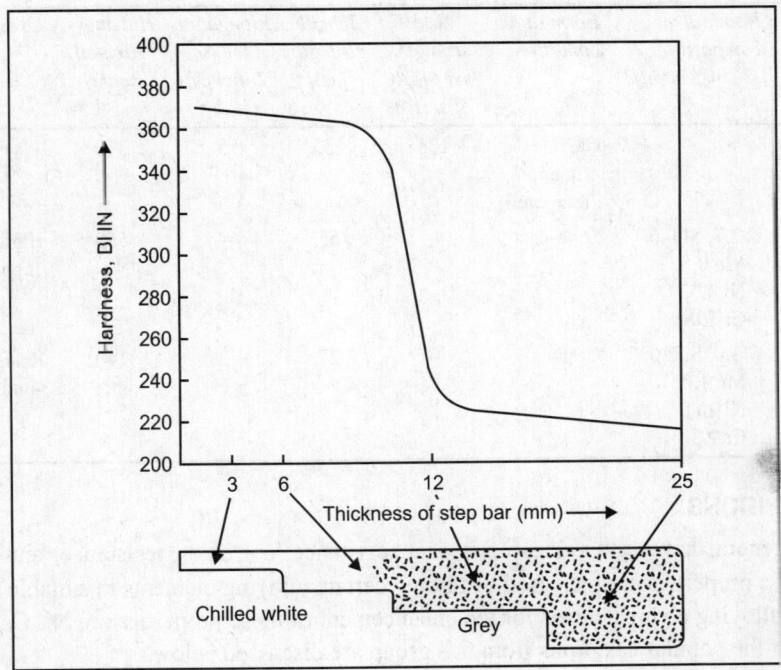

Fig. 8.9. The effect of thickness of cross-section on the rate of cooling, and subsequently upon the microstructure of a grey cast iron.

Table 8.2 gives comparative qualities of cast irons.

Table 8.2. Comparative qualities of cast irons.

Name	Nominal composition [% by weight]	Form and condition	Yield strength [ksi (0.2% offset)]	Tensile strength [ksi]	Elongation [% (in 2 inches)]	Hardness [Brinell scale]	Uses
Grey cast iron (ASTM A48)	C 3.4, Si 1.8, Mn 0.5	Cast	–	25	0.5	180	Engine cylinder blocks, flywheels cylinder blocks, flywheels, gears, machine-tool bases
White cast iron	C 3.4, Si 0.7, Mn 0.6	Cast (as cast)	–	25	0	450	Bearing surfaces
Malleable iron (ASTM A47)	C 2.5, Si 1.0, Mn 0.55	Cast (annealed)	33	52	12	130	Axle bearings, track wheels, automotive crankshafts
Ductile or nodular iron	C 3.4, P 0.1, Mn 0.4, Ni 1.0, Mg 0.06	Cast	53	70	18	170	Gears, camshafts, crankshafts

(Contd ...)

Name	Nominal composition [% by weight]	Form and condition	Yield strength [ksi (0.2% offset)]0	Tensile strength [ksi]	Elongation [% (in 2 inches)]	Hardness [Brinell scale]	Uses
Ductile or nodular iron (ASTM A339)	–	Cast (quench tempered)	108	135	5	310	–
Ni-hard type 2	C 2.7, Si 0.6, Mn 0.5, Ni 4.5, Cr 2.0	Sand-cast	—	55	—	550	High strength applications
Ni-resist type 2	C 3.0, Si 2.0, Mn 1.0, Ni 20.0, Cr 2.5	Cast	—	27	2	140	Resistance to heat and corrosion

ALLOY CAST IRONS

Cast irons in general have low values of impact resistance, corrosion resistance, and temperature resistance. These properties are increased by adding certain alloying elements in suitable amount. The most common alloying elements used for the enhancement of these properties are Ni, Cr, Mo, V, Cu, and Si. Some of the popular cast irons from this group are discussed below.

Ni-Hard

The hardness and wear resistance of white cast iron is increased by the addition of addition of nickel and, chromum with improvement in toughness. Due to increased, harden ability resulting from the addition of these elements, austenite transforms to martensite during solidification of the alloy. Because of more carbon and alloying elements in austenite, M_f is below room temperature and hence austenite-martensite transformation does not go to completion at room temperature. The microstructure shows massive carbides in martensite-austenite matrix with a morphology similar to that of white cast iron structure without the alloying additions.

If only nickel is added for the above purpose, there is a danger of graphitisation because nickel is a graphitiser. As a graphitiser, it is considered half as powerful as silicon. To, avoid the risk of graphitisation, chromium is added which is a carbide former. By proper adjustment of the amounts of nickel and chromium, graphitisation is prevented.

Ni-hard contains about 3 to 5 per cent nickel and 1 to 3 per cent chromium. Such a cast iron shows hardness in the range of 550 to 700 BHN as against 350 to 500 BHN of white cast irons.

Ni-hard contains continuous massive carbides and hence has poor impact strength. It also has poor fatigue resistance. To improve these properties, the continuous network of carbides is replaced by discontinuous carbides by increasing the amount of nickel and chromium. Such a cast iron contains 4 to 8 per cent nickel and 4 to 15 per cent chromium and is called modified Ni-hard. Increased amount of Ni and Cr give rise to increased amount of untransformed austenite in the cast condition. This untransformed austenite is transformed to martensite and bainite by a suitable heat treatment. The microstructure of modified Ni-hard after heat treatment shows discontinuous carbides in a matrix of tempered martensite and bainite.

Ni-Resist

Increase in corrosion resistance of a grey or nodular cast iron is obtained by adding large amount of nickel. Nickel is an austenite stabiliser and hence the matrix becomes austenitic. Therefore such cast irons are called as austenitic cast irons. Ni-resist contains 14 to 36 per cent nickel and 1 to 8 per cent chromium. Some of the grades contain copper between 5 to 8 per cent. The microstructure consists of flakes or nodules of graphite uniformly distributed in the matrix of austenite.

They have better corrosion resistance, excellent erosion resistance to the flow of liquids and fairly good were resistance. Also, they have good scaling and growth resistance upto about 800°C after a stabilising treatment. Typical properties of Ni-resist are as below:

T.S   15 to 36 kg/mm^2.
Hardness   100 to 250 BHN.
Elongation   5 to 20 per cent.

They are used in applications requiring high corrosion, erosion, and heat resistance. Some of the applications are generator and motor covers, pump 'bodies and impellers, valve seatings, exhaust manifolds, furnace parts, sewage pipes and cylinder liners.

Silal and Nicrosilal

Silicon in amounts 5 to 7 per cent is added to low carbon cast irons to increase oxidation resistance and to prevent growth of cast irons at elevated service temperatures. The microstructure of these cast irons consists of ferrite and fine graphite. Such a cast iron is called Silal.

The most serious drawback of Silal is its brittleness. Addition of nickel and chromium, reduces the brittleness by changing the ferritic matrix to austenitic matrix. Such cast irons are called Nicrosilal. The approximate range of composition of Nicrosilal is as below:

C   2.0 to 2.3 per cent.
Si   5 to 6 per cent.
Ni   18 to 22 per cent.
Cr   2 to 4 per cent.

They are used for exhaust manifolds, gas turbine components, aluminium melting crucibles, glass moulds, retorts, and such other applications.

HEAT TREATMENT OF CAST IRONS

Structure and properties of cast irons may be improved by suitable heat treatments. Some of the important heat treatments used to improve service behaviour of cast irons are as follows:

Stress Relieving

Internal stresses are developed due to uneven cooling which occurs during solidification or casting. These stresses increase the brittleness and also distort the component. The above drawbacks are eliminated by heating the castings to a temperature of 400°–500°C for few hours. This relieves the internal stresses and is called seasoning of castings.

Annealing

Machinability of some of the castings may be improved by annealing from a temperature of 800° to 900°C. This results in decomposition of cementite into ferrite and graphite, improving machinability. If cementite is not present in the casting, annealing does not produce any significant effect on properties except in lowering the internal stress level.

Malleablising heat treatment of white cast iron is an annealing process and hence, it is also called as *malleablise annealing*.

Hardening and Tempering

Cast irons can be hardened and tempered as steels because of their high carbon content and sufficient hardenability. Combined carbon dissolves rapidly whereas free carbon (i.e. graphite) dissolves very slowly in austenite and hence to bring substantial amount of carbon in austenitie within a reasonable soaking period for effective hardening, the cast iron must contain combined carbon, i.e. the matrix should be pearlitic. Ferritic cast irons show almost no response to hardening with the usual period of soaking.

The heat treatment consists of heating the pearlitic (or pearlitic + ferritic) cast iron to just above the upper critical temperature and cooling rapidly to room temperature, usually in oil. This results in increase in hardness and wear resistance due to the formation of martensite. Hardened castings are tempered at around 300°C for improvement in toughness and ductility.

Surface Hardening

Pearlitic cast irons may be surface hardened by flame hardening or induction hardening similar to that of steels to increase hardness, wear resistance and abrasion resistance of the surface. Cast irons may also be nitrided for the same purpose.

Chapter 9
Powder Metallurgy

INTRODUCTION

Powder metallurgy is that branch of fabrication which is concerned with the production of finished, or semi-finished products from basic materials in the form of powders. In general, the ability of the process to change these powders into solid metals depends firstly upon the principles of solid phase welding and secondly upon the transposition of matter by diffusion processes. Melting may or may not take place, depending upon the alloy system concerned.

Before the powder metallurgy product can be made, two conditions must be fulfilled:
1. It must be possible to form a continuously bonded matrix. If one metal constituent is to form a continuous matrix, then that metal, in powder form, must be able to respond to solid phase welding; or if an alloy is to be formed, the constituent powders must be able first of all to respond to solid phase welding and then must be capable of diffusion into one another.
2. The powders in which the basic materials are available must be capable of sufficiently close packing under pressure to permit welding to take place and, in the case of alloying, be capable of being sufficiently intimately mixed.

It must always be borne in mind that the size of product from powder metallurgy is bound to be limited, both by handling strength considerations during manufacture and by economic limitations upon equipment size. It must be further borne in mind that only relatively large numbers of a product will justify its manufacture by what is either a mass-production or continuous-production method.

METHODS

The method of powder metallurgical manufacture can be divided roughly into four stages; but each stage may have many subdivisions and variations. The four stages are:
1. Powder preparation.
2. Mixing.
3. Compacting.
4. Sintering.

Stages 3 and 4 may be performed simultaneously in some applications. The compacting process may include both drying and baking, and sintering may be subdivided into stages and may be followed by further fabrication in the form of mechanical working and/or heat treatment. Flow diagram for making powder metallurgy components is shown in Fig. 9.1.

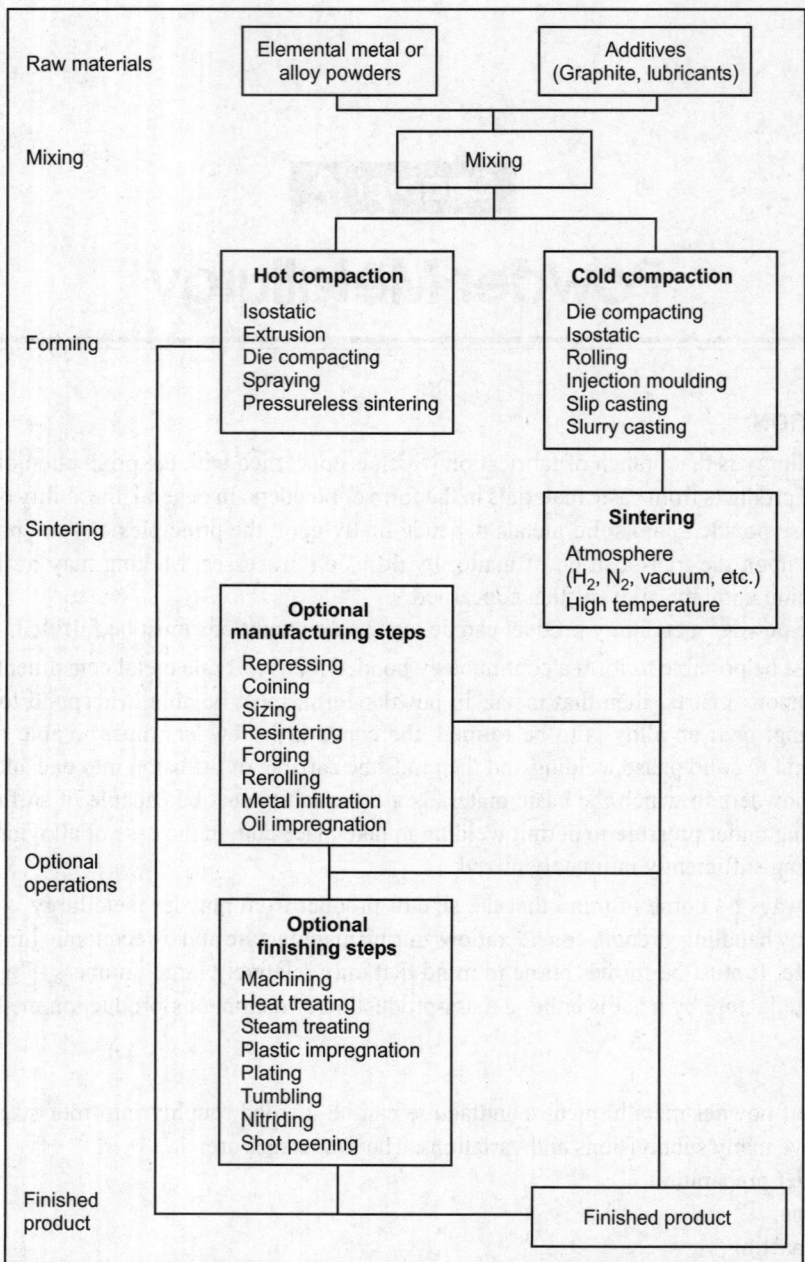

Fig. 9.1. Flow diagram for making powder metallurgy components.

Powders Preparation

Many methods are available for the production of metal powders. Unfortunately most are expensive and this is one, possibly the main reason why powder metallurgy is not more widely used. There are four general methods for producing powders. The first and most obvious method is to use mechanical means to break down metal from: a larger mass into the required powder. There are many ways for approaching this problem and the process may begin by using heavy crushing machines and then go on to use crushing rolls and finally a stamping mill or a ball mill to produce successively finer grades of powder. We need not concern ourselves here with the earlier stages of the process but we must give some consideration to the production of the finer powders. This is most often done in ball mills. A ball mill is a horizontal barrel-shaped container holding a quantity of balls which, being free to tumble about as the container rotates, crush and abrade any powder particles that are introduced into the container. It may be necessary to pass the powder through several stages of ball milling to obtain successively smaller and more uniformly sized particles.

It is often necessary, at this stage, to introduce some form of liquid into the container (e.g. distilled water or volatile oil) with the purpose of preventing particles from sticking to each other by pressure welding and so building up uneven masses. The liquid may also serve to reduce the amount of wear which is likely to occur on the balls and may help to prevent atmospheric attack upon the surface of the particles. There are two types of ball mill. The first is the rotary-type mill in which the container is rotated horizontally on rollers, so that the balls which it contains are tumbled about during the rotation. Then there is the vibratory mill, in which the containers are vibrated and the balls are shaken together under the motion. The most violent action is that of tumbling, and the gentlest action is that of vibration. Containers vary in design, according to the manufacturer, and may be made of different materials, stainless steel being used most often. Sometimes, containers may be lined with abrasion resisting materials. Chemical methods for powder production are frequently employed, sometimes to produce powder in a finely divided form, and sometimes to produce a basic powder which may subsequently be finished to a finer and more uniform size by mechanical means.

There are several chemical methods, one of the most common being the reduction of a metal oxide in an appropriate atmosphere, such as hydrogen, which combines with the oxygen and leaves the metal free. There are other methods similar to this in which a chemical in gaseous or liquid form is used to react with one or more of the constituents of a compound of the metal to be extracted. The reaction must occur in such a way that either the metal is freed or the compound is altered to some less complex compound which may be further broken down by similar treatment to release the metal in a later stage in the process.

Still another method for producing powder is by evaporating the metal and then precipitating it in a collecting area. The metal need not necessarily be melted to achieve this purpose, but may go direct from the solid state into the vapour stage by a process known as 'sublimation'. The use of a vacuum will markedly reduce the vapourisation temperature of a metal, and often makes powder production surprisingly easy, although still costly.

Vapourisation by feeding a rod of the metal into a high temperature flame may also be used for producing metal powders. The vapourised droplets are allowed to condense on to a cool surface of a material to which they will not adhere, or are solidified in a cooling stream of water or other suitable liquid. This method is not very useful for large-scale production of powder.

One other method is available for production of powder, namely electrolysis, which can be applied in several different ways. This method may be used to give deposition of metallic particles upon the surface of an electrode of a type to which the metal particles will not bond, or it may be used in such a way that the intercrystalline boundaries of a solid mass of metal are electrolysed out of the way, so leaving the individual grains free from each other.

This latter method is used for producing stainless steel powders from solid metal. The metal is first treated to cause precipitation of chromium carbide at the grain boundaries so that these chromium carbide layers may be subsequently electrolysed out of the way.

The shape of the individual particles of a powder can be a very important factor. Rough and angular shapes are more difficult to compact in such a way that the maximum amount of space is filled and the maximum density obtained. On the other hand, smooth shapes tend to interlock less positively, therefore the compacted powders do not hold together so firmly. Irregular surfaces on the particles may make it difficult to ensure sufficiently close and intimate contact between individual grains to effect the necessary welding and/or diffusion, although the smaller the points of contact the higher the local stress and the easier the welding. Much research has gone into this problem and each metal has to be treated on its own merits and in relation to the particular application for which it is intended.

Differing methods of preparation will produce differing types of particle. It will be noted that two are of irregular shape and one is of a more smoothly rounded shape. It must be remembered that these shapes are not necessarily basic but may vary with the same methods from metal to metal.

The range of particle sizes can also be very important. If all particles are of identical size and rounded form, then the packing system will be similar to that shown in Fig. 9.2(a) in which, it will be noted, there are relatively large spaces between the grains tending to produce a relatively porous structure of low density. Of course, if the material is of a type which deforms readily, this situation may be materially changed when the powder is subjected to pressure during compacting.

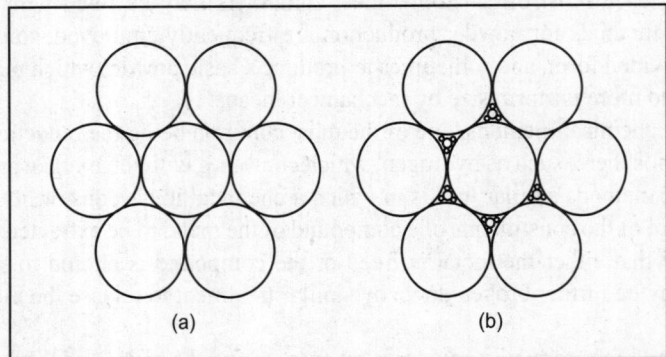

Fig. 9.2. Influence of particle size and distribution on density. (a) Packing of large spherical particles of one size, and (b) packing of large and small spherical particles by selection of sizes to give ordered distribution.

On the other hand, if a porous structure is desirable, then uniform granules subjected to sufficient pressure to give compacting but insufficient to cause marked deformation of particles, will give the desired effect. Again, if a high density is required with the minimum of porosity and if, at the same time, the granules are of a material which does not readily deform, then it will be an advantage to have a range of particle sizes, so that more intimate and uniform contact may be obtained between grains, accompanied by better filling of a given volume.

This effect can be seen in Fig. 9.2(b) which illustrates how granules of large size may have their interstices filled by relatively smaller granules. This latter type of packing may also have advantages when a continuous matrix of one constituent of low volume is required. If the matrix material is made of relatively small particle size then it can give a distribution similar to that of the smaller particles, as shown in Fig. 9.2(b), so that the matrix material is distributed in the correct position for manufacture into the final product. The production of desirable sizes and distributions is a very complex subject and beyond the scope of this present work.

Mixing

Mixing of powder preparatory to compacting is a very important aspect of the main process. If the material is all of one type, then the former's influence is not great; but if there is more than one kind of metal powder to be mixed, then the mixing must be done very carefully to ensure that the powders are uniformly distributed in the correct relationship throughout each other. For example, referring again to Fig. 9.2(b), if mixing is not effectively done, then the small particles will not be uniformly distributed around the larger particles and uniformity will not be obtained in the final product. There are cases, however, in which mixing might not be critical for dissimilar materials as, for example, when the matrix material is expected to melt and become very fluid during sintering. Then it can be expected that the matrix material will be capable of distributing itself correctly whilst in the molten state.

To ensure effective mixing of differing powders, it may be necessary to tumble the powders together for periods of several hours, depending upon the nature of the materials, the relative particle sizes and the particle shapes. This mixing may be done in containers of exactly the same type as the ball mills, and by the same methods of movement, but without any balls in the container. It may be necessary to incorporate some additive, in the form of a liquid, to the powder to prevent the granules from sticking together and to enable them to move freely against each other. An example of this is found in the preparation of tungsten carbides, or hard metal powders, to which a solution of paraffin wax, in a volatile solvent such as carbon tetrachloride, is added as a lubricant.

The solvent carries the wax throughout the powder, wets all the particle surfaces, then evaporates leaving behind a film of wax which serves as the lubricant. The amount of wax which is added is of the order of 2 per cent of that of the powder and has to be removed before the final sintering. Removal is effected by a preheating process, at temperatures up to 850°C, the heating being done slowly so that evaporation of the wax does not damage the compact.

Correct proportioning of the powders is extremely important, since the ratios of the quantities will govern the nature of the final product, as regards both mechanical efficiency and physical properties. This has to be linked up also with the efficiency of mixing which has already been considered. This question of proportioning of the constituents is one that cannot be overestimated, since the uniformity of the final products is governed by it and such products are made in large numbers.

Compacting

The next stage in powder metallurgical manufacture is that of compacting or pressing the powders into their semi-finished form, preparatory to sintering. High pressures are needed in this process because, if an adequate 'green' strength is to be obtained, appreciable plastic deformation of the powder particles is required, otherwise the necessary degree of cold welding will not occur, the unsintered compacts will be difficult to handle without causing damage and the final products will vary in quality. The degree of pressure that is required will depend on several factors, among which will be: (i) the required density of the final product, and (ii) the ease with which the particles will weld together.

Compacting pressure may be applied in several ways, the three commonest being: (i) die pressing, (ii) roll pressing, and (iii) extrusion. Die pressing is done in special presses which include a feed hopper for the powder, some form of shaping die to form the product, and a ram to apply the correct pressure in the right direction. Die pressing is essentially a limited process in relation to size and continuity of product and many efforts have been made to devise special systems of cyclic pressing to overcome this weakness, but with relatively little success.

Roll compacting is often used for production of continuous strip section, using a system similar to that illustrated diagrammatically in Fig. 9.3. The purpose is to replace the die and ram with two rolls of appropriate size into which a regulated stream of powder is guided, so that the rolls are able to apply the necessary compacting pressure in a continuous sequence. Roll diameter has to be relatively large if the powder is to be drawn in and effectively compressed. Small roll diameters make the entry angle of the powder too sharp; slipping occurs and the powder is not drawn efficiently into the rolls. This latter defect may be overcome by feeding powder in on a preformed thin sheet or foil.

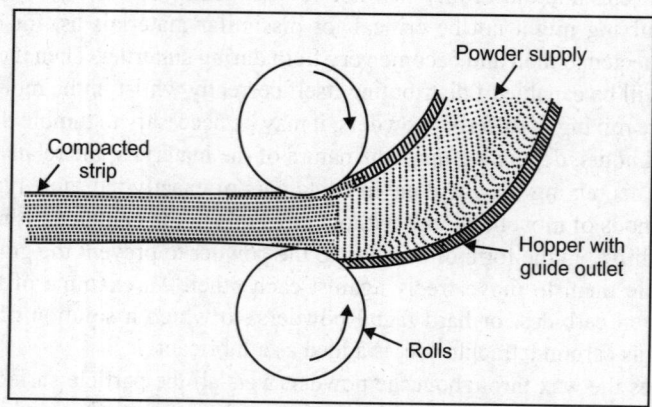

Fig. 9.3. Principle of roll compacting.

The extrusion method of compacting does not give such efficient control as that given by straightforward pressing or even by rolling. It is difficult to obtain high densities and some porosity is always left. It is also necessary to ensure some degree of plasticity in the compacted material, so that the extruded product may be transferred from the extrusion head (normally placed in the downward-acting vertical position), into a horizontal delivery position in which the extruded section may harden. Such plasticity may be developed in a compact by incorporating some form of plasticiser, which may take the form of a synthetic resin gum addition, although there are many other possibilities. It is necessary for extruded sections to be presintered to get rid of the plasticising material, an operation which requires very careful control to prevent cracking as the plasticiser is driven off.

As was suggested above, the compacting process is important in relation to handling of the product before sintering, as well as to the final result. The degree of pressure employed has a very material effect upon the density of the compact which, in turn, relates not only to the nature of the finished product but also to the 'green' strength, that is the strength of the compact after compacting but before sintering or presintering. This latter strength is important for several reasons. First of all, it is inevitable that the compact be handled between the compacting operation and succeeding stages in the process. Secondly, if the final product is of a type which is unmachinable, it may be necessary to machine to the correct shape in the 'green' stage or some intermediate stage between that and sintering, making due allowance for shrinkage. This aspect will be considered later in more detail. Reverting now to the question of compacting density and green strength, Fig. 9.4(a) shows the influence of differing pressures **on the densities of compacts made from various stainless steel powders, six different compositions in** all. (Although little industrial use is made of powder production of stainless steel, much fundamental research work on powder metallurgy has been done with it.) It will be noted that the density increases with increasing pressure, but with a tendency for the rate of increase to tail off as the maximum possible density, free from defects, is approached. Density, as we have already suggested, is closely associated with the green strength and the relationship between green strength and apparent density is shown in Fig. 9.4(b) for a number of stainless steel powders.

The relationship here is one of almost direct proportion between strength and density; but it should be remembered that these relations are not necessarily true in the same way for other materials and that each material will have its own characteristics.

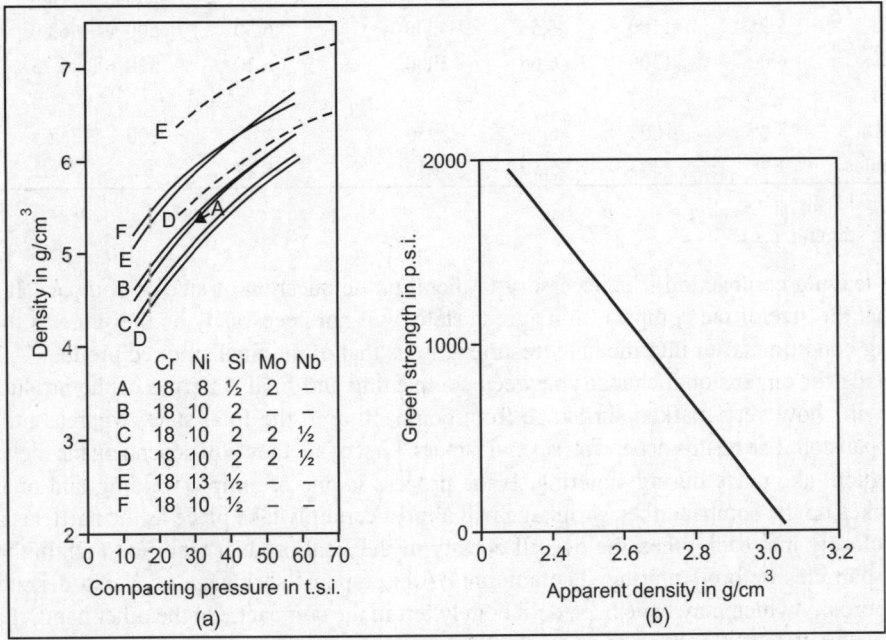

Fig. 9.4. Interrelationship between compacting pressure, green density and green strength of stainless-steel powder compacts: (a) relationship between compacting pressure and green density, (b) influence of apparent density upon the green strength of stainless-steel powders compacted at 30 t.s.i. No lubricant was added to powders.

Lubrication of the powders may influence, to a greater or lesser extent, the densities that are obtained with given pressures and the resulting densities are also affected by the nature of the powder particles. With an added lubricant, the powders may be able to move more readily against each other and so compact more firmly for a given pressure, whereas the state of the material may influence the plasticity of the powder particles, thus changing the density into which they will compact.

Some illustration of these effects may be seen in Table 9.1 which compares the green density and green strength for several stainless steel compacts at two different pressures: (i) without lubricant, and (ii) with lubricant. In addition, with the last powder listed in the table, comparison may be made of the effect of annealing the particles before compacting. It will be noted that in general the green density in the lubricated condition is markedly higher than in the unlubricated condition and that the density in the annealed condition, in which the particles are more plastic, is higher in both cases than that in the unannealed condition.

Table 9.1. The variation of green properties of stainless steel powder compacts with and without lubricant.

Brand of powder	No lubricant added				½% lithium stearate added			
	Compacting pressure, t.s.i.				Compacting pressure, t.s.i.			
	30		50		30		50	
	GD^a	GS^b	GD	GS	GD	GS	GD	GS
Cosint 304L	5.75	900	6.35	2600	6.05	240	6.60	900
Cosint 316L	5.95	1500	6.55	4000	6.30	500	6.80	1500
Cosint 347L	6.00	1300	6.65	3000	6.20	310	6.75	850
Cosint 410L								
Annealed	5.85	1000	6.55	2950	6.00	200	6.55	720
Not annealed	4.96	303	5.59	930	5.27	Nil	5.82	241

[a]GD = Green density, g/c.c.
[b]GS = Green strength, p.s.i.

Before leaving compacting it is necessary to mention the question of size of compact. It must be obvious that the size of the compact, in its green state, will not necessarily be the same as that in the presintering condition, after intermediate treatment, or as that of the final sintered product. Allowance must be made for dimensional changes between compacting and final sintering of the product. Many materials will show very marked shrinkage from compacting to the final state, whereas others may show an expansion. The results depend on several factors. First of all, they will depend on the metallurgical changes which take place during sintering. If the process is one of simple welding and one type of powder makes up the compact, then shrinkage will almost certainly take place as the particles set more and more closely into each other, the overall density of the final product tending to attain that of the individual particles before sintering. The amount of this type of shrinkage will also depend on the degree of porosity which may have been deliberately left in the compact. On the other hand, if alloying and diffusion are to take place during sintering, then the changes in dimensions will be governed by the nature of the final composition relative to that in the green condition. Changes which form an alloy of lower density than that of the constituents in their separate form will lead to an expansion. Dimensional changes are also dependent on the shape and size of the compact and there is no fixed rule that may be applied to all materials in all circumstances; each material and each product has to be considered on its own merits. The actual pressures used in compacting are dependent upon the nature of the material, the size of the compact and desired structure in the final product, and have to be individually decided, largely on an empirical basis, for each particular case. Thus, pressures may range from as low as 1 t.s.i. (travel services international) with one material, say a porous bronze, to as high as 50 t.s.i. for a maximum density product. It will be realised that the required pressure decides the size of compact which is obtainable from any given press. Generally speaking, the higher the pressure for a given product, other factors being neglected, the smaller the distortion, as distinct from shrinkage, which is likely to occur during the later stages of the process.

Before considering the application of sintering it is advisable to consider intermediate treatment which may be necessary between compacting and sintering proper.

If a lubricant is added to the powder to facilitate compacting, then it may be necessary to introduce a process to get rid of the lubricant before sintering or the lubricant may cause cracking, or may seriously modify the final metal structure. We have already mentioned one such treatment, for the removal of paraffin wax from cemented carbide compacts, but there are many other treatments varying with the lubricant. Some lubricants require no special treatment and, it is claimed, can actually improve the properties of the final product. This is the case with the lithium stearate which was added, as a lubricant, to the stainless steel powder listed in Table 9.1.

It will be noted that the lubricant causes a reduction in the green strength but not in that of the final product in which the improved density has the greater influence. We have mentioned products which are so hard in the sintered condition that they are then unmachinable and have suggested that these may be preformed after compacting but before sintering. This condition applies to the cemented carbide products used in the manufacture of tips for cutting tools. In this case, two procedures may be followed. In one, large blocks of uniform shape may be produced in quantity, and from these blocks smaller sections may be cut in the green state for differing products.

Before such green compacts can be treated in this way, they must be hardened to some extent to make them less brittle and weak. This is done by giving them a heat treatment at a temperature of about 1000°C to develop some bonding between the particles. This treatment is in addition to the treatment necessary to remove the lubricant. A second method of preparation is to press a semi-finished, standard shape and then to modify this shape in the green condition by machining, to bring it to the desired shape and pre-sinter dimensions.

Sintering

Sintering is not necessarily a simple straightforward operation. For many powder metallurgy products the process can take place in one simple stage; but, on the other hand, there are materials which require complicated sintering treatment in as many as five or six stages according to the desired metallurgical results. The process may be regarded as grouped under three general headings. First, where the treatment is being applied to a homogeneous material with the main purpose of achieving strength. Second is the group in which the purpose is again to achieve strength, but this time in a heterogeneous metal without alloying taking place. The third group is that in which the treatment is applied not only to give strength and bond, but also to produce metallurgical reactions between the constituents to achieve some particular type of structure. Each of these divisions will require individual sintering treatments appropriate to the particular materials concerned, but the treatments will tend to be similar within each group.

When the material is homogeneous and it is simply a matter of bonding strength, then, generally speaking, the higher the sintering temperature and the nearer it gets to the melting temperature of the material, the stronger the resulting product. This is illustrated in Fig. 9.5 which shows the effect of sintering temperature on a stainless steel powder compact.

If the material is not homogeneous but the purpose is to achieve strength without reaction between the differing materials in the compact, then the response of the compact to the sintering will not necessarily be as simple as that shown in Fig. 9.5. This is illustrated in Fig. 9.6 which shows graphs relating the sintering temperature to the hardness of the final product (in this case a hard metal containing tungsten carbide and cobalt). The general characteristic of the curves is that there is a peak temperature which gives optimum results. The curves also show the influence of the particle size, in that it is the finest particle which gives the quickest response. This effect is tied up with the higher densities that may be achieved with much lower compacting pressures on the finer powders.

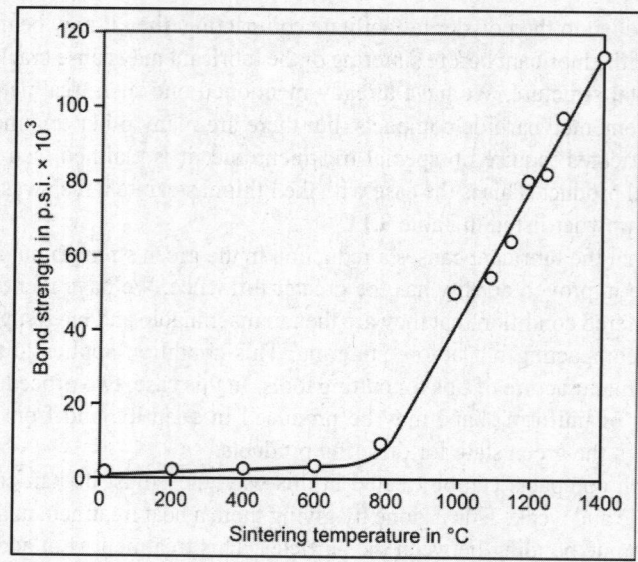

Fig. 9.5. Strength of a stainless steel compacted at 30 t.s.i. as a function of sintering temperature.

This is amplified in Table 9.2 which shows the compact hardnesses achieved for conditions of pressure similar to those used in the examples shown in Fig. 9.6. It will be noted from the latter that maximum hardness is achieved with the finest powder at the lowest pressure.

Table 9.2. Effects of compacting pressure on hardness of sintered WC-Co mixtures.

Coarse powder No. 4[a]		Fine powder No. 6[a]		Fine powder No. 7[b]	
Compacting pressure, t.s.i.	Hardness, R_A	Compacting pressure, t.s.i.	Hardness, R_A	Compacting pressure, t.s.i.	Hardness, R_A
21.3	71	0.7	87	0.15	89
28.4	72	1.4	87	0.3	92
35.5	75	2.8	87.5	0.5	90.5
42.6	77	4.2	87.5	0.7	91
56.8	78	4.9	88	1.4	91.5
71.0	76.5	5.7	89	14.2	89.5
106.5	75	6.4	88	–	–
–	–	7.1	87.5	–	–
–	–	14.2	86.5	–	–
–	–	21.3	86	–	–
–	–	35.5	85	–	–

For particle sizes see Fig. 9.6.
[a]Sintered at 1500°C (2730°F) for 30 min.
[b]Sintered at 1400°C (2550°F) for 30 min.

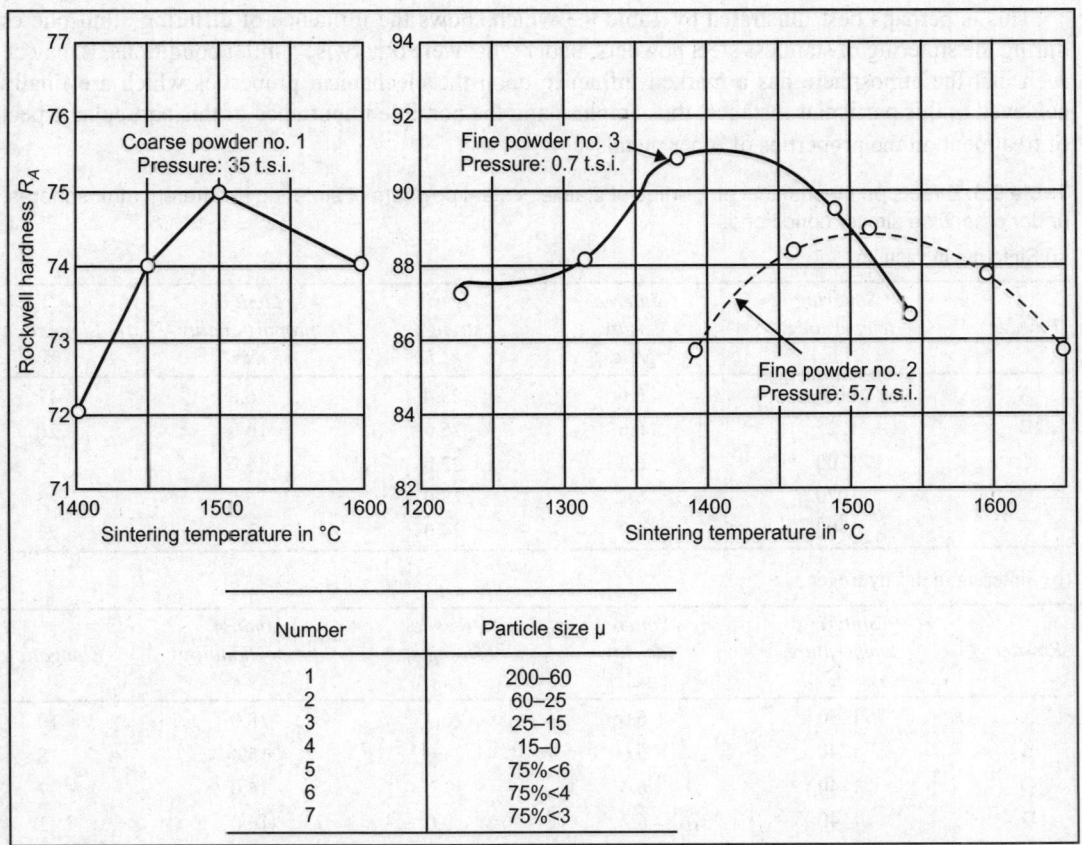

Fig. 9.6. Effect of sintering temperature on hardness of WC-8% Co prepared from different grades of powder.

When alloy or structural changes in the basic materials are to be achieved, then the situation becomes more complex; the single sintering treatments, which were effective in the two examples which have been quoted, are no longer sufficient in all cases and the process may have to be subdivided into stages. This whole field is beyond the scope of the present consideration, so one example will have to serve as illustration. This example is a nickel–iron–molybdenum magnetic alloy which requires no less than four sintering treatments to achieve maximum density and the required structure.

First of all, presintering at 900°C for one hour is required, followed by a second sintering for 12 hours at 1250°C, then a third sintering for 71 hours at 1350°C, then finally a fourth sintering for 4 hours at 1400°C before full density is achieved. In addition, to give the necessary homogeneity of structure, a hot rolling stage performed at 1100°C is given after the third sintering. All this procedure is required, in this particular case, to obtain the crystal orientation and structure necessary to achieve the maximum magnetic permeability in the final product; but it should be remembered that this material is rather complex.

Not only are the sintering sequence and temperature of importance, but also the atmosphere in which the sintering takes place. Invariably this atmosphere must be controlled in one way or another if oxidation and other undesirable reactions are to be avoided.

This is perhaps best illustrated by Table 9.3 which shows the influence of differing atmospheres during the sintering of stainless steel powders, under what were otherwise similar conditions. It may be seen that the atmosphere has a marked influence upon the mechanical properties which are finally achieved in this particular instance, thus emphasising the possible importance of this particular aspect of treatment on the properties of other metals.

Table 9.3. Effects on mechanical properties of stainless steel powders of sintering in different atmospheres, under otherwise similar conditions.

(a) Sintering in vacuum.

Powder	Sintering temperature, °C	Sintered density, g/c.c.	Tensile strength, t.s.i.	Limit of proportionality t.s.i.	Elongation %
A	1100	6.6	23.4	16.8	11
B	1225	6.6	25.5	16.0	20
C	1100	6.3	22.0	16.0	5
D	1070	6.2	18.0	16.5	3
E	1300	6.9	24.0	13.0	22

(b) Sintering in dry hydrogen.

Powder	Sintering temperature, °C	Sintered density, g/c.c.	Tensile strength, t.s.i.	Limit of proportionality t.s.i.	Elongation %
A	1150	6.6	26.4	18.0	10
B	1240	6.6	24.0	15.4	18
C	1140	6.3	22.0	15.0	7
D	1140	6.2	20.0	16.0	3
E	1320	6.9	24.0	16.0	18

(c) Specimens sintered in cracked ammonia at 1300°C for 1 hour.

Powder	Linear Shrinkage, %	Sintered density, g/c.c.	Tensile strength, t.s.i.	Limit of proportionality t.s.i.	Elongation %
A	1.4	6.5	28.8	22.4	10
B	1.0	6.4	26.5	19.5	11
C	1.4	6.3	26.8	20.0	12
D	1.4	6.2	29.0	23.6	5
E	0.7	6.7	27.8	20.5	10

The duration of the sintering treatment is an important factor, particularly in those materials which sinter readily. It will be seen that the prolonged treatment time has permitted the tungsten carbide crystals to merge together in one particular area, giving an excessively enlarged grain, a state of affairs which, if widespread throughout the material, could lead to very uneven performance in service of this cemented carbide. The importance and incidence of grain growth varies from material to material; but it is important that its effect should be controlled if optimum properties are to be achieved.

ADVANTAGES AND DISADVANTAGES OF POWDER METALLURGY (P/M)

Advantages of Powder Metallurgy

Powder metallurgy has several unique advantages which are as below:

1. Metal plus metal components can be manufactured by P/M. There is almost no need of referring to their equilibrium or phase diagrams. Components of any desired composition can be manufactured.
2. Metal plus non metal components can be manufactured which are quite impossible to manufacture by the usual methods.
3. Controlled porosity can be obtained in the components. This is essential for certain applications like liquid and gas filters, self-lubricating bearings and insulating bricks. The amount of porosity alongwith control over size, shape and distribution of pores can be obtained to achieve the desired properties in the component. This is not possible by any of the usual techniques.
4. It is possible to produce components with properties similar to the parent metals. Whereas, if the components are manufactured by melting, the alloy may have different properties from their parent metals. This advantage is unique for certain applications like electrical contact materials, where hardness and electrical conductivity of the parent metals is retained in the component. The metal powder of W or Mo which has high hardness is mixed with powder of Cu or Ag which has good electrical conductivity and processed by P/M. Such a component has good hardness and electrical conductivity which satisfies the requirements of electrical contact materials.
5. Production of refractory metals like W, Mo, Ti, Th, etc. is possible without melting, e.g. manufacture of ductile tungsten in wire form for incandescent lamp filaments.
6. Components from metals which are completely insoluble in the liquid state can be manufactured with uniform distribution of one metal into the other. However, if they are manufactured by melting and casting, the distribution of one phase into the other is nonuniform, e.g. the material for journal bearing should have soft and hard phases. Copper is hard and lead is soft but they are completely insoluble in the liquid state and hence, if Cu-Pb bearing is manufactured by melting and casting, it will show non uniform distribution of Pb in Cu. However, powder metallurgical processing of this bearing shows better homogeneity.
7. Manufacture of cemented carbide cutting tools is only possible by P/M. The melting points of the carbides which are used for the manufacture of these cutting tools are extremely high and hence melting is not possible. Therefore, the usual techniques of shaping are not applicable. Hence, such cutting tools and diamond impregnated tools for cutting of porcelain, glass, and tungsten alloys are only made by P/M.
8. Components containing metallic as well as non-metallic materials, non-metallic components having metallic base, and also those composed of two or more layers of different metals can only be produced by P/M.
9. Composite and dispersion hardened materials can be manufactured, e.g. cermets and thoria dispersed tungsten filaments.
10. There is a little chance for contamination of metal powders during processing by P/M and hence the purity of the component remains the same as the original purity of metal powders.
11. P/M parts may be welded, brazed, machined, heat treated, plated or impregnated with lubricants or other materials.

12. Some of the metal powders find application in other fields such as painting, welding, pyrotechniques, explosives, plastics and RCC, e.g. Al powder is used in painting, thermit welding and RCC construction whereas Al and Mg powders are used for explosives.
13. Close control over the dimensions of the finished component can easily be obtained.
14. No machining or minimum machining is required and hence the scrap is minimum. This gives yield of over 99.0 per cent.
15. Fast production of simple shaped components is possible due to lesser number of steps involved in P/M. This is very useful to manufacture large number of components in a short time. Due to fast production on mass scale, the cost of the component may come down.
16. Highly qualified or skilled personnel is not required for plant operation and maintenance.

Disadvantages of Powder Metallurgy

Powder metallurgy has some drawbacks as given below which limits its application in some of the situations.
1. Most of the powders used in P/M are fine and fine powders of some of the metals like Mg, Al, Zr, Ti, etc. are likely to explode and cause fire hazards when they come in contact with air and hence, they should be preserved carefully. Other metal powders are also likely to get oxidised slowly in air and hence, they must be stored properly to avoid their deterioration.
2. It is not suitable to manufacture small number of components because of high initial investment on tooling and equipment.
3. Large sized components cannot be manufactured because of the limited capacity of presses available for compaction.
4. Complex shaped parts cannot be manufactured with ease by P/M.
5. P/M parts have poor corrosion resistance because they are porous. Due to this porosity, large internal surface area gets exposed to corrosive environment.
6. Components with theoretical density cannot be manufactured.
7. Due to the presence of porosity, mechanical properties such as ductility, UTS and toughness are poor as compared to components manufactured by conventional methods. The surface finish is also poor.

CHARACTERISATION AND TESTING OF METAL POWDERS

The success of obtaining the desired properties in the component depends on the properties of metal powders used for its manufacture. Therefore, it is essential to test these powders for their properties which helps in the selection of right type of powder for a given application. The following powder properties should be evaluated:
1. Chemical composition with type and amount of impurity.
2. Shape, size and distribution.
3. Porosity.
4. Microstructure.

Specific surface, density, flow rate, and compacting and sintering characteristics are the other properties which are dependent entirely or to a large extent on the above basic properties of metal powders.

Chemical Composition

Chemical composition and impurities in metal powders are determined by standard techniques of chemical analysis such as gravimetric, volumetric, colourometric, etc. or they can be determined by spectroscopy. The choice of a particular method depends upon the type of the element, its amount, and the accuracy with which it is to be determined. The impurities not only have undesirable effect on component properties but also strongly influence pressing and sintering characteristics, and hence their determination with high accuracy is essential.

Shape, Size and Distribution

Powder shape, size and distribution can be measured by using one or more of the following methods:

Sieve method

It is the most simple method for the determination of size and distribution of powder particles. Standard sieves of different mesh numbers are used for this purpose. The opening of a screen is expressed by the number of meshes per linear inch. In almost all the cases, mesh number indicates the number of apertures per linear inch. The procedure used is simple and is described below:

> Different sieves are arranged one below the other as per their mesh numbers, the coarsest being at the top. 100 gm of metal powder is placed on the top sieve and the entire stack of sieves is vibrated for 15 minutes by a standard shaking machine which gives circular and translatory motions to the screens. After this, the amount of powder retained on each sieve is accurately measured. From these weights, size and size distribution can be found out.

The particles which pass through the size are denoted by minus number and the particles which are retained on the sieve are denoted by plus number of that particular sieve. Size distribution is expressed by weight fraction of powder retained on each sieve.

Sieve method gives fairly accurate result when the powder is in the size range of 44 to 840 microns.

Microscopic method

Optical and electron microscopes are used for measurement of size and distribution of particles. Optical microscopes can magnify up to 2000X and electron microscopes up to 1,00,000X.

Depending on the size range of particles in powder, a suitable magnification is employed and individual size of particles is measured. Since the particles encountered in P/M are of different sizes, large number of readings should be taken and average size should be found out. Also, the shape, size variation and porosity in powder particles can be directly observed by the microscopes.

Optical or electron microscopy can be used for the measurement of particle sizes above 0.1 micron and electron microscopy is used for particle sizes of smaller than 0.1 micron (1 micron = 10^{-3} mm).

Sedimentation method

In this method, classification on the basis of size and size distribution of powder particles is done according to their settling velocities in a fluid. This involves suspending a small quantity of powder sample in a fluid medium and allowing the particles to settle for a suitable time. Settling velocity of a spherical particle is proportional to the square of the particle diameter and hence particles of equal sizes can be separated on the basis of equal settling velocities. This is done by measuring the amount of particles settling at different intervals of time. For irregularly shaped particles, particle size is assumed to be the same as that of spherical particle having the same settling velocity as that of irregularly shaped

particle under similar conditions of testing. Some of the other techniques make use of the following properties for finding out size and size distribution of particles:
1. Changes in specific gravity of the suspension at various depths (hydrometer or specific gravity method).
2. Changes in density of suspension by changes in pressure at various heights with fixed time or at fixed height with varying times (manometric method).
3. Changes in intensity of transmitted light through the dilute suspension at a certain depth by photoelectric cells (turbidimetric method).

These methods are suitable for the measurement of particle sizes in the range of 0.05 to 50 microns.

Elutriation method

This method is used for determination of size distribution of fine particles. Here, the metal powder is allowed to settle in a moving liquid or gas of a constant velocity.

The particles with settling velocity of less than the velocity of rising fluid will be carried upwards and those with higher settling velocities will settle at the bottom. By altering the velocity of medium, the particles can be separated according to their sizes.

This is a fractioning method and is used for determination and separation of size fractions of the powder. This method is also used to remove unwanted fine materials from the powder. The method is suitable for powder sizes in the range of 5 to 100 microns.

It is important to note that the particle shape is evaluated only by microscopic method. The shape of the particle can be directly seen by either optical or electron microscopes. For non spherical particles, shape factor is specified which is the ratio of its length to breadth.

Usual particle size range of powders used in P/M is between 4 to 200 microns. Therefore, the choice of a particular method will depend on the exact size of particles in a given powder.

Particle Porosity and Microstructure

For the determination and observation of these properties, microscopy is used. The powder is mounted in some suitable medium for observation under microscope. Depending on its suitability, either hot mounting or cold setting method is used. These methods are described in detail in chapter 21 on metallography. The brief steps in these methods are as below.

Hot mounting

The metal powder in small quantity is mixed with bakelite powder, mounted using a standard specimen mounting press, polished carefully, etched in a suitable etchant, washed with water and alcohol, and dried using blast of hot air and examined under microscope.

Cold mounting

Small quantity of metal powder is mixed with some suitable polymeric liquid and hardener. This medium is poured in a steel tube of a suitable size. This liquid from the medium polymerises and becomes hard in a period of 10 to 15 min. Subsequently the sample is removed and polished, etched, washed, and examined under the microscope.

The metallographic examination of these powders will reveal not only the various phases, inclusions, impurities, internal porosity, etc. but also the particle size, shape and distribution.

Other Properties

Specific surface

It is defined as the total surface area of a powder per unit weight (cm^2/gm). It depends on size, shape, density and surface conditions of the particles. It is evaluated either by permeability method or adsorption method. However, permeability method is widely used because of its simplicity and rapidity. Here, a fluid is passed with constant pressure through a bed of packed powder contained in a chamber and the pressure drop across the bed of the powder is measured. From the observed drop of pressure, surface area is calculated.

The compacting and sintering characteristics are strongly influenced by the contact area between the metal particles. Fine particles have large surface area and give high sintering rate which reduces the time of sintering. However, this results in the entrapment of air and other gases and also causes bridging effects. Due to this, the compact is likely to crack either before or during sintering. Coarse particles have smaller surface area and hence sintering characteristics are poor; and also these components show poor mechanical properties.

Density

Apparent density

The apparent density (or packing density) of a powder is defined as the mass per unit volume of loose or unpacked powder. Thus it includes internal pores but excludes external pores. It is governed by chemical composition, particle shape, size distribution, method of manufacture of metal powders and surface conditions.

This strongly influences the pressing characteristics. The lower the apparent density, the longer will be the compression stroke and deeper dies will be required to produce a compact of given thickness and density.

Tap density

The tap density is the apparent density of the powder after it has been mechanically shaked or tapped until the level of the powder remains constant. This has a similar effect as apparent density on pressing characteristics. Apparent density is measured by using a standard flowmeter funnel or volumeter and tap density by Ro tap machine.

Flow rate

The flow-rate is a very important characteristic of powders which measures the ability of a powder to be transferred. It is defined as the rate at which a metal powder will flow under gravity from a container through an orifice having a specific shape and size. Such an apparatus which is used to determine flow rate is called flow meter.

Flowmeter consists of a standard and accurately machined conical funnel made of brass with smooth surface finish having an internal angle of 60°. The orifice situated at the bottom of the funnel is either 1/8" (for ferrous powders) or 1/10" in diameter (for nonferrous powders) and has a length of 1/8". The time required to flow 50 gm powder from this funnel is measured and reported as flow rate in gms/minute.

Flow rate depends on particle size, shape, distribution, amount of absorbed-gases, amount of moisture, and coefficient of friction. In general, fine or irregular particles have poor flowability and coarse or spherical particles have better flow ability. Flow rate increases with decreased particle irregularity and increased particle size.

For rapid filling of the die and uniform density of the cold compact, the powder must have high flowability. There is a close relationship between apparent density and flow ability and hence it is very difficult to vary anyone without altering the other. Flow rate, apparent density, and tap density are important properties because they affect transporting and pressing characteristics of powders.

Compacting or pressing properties

These are represented by the terms compressibility and compactibility. Compressibility is defined as the powders ability to deform under applied pressure and is measured by many ways as below:
1. Ratio of the green density of compact to the apparent density of the powder.
2. Ratio of the height of the uncompacted powder in the die to the height of the pressed compact.
3. Ratio of the volume of powder poured into the die to the volume of the pressed compact (i.e. compression ratio).

Compactibility

Compactibility is defined as the minimum pressure required to produce a compact of given green strength. Both these terms are important in densification of powder particles and are dependent on particle size, shape, porosity or density, hardness, surface properties, chemical composition and previous history of powder.

Green density

It is the density of a cold compact [= weight of the compact/volume of the compact] and largely depends on the basic properties of powder particles. Green density increases with: (i) increase of compaction pressure, (ii) increase of particle size, (iii) increase of apparent density, (iv) decrease of particle irregularity, (v) decrease of particle hardness or strength, and (vi) decrease of compacting speed. The general dependence of green density on other factors is shown schematically in Fig. 9.7.

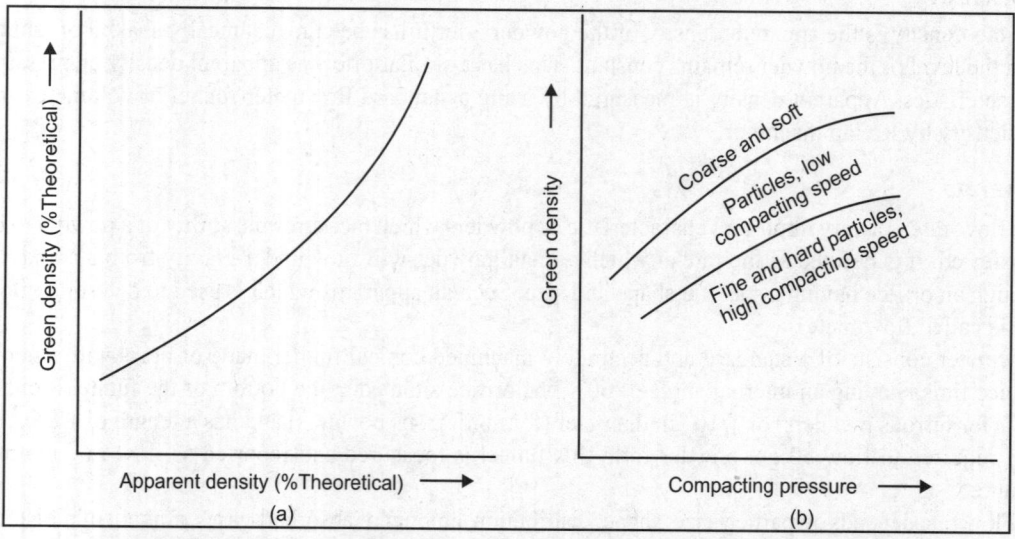

Fig. 9.7. Variation of green density with (a) apparent density, and (b) compacting pressure.

Green strength

It is the mechanical strength of a green compact and is expressed in kg per square mm. This property is determined by conducting transverse rupture test or radial crushing test on green powder compacts of suitable size and shape using standard testing machines.

The strength of a green compact depends on the shape, size, distribution, surface condition, hardness, yield strength, etc. of powder particles and pressure applied during compaction. The strength is developed mainly due to cold welding and mechanical interlocking of particles because of application of pressure. The green compacts should not fracture during their ejection from the dies and should not loose the sharp edges during handling or transferring to the sintering furnace. This can be achieved by a proper green strength of the compacts. Hence, it is necessary to control the green strength of the compacts.

Green spring

The compacts expand as soon as they are ejected out of the die cavity and this effect is called as Green spring. It is necessary to determine the amount of green spring for the manufacture of components with close dimensional tolerances. The die should be properly designed so that the ejected component has exactly the same dimensions as desired or specified

In general, the green spring amounts to about 0.2 per cent on the diameter side and 0.5 per cent on the length side. It depends on the powder material, compacting pressure, elastic recovery of the tools, and design of the dies.

Sintering characteristics

The idea about sintering characteristics and quality can be obtained from the properties of the sintered compacts. Therefore, they are tested for the following properties.

Dimensional change during sintering

$$\% \text{ Shrinkage (or growth)} = \frac{\text{Change in length}}{\text{Sintered length}} \times 100 \qquad \ldots (9.1)$$

$$\% \text{ Shrinkage (or growth)} = \frac{\text{Change in length}}{\text{Unsintered length}} \times 100 \qquad \ldots (9.2)$$

Equation 9.1 is used in carbide industries and Eq. 9.2 is used in bearing and other industries. The die should be properly designed so as to obtain exact sized final components.

Density and porosity

By the measurement of density, the total amount of porosity can be calculated from the following relationship:

$$\rho = 1 - \frac{\rho_v}{\rho_s} \qquad \ldots (9.3)$$

where, ρ is the fractional porosity, ρ_v is the density of sintered component, and ρ_s is the density of the solid material.

The total porosity consists of interconnected porosity and closed porosity. These two can be found out separately by standard techniques. It is very difficult to produce P/M components without porosity. **The porosity has undesirable effects on mechanical properties and corrosion resistance. Complete account** of porosity in respect of its type, amount, size, shape and distribution is required for correct understanding of the effects of porosity on mechanical properties.

Mechanical properties
Mechanical properties of sintered compacts such as compressive strength, hardness, etc. are determined by using appropriate methods of testing. These results are necessary for deciding the suitability of the component for a particular service application.

Microstructure
Metallographic examination of sintered components will not only reveal the size, shape, distribution and amount of porosity but also the amount of phases, their distribution, grain size, inclusions and homogeneity of components. Because of the presence of porosity, due cares should be taken during polishing and etching of samples to avoid erroneous observations and results.

MANUFACTURE OF SOME TYPICAL POWDER METALLURGY (P/M) COMPONENTS

Oil Impregnated Porous Bearings (Self-lubricating Bearings)

These bearings are manufactured from either bronze, brass, iron or aluminium alloy powders with or without graphite. However, bronze bearings are widely used and are made from Cu and Sn (90:10) with addition of graphite. Graphite increases porosity and also improves pressing characteristics. Some amount of free graphite is desirable because it is a solid lubricant and takes care under severe loading conditions. However, large amounts of graphite will reduce the strength of bearing. The steps in the production of a porous bronze bearing are as below:

1. Mixing.
2. Cold compaction.
3. Sintering.
4. Repressing (i.e. sizing) or machining.
5. Impregnation.

Metal powders of Cu and Sn with small amount of fine natural graphite are blended or mixed to obtain the desired alloy composition (90 Cu:10 Sn). This powder is cold compacted at pressures between 20 to 50 kg/mm^2 to form green compacts of desired shape and size.

These compacts are sintered in a reducing atmosphere at a temperature of about 800°C. A typical sintering cycle consists of holding the compact at 400°–450°C for the removal of part of the graphite and diffusion of molten Sn into the copper, followed by further heating to 800°C for periods as short as 5 minutes. At this temperature, a tin-rich liquid phase is formed which is absorbed by the copper.

Distortions occurring during sintering can be eliminated by repressing (i.e. sizing) or machining. If the pore size is large, sizing can be done and if it is small, machining should be done. For small pore sizes, sizing should not be done because it may result in closure of pores.

The repressed or machined components are impregnated with oil or hot oil using pressure, vacuum or a combination of these. Such an oil impregnated bearing is called self lubricating bearing because it does not require external lubrication. These bearings must have the following characteristics for their efficient working:

1. Sufficient porosity (30 to 50 per cent) to retain the maximum possible amount of oil.
2. Inter connected porosity in the largest proportion and should be uniformly distributed throughout the material.

3. Sufficient strength to sustain the loads.
4. Good dimensional accuracy.

When the porosity is more, the strength of the bearing is less. Such bearings have more oil retaining capacity but less load sustaining ability and hence they are suitable for high speeds and low load conditions. When the porosity is less, the strength of the bearing is more. Such bearing have less oil retaining capacity but more load bearing ability and hence they are widely used for low speeds and high load conditions. These bearings contain more amount of free graphite which compensates for the less quantity of oil.

The working of the bearing is as below:

> As the speed of shaft increases, the temperature of bearing rises due to frictional heat. This results in decrease of viscosity and increase in volume of the oil. Due to this, the oil is pulled out from the pores and gets rapidly circulated alongwith the rotating shaft. With decrease of shaft speed, pressure decreases and temperature also decreases; and due to this, the oil goes back to pores by capillary action. There is no wastage of oil and working of the bearing is smooth and silent.

These bearings find applications in places which are inaccessible or difficult to accessible. These are the places which are impossible or difficult for regular lubrication. They are also used in certain applications where it is desirable that the oil should not come in contact and contaminate the products (e.g. in food and textile industries).

Cemented Carbides

These are important products of P/M and find wide applications as cutting tools, wire drawing and deep drawing dies, drills and stone working tools. They are manufactured from carbides of refractory metals such as W, Mo, Ti, Ta or Nb. These carbides are extremely hard (hardness more than 3000 VPN) and retain their hardness upto a very high temperature. However, they are extremely brittle and hence are likely to fail with slight shock loading. To increase their shock resisting ability, metals such as Co, Ni, Cr or alloys of Co–Cr or Co–Ni–Cr are used up to 20 per cent and the processing is done by P/M. The hard carbide powders are bonded or cemented together by these metals or alloys. The actual proportion of the various carbides and the metal or alloy used depend on the specific application. For most of the common applications, carbides of W and Mo are used and the binder is Co. The steps in the manufacture of cemented carbides are as below.

Powder manufacture

Carbide powders of the refractory metals are produced either from their respective oxides or metals. Metal oxides can be reduced to metals by carbon or hydrogen and subsequently the metals can be converted to carbides by direct reaction with the carbon, or the metal oxides can be directly converted to carbides in a single step by reaction with carbon. In the former method, close control of composition is possible whereas in the later, it is difficult because of combination of reduction and carburisation reactions in a single operation. Co powder is obtained by the reduction of the oxide or oxalate by H_2 at temperatures of 600° to 700°C.

Milling

Carbide powders are mixed in the required proportion alongwith the powder of metallic binder by a wet mixing method. Lubricants such as paraffin wax dissolved in gasoline, camphor in ether or light hydrocarbons and glycerine in alcohol are mixed to these powders just prior to compaction which facilitates pressing and avoids defects and cracks in the compacts.

Cold pressing and sintering

This mixture is compacted at a pressure of 35 to 45 kg/mm² and the compacts are heated to about 400°C for a sufficient period to remove the lubricant by volatilisation. Sintering of these compacts is earned out in two stages. The preliminary sintering is done using H_2 atmosphere at a temperature between 900° to 1150°C. This is done to impart sufficient strength to the compacts. At this stage, they can be machined or cut to a shape and size to obtain exact dimensions of the component after final sintering. Final sintering is done in the temperature range of 1350° to 1550°C for about two hours using H_2 atmosphere or vacuum. The liquid phase formed at this temperature binds the particles and hence the name is cemented carbides. During this stage of sintering, large amount of shrinkage occurs in the component and hence to obtain the final dimensions within tolerance limit, the component must have oversized dimensions before sintering. Cemented carbides may also be produced by infiltration of porous carbide skeletons with liquid cobalt.

Machining

It should be done to the extremely close tolerances and is done in two steps. First it is ground rough using silicon carbide grinding wheels and finally with metal bonded diamond wheels. Electrospark or ultrasonic machining has also been used for threading, boring or engraving of these cemented carbide components. The flow sheet for the manufacture of sintered cemented carbides is shown in Fig. 9.8.

Cermets

They are manufactured from the powders of ceramics and metals by powder metallurgy. Cermet is a short form of ceramic plus metal. Ceramics have excellent high temperature strength and hardness whereas metals have good shock resisting ability. The above properties are combined together by mixing the powders of ceramics and metals and processing by P/M. Ceramic particles are bonded by metal particles and hence the properties of cermets depend upon the type of ceramic, type and amount of metallic binder and other powder metallurgical parameters. Some cermets are also made by impregnation of a porous ceramic structure with a metallic binder. The amount of binder usually varies between 20 to 70 per cent. The most common ceramics are oxides, carbides or borides of metals such as W, Cr, Ti, Ta, Be, Al and Si, and the bonding metals are Fe, Ni, Cr and Co.

Cermets find applications in rocket and jet engines, as spinning tools for hot metals, hot forging dies and other similar high temperature applications. They are also suitable for cutting of metals at high speeds with medium to light chip loads.

Cemented Carbide Tipped Tools (Sintered Carbide Cutting Tools)

These tools are superior to all other tools in respect of cold and hot hardness, compressive strength, modulus of elasticity, abrasion resistance and cutting ability. Their cold hardness exceeds 1500 VPN and they maintain high hardness up to approximately 1200°C. Hence, they are highly suitable for fast cutting of metals. The cutting speed with the use of carbide tipped tools is increased from 6 to 8 times over that with the customary high speed steels. Because of the high cost of these materials only the cutting edge is made from them and brazed or mechanically clamped to the ordinary steel shank. Tools are brazed with silver solders, electrolytic copper and copper–nickel alloys for low, moderate and high operating temperatures respectively. The brazing is done by using a small piece of sheet or wire of brazing metal and heating by gas or electricity using a suitable flux such as borax. The tool should be cooled slowly after brazing either in charcoal dust or ash or in still air in order to avoid cracking of the joint.

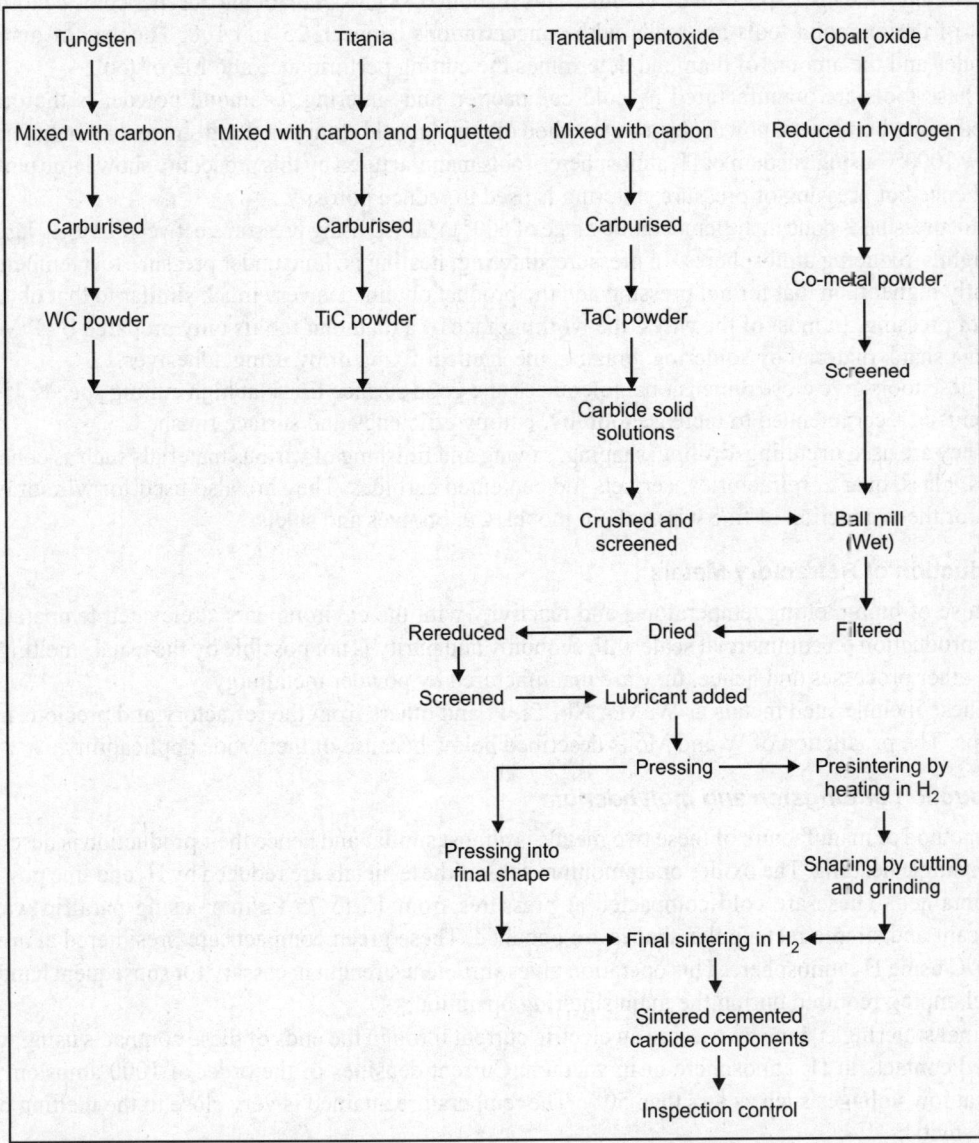

Fig. 9.8. Steps for the manufacture of cemented carbides.

Diamond Impregnated Tools

These tools are manufactured from a mixture of diamond dust and powder of a bonding material such as mild steel, Co, or cemented carbides by P/M. The size of diamond particles varies between 60 to 400 mesh depending upon the specific application. The finer sizes are mainly used for finishing operation such as honing, lapping and polishing where as medium and coarse sizes are used for grinding and cutting wheels. The amount of diamond dust in the tool is expressed by a concentration number and 100 concentration means 25 per cent by volume. This is about 0.88 gms of diamond dust per cubic centimetre. Most of the diamond tools are made with concentrations between 25 and 100. The size of diamond particles and the amount of diamond determines the cutting performance and life of tool

These tools are manufactured by cold compaction and sintering. Diamond powder is thoroughly mixed with a bond metal powder by a wet method of mixing, cold compacted and sintered at a temperature below 1000°C using vacuum or H_2 atmosphere. Tools manufactured by this procedure show large porosity and hence hot pressing or pressure sintering is used to reduce porosity.

Hot pressing is done in the temperature range of 600° to 900°C using pressures between 12 to 20 kg/mm^2 in slightly reducing atmospheres. In pressure sintering, heating is done under pressure to a temperature slightly higher than that for hot pressing and the product obtained is very much similar to that obtained by hot pressing. In most of the cases, the working face of a diamond tool is only prepared by P/M and set in a shank material by soldering, brazing, mechanical fixing or by using adhesives.

These tools give close dimensional tolerances and good surface finish at high cutting speeds. Use of coolents is recommended to increase tool life, cutting efficiency and surface finish.

They are used in cutting, drilling, shaping, sawing and finishing of various materials such as concrete, rocks, glass, quartz, refractories, cermets md cemented carbides. They are also used for wire drawing dies for the production of fine wires of Ni, monel, Cu, bronzes and steels.

Production of Refractory Metals

Because of high melting temperatures and reactivity with the environments at elevated temperatures, their production on commercial scale with economy and purity is not possible by the usual smelting and such other processes and hence, they are manufactured by powder metallurgy.

These include such metals as W, Mo, Nb, Ta, Pt and others from the refractory and precious metal groups. The production of W and Mo is described below because of their wide applicability.

Production of tungsten and molybdenum

The method of manufacture of these two metals is almost similar and hence their production is described under single heading. The oxides or ammonium salts of these metals are reduced by H_2 and fine powders are obtained. These are cold compacted at pressures from 15 to 75 kg/mm^2 using paraffin wax as lubricant and simple rectangular shapes are obtained. These green compacts are presintered at around 1000°C using H_2 atmosphere. This operation gives sufficient strength necessary for subsequent handling and clamping required during the main sintering operation.

Final sintering is done by passing an electric current through the ends of these compacts using water cooled contacts in H_2 atmosphere or in vacuum. Current densities of the order of 1000 amps/cm^2 are used at low voltages such as less than 50 V. The temperature attained is very close to the melting point of the metal.

After this treatment, the bars still have appreciable porosity which makes them brittle. The porosity is reduced by rolling, forging or swaging at temperatures between 1300° to 1700°C for tungsten and 1000° to 1400°C for molybdenum. As the deformation continues, the working temperature is gradually reduced. Tungsten can be drawn into fine wires at about 400°C whereas molybdenum can be rolled to thin sheets at room temperature.

Tungsten manufactured by the above technique is called ductile tungsten. It is used for applications such as thoriated tungsten filaments for electric bulbs, electrical contacts, heating elements for high temperature furnaces, radiation shields in nuclear applications and rocket nozzles.

Molybdenum is used for applications such as heating elements for high temperature furnaces, hooks and grids in thermionic valves in the electronic industry, electric lamp filament supports in wire form, valves to be used in hot H_2SO_4, electrodes and stirrers for glass melting equipment, moulds and cores for die casting, and hot working tools and dies.

Electrical Contact Materials

Electrical contact materials should have the following properties:
1. High electrical conductivity.
2. High thermal conductivity to dissipate heat resulting from the passage of electric current.
3. High melting temperature.
4. High resistance to wear and abrasion from the mechanical motion at the contact interface.
5. High resistance to sparking which can occur on breaking the contact surfaces.
6. Low vapour pressure.
7. Low temperature coefficient of resistance; due to this the current carrying ability does not decrease much due to rise of temperature.
8. High resistance to welding at the contact surfaces.
9. Low contact resistance; due to this overheating will be less.

No one material satisfies all the above requirements and hence two materials are mixed together in the desired proportions and processed by P/M. Each individual material has few of the above properties at the optimum level and the two together give all the properties at the best possible level, e.g. for high hardness, wear resistance, resistance to sparking and high melting temperature, refractory metals such as W or Mo and for high electrical and thermal conductivity, metals such as Cu or Ag are used.

Manufacturing processes

Two main P/M manufacturing processes are used. They are :
1. Conventional pressing and sintering followed by further cold or hot or working.
2. Pressing, sintering and infiltration.

In the first technique the metal powders of W or Mo are mixed with Cu or Ag in the required proportion and compacted at a pressure between 50 to 130 kg/mm^2. These cold compacts are sintered in a strongly reducing atmosphere at a temperature just below the melting point of the low melting metal. These sintered compacts have low density and hence they are further cold or hot compacted to develop high densities which are required for a good contact material. The properties of these components may also be controlled, to some extent, by controlling the particle size and shape of metal powders used in the manufacture of these components.

Liquid phase sintering, i.e. sintering at a temperature above the melting point of the high-conductivity constituent gives better physical properties and electrical conductivity. However, this results in considerable shrinkage and hence final forming or machining is required for obtaining exact dimensions.

The second technique involves the step of infiltrating the porous refractory metal powder skeleton with a second metal of high electrical conductivity. If impregnation is done correctly and the exact amount of impregnant is used, a component of very high density may be produced. On the other hand, if the component is only partly impregnated, it may be further densified by repressing.

These electrical contact materials are joined to conductors by brazing or soldering and used. The brazing operation is done either in a controlled atmosphere or in vacuum. The conductor material may also be cast on to the contact material and it has been observed that such a material shows good bond strength. The sintered contact materials are as below:

Simple refractory metals such as W and Mo, W-Cu, WC-Cu, W-Ag, WC-Ag, Mo-Ag, Ni-Ag, Ag-graphite and Cu-graphite.

Sintered Metal Friction Materials

Modern friction materials are used in devices such as clutches and brakes in which elements of a controlled friction level are necessary. For a satisfactory performance, the friction materials should have the following characteristics:

1. Sufficient coefficient of friction.
2. Minimum reduction in coefficient of friction with increasing temperature.
3. Smoothness of engagement.
4. Should not cause undue wear or damage to the opposing plate.
5. Good thermal conductivity.
6. Sufficient corrosion resistance.
7. Distorting ability which makes it possible to adjust with the actual working conditions.

No single material satisfies all the above requirements and hence many materials are mixed together in the powder form and processed by P/M to obtain all these properties in the component. As an example, the manufacturing process of a copper-based friction material is described below.

Blending of the raw materials

A typical composition of a copper based friction material is given below:

Metals	Weight %
Copper	68
Tin	8
Lead	7
Graphite	6
Silica	4
Iron	7

This is basically a 90/10 bronze material with additions of Pb, graphite, Silica and Fe. On weight% basis only 10 per cent is the amount of nonmetals. However, on volume basis it is about 30 per cent and hence care must be taken during mixing and blending for obtaining uniform distribution of these constituents throughout the mix. Silica is used for friction and hence its amount depends on the coefficient of friction required in the material. Mixing is carried out in conventional types of equipment such as double cone or Y-cone blenders. During mixing of the powders, gravity segregation is likely to occur because of large differences in the specific gravities of these powders. This is minimised by the addition of small amounts of light—fraction oils which volatilise at an early stage of sintering process.

Compacting

The powder is compacted at a pressure usually not exceeding 30 kg/mm^2. The compact is fragile and hence it should be handled carefully prior to its sintering.

Sintering

Sintering is done at about 800°C under load using a protective atmosphere. The heating cycle is between 4 to 6 hours depending on the size of the component. After sintering, they are machined to the exact shape and size.

TYPES OF METALS AND APPLICATIONS

Although the field of powder metallurgy is so widespread in application and varied in its nature, it is possible to classify the types of structure, in a general sort of way, under six headings. These headings are:
1. Porous metals.
2. Alloys with excessively high melting temperatures.
3. Alloys of metals which are mutually insoluble in the liquid state.
4. Alloys with poor casting qualities.
5. Alloys containing insoluble constituents required in a fine dispersion.
6. Alloys not readily machinable in their finished form and yet required to be more dimensionally accurate than they would be in a casting, or alternatively, alloys which can be produced in their finished shape more cheaply by this method.

Porous Metals

Porous metals are required in three applications, the first two being very common and the third somewhat rare. The first and probably the main application, is for self-lubricating bearings in which the porosity is used to hold a supply of lubricating oil which is then available for feeding directly to the bearing face. The second application is for filters for the separation of very fine sediment from different liquids. The third application is for low density metals. In the first two cases, the pores have to be interconnected throughout the structure, so that the respective liquids may travel through the material; but, in the third group, it is generally desirable that the pores should not be interconnected so that the overall density is not disturbed by infiltration. The degree of porosity in the first two cases can be governed both by the size of particle used in the compact and by the degree of pressure which is applied during compacting. In the case of the bearing metal the control is not so critical as it is for the filter, where uniformity of filtering is of primary importance. Because of the porosity, the strength of a porous metal must inevitably be considerably less than that of the nonporous basis material, a factor for which due allowance must be made. In this connection it is preferable to keep the thickness of a self-lubricating shell down to a minimum and to rely on the support of the bearing housing to give strength and rigidity.

Alloys with Excessively High Melting Temperatures

The group of alloys in which are included those metals with exceptionally high melting points is of growing importance, both in the development of heat resisting metals of the more highly alloyed type and in the preparation of sections of pure metals of basically high melting temperature. Naturally, a metal with a high melting temperature will tend to be relatively strong when stressed in a high temperature range. This fact is exemplified by the incorporation in heat-resisting alloys of metals with high melting points. Typical of these are molybdenum, with a melting temperature of about 2620°C, tungsten, with a melting temperature of about 3410°C, and niobium, with a melting temperature of about 2000°C. If solid pieces of such metals are required, it is exceedingly difficult to obtain them by casting methods, and powder metallurgical methods have to be used in many instances. A high melting point compound best prepared by powder metallurgical methods, is tungsten carbide which, when incorporated in an alloy, perhaps as the main constituent, is often required in a prefabricated form suitable for its incorporation in those alloys since, prior to its application, it has to be present as an insoluble constituent.

An illustration of this type of application is provided by the preparation of tungsten carbide particles for incorporation in a welded surface-facing, for the cutting edge of a coal cutter, or for some similar application. In this instance the weld cannot be cast as a homogeneous alloy, or from a homogeneous alloy, so the carbide particles are enclosed in an iron or steel tube, which is then used as a welding filler rod. The enclosed carbide particles are thus deposited together with the melting tube material, giving a deposit of abrasive tungsten carbide particles embedded in a matrix of iron, firmly bonded to the body of the cutter. Such tungsten carbide, if required in rough form, may be prepared by arc melting but it is frequently desirable that the particles should be angular in shape to make their cutting action more efficient. Such shapes are best produced by powder metallurgical methods, by preparing, for example, a long prism of triangular section and then subdividing the prism into short lengths to form the particles.

Other applications which may be included in this group are those in which certain nonmetals, having high melting points, have to be incorporated in a metal matrix to form what has come to be known as a 'cermet' or a metal-bonded ceramic. The type of application for which this class of material is most commonly prepared is for the turbine blades in a gas turbine where the temperature of operation is in the range 900°–1000°C. Some heat resisting metal alloys may be prepared in the same way for the same purpose.

Alloys of Metals which are Mutually Insoluble in the Liquid State

Those alloys whose constituents are mutually insoluble in the liquid state offer a serious problem to casting and, indeed, may be almost impossible to cast effectively. This is particularly true if the constituents are also insoluble in the solid condition. For such alloys, powder metallurgical methods offer the only practical solution if reasonably uniform structures are to be obtained. It will be appreciated that such alloys like copper-molybdenum series must be difficult to cast since the liquids will tend to separate under gravity. In such cases, if a finely divided uniform structure is to be obtained, the only feasible approach is by powder metallurgical methods. Another equilibrium relationship which gives rise to trouble in casting is that known as a monotectic which we will not consider in detail but which is illustrated in Fig. 9.9, in the copper–lead equilibrium diagram. The relevant portion of the diagram is the horizontal line BCD (which represents the temperature of the monotectic change) at which the temperature is, arrested until the copper has crystallised out to the composition represented by point D. This means that there is almost complete segregation of the constituents and casting of a uniform alloy is practically impossible. If a lead bronze is required to have a reasonably uniform structure, then powder metallurgical methods offer the only sure means of obtaining this.

Alloys with Poor Casting Qualities

Many metals are very difficult to cast because of the complex nature of the phase changes which tend to take place during solidification, and such changes often give rise to marked segregation in the alloy structure. If it is important that segregation be severely limited, then powder metallurgy is the only possible solution. The heat resisting alloy, which has been used for high temperature gas turbine components, based on a primary alloy of 70 per cent cobalt and 30 per cent chromium which has been modified by adding 5 per cent niobium carbide. The marked segregation in the cast structure is clearly apparent and can be compared with the uniformity of the powder metallurgy type. In the latter case, the powder constituents were 70 per cent cobalt, 30 per cent chromium alloy powder, mixed with 5 per cent of niobium carbide powder. Some of the alloys, specially developed for their magnetic properties, are subject to similar difficulties in casting and powder metallurgical preparation offers the best fabricating method for them.

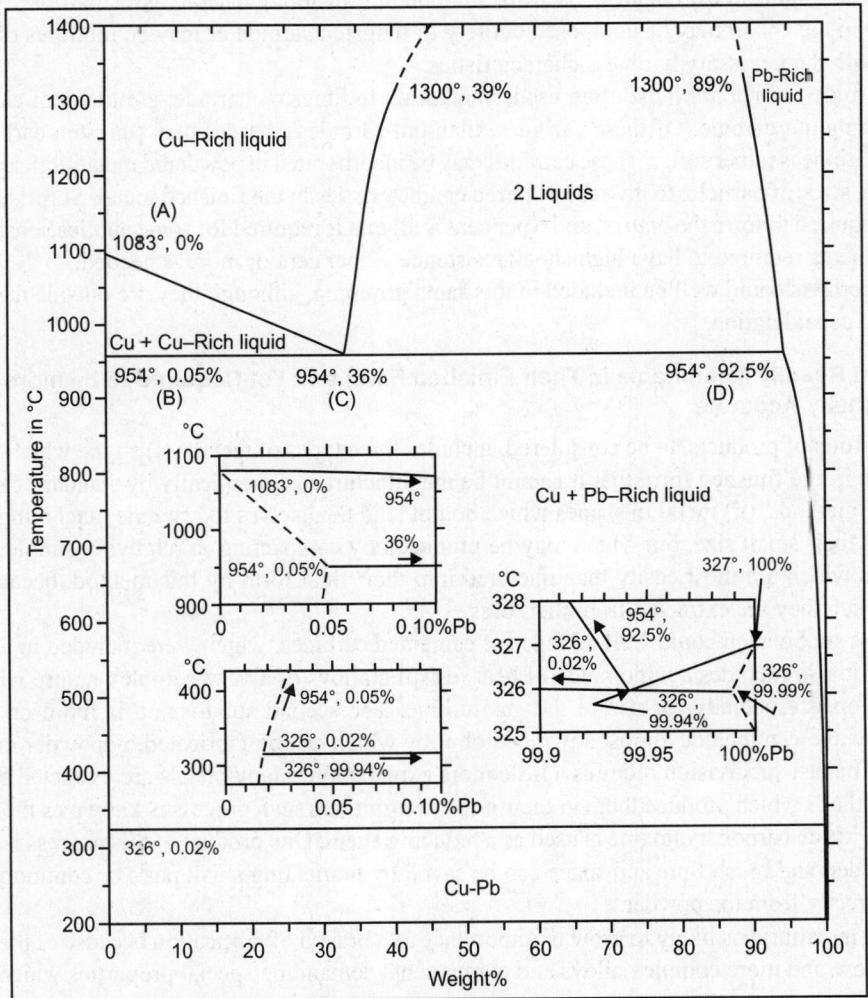

Fig. 9.9. Copper–lead equilibrium diagram.

Alloys Containing Insoluble Constituents Required in a Fine Dispersion

Hard, abrasive material such as tungsten carbide, despite its great hardness, tends to be excessively brittle and therefore relatively useless for machining operations or other applications where any shock loading is likely to be applied. To overcome this difficulty a range of hard metals, known as 'cemented carbides', have been developed and these form the main division of the fifth group of powder metallurgical applications. This group includes those alloys which contain finely dispersed, insoluble constituents embedded in a continuous matrix.

The method of fabrication which is adopted for these cemented carbides is to incorporate in the mix some relatively soft material in sufficient amounts to form a ductile matrix in which the hard particles can be located. This matrix has to be able to withstand relatively high temperatures and so, for most cutting metal applications, cobalt is used for the bonding material. The abrasive particles which ate embedded in the cobalt may be composed entirely of tungsten carbide or may be mixtures of different carbides with the necessary hardness characteristics.

The carbides which are most often used, in addition to tungsten carbide, are titanium carbide and possibly tantalum carbide. Of these carbides, titanium carbide is harder than tungsten carbide while tantalum carbide is rather softer. These carbides may be incorporated in powdered metallurgical products, in differing sizes of particle, to give the required characteristics in the finished metal. Surprisingly little cobalt is required to form the matrix, and 6 per cent is all that is required for some applications, although for components required to have high shock resistance 12 per cent or more is needed.

Some cermets could well be included in this same grouping, although they are outside the scope of the present consideration.

Alloys Not Readily Machinable in Their Finished Form and Yet Required to be more Dimensionally Accurate

The final group of products, to be considered, includes three types of metals: (i) a type which is so hard to machine in the finished form that it cannot be manufactured economically by standard casting and machining methods, (ii) metal in shapes which do not lend themselves to accurate machining, perhaps because of their small size, but which may be produced by compacting in relatively simple dies, and (iii) metals which are most easily manufactured into their final form by this method, because of the form in which they are extracted from their ores.

The first subdivision could well include the cemented carbides, which were included in a previous group, but it also includes a wide range of heat resisting alloys of a very complex nature which have been developed especially for use in the gas turbine. The second subdivision is more or less self-explanatory and can include almost any metal or alloy which can be fabricated by powder metallurgy methods. The last subdivision requires a little more explanation. Many metals are extracted from their ores by methods which produce them in their powder form; one such process is known as the carbonyl process, in which carbon monoxide is used as a reducing agent. One product of this process is carbonyl nickel powder, and much time and space can be saved by fabricating small parts or continuous small sections directly from the powder.

Powder metallurgy is likely to grow in importance as a branch of fabrication because of the growing need for more and more complex alloys and components demanding special properties which are only obtainable by these means.

Chapter 10

Aluminium and Aluminium Alloys

INTRODUCTION

Aluminium alloys are alloys in which aluminium (Al) is the predominant metal. The typical alloying elements are copper, magnesium, manganese, silicon, and zinc. There are two principal classifications, namely casting alloys and wrought alloys, both of which are further subdivided into the categories heat-treatable and non-heat-treatable. About 85 per cent of aluminium is used for wrought products, for example rolled plate, foils and extrusions. Cast aluminium alloys yield cost effective products due to the low melting point, although they generally have lower tensile strengths than wrought alloys. The most important cast aluminium alloy system is Al-Si, where the high levels of silicon (4.0 to 13 per cent) contribute to give good casting characteristics. Aluminium alloys are widely used in engineering structures and components where light weight or corrosion resistance is required.

Alloys composed mostly of the two lightweight metals aluminium and magnesium have been very important in aerospace manufacturing since somewhat before 1940. Aluminium-magnesium alloys are both lighter than other aluminium alloys and much less flammable than alloys that contain a very high percentage of magnesium.

Aluminium alloy surfaces will keep their apparent shine in a dry environment due to the formation of a clear, protective layer of aluminium oxide. In a wet environment, galvanic corrosion can occur when an aluminium alloy is placed in electrical contact with other metals with more negative corrosion potentials than aluminium.

ENGINEERING USES OF ALUMINIUM ALLOYS

Aluminium alloys with a wide range of properties are used in engineering structures. Alloy systems are classified by a number system (ANSI) or by names indicating their main alloying constituents (DIN and ISO). Selecting the right alloy for a given application entails considerations of its tensile strength, density, ductility, formability, workability, weldability, and corrosion resistance, to name a few. Aluminium alloys are used extensively in aircraft due to their high strength-to-weight ratio. On the other hand, pure aluminium metal is much too soft for such uses, and it does not have the high tensile strength that is needed for airplanes and helicopters.

Aluminium Alloys Versus Types of Steel

Aluminium alloys typically have an elastic modulus of about 70 GPa, which is about one-third of the elastic modulus of most kinds of steel and steel alloys. Therefore, for a given load, a component or unit made of an aluminium alloy will experience a greater elastic deformation than a steel part of the identical size and shape. Though there are aluminium alloys with somewhat-higher tensile strengths than the commonly-used kinds of steel, simply replacing a steel part with an aluminium alloy might lead to problems.

With completely-new metal products, the design choices are often governed by the choice of manufacturing technology. Extrusions are particularly important in this regard, owing to the ease with which aluminium alloys, particularly the Al-Mg-Si series, can be extruded to form complex profiles.

In general, stiffer and lighter designs can be achieved with aluminium alloys than is feasible with steels. For instance, consider the bending of a thin-walled tube: the second moment of area is inversely related to the stress in the tube wall, i.e. stresses are lower for larger values. The second moment of area is proportional to the cube of the radius times the wall thickness, thus increasing the radius (and weight) by 26 per cent will lead to a halving of the wall stress. For this reason, bicycle frames made of aluminium alloys make use of larger tube diameters than steel or titanium in order to yield the desired stiffness and strength. In automotive engineering, cars made of aluminium alloys employ space frames made of extruded profiles to ensure rigidity. This represents a radical change from the common approach for current steel car design, which depend on the body shells for stiffness, that is a unibody design.

Aluminium alloys are widely used in automotive engines, particularly in cylinder blocks and crankcases due to the weight savings that are possible. Since aluminium alloys are susceptible to warping at elevated temperatures, the cooling system of such engines is critical. Manufacturing techniques and metallurgical advancements have also been instrumental for the successful application in automotive engines.

An important structural limitation of aluminium alloys is their lower fatigue strength compared to steel. In controlled laboratory conditions, steels display a fatigue limit, which is the stress amplitude below which no failures occur. Aluminium alloys are therefore sparsely used in parts that require high fatigue strength in the high cycle regime (more than 10^7 stress cycles).

Heat Sensitivity Considerations

Often, the metal's sensitivity to heat must also be considered. Even a relatively routine workshop procedure involving heating is complicated by the fact that aluminium, unlike steel, will melt without first glowing red. Forming operations where a blow torch is used therefore require some expertise, because no visual signs reveal how close the material is to melting.

Aluminium also is subject to internal stresses and strains when it is overheated; the tendency of the metal to creep under these stresses tends to result in delayed distortions. For example, the warping or cracking of overheated aluminium automobile cylinder heads is commonly observed, sometimes years later, as is the tendency of welded aluminium bicycle frames to gradually twist out of alignment from the stresses of the welding process. Thus, the aerospace industry avoids heat altogether by joining parts with adhesives or mechanical fasteners. Adhesive bonding was used in some bicycle frames in the 1970s, with unfortunate results when the aluminium tubing corroded slightly, loosening the adhesive and collapsing the frame.

Stresses in overheated aluminium can be relieved by heat-treating the parts in an oven and gradually cooling it — in effect annealing the stresses. Yet these parts may still become distorted, so that heat-treating of welded bicycle frames, for instance, can result in a significant fraction becoming misaligned. If the misalignment is not too severe, the cooled parts may be bent into alignment. Of course, if the frame is properly designed for rigidity, that bending will require enormous force.

Aluminium's intolerance to high temperatures has not precluded its use in rocketry; even for use in constructing combustion chambers where gases can reach 3500 K. The Agena upper stage engine used a regeneratively cooled aluminium design for some parts of the nozzle, including the thermally critical throat region; in fact the extremely high thermal conductivity of aluminium prevented the throat from reaching the melting point even under massive heat flux, resulting in a reliable lightweight component.

Household Wiring

Because of its high conductivity and relatively low price compared with copper in the 1960s, aluminium was introduced at that time for household electrical wiring in the United States, even though many fixtures had not been designed to accept aluminium wire. But the new use brought some problems:
1. The greater coefficient of thermal expansion of aluminium causes the wire to expand and contract relative to the dissimilar metal screw connection, eventually loosening the connection.
2. Pure aluminium has a tendency to 'creep' under steady sustained pressure (to a greater degree as the temperature rises), again loosening the connection.
3. Galvanic corrosion from the dissimilar metals increases the electrical resistance of the connection.

All of this resulted in overheated and loose connections, and this in turn resulted in some fires. Builders then became wary of using the wire, and many jurisdictions outlawed its use in very small sizes, in new construction.

Another way to forestall the heating problem is to crimp the aluminium wire to a short 'pigtail' of copper wire. A properly done high-pressure crimp by the proper tool is tight enough to reduce any thermal expansion of the aluminium. Today, new alloys, designs, and methods are used for aluminium wiring in combination with aluminium terminations.

Alloy Designations

Wrought and cast aluminium alloys use different identification systems. Wrought aluminium is identified with a four digit number which identifies the alloying elements.

Cast aluminium alloys use a four to five digit number with a decimal point. The digit in the hundreds place indicates the alloying elements, while the digit after the decimal point indicates the form (cast shape or ingot).

Temper designation

The temper designation follows the cast or wrought designation number with a dash, a letter, and potentially a one to three digit number, e.g. 6061-T6.

Wrought alloys

The International alloy designation system is the most widely accepted naming scheme for wrought alloys. Each alloy is given a four-digit number, where the first digit indicates the major alloying elements:
1. 1000 series are essentially pure aluminium with a minimum 99 per cent aluminium content by weight and can be work hardened.
2. 2000 series are alloyed with copper, can be precipitation hardened to strengths comparable to steel. Formerly referred to as duralumin, they were once the most common aerospace alloys, but were susceptible to stress corrosion cracking and are increasingly replaced by 7000 series in new designs.
3. 3000 series are alloyed with manganese, and can be work hardened.
4. 4000 series are alloyed with silicon. They are also known as silumin.
5. 5000 series are alloyed with magnesium.

6. 6000 series are alloyed with magnesium and silicon, are easy to machine, and can be precipitation hardened, but not to the high strengths that 2000 and 7000 can reach.
7. 7000 series are alloyed with zinc, and can be precipitation hardened to the highest strengths of any aluminium alloy.
8. 8000 series is a category mainly used for lithium alloys.

Cast alloys

The aluminium association (AA) has adopted a nomenclature similar to that of wrought alloys. British Standard and DIN have different designations. In the AA system, the second two digits reveal the minimum percentage of aluminium, e.g. 150.x correspond to a minimum of 99.50 per cent aluminium. The digit after the decimal point takes a value of 0 or 1, denoting casting and ingot respectively. The main alloying elements in the AA system are as follows:

1. 1xx.x series are minimum 99 per cent aluminium.
2. 2xx.x series copper.
3. 3xx.x series silicon, copper and/or magnesium.
4. 4xx.x series silicon.
5. 5xx.x series magnesium.
6. 7xx.x series zinc.
7. 8xx.x series lithium.

Minimum tensile requirements for cast aluminium alloys is shown in Table 10.1.

Table 10.1. Minimum tensile requirements for cast aluminium alloys.

Alloy type		Temper	Tensile strength (min) [ksi]	Yield strength (min) [ksi]	Elongation in 2 in [%]
ANSI	UNS				
201.0	A02010	T7	60.0	50.0	3.0
204.0	A02040	T4	45.0	28.0	6.0
242.0	A02420	O	23.0	N/A	N/A
		T61	32.0	20.0	N/A
A242.0	A12420	T75	29.0	N/A	1.0
		T4	29.0	13.0	6.0
		T6	32.0	20.0	3.0
295.0	A029550	T62	36.0	28.0	N/A
		T7	29.0	16.0	3.0
319.0	A03190	F	23.0	13.0	1.5
		T5	25.0	N/A	N/A
		T6	31.0	20.0	1.5
328.0	A03280	F	25.0	14.0	1.0
		T6	34.0	21.0	1.0
355.0	A03550	T6	32.0	20.0	2.0
		T51	25.0	18.0	N/A
		T71	30.0	22.0	N/A
C355.0	A33550	T6	36.0	25.0	2.5

(Contd ...)

Alloy type		Temper	Tensile strength (min) [ksi]	Yield strength (min) [ksi]	Elongation in 2 in [%]
ANSI	UNS				
356.0	A03560	F	19.0	9.5	2.0
		T6	30.0	20.0	3.0
		T7	31.0	N/A	N/A
		T51	23.0	16.0	N/A
		T71	25.0	18.0	3.0
A356.0	A13560	T6	34.0	24.0	3.5
		T61	35.0	26.0	1.0
443.0	A04430	F	17.0	7.0	3.0
B443.0	A24430	F	17.0	6.0	3.0
512.0	A05120	F	17.0	10.0	N/A
514.0	A05140	F	22.0	9.0	6.0
520.0	A05200	T4	42.0	22.0	12.0
535.0	A05350	F	35.0	18.0	9.0
705.0	A07050	T5	30.0	17.0†	5.0
707.0	A07070	T7	37.0	30.0†	1.0
710.0	A07100	T5	32.0	20.0	2.0
712.0	A07120	T5	34.0	25.0†	4.0
713.0	A07130	T5	32.0	22.0	3.0
771.0	A07710	T5	42.0	38.0	1.5
		T51	32.0	27.0	3.0
		T52	36.0	30.0	1.5
		T6	42.0	35.0	5.0
		T71	48.0	45.0	5.0
850.0	A08500	T5	16.0	N/A	5.0
851.0	A08510	T5	17.0	N/A	3.0
852.0	A08520	T5	24.0	18.0	N/A

† Only when requested by the customer.

Named alloys

1. Alclad Aluminium sheet formed from high-purity aluminium surface layers bonded to high strength aluminium alloy core material.
2. Birmabright (aluminium, magnesium) a product of The Birmetals Company, basically equivalent to 5251.
3. Duralumin (copper, aluminium).
4. Magnalium.
5. Magnox (magnesium, aluminium).
6. Silumin (aluminium, silicon).
7. Titanal (aluminium, zinc, magnesium, copper, zirconium) a product of Austria Metall AG. Commonly used in high performance sports products, particularly snowboards and skis.

8. Y alloy, Hiduminium, R. R. alloys: pre-war nickel-aluminium alloys, used in aerospace and engine pistons, for their ability to retain strength at elevated temperature.

Applications

Aerospace alloys

Scandium-aluminium

The addition of scandium to aluminium creates nanoscale Al_3Sc precipitates which limit the excessive grain growth that occurs in the heat-affected zone of welded aluminium components. This has two beneficial effects: the precipitated Al_3Sc forms smaller crystals than are formed in other aluminium alloys and the width of precipitate-free zones that normally exist at the grain boundaries of age-hardenable aluminium alloys is reduced. Scandium is also a potent grain refiner in cast aluminium alloys, and atom for atom, the most potent strengthener in aluminium, both as a result of grain refinement and precipitation strengthening. However, titanium alloys, which are stronger but heavier, are cheaper and much more widely used.

The main application of metallic scandium by weight is in aluminium-scandium alloys for minor aerospace industry components. These alloys contain between 0.1 per cent and 0.5 per cent (by weight) of scandium. They were used in the Russian military aircraft Mig 21 and Mig 29.

Some items of sports equipment, which rely on high performance materials, have been made with scandium-aluminium alloys, including baseball bats, lacrosse sticks, as well as bicycle frames and components. US gunmaker Smith and Wesson produces revolvers with frames composed of scandium alloy and cylinders of titanium.

List of aerospace aluminium alloys

The following aluminium alloys are commonly used in aircraft and other aerospace structures:
1. 7075 aluminium.
2. 6061 aluminium.
3. 6063 aluminium.
4. 2024 aluminium.
5. 5052 aluminium.

Note that the term aircraft aluminium or aerospace aluminium usually refers to 7075.

Marine alloys

These alloys are used for boat building and shipbuilding, and other marine and salt-water sensitive shore applications.:
1. 5052 aluminium.
2. 5083 aluminium.
3. 5086 aluminium.
4. 6061 aluminium.
5. 6063 aluminium.

Cycling alloys

These alloys are used for cycling frames and components:
1. 2014 aluminium.
2. 6061 aluminium.

3. 6063 aluminium.
4. 7005 aluminium.
5. 7075 aluminium.
6. Scandium aluminium.

Automotive alloys

6111 aluminium is extensively used for automotive body panels.

HEAT TREATING OF ALUMINIUM AND ALUMINIUM ALLOYS

Heat treating processes for aluminium are precision processes. They must be carried out in furnaces properly designed and built to provide the thermal conditions required, and adequately equipped with control instruments to insure the desired continuity and uniformity of temperature-time cycles. To insure the final desired characteristics, process details must be established and controlled carefully for each type of product. The general types of heat treatments applied to aluminium and its alloys are:
1. Preheating or homogenising, to reduce chemical segregation of cast structures and to improve their workability.
2. Annealing, to soften strain-hardened (work-hardened) and heat treated alloy structures, to relieve stresses, and to stabilise properties and dimensions.
3. Solution heat treatments, to effect solid solution of alloying constituents and improve mechanical properties.
4. Precipitation heat treatments, to provide hardening by precipitation of constituents from solid solution.

INGOT PREHEATING TREATMENTS (HOMOGENISING)

The initial thermal operation applied to ingots prior to hot working is referred to as 'ingot preheating', which has one or more purposes depending upon the alloy, product, and fabricating process involved. One of the principal objectives is improved workability. The microstructure of most alloys in the as-cast condition is quite heterogeneous. This is true for alloys that form solid solutions under equilibrium conditions, and even for relatively dilute alloys.

Annealing

The distorted, dislocated structure resulting from cold working of aluminium is less stable than the strain-free, annealed state, to which it tends to revert. Lower-purity aluminium and commercial aluminium alloys undergo these structural changes only with annealing at elevated temperatures. Accompanying the structural reversion are changes in the various properties affected by cold working. These changes occur in several stages, according to temperature or time, and have led to the concept of different annealing mechanisms or processes.

Recovery: The reduction in the number of dislocations is greatest at the center of the grain fragments, producing a subgrain structure with networks or groups of dislocations at the subgrain boundaries. With increasing time and temperature of heating, polygonisation becomes more nearly perfect and the subgrain size gradually increases. In this stage, many of the subgrains appear to have boundaries that are free of dislocation tangles and concentrations. Recovery annealing is also accompanied by changes in other properties of cold worked aluminium. Complete recovery from the effects of cold working is obtained only with recrystallisation.

Recrystallisation: Recrystallisation is characterised by the gradual formation and appearance of a microscopically resolvable grain structure. The new structure is largely strain-free—there are few if any dislocations within the grains and no concentrations at the grain boundaries.

Grain growth after recrystallisation: Heating after recrystallisation may produce grain coarsening. This can take one of several forms.

Precipitation Hardening

General principles of precipitation hardening: The heat treatable alloys contain amounts of soluble alloying elements that exceed the equilibrium solid solubility limit at room and moderately higher temperatures. The amount present may be less or more than the maximum that is soluble at the eutectic temperature.

Nature of precipitates and sources of hardening: Intensive research during the past forty years has resulted in a progressive accumulation of knowledge concerning the atomic and crystallographic structural changes that occur in supersaturated solid solutions during precipitation and the mechanisms through which the structures form and alter alloy properties. In most precipitation-hardenable systems, a complex sequence of time-dependent and temperature-dependent changes is involved.

Kinetics of solution and precipitation: The relative rates at which solution and precipitation reactions occur with different solutes depend upon the respective diffusion rates, in addition to solubilities and alloy contents. Bulk diffusion coefficients for several of the commercially important alloying elements in aluminium were determined by various experimental methods.

Nucleation: The formation of zones can occur in an essentially continuous crystal lattice by a process of homogeneous nucleation. Recent investigations provide evidence that a critical vacancy concentration is required for this process and that a nucleation model involving vacancy-solute atom clusters is consistent with certain effects of solution temperature and quenching rate.

The nucleation of a new phase is greatly influenced by the existence of discontinuities in the lattice. Since in polycrystalline alloys grain boundaries, subgrain boundaries, dislocations, and interphase boundaries are locations of greater disorder and higher energy than the solid-solution matrix, they are preferred sites for nucleation of precipitates.

Quenching

Quenching is in many ways the most critical step in the sequence of heat treating operations. The objective of quenching is to preserve as nearly intact as possible the solid solution formed at the solution heat treating temperature, by rapidly cooling to some lower temperature, usually near room temperature.

Critical temperature range: The fundamentals involved in quenching precipitation-hardenable alloys are based on nucleation theory applied to diffusion-controlled solid state reactions. The effects of temperature on the kinetics of isothermal precipitation depend principally upon degree of supersaturation and rate of diffusion.

Quenching medium: Water is not only the most widely used quenching medium but also the most effective. It is apparent that in immersion quenching, cooling rates can be reduced by increasing water temperature. Conditions that increase the stability of a vapour film around the part decrease the cooling rate; various additions to water that lower surface tension have the same effect.

Ageing at room temperature (natural ageing)

Most of the heat treatable alloys exhibit age hardening at room temperature after quenching, the rate and extent of such hardening varying from one alloy to another. No discernible microstructural changes accompany the room-temperature ageing, since the hardening effects are attributable solely to the formation of zone structure within the solid solution.

Since the alloys are softer and more ductile immediately after quenching than after ageing, straightening or forming operations may be performed more readily in the freshly quenched condition.

Precipitation heat treating (artificial ageing)

The effects of precipitation on mechanical properties are greatly accelerated, and usually accentuated, by reheating the quenched material to about 100° to 200°C. The effects are not entirely attributable to a changed reaction rate; as mentioned previously, the structural changes occurring at the elevated temperatures differ in fundamental ways from those occurring at room temperature. These differences are reflected in the mechanical characteristics and some physical properties. A characteristic feature of elevated-temperature ageing effects on tensile properties is that the increase in yield strength is more pronounced than the increase in tensile strength. Also ductility, as measured by percentage elongation, decreases. Thus, an alloy in the T6 temper has higher strength but lower ductility than the same alloy in the T4 temper.

Precipitation heat treating without prior solution heat treatment

Certain alloys that are relatively insensitive to cooling rate during quenching can be either air cooled or water quenched directly from a final hot working operation. In either condition, these alloys will respond strongly to precipitation heat treatment.

Precipitation heat treating cast products

The mechanical properties of permanent mould, sand, and plaster castings of most alloys are greatly improved by solution heat treating, quenching, and precipitation heat treating, using practices analogous to those employed for wrought products.

Chapter 11

Cast Iron Alloys

INTRODUCTION

Cast iron usually refers to grey iron, but also identifies a large group of ferrous alloys, which solidify with a eutectic. The colour of a fractured surface can be used to identify an alloy. White cast iron is named after its white surface when fractured, due to its carbide impurities which allow cracks to pass straight through. Grey cast iron is named after its grey fractured surface, which occurs because the graphitic flakes deflect a passing crack and initiate countless new cracks as the material breaks. Carbon (C) and silicon (Si) are the main alloying elements, with the amount ranging from 2.1 to 4 wt% and 1 to 3 wt%, respectively. While this technically makes these base alloys ternary Fe-C-Si alloys, the principle of cast iron solidification is understood from the binary iron-carbon phase diagram. Since the compositions of most cast irons are around the eutectic point of the iron-carbon system, the melting temperatures closely correlate, usually ranging from 1150° to 1200°C (2102° to 2192°F), which is about 300°C (572°F) lower than the melting point of pure iron. Cast iron tends to be brittle, except for malleable cast irons. With its relatively low melting point, good fluidity, castability, excellent machinability, resistance to deformation and wear resistance, cast irons have become an engineering material with a wide range of applications and are used in pipes, machines and automotive industry parts, such as cylinder heads (declining usage), cylinder blocks and gearbox cases (declining usage). It is resistant to destruction and weakening by oxidisation (rust).

PRODUCTION OF CAST IRON ALLOYS

Cast iron is made by re-melting pig iron, often along with substantial quantities of scrap iron and scrap steel and taking various steps to remove undesirable contaminants such as phosphorus and sulphur. Depending on the application, carbon and silicon content are reduced to the desired levels, which may be anywhere from 2 to 3.5 per cent and 1 to 3 per cent respectively. Other elements are then added to the melt before the final form is produced by casting. Iron is sometimes melted in a special type of blast furnace known as a cupola, but more often melted in electric induction furnaces. After melting is complete, the molten iron is poured into a holding furnace or ladle.

Types

Alloying elements

Cast iron's properties are changed by adding various alloying elements, or alloyants. Next to carbon, silicon is the most important alloyant because it forces carbon out of solution. Instead the carbon forms graphite which results in a softer iron, reduces shrinkage, lowers strength, and decreases density. Sulphur, when added, forms iron sulphide, which prevents the formation of graphite and increases hardness. The problem with sulphur is that it makes molten cast iron sluggish, which causes short run defects. To counter the effects of sulphur, manganese is added because the two form into manganese sulphide instead of iron sulphide. The manganese sulphide is lighter than the melt so it tends to float out of the melt and into the slag. The amount of manganese required to neutralise sulphur is $1.7 \times$ sulphur content $+0.3$ per cent. If more than this amount of manganese is added, then manganese carbide forms, which increases hardness and chilling, except in grey iron, where up to 1 per cent of manganese increases strength and density. Nickel is one of the most common alloyants because it refines the pearlite and graphite structure, improves toughness, and evens out hardness differences between section thicknesses. Chromium is added in small amounts to the ladle to reduce free graphite, produce chill, and because it is a powerful carbide stabiliser; nickel is often added in conjunction. A small amount of tin can be added as a substitute for 0.5 per cent chromium. Copper is added in the ladle or in the furnace, on the order of 0.5 to 2.5 per cent, to decrease chill, refine graphite, and increase fluidity. Molybdenum is added on the order of 0.3 to 1 per cent to increase chill and refine the graphite and pearlite structure; it is often added in conjunction with nickel, copper, and chromium to form high strength irons. Titanium is added as a degasser and deoxidiser, but it also increases fluidity. 0.15 to 0.5 per cent vanadium are added to cast iron to stabilise cementite, increase hardness, and increase resistance to wear and heat. 0.1 to 0.3 per cent zirconium helps to form graphite, deoxidise, and increase fluidity. In malleable iron melts, bismuth is added, on the scale of 0.002 to 0.01 per cent, to increase how much silicon can be added. In white iron, boron is added to aid in the production of malleable iron; it also reduces the coarsening effect of bismuth.

Grey cast iron

Grey cast iron is characterised by its graphitic microstructure, which causes fractures of the material to have a grey appearance. It is the most commonly used cast iron and the most widely use cast material based on weight. Most cast irons have a chemical composition of 2.5 to 4.0 per cent carbon, 1 to 3 per cent silicon, and the remainder is iron. Grey cast iron has less tensile strength and shock resistance than steel, however its compressive strength is comparable to low and medium carbon steel.

White cast iron

With a lower silicon content and faster cooling, the carbon in white cast iron precipitates out of the melt as the metastable phase cementite, Fe_3C, rather than graphite. The cementite which precipitates from the melt forms as relatively large particles, usually in a eutectic mixture, where the other phase is austenite (which on cooling might transform to martensite). These eutectic carbides are much too large to provide precipitation hardening (as in some steels, where cementite precipitates might inhibit plastic deformation by impeding the movement of dislocations through the ferrite matrix). Rather, they increase the bulk hardness of the cast iron simply by virtue of their own very high hardness and their substantial volume fraction, such that the bulk hardness can be approximated by a rule of mixtures. In any case, they offer hardness at the expense of toughness. Since carbide makes up a large fraction of the material, white cast iron could reasonably be classified as a cermet. White iron is too brittle for use in many structural components, but with good hardness and abrasion resistance and relatively low cost, it finds use in such applications as the wear surfaces (impeller and volute) of slurry pumps, shell liners and lifter bars in ball mills and autogenous grinding mills, balls and rings in coal pulverisers, and the teeth of a backhoe's digging bucket (although cast medium-carbon martensitic steel is more common for this application).

It is difficult to cool thick castings fast enough to solidify the melt as white cast iron all the way through. However, rapid cooling can be used to solidify a shell of white cast iron, after which the remainder cools more slowly to form a core of grey cast iron. The resulting casting, called a chilled casting, has the benefits of a hard surface and a somewhat tougher interior. High-chromium white iron alloys allow massive castings (for example, a 10 ton impeller) to be sand cast, i.e. a high cooling rate is not required, as well as providing impressive abrasion resistance.

Malleable cast iron

Malleable iron starts as a white iron casting that is then heat treated at about 900°C (1650°F). Graphite separates out much more slowly in this case, so that surface tension has time to form it into spheroidal particles rather than flakes. Due to their lower aspect ratio, spheroids are relatively short and far from one another, and have a lower cross section vis-*a*-vis a propagating crack or phonon. They also have blunt boundaries, as opposed to flakes, which alleviates the stress concentration problems faced by grey cast iron. In general, the properties of malleable cast iron are more like mild steel. There is a limit to how large a part can be cast in malleable iron, since it is made from white cast iron.

Ductile cast iron

A more recent development is nodular or ductile cast iron. Tiny amounts of magnesium or cerium added to these alloys slow down the growth of graphite precipitates by bonding to the edges of the graphite planes. Along with careful control of other elements and timing, this allows the carbon to separate as spheroidal particles as the material solidifies. The properties are similar to malleable iron, but parts can be cast with larger sections. Table 11.1 compares the qualities of cast irons.

Table 11.1. Comparative qualities of cast irons

Name	Nominal composition [% by weight]	Form and condition	Yield strength [ksi (0.2% offset)]	Tensile strength [ksi]	Elongation [% (in 2 inches)]	Hardness [brinell scale]	Uses
Grey cast iron (ASTM A48)	C 3.4, Si 1.8, Mn 0.5	Cast	–	25	0.5	180	Engine cylinder blocks, flywheels gears, machine tool bases
White cast iron	C 3.4, Si 0.7, Mn 0.6	Cast (as cast)	–	25	0	450	Bearing surfaces
Malleable iron (ASTM A47)	C 2.5, Si 1.0, Mn 0.55	Cast (annealed)	33	52	12	130	Axle bearings, track wheels, automotive crankshafts
Ductile or nodular iron	C 3.4, P 0.1, Mn 0.4, Ni 1.0, Mg 0.06	Cast	53	70	18	170	Gears, camshafts crankshafts
Ductile or nodular iron (ASTM A339)	–	Cast (quench tempered)	108	135	5	310	–

(Contd ...)

Name	Nominal composition [% by weight]	Form and condition	Yield strength [ksi (0.2% offset)]	Tensile strength [ksi]	Elongation [% in 2 inches)]	Hardness [brinell scale]	Uses
Ni-hard type 2	C 2.7, Si 0.6, Mn 0.5, Ni 4.5, Cr 2.0	Sand–cast	–	55	–	550	High strength applications
Ni-resist type 2	C 3.0, Si 2.0, Mn 1.0, Ni 20.0, Cr 2.5	Cast	–	27	2	140	Resistance to heat and corrosion

HEAT TREATING IRON CASTINGS

Many metal castings are designed with relatively uniform wall thickness and section size and therefore experience little significant residual stress and structural variation after solidification. However, iron castings can be prone to retain residual stresses and structural variations after cooling, especially when they have a complex shape with many interconnected thick and thin sections. This variation can cause distortion and non-uniform mechanical properties. Dimensional instability is most likely to become evident during machining. Annealing, stress relieving and normalised are thermal treatments that can reduce the residual stress and non-uniform mechanical properties likely to be found in certain iron casting geometries.

STEPS IN HEAT TREATING
Annealing Treatments

Annealing is a thermal treatment process that softens cast iron by slow-cooling the austenitic matrix (the phase where the iron is composed of a solid solution of cementite through its critical temperature range. This creates a ferritic microstructure. Annealing can relieve residual stresses in castings if the slow cooling is continued to a low enough temperature.

There are three types of annealing for iron castings, high, medium and low (sub-critical). In high-temperature annealing, a casting is heated above the critical range to a temperature (1650°–1750°F/ 900°–950°C) at which both primary carbides and free cementite decompose to ferrite and graphite. A ferritic structure is produced and minimum hardness is obtained if the casting is cooled slowly to below the critical range. This slow cooling often is referred to as 'furnace cooled'.

In the absence of massive carbides or if minute quantities of well-dispersed carbides are present, medium-temperature annealing (also known as full annealing) is used. In this process, a casting is heated to just above the critical range (1500°–1650°F/820°–900°C), depending mainly on the silicon content, then slow-cooled. Low-temperature (or subcritical) annealing, also known as ferritising, is accomplished by heating to just below the critical range, followed by slow cooling. The purpose is to convert pearlitic carbides, in the absence of free cementite, to ferrite and graphite by a gradual diffusion process, rather than by transformation.

Stress-relieving Treatments

Stress relieving is a heat treatment used to relieve stress in the subcritical stage and thus minimise distortion. Sand castings slowly cooled in the mould are largely free of residual stresses. However, this slow cooling could result in a casting that is too soft and has mechanical properties that are out of specification. Selecting the proper stress-relieving temperature-time cycle is a compromise that reduces residual stress while allowing the desired mechanical properties to be maintained in the casting.

Normalising Treatments

A normalising heat treatment typically is applied to iron castings in order to obtain a higher hardness and strength than is obtained in the as-cast or annealed condition. In normalising treatments, ferrous alloys are heated to a suitable temperature above the transformation range and then air-cooled to room temperature, thus creating a pearlitic structure.

The heating rate for normalising is not important. The casting can be cooled in still air or with large fans. However, large differences in temperature in a complex casting below 1000°F (540°C) can cause distortion or, possibly, cracking. Because the carbon diffusion rate in iron is rapid at normalised temperatures, the required holding time is the time needed to obtain a uniform temperature throughout the casting.

Typical holding temperatures are about 100°F (40°C) above the critical temperature range as shown in Table 11.2. The determining factor is the silicon content, since increasing silicon content increases the critical temperature range.

Table 11.2. Normalising temperature range and silicon range (in weight percentage) for each iron family.

Iron family	Normalising Temperature, [°F (°C)]	Silicon range, (wt. %)
Malleable iron	1475–1525 (800–830)	1.2–1.9
High strength grey iron	1500–1600 (810–870)	1.0–3.0
Lower strength grey iron	1550–1650 (840–900)	1.5–3.0
Ductile iron	1600–1650 (870–900)	1.8–3.0

Austempering

In the 1930s, a fine, feathery, needle-like microstructure unlike ferrite, pearlite and martensite was found in steels when they were cooled rapidly from austenitising temperatures and held at intermittent temperatures. This structure, called bainite, formed above the martensite start temperature (M) but below the pearlite formation region found in isothermal transfomation (IT) diagrams. Years later, this same heat treating process, called 'austempering,' was applied to cast iron. A similar needle-like microstructure was formed. However, X-ray diffraction determined this structure to be acicular ferrite and carbon-enriched austenite or ausferrite. Austempering is valuable because it is stronger and tougher than tempered martensitic structures obtained with conventional heat treatment of cast iron.

The procedure consists of three basic steps.
1. Heat the part to austenitise in the temperature range of 1550°–1700°F (843°–927°C) for a time sufficient to produce a fully austenitic matrix that is saturated with the equilibrium carbon content.
2. Cool the part rapidly enough (quench) to avoid the formation of ferrite and pearlite to a temperature above M in the range of 450°–750°F (230°–400°C).

3. Hold at the austempering temperature to produce ausferrite. In the higher-silicon grey and ductile irons, the resultant structure is ausferrite. If low quench temperatures are used, then a small amount of martensite may be present with the ausferrite. In the lower-silicon malleable irons, the structure may contain some bainite along with the ausferrite.

The austenitising temperature is a function of the chemical composition of the iron. The austenitising tinge is largely a function to the section size of the part, though the chemical composition of the iron and the graphite morphology play small roles as well. The final properties determine the choice of austempering (quench) temperature. Higher austempering temperatures result in coarser structures that exhibit good ductility and dynamic properties. Lower austempering temperatures produce freer structures that have higher tensile and yield strengths and superior wear resistance. The austempering time is dependent upon austempering temperature. Longer times require lower temperatures. It should be noted that austempering is not a band-aid for poor-quality cast iron. Because ausferrite is stronger than conventional cast iron microstructures, it is more sensitive to defects within the iron. In order to successfully austemper cast iron, it should have a consistent chemical analysis, consistent graphite shape and distribution, and a matrix structure essentially free of porosity and carbides. The casting and austempering processes are specific to the casting supplier and the heat treater. To achieve the desired properties in a component, both the casting process and the type of austempering process must be established and documented at the outset of production.

Martempering

Since the 1950s, hot oil (410°F [210°C]) quenching has been routinely applied to cast irons to minimise distortion and cracking in cast iron parts. This process, known as marquenching, or martempering, also may require a subsequent tempering operation. The highest temperature quench oils are used to restrict the quenching process to temperatures just at or below [M_s]. Thus, mixed microstructures of martensite, bainite, and ausferrite are produced. When austempering, components are from the austenitising temperature to a temperature above the martensite start temperature (M) and then held for a time sufficient to form the desired microstructure (ausferrite). Because ausferrite forms over many minutes or hours at one temperature, no cracking occurs. Furthermore, unlike martempering, no subsequent tempering operation is required.

SPHEROIDAL GRAPHITE CAST IRON

It is produced by treating the molten alloy with magnesium or cerium or a combination of two elements, or such elements like Ca, Ba, Li, Zr causing spheroidal graphite to grow during solidification. Use of magnesium to have 0.04–0.06 per cent residual content is more easy to adopt and economical, which is followed by addition of ferro-silicon. Certain elements, if present, like 0.1 per cent Ti, 0.009 per cent Pb, 0.003 per cent Bi, 0.004 per cent Sb prevent the production of SG iron, but their effect can be removed by adding 0.005–0.01 per cent Ce. For most raw materials, combined use of Mg and Ce (it improves magnesium recovery) followed by ferro silicon as inoculant is made to produce Spheroidal Graphite Cast Iron (SG iron).

Steps in Production of SG Iron

Desulphurisation

Sulphur helps to form graphite as flakes. Thus, the raw material for producing SG Iron should have low sulphur (less than 0.1 per cent) or remove sulphur from iron during melting or by mixing iron with a desulphurising agent such as calcium carbide or soda ash (sodium carbonate).

Nodulising

Magnesium is added to remove sulphur and oxygen still present in the liquid alloy and provides a residual 0.04 per cent magnesium, which causes growth of graphite to be spheroidal, probably the interface energy becomes high to have a dihedral angle of 180°, (in simple term the graphite does not wet the liquid alloy.). Magnesium treatment desulphurises the iron to below 0.02 per cent S, before alloying it. Magnesium and such elements have strong affinity for sulphur, and thus scavenge sulphur from the molten alloy as an initial stage for producing SG iron. These additions are expensive to increase the cost of SG iron produced. Thus sulphur of molten alloy (or the raw material used), before nodulising, should be kept low.

Magnesium is added when melt is near 1500°C, but magnesium vapourises at 1150°C. Magnesium being lighter floats on the top of the bath, and being reactive burn off at the surface. In such cases magnesium is added as Ni-Mg, Ni-Si-Mg alloy or magnesium coke to reduce the violence of the reaction and to have saving in Mg.

Inoculation

As magnesium is carbide former, ferrosilicon is added immediately as innoculant. Remelting causes reversion to flake graphite due to loss of magnesium.

Stirring of molten alloy after addition of nodulising element evolves a lot of gas, which gets dissolved in liquid alloy, and forms blow-holes in solid casting. The contraction during solidification of nodular cast iron castings is much greater than that of grey iron castings, which needs careful design of moulds to avoid shrinkage cavities in solidified castings.

Average composition of SG cast iron is given below:
1. Carbon – 3.0–4.0 per cent.
2. Silicon – 1.8 – 2.8 per cent.
3. Manganese – 0.1–1.00 per cent.
4. Sulphur – 0.03 per cent max.
5. Magnesium – 0.01–0.10 per cent.

Properties of SG Cast Iron

A number of properties such as mechanical, physical and service properties are of important in assessing materials suitably for any application. The mechanical properties of interest are tensile strength, proof stress, elongation, hardness, impact strength, elastic modulus, and fatigue strength, notch sensitivity while the physical properties of interest are damping capacity, machinability and conductivity. The service properties generally involved are wear resistance, heat resistance, corrosion resistance.

Easy to cast

The high fluidity of the metal in its molten state makes it ideal for the casting process.

Strength

Tensile strengths of up to 900 N/mm^2 (ADI gives the option of higher strengths).

Ductility

Elongations of in excess of 20 per cent (lower grades only).

Excellent corrosion resistance
When compared to other ferrous metals.

Ease of machining
Free graphite in the structure also lends itself to machining (chip formation).

Cost per unit strength
Significantly cheaper than most materials

Effect of Alloying Elements on the Properties of Ductile Iron

Manganese
As it is a mild pearlite promoter, with some required properties like proof stress and hardness to a small extent. As Mn retards the onset of the eutectoid transformation, decreases the rate of diffusion of C in ferrite and stabilise cementite (Fe_3C). But the problem here is the embrittlement caused by it, so the limiting range would be 0.3–1.0.

Silicon
As the Si in the ductile iron matrix provides the ferritic matrix with the pearlitic one. Silicon enhances the performance of ductile iron at elevated temperature by stabilising the ferritic matrix and forming the silicon reach surface layer, which inhibits the oxidation. The potentially objectionable influences of increasing silicon content are:
1. Reduced impact test energy.
2. Increased impact transition temperature.
3. Decreased thermal conductivity.

Si is used to promote ferrite and to strengthen ferrite. So Si is generally held below 2.2 per cent when producing the ferritic grades and between 2.5 per cent and 2.8 per cent when producing pearlitic grades.

Copper
It is a strong pearlite promoter. It increases the proof stress with also the tensile strength and hardness with no embrittlement in matrix. So in the pearlitic grade of the ductile iron the copper is kept between 0.4–0.8 per cent and is a contaminant in the ferritic grade.

Nickel
As it helps in increasing the UTS without affecting the impact values. So it can be in the range of 0.5–2.0. It strengthens ferrite, but has much less effect than silicon in reducing ductility. But there is the danger of embrittlement with the large additions; in excess of 2 per cent. Due to the high cost it is generally present as traces in the matrix.

Molybdenum
It is a mild pearlite promoter. Forms intercellular carbides especially in heavy sections. Increases proof stress and hardness. Danger of embrittlement, giving low tensile strength and elongation value. And it also improves elevated temperature properties.

Chromium

It prevents the corrosion by forming the layer of chromium oxide on the surface and stops the further exposition of the surface to the atmosphere. But as it is a strong carbide former so not required in carbide free structure and <1 per cent required in the grade of GGG 50 it is kept around 0.05 per cent maximum.

Sulphur and phosphorus

As P is kept intentionally very low, as it is not required because it causes cold shortness and so the property of ductile iron will be ruined. But the addition of S is done for better machinability, but it is kept around 0.009 and maximum 0.015 per cent. As the larger additions of sulphur may cause the hot (red) shortness.

Magnesium Treatment

Research work has shown that on a laboratory scale additions of a number of elements are capable of producing spheroidal graphite structures in the cast irons. These elements include magnesium, cerium, calcium and yttrium. However, owing to a number of factors the application of these elements on a production scale has been restricted to the element magnesium, although it is claimed that in Japan calcium based alloys are used for producing ductile iron castings. It is generally supposed that magnesium removes impurities such as sulphur and oxygen, which may tend to segregate to free surfaces of molten metal, thereby lowering surface tension.

Similarly, these impurities lower the interfacial tension between the graphite and metal. When they are removed, this interfacial tension rises to a higher value and it is often presumed that it constrains the graphite to reduce its surface area per unit volume, which it does by assuming a spherical shape. The use of cerium results in nodular graphite structures, with certain type of metal compositions, but these restrictions and the general inconsistency of the process again makes it unsuitable for large-scale application.

However, the benefits of including a small amount of cerium in the nodularising process in order to offset the subversive nature of contaminating elements such as lead, antimony and titanium are well known, and the majority of ductile iron is produced using the ceriumbearing magnesium alloys.

Carbide in the structure

SG iron castings are more prone to contain carbides than flake-graphite castings of similar section and size and carbon and silicon contents. This occurs partly because the spherodising process generally involves the addition of magnesium and/or cerium, which are both elements that to promote the formation of eutectic carbide; and partly because the sequence of solidification produced by the growth of nodular graphite tend to promote undercooling during solidification to temperatures at which white iron structure is likely to form by heat treatment. The presence of carbide in ductile iron is undesirable for a number of reasons:

1. It increases the tendency to form shrinkage porosity and thus increases the feeding requirements during casting.
2. It increases the risk of cracking during knockout and fettling.
3. It decreases the ductility of the iron.

4. It drastically reduces the impact resistance.
5. It increases hardness and reduces machinability.
6. It requires heat treatment to 900°–920°C to remove the carbide.

High silicon levels are also beneficial but the potential embrittling action of silicon contents much above about 2.6 per cent should not be overlooked.

Factors that Affect the Properties of the SG Cast Iron

Graphite structure

Graphite occupies about 10–15 per cent of the total material volume. And its presence is to reduce the effective cross sectional area. The amount and form of the graphite in the ductile iron are determined during solidification and cannot be altered by subsequent heat treatment. All of the mechanical and physical properties of this class of materials are a result of the graphite being substantially or wholly in the spheroidal nodular shape, and any departure from this shape in a proportion of the graphite will cause some deviation from these properties. All properties relating to the strength and ductility decreases as the proportion of non-nodular graphite increases, and those relating to the failure, such as proof strength. The form of non-nodular graphite is important because thin flakes with sharp edges have a more adverse effect on the strength properties than compacted forms of graphite with round ends. For this reason, visual estimates of percentage of nodularity are rough guide to properties.

Graphite amount

As the amount of graphite increases, there is relatively small decrease in strength and elongation, in modulus of elasticity, and in density. In general these effects are small compared with the effects of other variables because the carbon equivalent content of spheroidal graphite iron is not a major variable and is generally maintained close to the eutectic value.

Matrix structure

The principal factor in determining the different grades of ductile iron in the specifications is the matrix structure. In the as-cast condition, the matrix will consist of varying proportions of pearlite and ferrite, and as the amount of pearlite increases, the strength and hardness of the iron also increases. The proportions of ferrite and pearlite in the matrix principally determine ductility and impact properties. The matrix structure can be change by heat treatments, and those most often carried out are annealing to produce a fully ferritic matrix, and normalising to produce a substantially pearlitic matrix. In general annealing produces a more ductile matrix with a lower impact transition temperature than is obtained in as-cast ferritic irons.

Section size

As the section size decreases, the solidification and cooling rates in the mould increases. This results in a fine grain structure that can be annealed more rapidly. In thinner sections, however, carbides may be present, which will increase hardness, decrease machinability, and lead to brittleness. To achieve soft ductile structures in thin sections, heavy inoculation, probably at a last stage, is desirable to promote graphite formation through a high nodule number. As the section size increases, the nodule number decreases, and micro segregation becomes more pronounced. This results in a large size of nodule size, a reduction in the proportion of as cast ferrite, and increasing resistance to the formation of a fully ferritic structure upon annealing.

Composition

In addition to the effects of elements in stabilising pearlite or retarding transformation (which facilitates heat treatment to change matrix structure and properties), certain aspects of composition have an important influence on some properties. Silicon hardens and strengthens ferrite and raises its impact transition temperature; therefore, silicon content should be kept low as practical, even below 2 per cent, to achieve maximum ductility and toughness. Nickel also strengthens ferrite, but has much less effect than silicon in reducing ductility. When producing as-cast grades of iron requiring fairly ductility and strength such as ISO GRADE 5007, it is necessary to keep silicon low to obtain high ductility, but it may also be necessary to add some nickel to strengthen the iron sufficiently to obtain the required tensile strength. Almost all elements present in trace amounts combine to reduce ferrite formation, and high-purity charges must be used for irons to be produced in the ferritic as-cast condition. Similarly, all carbide forming elements and manganese must be kept low to achieve maximum ductility and low hardness. Silicon is added to avoid carbides and to promote ferrite as-cast in thin sections. The electrical, magnetic, and thermal properties of Ductile irons are influenced by the composition of the matrix. In general, as the amount of alloying elements increases and thermal conductivity deceases.

Applications of SG Iron

The possible applications of SG iron are very wide. The properties are such as to extend the field of usefulness of cast iron and enable it, for some purpose, to replace steel casting, malleable cast iron, and non-ferrous alloys. But SG iron is not recommended as a replacement for all castings at present made in flake graphite irons, sometimes the inherent properties of the flake graphite iron are adequate for the purpose of exiting designs. The use of SG iron is suggested where improved properties are dictate a replacement of other material or where the use of SG iron will permit an improvement in the design. Some popular uses of SG iron for various engineering application are for:

1. Support bracket for agricultural tractor.
2. Tractor life arm.
3. Check beam for lifting track.
4. Mine cage guide brackets.
5. Gear wheel and pinion blanks and brake drum.
6. Machines worm steel.
7. Flywheel.
8. Thrust bearing.
9. Frame for high speed diesel engine.
10. Four throw crankshaft.
11. Fully machined piston for large marine diesel engine.
12. Bevel wheel.
13. Hydraulic clutch on diesel engine for heavy vehicle.
14. Fittings overhead electric transmission lines.
15. Boiler mountings, etc.

HEAT TREATMENT OF SG CAST IRON

The most important heat treatments and their purposes are:

1. Stress relieving: A low-temperature treatment, to reduce or relieve internal stresses remaining after casting.

2. Annealing: To improve ductility and toughness, to reduce hardness and to remove carbides.
3. Normalised: To improve strength with some ductility.
4. Hardening and tempering: To increase hardness or to give improved strength and higher proof stress ratio.
5. Austempering: To yield bainitic structures of high strength, with significant ductility and good wear resistance.
6. Surface hardening: By induction, flame, or laser to produce a local wear resistant hard surface.

Although ductile iron and steel are superficially similar metallurgically, the high carbon and silicon levels in ductile iron result in important differences in their response to heat treatment. The higher carbon levels in ductile iron increase hardenability, permitting heavier sections to be heat treated with lower requirements for expensive alloying or severe quenching media. These higher carbon levels can also cause quench cracking due to the formation of higher carbon martensite, and/or the retention of metastable austenite. These undesirable phenomena make the control of composition, austenitising temperature and quenching conditions more critical in ductile iron. Silicon also exerts a strong influence on the response of ductile iron to heat treatment. The higher the silicon content, the lower the solubility of carbon in austenite and the more readily carbon is precipitated as graphite during slow cooling to produce a ferritic matrix.

Although remaining unchanged in shape, the graphite spheroids in ductile iron play a critical role in heat treatment, acting as both a source and sink for carbon. When heated into the austenite temperature range, carbon readily diffuses from the spheroids to saturate the austenite matrix. On slow cooling the carbon returns to the graphite 'sinks', reducing the carbon content of the austenite. This availability of excess carbon and the ability to transfer it between the matrix and the nodules makes Ductile Iron easier to heat treat and increases the range of properties that can be obtained by heat treatment.

Austempered ductile irons (ADI) are the most recently developed materials of the DI family. By adapting the austempering treatment initially introduced for steels to DI, it has been shown that the resulting metallurgical structures provide properties that favorably compare to those of steel while taking advantage of a near-net-shape manufacturing process.

Austenitising Ductile Cast Iron

The usual objective of austenitising is to produce an austenitic matrix with as uniform carbon content as possible prior to thermal processing. For a typical hypereutectic ductile cast iron, an upper critical temperature must be exceeded so that the austenitising temperature is in two-phase (austenite and graphite) field. This temperature varies with alloy content. The 'equilibrium' austenite carbon content in equilibrium with graphite increases with an increase in austenitising temperature. This ability to select (within limits) the matrix austenite carbon content makes austenitising temperature control important in processes that depend on carbon in the matrix to drive a reaction. This is particularly true in structures to be austempered, in which the hardenability (or austemperability) depends to a significant degree on matrix carbon content. In general, alloy content, the original microstructure, and the section size determine the time required for austenitising.

Annealing Ductile Cast Iron

When maximum ductility and good machinability are desired and high strength is not required, ductile iron castings are generally given a full ferritising anneal. The microstructure is thus converted to ferrite, and the excess carbon is deposited on the existing nodules. Amounts of manganese, phosphorus, and alloying elements such as chromium and molybdenum should be as low as possible if superior machinability is desired because these elements retard the annealing process. Recommended practice for annealing ductile iron castings is given below for different alloy contents and for castings with and without eutectic carbides:

1. Full anneal for unalloyed 2 to 3 per cent Si iron with no eutectic carbide: Heat and hold at 870° to 900°C (1600° to 1650°F) for 1 hr per inch of section. Furnace cool at 55°C/hr (100°F/hr) to 345°C (650°F). Air cool.
2. Full anneal with carbides present: Heat and hold at 900° to 925°C (1650° to 1700°F) for 2 hr minimum, longer for heavier sections. Furnace cool at 110°C/hr (200°F/hr) to 700°C (1300°F). Hold 2 hr at 700°C (1300°F). Furnace cool at 55°C/hr (100°F/hr) to 345°C (650°F). Air cool.
3. Subcritical anneal to convert pearlite to ferrite: Heat and hold at 705° to 720°C (1300° to 1330°F), 1 hr per inch of section. Furnace cool at 55°C/hr (100°F/hr) to 345°C (650°F). Air cool. When alloys are present, controlled cooling times through the critical temperature range down to 400°C (750°F) must be reduced to below 55°C/hr (100°F/hr).

Normalising Ductile Cast Iron

Normalising (air cooling following austenitising) can result in a considerable improvement in tensile strength and may be used in the production of ductile iron of ASTM type 100–70–03. The microstructure obtained by normalising depends on the composition of the castings and the cooling rate. The composition of the casting dictates its hardenability that is, the relative position of the fields in the time-temperature CCT diagram. The cooling rate depends on the mass of the casting, but it also may be influenced by the temperature and movement of the surrounding air, during cooling. Normalising generally produces a homogeneous structure of fine pearlite, if the iron is not too high in silicon content and has at least a moderate manganese content (0.3 to 0.5 per cent or higher). Heavier castings that require normalising usually contain alloying elements such as nickel, molybdenum, and additional manganese, for higher hardenability to ensure the development of a fully pearlitic structure after normalising. Lighter castings made of alloyed iron may be martensitic or may contain an acicular structure after normalising. The normalising temperature is usually between 870° and 940°C (1600° and 1725°F). The standard time at temperature of 1 hr per inch of section thickness or 1 hr minimum is usually satisfactory. Longer times may be required for alloys containing elements that retard carbon diffusion in the austenite.

Quenching and Tempering Ductile Cast Iron

An austenitising temperature of 845° to 925°C (1550° to 1700°F) is normally used for austenitising commercial castings prior to quenching and tempering. Oil is preferred as a quenching medium to minimise stresses and quench cracking, but water or brine may be used for simple shapes. Complicated castings may have to be oil quenched at 80° to 100°C (180° to 210°F) to avoid cracks.

The influence of the austenitising temperature on the hardness of waterquenched cubes of ductile iron shows that the highest range of hardness (55 to 57 HRC) was obtained with austenitising temperatures between 845° and 870°C (1550° and 1600°F). At temperatures above 870°C, the higher matrix carbon content resulted in a greater percentage of retained austenite and therefore a lower hardness.

Castings should be tempered immediately after quenching to relieve quenching stresses. Tempered hardness depends on as-quenched hardness level, alloy content, and tempering temperature, as well as time. Tempering in the range from 425° to 600°C (800° to 1100°F) results in a decrease in hardness, the magnitude of which depends upon alloy content, initial hardness, and time.

Austempering Ductile Cast Iron

When optimum strength and ductility are required, the heat treater has the opportunity to produce an austempered structure of austenite and ferrite. The austempered matrix is responsible for a significantly better tensile strength-to-ductility ratio than is possible with any other grade of ductile cast iron. The production of these desirable properties requires careful attention to section size and the time-temperature exposure during austenitising and austempering, times vary from 1 to 4 hr (Fig. 11.1).

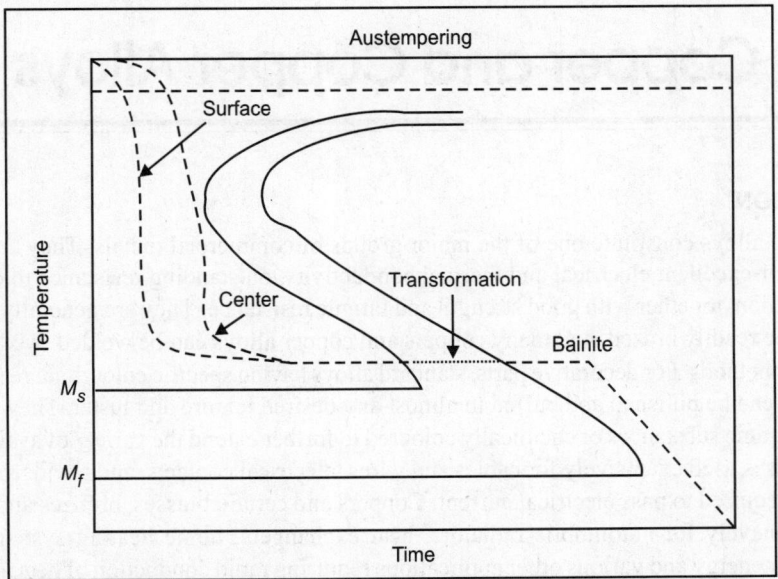

Fig. 11.1. Schematic diagram for austempering superimposed on TTT diagram.

The Austempering process consists of the following stages.
1. Transformation of matrix to austenite, i.e. austenitisation.
2. Quenching to the austempering temperature.
3. Holding at the austempering temperature to effect isothermal transformation to acicular bainite + stabilised austenite.
4. Cooling to room temperature after the proper holding time.

Chapter 12

Copper and Copper Alloys

INTRODUCTION

Copper and its alloys constitute one of the major groups of commercial metals. They are widely used because of their excellent electrical and thermal conductivity, outstanding resistance to corrosion, and ease of fabrication, together with good strength and fatigue resistance. They are generally nonmagnetic.

They can be readily brazed, and many coppers and copper alloys can be welded by various gas, arc and resistance methods. For decorative parts, standard alloys having specific colours are readily available. Copper alloys can be polished and buffed to almost any desired texture and luster. They can be plated, coated with organic substances or chemically coloured to further extend the variety of available finishes.

Pure copper is used extensively for cables and wires, electrical contacts, and a wide variety of other parts that are required to pass electrical current. Coppers and certain brasses, bronzes and cupronickels are used extensively for automobile radiators, heat exchangers, home heating systems, panels for absorbing solar energy and various other applications requiring rapid conduction of heat across or along a metal section. Because of their outstanding ability to resist corrosion, coppers, brasses, some bronzes, and cupronickels are used for pipes, valves and fittings in systems carrying potable water, process water or other aqueous fluids.

In all classes of copper alloys, certain alloy compositions for wrought products have counterparts among the cast alloys, which enables the designer to make an initial alloy selection before deciding on the manufacturing process.

Most wrought alloys are available in various cold worked conditions, which have room temperature strengths and fatigue resistances that depend on the amount of cold work more than on alloy content. Typical applications of cold worked conditions (cold worked tempers) include springs, fasteners, hardware, small gears, and cams. Certain types of parts—most notably plumbing fittings and valves—are produced by hot forging simply because no other fabrication process can produce the required shapes and properties as economically.

Copper alloys containing 1 to 6 per cent Pb are free machining grades, and are used widely for machined parts especially those produced in screw machines.

Copper and its alloys are relatively good conductors of electricity and heat. In fact, copper is used for these purposes more often than any other metal. Alloying invariably decreases electrical conductivity and, to a lesser extent, thermal conductivity. For this reason, coppers and high copper alloys are preferred over copper alloys containing more than a few percent total alloy content when high electrical or thermal conductivity is required for the application. The amount of reduction due to alloying does not depend on conductivity or any other bulk property of the alloying element, but only on the effect that the particular foreign atoms have on the copper lattice.

Electrical coppers: Commercially pure copper is represented by UNS numbers C10100 to C13000. The various coppers within this group have different degrees of purity, and therefore different metal characteristics. Fire refined tough pitch copper C12500 is made by deoxidising anode copper until the oxygen content has been lowered to the optimum value of 0.02 to 0.04 per cent.

Electrolytic tough pitch copper C11000 is made from cathode copper—that is, copper that has been refined electrolytically C11000 is the most common of all the electrical coppers. It has high electrical conductivity, in excess of 100 per cent IACS. It has the same oxygen content as C12500, but differs in sulphur content and in overall purity. C11000 has less than 50 ppm total metallic impurities (including sulphur). Oxygen-free coppers C10100 and C10200 are made by induction melting prime-quality cathode copper under nonoxidising conditions produced by a granulated graphite bath covering and a protective reducing atmosphere that is low in hydrogen.

If resistance to softening at slightly elevated temperature is required, C11100 is often specified. This copper contains a small amount of cadmium, which raises the temperature at which recovery and recrystallisation occurs.

High purity copper is a very soft metal. It is softest in its undeformed, single-crystal form, requiring a shear stress of only 3.9 MPa. Annealed tough pitch copper is almost as soft as high purity copper, but many of the copper alloys are much harder and stiffer, even in annealed tempers.

CLASSIFICATION OF COPPER ALLOYS

The most common way to catalog copper and its alloys is to divide them into six families: coppers, dilute copper alloys, brasses, bronzes, copper nickels and nickel silvers. The first family, the coppers, is essentially commercially pure copper, which ordinarily is soft and ductile and contains less than about 0.7 per cent total impurities. The dilute copper alloys contain small amounts of various alloying elements that modify one or more of the basic properties of copper.

Solid Solution Alloys

The most compatible alloying elements with copper are those that form solid-solution fields. These include all elements forming useful alloy families (Zn, Sn, Al, Si). Hardening in these systems is great enough to make useful objects without encountering brittleness associated with second phases or compounds. Cartridge brass is typical of this group, consisting of 30 per cent Zn in copper and exhibiting no beta phase except an occasional small amount due to segregation, which normally disappears after the first anneal. Provided that there are no elements such as Fe, cold working and grain growth relation ships are easily reproduced in practice.

Age-hardenable Alloys

Age hardening produces very high strengths, but is limited to those few copper alloys in which the solubility of the alloying element decreases sharply with decreasing temperature. The beryllium coppers can be considered typical of the age-hardenable copper alloys. Other age-hardenable alloys include C15000 (zirconium copper); C18200, C18400 and C18500 (chromium coppers); C19000 and C19100 (copper nickel phosphorus alloys); and C64700 (copper nickel silicon alloy).

By combining cold working with heat treatment, higher strengths can be obtained than can be achieved by either cold working or age hardening alone. Beryllium copper illustrates well the effects of heat treatment and cold working: in the soft, solution treated condition, the tensile strength is about 500 MPa, solution treated and aged, about 1000 MPa, and solution treated, cold worked and aged, about 1400 MPa. Some age-hardening alloys have different desirable characteristics, such as high strength combined with better electrical conductivity than the beryllium coppers.

Insoluble Alloying Elements

Lead, tellurium and selenium are added to copper and its alloys to improve machinability. They, along with bismuth, make hot rolling and hot forming nearly impossible and severely limit the useful range of cold working. An exception here are the high-zinc brasses, which become fully beta phase at high temperature. The beta phase can dissolve lead, thus avoiding a liquid grain-boundary phase at hot forging or extrusion temperatures. Most free-cutting brass rod is made by beta extrusion. C37700, one of the leading high-zinc brasses, is so readily hot forged that it is the standard alloy against which the forgeability of all copper alloys is judged.

Deoxidisers

Li, Na, Be, Mg, B, Al, C, Si and P can be used to deoxidise copper. Ca, Mn and Zn can sometimes be considered deoxidisers, although they normally fulfil different roles.

The first requirement of a deoxidiser is that it have an affinity for oxygen in molten copper. Probably the second most important requirement is that it be relatively inexpensive compared to copper and any other additions. Thus, although zinc normally functions as a solid-solution strengthener, it is sometimes added in small amounts to function as a deoxidiser, because it has high affinity for oxygen and is relatively low in cost. In tin bronze, phosphorus has traditionally been the deoxidiser, hence the name 'phosphor bronzes' for these alloys.

Silicon instead of phosphorus is the deoxidiser for chromium coppers because phosphorus severely reduces electrical conductivity. Most deoxidisers contribute to hardness and other qualities, which often makes classification as a deoxidiser indistinct.

COPPER–ZINC ALLOYS: THE BRASSES

The copper alloys may be endowed with a wide range of properties by varying their composition and the mechanical and heat treatment to which they are subjected. For this reason they probably rank next to steel in importance to the engineer. The important alloys of copper and zinc from an industrial point of view are the brasses comprised within certain limits of zinc content. That portion of the constitutional diagram which refers to these alloys is given in the Fig. 12.1.

The addition of zinc to copper results in the formation of a series of solid solutions which, in accordance with usual practice, are referred to in order of diminishing copper content as the α, β, γ, etc. constituents. The diagram may be summarised as shown in Table 12.1.

Further changes in composition of the α and β' phases below 400°C are only observed after prolonged annealing. There is a certain connection between the properties and the microstructure which may be expressed in general terms.

The tensile strength increases with increase in zinc content, rises somewhat abruptly with the appearance of β, and reaches a maximum at a composition corresponding roughly to equal parts of α and β. It falls off rapidly at the appearance of the γ constituent.

Table 12.1. The important alloys of copper and zinc from an industrial point of view.

Percentage composition		Constituent just below the freezing point	Constituent after slow cooling to 400°C
Copper	Zinc		
100 to 67.5	0 to 32.5	α	α
67.5 to 63	32.5 to 37	α + β	α
63 to 61	37 to 39	β	α
61 to 55.5	39 to 45.5	β	α + β′
55.5 to 50	45.5 to 50	β	β′
50 to 43.5	50 to 56.5	β	β′ + γ
43.5 to 41	56.5 to 59	β + γ	β′ + γ

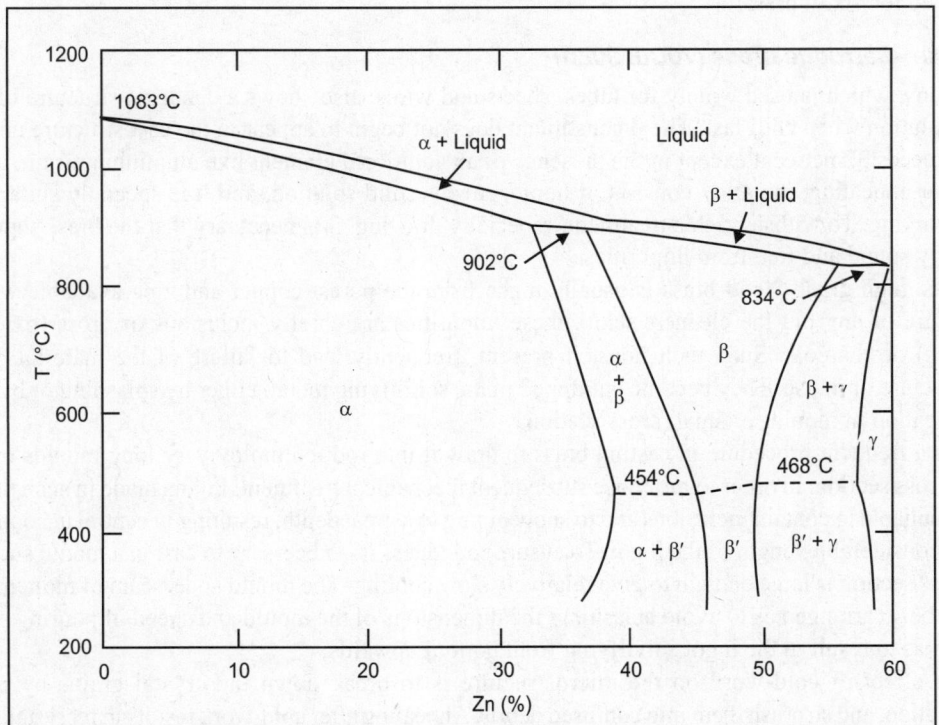

Fig. 12.1. Constitutional diagram of the copper–zinc alloys.

Elongation rises to a maximum and begins to fall again before the composition reaches the limit of the α solution. It falls considerably as the amount of β increases, and is very small in the presence of γ.

The α constituent shows the greatest resistance to shock. This is diminished by the presence of β, and the alloy becomes extremely brittle when γ is present.

Hardness is greatly increased by the presence of β and still further when γ appears.

Alloys containing α phase only are specially suitable for cold working, and may be hot- or cold-rolled. Those containing α and β will suffer very little deformation without rupture in the cold rolling and may only be hot rolled. The β constituent may also be forged, rolled or hot extruded, but alloys containing γ should invariably be avoided for any mechanical treatment.

Designation System of Brasses

The brasses of industrial importance are often designated by their copper and zinc content.

C23000—Red brass (85Cu, 15Zn)

This alloy is used for ornaments and for cheap jewellery which is to be gilded: it withstands cold-work, cupping, etc. On account of the range of solidification, the cast material has a dendritic structure.

If cooled very slowly or annealed, diffusion takes place, yielding polyhedral grains of uniform composition. The process of diffusion is assisted by mechanical deformation of the grains by hot- or cold-work followed by annealing. The changes which occur in rolling and annealing are similar to those described for 70:30 brass.

C26000—Cartridge brass (70Cu: 30Zn)

This alloy, which is used widely for tubes, sheets and wires, also shows a dendritic structure of the a solid solution when chill fast. The β constituent does not begin to appear in the cast structure until the zinc exceeds 32 per cent except in the presence of an additional element like aluminium or tin.

After annealing, the alloy consists of homogeneous solid solution, and it is specially suitable for cold-working. To withstand this treatment, especially drawing, it is necessary that the brass should be perfectly sound and free from impurities.

Since high grade 70:30 brass is usually made from the purest copper and zinc available without admixture of any but the cleanest scrap, these impurities are chiefly inclusions of dross (oxides or silicates) or charcoal. Such inclusions, if present, frequently lead to failure of the material during manufacture or in use. They become entrapped in the solidifying metal, either by splashing or by rapid solidification in moulds of small cross section.

It is a frequent procedure in casting brass to draw it into rod to employ very long moulds of very small cross section, in order to minimise subsequent mechanical treatment. Ingots made in such moulds are most liable to contain inclusions and to show piping to a great depth, resulting in central unsoundness over a considerable length of the ingot. To ensure soundness it is necessary to cast in a mould such that the cross section is large enough to give relatively slow cooling. The mould and stream of molten metal should be so arranged as to avoid splashing; the dimensions of the mould and speed of pouring should be such as to result in the ingot solidifying from bottom upwards.

The effect of cold-work on the microstructure is to break down the crystal grains by plastic deformation, and so crush them into confused debris. Annealing after cold-work results in recrystalisation and subsequent crystal growth.

C28000—Muntz metal (60Cu: 40Zn)

The molten metal begins to freeze at about 905°C, and dendrites of the β solution are formed. With sufficiently slow cooling through the range of solidification the alloy consists of homogeneous β constituent when just solid, but, on cooling, this solution retains less copper and at 770°C the α constituent separates from the homogeneous β and increases in amount as the temperature falls. The structure on reaching atmospheric temperature is therefore a mixture of α and β, the relative proportions of which may be controlled to some extent by the rate of cooling.

For example, a thin section of 60:40 brass quenched from 800°C consists of homogeneous β. With a larger section it is impossible to suppress completely the separation of α, but a specimen rapidly cooled from this temperature always contains more β than a specimen more slowly cooled. These microstructural characteristics are accompanied by changes in mechanical properties which can be deduced from the known hardness and brittleness of the β constituent and the softness and ductility of the α constituent.

Hot-rolled 60:40 brass, the rolling of which has been stopped above 700°C, shows a uniform structure in longitudinal and transverse directions. After the separation, the α and β constituents are each elongated in the direction of rolling, giving the normal structure of rolled 60:40 brass. The lower temperature of finishing, the smaller will be the grain size. If, however, rolling is continued much below 600°C, recrystalisation does not keep pace with the deformation and the metal is cold-worked.

Brazing solder (50Cu: 50Zn)

This alloy, if cooled sufficiently slowly through the range of solidification, consists of homogeneous β solution, which, however, may decompose on cooling if the copper content is less than 50 per cent. At atmospheric temperature the β solution will retain a maximum of just 50 per cent of zinc if no impurities are present, but any content of zinc over 50 per cent causes the separation of the γ constituent, which increases in amount as the temperature falls. Its presence renders the alloy extremely hard and brittle.

BRONZE

Bronze is a metal alloy consisting primarily of copper, usually with tin as the main additive, but sometimes with other elements such as phosphorus, manganese, aluminium, or silicon. It is hard and brittle, and it was particularly significant in antiquity, so much so that the Bronze Age was named after the metal. However, since 'bronze' is a somewhat imprecise term, and historical pieces have variable compositions, in particular with an unclear boundary with brass, modern museum and scholarly descriptions of older objects increasingly use the more cautious and inclusive term 'copper alloy' instead.

Though bronze is generally harder than wrought iron, with Vickers hardness of 60–258 vs. 30–80, the Bronze Age gave way to the Iron Age; this happened because iron was easier to find. Bronze was still used during the Iron Age, but, for many purposes, the weaker wrought iron was found to be sufficiently strong. Archaeologists suspect that a serious disruption of the tin trade precipitated the transition. The population migrations around 1200–1100 BC reduced the shipping of tin around the Mediterranean (and from Great Britain), limiting supplies and raising prices. As ironworking improved, iron became cheaper; and as cultures advanced from wrought iron to forged iron, they learned how to make steel, which is stronger than bronze and holds a sharper edge longer.

Composition

There are many different bronze alloys but modern bronze is typically 88 per cent copper and 12 per cent tin. Alpha bronze consists of the alpha solid solution of tin in copper. Alpha bronze alloys of 4–5 per cent tin are used to make coins, springs, turbines and blades. Historical 'bronzes' are highly variable in composition, as most metalworkers probably used whatever scrap was to hand; the metal of the 12th century English Gloucester Candlestick is bronze containing a mixture of copper, zinc, tin, lead, nickel, iron, antimony, arsenic with an unusually large amount of silver—between 22.5 per cent in the base and 5.76 per cent in the pan below the candle. The proportions of this mixture may suggest that the candlestick was made from a hoard of old coins. The Benin Bronzes are really brass, and the Romanesque Baptismal font at St Bartholomew's Church, Liège is described as both bronze and brass. Commercial bronze (90 per cent copper and 10 per cent zinc) and Architectural bronze (57 per cent copper, 3 per cent lead, 40 per cent zinc) are more properly regarded as brass alloys because they contain zinc as the main alloying ingredient. They are commonly used in architectural applications.

Bismuth bronze is a bronze alloy with a composition of 52 per cent copper, 30 per cent nickel, 12 per cent zinc, 5 per cent lead, 1 per cent bismuth. It is able to hold a good polish and so is sometimes used in light reflectors and mirrors. Other bronze alloys include aluminium bronze, phosphor bronze, manganese bronze, bell metal, speculum metal and cymbal alloys.

Properties

Bronze is considerably less brittle than iron. Typically bronze only oxidises superficially; once a copper oxide (eventually becoming copper carbonate) layer is formed, the underlying metal is protected from further corrosion. However, if copper chlorides are formed, a corrosion-mode called 'bronze disease' will eventually completely destroy it. Copper-based alloys have lower melting points than steel or iron, and are more readily produced from their constituent metals. They are generally about 10 per cent heavier than steel, although alloys using aluminium or silicon may be slightly less dense. Bronzes are softer and weaker than steel—bronze springs, for example, are less stiff (and so store less energy) for the same bulk. Bronze resists corrosion (especially seawater corrosion) and metal fatigue more than steel and is also a better conductor of heat and electricity than most steels. The cost of copper-base alloys is generally higher than that of steels but lower than that of nickel-base alloys.

Copper and its alloys have a huge variety of uses that reflect their versatile physical, mechanical, and chemical properties. Some common examples are the high electrical conductivity of pure copper, the excellent deep drawing qualities of cartridge case brass, the low-friction properties of bearing bronze, the resonant qualities of bell bronze, and the resistance to corrosion by sea water of several bronze alloys. The melting point of Bronze varies depending on the actual ratio of the alloy components and is about 950°C.

Uses

Bronze was especially suitable for use in boat and ship fittings prior to the wide employment of stainless steel owing to its combination of toughness and resistance to salt water corrosion. Bronze is still commonly used in ship propellers and submerged bearings.

It is also widely used for cast bronze sculpture. Many common bronze alloys have the unusual and very desirable property of expanding slightly just before they set, thus filling in the finest details of a mould. Bronze parts are tough and typically used for bearings, clips, electrical connectors and springs.

Spring bronze weatherstripping comes in rolls of thin sheets and is nailed or stapled to wood windows and doors. There are two types, flat and v-strip. It has been used for hundreds of years because it has low friction, seals well and is long lasting. It is used in building restoration and custom construction.

Bronze also has very little metal-on-metal friction, which made it invaluable for the building of cannon where iron cannonballs would otherwise stick in the barrel. It is still widely used today for springs, bearings, bushings, automobile transmission pilot bearings, and similar fittings, and is particularly common in the bearings of small electric motors. Phosphor bronze is particularly suited to precision-grade bearings and springs. It is also used in guitar and piano strings. Unlike steel, bronze struck against a hard surface will not generate sparks, so it (along with beryllium copper) is used to make hammers, mallets, wrenches and other durable tools to be used in explosive atmospheres or in the presence of flammable vapours. Bronze is used to make bronze wool for woodworking applications where steel wool would discolour oak.

PHOSPHOR BRONZE

Phosphor bronze is an alloy of copper with 3.5 to 10 per cent of tin and a significant phosphorus content of up to 1 per cent. The phosphorus is added as deoxidising agent during melting.

These alloys are notable for their toughness, strength, low coefficient of friction, and fine grain. The phosphorus also improves the fluidity of the molten metal and thereby improves the castability, and improves mechanical properties by cleaning up the grain boundaries.

Industrial Uses

Phosphor bronze is used for springs, bolts and various other items used in situations where resistance to fatigue, wear and chemical corrosion are required, e.g. ship's propellers in a marine environment. The alloy is also used in some dental bridges. Grades A, C and E – C51000, 52100, 50700 are commonly used nonferrous spring alloys. The combination of good physical properties, fair electrical conductivity and moderate cost make phosphor bronze round, square, flat and special shaped wire desirable for many springs and electrical contacts and a wide variety of wire forms where cost of properties does not prescribe beryllium copper. Oxygen-free copper can be alloyed with phosphorus (CuOFP alloy) to better withstand oxidising conditions. This alloy has application as thick corrosion-resistant overpack for spent nuclear fuel disposal in deep crystalline rocks.

Musical Instruments

Additionally, phosphor bronze is sometimes used in brass instruments (e.g. Flugelhorns), plus percussion instruments such as cymbals and snare drums. Some acoustic instrument strings for acoustic guitars, mandolins and violins are wrapped with this metal. Some harmonica reeds are made of phosphor bronze, such as those by the Suzuki brand.

Variants

Further increasing the phosphorus content leads to formation of a very hard compound Cu_3P (copper phosphide), resulting in a brittle form of phosphor bronze, which has a narrow range of applications.

Around 2001, the Olin Corporation developed another phosphor bronze alloy comprising:
1. Zinc – 9.9 per cent.
2. Tin – 2.2 per cent.
3. Iron – 1.9 per cent.
4. Phosphorus – 0.03 per cent.
5. Copper – 85.97 per cent.

Olin developed this new alloy for use in electrical and electronic connectors. When assessed in strictly metallurgical terms it is not true phosphor bronze, but a form of iron-modified tin brass.

ALUMINIUM BRONZE

Aluminium bronze is a type of bronze in which aluminium is the main alloying metal added to copper. A variety of aluminium bronzes of differing compositions have found industrial use, with most ranging from 5 to 11 per cent aluminium by weight, the remaining mass being copper; other alloying agents such as iron, nickel, manganese, and silicon are also sometimes added to aluminium bronzes.

Compositions

The following table lists the most common standard aluminium bronze wrought alloy compositions, by ISO 428 designations. The percentages show the proportional composition of the alloy by weight. Copper is the remainder by weight and is not listed (Table 12.2).

Table 12.2. The percentages show the proportional composition of the alloy by weight.

Alloy	Aluminium	Iron	Nickel	Manganese	Zinc	Arsenic
$CuAl_5$	4.0%–6.5%	0.5% max.	0.8% max	0.5% max	0.5% max	0.4% max
$CuAl_8$	7.0%–9.0%	0.5% max.	0.8% max	0.5% max	0.5% max	–
$CuAl_8Fe_3$	6.5%–8.5%	1.5%–3.5%	1.0% max	0.8% max	0.5% max	–
$CuAl_9Mn_2$	8.0%–10.0%	1.5% max	0.8% max	1.5%–3.0%	0.5% max	–
$CuAl_{10}Fe_3$	8.5%–11.0%	2.0%–4.0%	1.0% max	2.0% max	0.5% max	–
$CuAl_{10}Fe_5Ni_5$	8.5%–11.5%	2.0%–6.0%	4.0%–6.0%	2.0% max	0.5% max	–

Material Properties

Aluminium bronzes are most valued for their higher strength and corrosion resistance as compared to other bronze alloys. These alloys are tarnish-resistant and show low rates of corrosion in atmospheric conditions, low oxidation rates at high temperatures, and low reactivity with sulphurous compounds and other exhaust products of combustion.

They are also resistant to corrosion in sea water. Aluminium bronzes' resistance to corrosion rests in the aluminium component of the alloys, which reacts with atmospheric oxygen to form a thin, tough surface layer of alumina (aluminium oxide) which acts as a barrier to corrosion of the copper-rich alloy. The addition of tin can improve corrosion resistance.

Another notable property of aluminium bronzes are their biostatic effects. The copper component of the alloy prevents colonisation by marine organisms including algae, lichens, barnacles, and mussels, and therefore can be preferable to stainless steel or other non-cupric alloys in applications where such colonisation would be unwanted. Aluminium bronzes tend to have a golden colour.

Applications

Aluminium bronzes are most commonly used in applications where their resistance to corrosion makes them preferable to other engineering materials. These applications include plain bearings and landing gear components on aircraft, engine components (especially for seagoing ships), underwater fastenings in naval architecture, and ship propellers.

Aluminium bronzes are in the highest demand from the following industries and areas:
1. General sea water-related service.
2. Water supply.
3. Oil and petrochemical industries (i.e. tools for use in non-sparking environments).
4. Specialised anti-corrosive applications.
5. Certain structural retrofit building applications.

Aluminium bronze can be welded using the MIG welding technique with an aluminium bronze core and pure argon gas. Aluminium bronze is used to replace gold for the casting of dental crowns. The alloys used are chemically inert and have the appearance of gold.

WROUGHT PHOSPHOR BRONZES

Phosphor bronzes are copper alloys, containing 1–13 per cent of tin (Sn) and up to 0.3 per cent of phosphorous (P) as the major alloying elements. Wrought phosphor bronzes (1.25 per cent E, 5 per cent A, 8 per cent C, 10 per cent D) are designated with the numbers from C50000 through C54999 (including lead phosphor bronzes).

Lead phosphor bronzes contain tin (Sn) and phosphorous (P) as the major alloying elements and up to 4 per cent of lead (Pb) as additional alloying element. Wrought lead phosphor bronzes are designated with the numbers from C53000 through C54999. Phosphor bronzes containing up to 13 per cent of tin have mono-phase structure (α-phase). Such alloys have excellent formability in cold state and good corrosion resistance. Phosphorous is added to the phosphor bronzes as deoxidising agent during melting; however it also improves mechanical properties of the alloys. Alloys, containing more than 13 per cent of tin, have significant amount of brittle δ-phase. These bronzes have very low formability and cannot be used as wrought alloys.

Wrought phosphor bronzes are strengthened by cold work (strain hardening). Ductility of the alloys decreases as a result of cold work.

Wrought phosphor bronzes are used for manufacturing sleeve bushings, springs, clutch discs, fittings, wear resistant parts, electrical contacts, sliding bearings, screw products, valve parts, pressure vessels, pump body castings, impellers for chemical plants. Chemical compositions of some wrought phosphor bronzes is given in Table 12.3.

Table 12.3. Chemical compositions of some wrought phosphor bronzes.

UNS designation	Trade mark	Sn,%	Pb,%	P,%	Zn,%	Cu,%
C50500	Phosphor bronze 1.25% E	1.0–1.7	0.05 max.	0.03–0.35	0.30 max.	Balance
C51000	Phosphor bronze 5% A	4.2–5.8	0.05 max.	0.03–0.35	0.30 max.	Balance
C52100	Phosphor bronze 8% C	7.0–9.0	0.05 max.	0.03–0.35	0.20 max.	Balance
C52400	Phosphor bronze 10% D	9.0–11.0	0.05 max.	0.03–0.35	0.20 max.	Balance
C54400	Lead phosphor bronze B-2	3.5–4.5	3.5–4.5	0.01–0.50	1.5–4.5	Balance

Properties of some wrought phosphor bronzes are given below:
1. Wrought copper alloy C50500 (Phosphor bronze 1.25 per cent E).
2. Wrought copper alloy C51000 (Phosphor bronze 5 per cent A).
3. Wrought copper alloy C52100 (Phosphor bronze 8 per cent C).
4. Wrought copper alloy C52400 (Phosphor bronze 10 per cent D).
5. Wrought copper alloy C54400 (Lead phosphor bronze B-2).

WROUGHT COPPER–NICKEL ALLOYS AND NICKEL SILVERS

Copper–nickel alloys (copper–nickels, cupro-nickels) are copper alloys, containing 1.5–45 per cent of nickel (Ni) as the major alloying element. Wrought Copper-Nickel alloys are designated with the numbers from C70000 through C73499. Wrought copper–nickel alloys may contain up to 8 per cent of tin (Sn), up to 4.5 per cent of manganese (Mn), up to 2 per cent of iron (Fe), up to 2.5 per cent of chromium (Cr) and up to 1 per cent of silicon (Si) as additional alloying elements. Copper-nickel-zinc alloys form a separate group called nickel silvers.

Copper–nickel–zinc alloys (nickel silvers) are copper alloys containing 8–25 per cent of nickel (Ni) and 17–45 per cent of zinc (Zn) as the major alloying elements. Wrought copper–nickel–zinc alloys are designated with the numbers from C73500 through C79999. Wrought copper–nickel–zinc alloys may contain up to 6 per cent of manganese (Mn) as additional alloying element.

Copper–nickel alloys and most of copper–nickel–zinc alloys have monophase structure (α-phase) and possess very good formability in cold and hot states.

Wrought copper–nickel alloys have moderate mechanical strength and high ductility combined with very good corrosion resistance (particularly in sea water). Iron, manganese and chromium are added to the wrought copper–nickel alloys for increasing their hardness and strength. The alloys are strengthened by cold work (strain hardening). Ductility of the alloys decreases as a result of cold work. Separate group of copper–nickel alloys is Spinodal bronzes: copper–nickel–tin alloys possessing high mechanical strength due to a controlled heat treatment called Spinodal decomposition.

Copper–nickel alloys are used for manufacturing coins, sea water equipment, evaporators, heat exchanger tubes, automotive hydraulic and cooling systems.

Copper–nickel alloys (nickel silvers) are used in decorative applications and for manufacturing resistance wire, optical parts, screws, rivets, clips, tableware, electrical contacts. Chemical compositions of some wrought copper–nickel alloys and nickel silvers is given in Table 12.4.

Table 12.4. Chemical compositions of some wrought copper–nickel alloys and nickel silvers.

UNS designation	Trade mark	Ni,%	Zn,%	Mn,%	Fe,%	Cu,%
C70400	Copper–Nickel 5%	4.8–6.2	1.0 max.	0.3–0.8	1.3–1.7	Balance
C70600	Copper–Nickel 10%	9.0–11.0	1.0 max.	1.0 max.	1.0–1.8	Balance
C71000	Copper–Nickel 20%	19–23	1.0 max.	1.0 max.	1.0 max.	Balance
C71500	Copper–Nickel 30%	29–33	1.0 max.	1.0 max.	0.4–1.0	Balance
C74500	Nickel Silver 65–10	9.0–11.0	Balance	0.5 max.	0.25 max.	63.5–66.5
C75200	Nickel Silver 65–18	16.5–19.5	Balance	0.5 max.	0.25 max.	63.0–66.5
C75400	Nickel Silver 65–15	14.0–16.0	Balance	0.5 max.	0.25 max.	63.5–66.5
C75700	Nickel Silver 65–12	11.0–13.0	Balance	0.5 max.	0.25 max.	63.5–66.5
C77000	Nickel Silver 55–18	16.5–19.5	Balance	0.5 max.	0.25 max.	53.5–56.5

Properties of some wrought copper-nickel alloys and nickel silvers are given below:
1. Wrought copper alloy C70400 (Copper–Nickel 5 per cent).
2. Wrought copper alloy C70600 (Copper–Nickel 10 per cent).
3. Wrought copper alloy C71000 (Copper–Nickel 20 per cent).
4. Wrought copper alloy C71500 (Copper–Nickel 30 per cent).
5. Wrought copper alloy C74500 (Nickel Silver 65–10).
6. Wrought copper alloy C75200 (Nickel Silver 65–18).
7. Wrought copper alloy C75400 (Nickel Silver 65–15).
8. Wrought copper alloy C75700 (Nickel Silver 65–12).
9. Wrought copper alloy C77000 (Nickel Silver 55–18).

COPPER–NICKEL–ZINC ALLOYS

The alloys containing copper, nickel and zinc are known as 'Nickel Silvers' and were made at least 2000 yr. before nickel was isolated. Known under the name of Partong these alloys were produced in China by mixing a copper–nickel ore with zinc and smelting the mixture. It was not until 1894 that the alloy was made in Europe by mixing the constituent metals. Until 1914 such alloys were generally called 'German Silver'. The name was later changed to nickel silver. The term nickel brass was also used as it indicated the constituents more accurately.

Nickel silver does not contain silver and may be regarded as a brass to which nickel has been added. Nickel contents vary considerably but usually lie between 9–30 per cent depending on its application. The copper content tends to remain the same, approx. 60–65 per cent and the zinc is reduced as the nickel is increased. The higher the nickel content the whiter is the colour and although more corrosion resistant the ductility is reduced.

Note: Due to the way the copper and nickel combine, the nickel substitutes for the copper and the alloy is equivalent to 70/30 type brass in structure.

The alloys may be readily cold worked, but annealing is necessary at intermediate stages. Cold working increases the strength of nickel silver but reduces its ductility. In higher nickel content alloys a maximum stress of 55–60 tons may be obtained by cold working. This is a very high strength for a nonferrous alloy.

During the initial cold working slip occurs between the faces of the crystal structure within the material. Further deformation starts to split the crystals down into smaller crystals. This process continues until the structure has broken down into small crystals. The material is now fully work hardened and further deformation in this state would cause cracking. If further cold working is necessary then material should first be annealed. It is not good practise to leave a finished item in the fully work hardened state as inter granular cracking can occur at a later date.

The temperature for full annealing depends on the composition of the alloy and the amount of cold working the alloy has received. In practise temperatures between 650°–750°C are employed. The higher temperature is used with the alloys of the higher nickel content. On no account should the temperature exceed 800°C as the zinc is burnt out and the material rendered useless due to its loss of ductility.

The machining properties of nickel silver are greatly improved by the introduction of 1–2 per cent of lead. The addition of lead however lowers the strength of the alloy and in particular its ductility and malleability. The lead is not taken into solution with the alloy and stays in its original form around the edges of the nickel silver crystals making the material susceptible to cracking.

Both brass and nickel silver can be supplied in different grades of temper (hardness), from soft (fully annealed) to hard (fully cold worked). The reason for the different tempers is the wide range of uses of the material and the different manufacturing processes involved. Material to be deformed by pressing and forging would be required fully annealed in a soft condition. Material to be cut and machined would be better in a hard condition.

The temper grades are produced by varying the amount of cold working the material receives during the final stages of manufacture.

Brass and nickel silver cannot be hardened by heat treatment. This group of materials only hardens by working, after which the material may require annealing depending on the next manufacturing process.

Nickel silver has been widely used for numerous applications due to its corrosion resistance, colour and cold forming qualities. Items made from nickel silver range through car radiators, ball pens, musical instrument keys, transistor casings, electrical contacts, architectural ironmongery, cutlery, etc. If you have ever come across cutlery marked EPNS, this stands for Electro Plated Nickel Silver and is usually finished with silver or nickel plate.

Due to technological changes nickel silver is not as widely used today. The cutlery trade and musical instrument trade are probably the largest users today. Even the cutlery trade has significantly reduces it use of nickel silver in recent years because of the increasing cheapness and popularity of stainless steal (Table 12.5).

Table 12.5. Copper, nickel and zinc alloy specifications.

Material designation		Application
CZ 106	70/30 Brass	Cold working
CZ 109	60/40 Lead free	Hot working
CZ 122	58% Copper 2% Lead	Free machining
NS 103	10% Nickel 60–65% Copper	Cold working
NS 104	12% Nickel 60–65% Copper	Cold working
NS 105	15% Nickel 60–65% Copper	Cold working
NS 106	18% Nickel 60–65% Copper	Cold working
NS 111	10% Nickel 1–2% Lead	Free machining

Note: NS 106 is recommended for severe deep drawing applications. Nickel silver of a similar spec was used for unplated keys on early woodwind instruments due to its superior corrosion resistance, strength and colour.

The designation codes given have now been officially superseded by the ISO code, but most suppliers in some countries still use the original NS codes.

BERYLLIUM COPPER

Beryllium copper, also known as copper beryllium, BeCu or beryllium bronze, is a metal alloy of copper and 0.5 to 3 per cent beryllium, and sometimes with other alloying elements. Beryllium copper combines high strength with nonmagnetic and non-sparking qualities. It has excellent metalworking, forming and machining qualities. It has many specialised applications in tools for hazardous environments, musical instruments, precision measurement devices, bullets, and aerospace. Beryllium-containing alloys create an inhalation hazard during manufacturing due to their toxic properties.

Properties

Beryllium copper is a ductile, weldable, and machinable alloy. It is resistant to nonoxidising acids (for example, hydrochloric acid, or carbonic acid), to plastic decomposition products, to abrasive wear and to galling. Furthermore, it can be heat-treated to improve its strength, durability, and electrical conductivity. Beryllium copper attains the highest strength [to 1400 MPa (2,00,000 psi)] of any copper-based alloy.

As beryllium compounds are toxic there are some safety concerns for handling its alloys. In solid form and as finished parts, beryllium copper presents no particular health hazard. However, breathing its dust, as formed when machining or welding may cause serious lung damage. Beryllium compounds are known human carcinogens when inhaled. As a result, beryllium copper is sometimes replaced by safer copper alloys such as Cu-Ni-Sn bronze.

Uses

Beryllium copper is a nonferrous alloy used in springs, spring wire, load cells and other parts that must retain their shapes during periods in which they are subjected to repeated stress and strain. Due to its electrical conductivity, it is used in low-current contacts for batteries and electrical connectors. Because Beryllium copper is non-sparking but physically tough and nonmagnetic, it is used to make tools that can safely be used in environments where there are explosive vapours and gases e.g. oil rigs. Beryllium copper fulfils the demands of ATEX directive for use in zone 0, 1, and 2. Various tool types are available, e.g. screwdrivers, pliers, spanners, cold chisels and hammers. Another metal sometimes used for non-sparking tools is aluminium bronze. Compared to tools made of steel, beryllium copper tools are more expensive, not as strong and wear out more quickly. However, the advantages of using beryllium copper in hazardous environments outweigh these disadvantages.

Alloy 25 beryllium copper (C17200 and C17300) is an age-hardening alloy which attains the highest strength of any copper base alloy. It may be age hardened after forming into springs, intricate forms or complex shapes. It has superb spring properties, corrosion resistance and stability as well as good conductivity and low creep. Tempered beryllium copper is Alloy 25 (C17200 and C17300) which has been age hardened and cold drawn. No further heat treatment is necessary except for a possible light stress relief. It is sufficiently ductile to wind on its own diameter and can be formed into springs and most shapes. Tempered wire is most useful where the properties of beryllium copper are desired but age hardening of finished parts is not practical.

Alloys 3 (C17510) and 10 (C17500) beryllium copper are age-hardenable and provide excellent electrical conductivity in combination with good physical properties and endurance strength. Provided in either the age-hardenable condition or as tempered ware, they are used in springs and wire forms which are electrical conductors or where retention of properties at elevated temperatures is important.

Beryllium copper is also frequently used in the manufacture of professional-quality percussion instruments, especially tambourine and triangle, where it is prized for its clear tone and strong resonance. Unlike most other materials, an instrument composed of beryllium copper will maintain a consistent tone and timbre for as long as the material resonates. The 'feel' of such instruments is rich and melodious to the point that they seem out of place when used in darker, more rhythmic pieces of classical music.

Beryllium copper has also found use in ultra-low temperature cryogenic equipment, such as dilution refrigerators, because of its combination of mechanical strength and relatively high thermal conductivity in this temperature range. Beryllium copper has also been used for armour piercing bullets, though any such usage is unusual because bullets made from steel alloys are much less expensive, but have similar properties. Beryllium copper is also used for measurement-while-drilling tools in the directional (slant drilling) drilling industry. A nonmagnetic alloy is required as magnetometers are used for calculations received from the tool.

Beryllium copper is also used to create an RF tight, electronic seal on doors used with EMC and anechoic chambers.

For a time, beryllium copper was also used in the manufacture of golf clubs, with emphasis on wedges and putters. Many golfers prefer the soft feel of BeCu club heads, particularly for chip shots and putts around and on the green, where an extra measure of control is desired. Due to regulatory issues and high costs, BeCu clubs are hard to find in current production. Vintage and preowned examples remain in demand at used club shops and on Internet auction sites.

Alloys

High strength beryllium copper alloys contain up to 2.7 per cent of beryllium (cast), or 1.6–2 per cent of beryllium with about 0.3 per cent cobalt (wrought). The high mechanical strength is achieved by precipitation hardening or age hardening. The thermal conductivity of these alloys lies between steel and aluminium. The cast alloys are frequently used as material for injection moulds. The wrought alloys are designated by UNS as C17200 to C17400, the cast alloys are C82000 to C82800. The hardening process requires rapid cooling of the annealed metal, resulting in a solid state solution of beryllium in copper, which is then kept at 200°–460°C for at least an hour, facilitating precipitation of metastable beryllide crystals in the copper matrix. Overageing is avoided, as an equilibrium phase forms that depletes the beryllide crystals and reduces the strength enhancement. The beryllides are similar in both cast and wrought alloys.

High conductivity beryllium copper alloys contain up to 0.7 per cent beryllium, together with some nickel and cobalt. Their thermal conductivity is better than of aluminium, only a bit less than pure copper. They are usually used as electric contacts in connectors.

HEAT TREATING OF COPPER AND COPPER ALLOYS

The end products of copper fabricators can be generally described as mill products and foundary products. They consist of wire and cable, sheet, strip, plate, rod, bars, tubing, forgings, castings and powder metallurgy shapes. These products made from copper and copper alloys may be heat treated for several purposes such as homogenising, annealing, stress relieving and precipitation hardening.

Homogenising

Homogenising is applied to dissolve and absorb segregation and coring found in some cast and hot worked materials, chiefly those containing tin and nickel.

Diffusion and homogenisation are slower and more difficult in tin bronzes, silicon bronzes and copper nickels than in most other copper alloys. Therefore, these alloys usually are subjected to prolonged homogenising treatments before hot or cold working operations. The high-tin phosphor bronzes (above 8 per cent Sn) are noted for extreme segregation. Although these alloys sometimes are hot worked, usual practice is to roll them cold, making it necessary to first diffuse the brittle segregated tin phase, thereby increasing strength and ductility and decreasing hardness before rolling. These objectives are accomplished by homogenising at about 760°C.

Annealing

Softening or annealing of cold worked metal is accomplished by heating to a temperature that causes recrystallisation and, if maximum softening is desired, by heating well above the recrystallisation temperature to cause grain growth. Method of heating, furnace design, furnace atmosphere, and shape of work piece are important, because they affect uniformity of results, finish, and cost of annealing.

For copper and brass mill alloys, grain size is the standard means of evaluating a recrystallising anneal. Because many inter-reacting variables influence the annealing process, it is difficult to predict a specific combination of time and temperature that will always produce a given grain size in a given metal. Several copper alloys have been developed in which the grain size is stabilised by the presence of a finely distributed second phase.

Examples include copper-iron alloys such as C19200, C19400 and C19500, and aluminium-containing brasses and bronzes such as C61500, C63800, C68800 and C69000. These alloys will maintain an extremely fine grain size at temperatures well beyond their recrystallisation temperature, up to the temperature where the second phase finally dissolves or coarsens, which allows grain growth to proceed.

Generally, two annealed tempers are available: light anneal, which is performed at a temperature slightly above the recrystallisation temperature, and soft anneal, which is performed several hundred degrees higher, at a temperature just below the point at which rapid grain growth begins.

When annealing copper that contains oxygen, the hydrogen in the atmosphere must be kept to a minimum to avoid embrittlement. For temperatures lower than about 480°C, hydrogen preferably should not exceed 1 per cent.

Stress Relieving

Stress relieving is aimed to reduce or eliminate residual stress, thereby reducing the likelihood that the part will fail by cracking or corrosion fatigue in service. Parts are stress-relieved at temperatures below the normal annealing range that do not cause recrystallisation and consequent softening of the metal.

Residual stresses contribute to this type of failure, which is frequently seen in brasses containing 15 per cent zinc or more. Even higher-copper alloys such as aluminium bronzes and silicon bronzes may crack under critical combinations of stress and specific corroding, and all copper alloys are susceptible to more rapid corrosion attack when in the stressed condition.

Stressed phosphor bronzes and copper nickels have comparatively slight tendencies toward stress-corrosion cracking; these alloys are more susceptible to fire cracking, which is cracking caused when stressed metal is heated too rapidly to the annealing temperature. Slow heating provides a measure of stress relief and minimises nonuniform temperature distributions, which lead to thermal stress. Using a high stress-relieving temperature for a short time is generally considered best for keeping processing time and cost to a practical minimum, even though there is usually some sacrifice in mechanical properties. Using a lower temperature for a longer time will provide complete stress relief with no decrease in mechanical properties. Actually, the hardness and strength of severely cold worked alloys will increase slightly when low stress-relieving temperatures are used.

An additional benefit of a thermal stress relieving is dimensional stability of cold-formed parts. Also, it is often advisable to stress relieve welded or cold formed structures. For these structures, stress-relieving temperature is 85° to 110°C above that used for mill products of the same alloy.

Precipitation Hardening

High strength in most copper alloys is achieved by cold working. Solution treating and precipitation hardening is applied to strengthen special types of copper alloys above the levels ordinarily obtained by cold working. Examples of precipitation hardening copper alloys include the beryllium coppers, some of which also contain nickel, cobalt or chromium; the copper-chromium alloys; the copper-zirconium alloys; the copper-nickel-silicon alloys and the copper-nickel-phosphorus alloys.

All precipitation-hardening copper alloys have similar metallurgical characteristics: they can be solution treated to a soft condition by quenching from a high temperature, and then subsequently precipitation hardened by ageing at a moderate temperature for a time usually not exceeding 3 hr.

The main advantages of these alloys are:
1. Customer fabrication is easily performed in the soft, solution-annealed condition.
2. The precipitation-hardening heat treatment performed by the fabricator is relatively simple. It is carried out at moderate temperatures, usually in air. Controlled cooling is not needed, and time of treatment is not of critical importance.
3. Different combinations of properties—including strength, hardness, ductility, conductivity, impact resistance and inelasticity—can be obtained by varying hardening times and temperatures. The particular requirements of the application determine the type of hardening treatment.

Age-hardenable alloys are furnished in the solution-treated condition, in the solution treated and cold worked condition or in the age-hardened condition.

Beryllium coppers

Wrought beryllium coppers, C17000, C17200 and C17500, can develop wide ranges of mechanical properties, depending on solution treating and ageing conditions, on the amount of cold work imparted to the alloy and on whether the alloy is cold worked after solution treating and before ageing or is cold worked after ageing.

Copper–nickel–phosphorus alloys

Alloys containing about 1 per cent nickel and about 0.25 per cent phosphorus, typified by C19000, are used for a wide variety of small parts requiring, high strength, such as springs, clips, electrical connectors and fasteners. C19000 is solution treated at 700° to 800°C. If the metal must be softened between cold working steps prior to ageing, it may be satisfactorily annealed at temperatures as low as 620°C. Rapid cooling from the annealing temperature is not necessary. For ageing, the material is held at 425° to 475°C for 1 to 3 hr.

Chromium coppers

Chromium coppers containing about 1 per cent Cr, such as C18200, C18400 and C18500, are solution treated at 950° to 1010°C and rapidly quenched. Solution treating usually is done in molten salt, but may be done in a controlled-atmosphere furnace to prevent surface scaling and internal oxidation. Solution treated chromium copper is aged at 400° to 500°C for several hours to produce the desired mechanical and physical properties. A typical ageing cycle is 455°C for 4 hr or more.

Zirconium copper

Zirconium copper C15000 (99.8 Cu–0.2 Zr) is solution treated at 900° to 925°C, then quenched in water. Time at the solution treating temperature should be minimised to limit grain growth and possible internal oxidation by reaction of zirconium with the furnace atmosphere. Because solution and diffusion of the zirconium occur rapidly at the solution treating temperature, holding at temperature is not required. Ageing is done at 500° to 550°C (930° to 1020°F) for 1 to 4 hr. If the material has been cold worked, following solution treating, ageing temperature may be reduced to 375° to 475°C.

Alpha aluminium bronzes

The structure and consequent heat treatability of aluminium bronze varies greatly with composition. Single-phase (alpha) aluminium bronzes, which contain only copper and aluminium (up to about 10 per cent Al), can be strengthened only by cold working. They can be softened by annealing at 425° to 760°C.

Chapter 13

Titanium Alloys

INTRODUCTION

Titanium alloys are metallic materials which contain a mixture of titanium and other chemical elements. Such alloys have very high tensile strength and toughness (even at extreme temperatures), light weight, extraordinary corrosion resistance, and ability to withstand extreme temperatures. However, the high cost of both raw materials and processing limit their use to military applications, aircraft, spacecraft, medical devices, connecting rods on expensive sports cars and some premium sports equipment and consumer electronics. Auto manufacturers Porsche and Ferrari also use titanium alloys in engine components due to its durable properties in these high stress engine environments.

Although 'commercially pure' titanium has acceptable mechanical properties and has been used for orthopedic and dental implants, for most applications titanium is alloyed with small amounts of aluminum and vanadium, typically 6 per cent and 4 per cent respectively, by weight. This mixture has a solid solubility which varies dramatically with temperature, allowing it to undergo precipitation strengthening. This heat treatment process is carried out after the alloy has been worked into its final shape but before it is put to use, allowing much easier fabrication of a high-strength product.

TRANSITION TEMPERATURE

The crystal structure of titanium at ambient temperature and pressure is close-packed hexagonal α phase with a c/a ratio of 1.587. At about 890°C, the titanium undergoes an allotropic transformation to a body-centred cubic β phase which remains stable to the melting temperature. Some alloying elements raise the alpha-to-beta transition temperature (i.e. alpha stabilisers) while others lower the transition temperature (i.e. beta stabilisers). Aluminium, gallium, germanium, carbon, oxygen and nitrogen are alpha stabilisers. Molybdenum, vanadium, tantalum, niobium, manganese, iron, chromium, cobalt, nickel, copper and silicon are beta stabilisers.

CLASSIFICATION OF TITANIUM ALLOYS

Titanium Alloys are generally classified into four main categories:
1. Alpha alloys which contain neutral alloying elements (such as tin) and/or alpha stabilisers (such as aluminium or oxygen) only. These are not heat treatable.
2. Near-alpha alloys contain small amount of ductile beta-phase. Besides alpha-phase stabilisers, near-alpha alloys are alloyed with 1–2 per cent of beta phase stabilisers such as molybdenum, silicon or vanadium.

3. Alpha and beta Alloys, which are metastable and generally include some combination of both alpha and beta stabilisers, and which can be heat treated.
4. Beta Alloys, which are metastable and which contain sufficient beta stabilisers (such as molybdenum, silicon and vanadium) to allow them to maintain the beta phase when quenched, and which can also be solution treated and aged to improve strength.

Properties

Generally, beta-phase titanium is stronger yet less ductile and alpha-phase titanium is more ductile. Alpha-beta-phase titanium has a mechanical property which is in between both. Titanium dioxide dissolves in the metal at high temperatures, and its formation is very energetic. These two factors mean that all titanium except the most carefully purified has a significant amount of dissolved oxygen, and so may be considered a Ti-O alloy. Oxide precipitates offer some strength, but are not very responsive to heat treatment and can substantially decrease the alloy's toughness.

Many alloys also contain titanium as a minor additive, but since alloys are usually categorised according to which element forms the majority of the material, these are not usually considered to be 'titanium alloys' as such.

Titanium alone is a strong, light metal. It is as strong as steel, but 45 per cent lighter. It is also twice as strong as aluminium but only 60 per cent heavier. Titanium is not easily corroded by sea water, and thus is used in propeller shafts, rigging and other parts of boats that are exposed to sea water. Titanium and its alloys are used in airplanes, missiles and rockets where strength, low weight and resistance to high temperatures are important. Further, since titanium does not react within the human body, it and its alloys are used to create artificial hips, pins for setting bones, and for other biological implants.

Grades

The ASTM defines a number of alloy standards with a numbering scheme for easy reference:
1. Grade 1–4 are unalloyed and considered commercially pure or 'CP'. Generally the tensile and yield strength goes up with grade number for these 'pure' grades. The difference in their physical properties is primarily due to the quantity of interstitial elements. They are used for corrosion resistance applications where cost and ease of fabrication and welding are important.
2. Grade 5, also known as Ti6Al4V, Ti-6Al-4V or Ti 6-4, is the most commonly used alloy. It has a chemical composition of 6 per cent aluminium, 4 per cent vanadium, 0.25 per cent (maximum) iron, 0.2 per cent (maximum) oxygen, and the remainder titanium. Grade 5 is used extensively in Aerospace, Medical, Marine, and Chemical Processing. It is used for connecting rods in ICEs. It is significantly stronger than commercially pure titanium while having the same stiffness and thermal properties (excluding thermal conductivity, which is about 60 per cent lower in Grade 5 Ti than in CP Ti). Among its many advantages, it is heat treatable. This grade is an excellent combination of strength, corrosion resistance, weld and fabricability. In consequence, its uses are numerous such as for military aircraft or turbines. It is also used in surgical implants. Generally, it is used in applications up to 400 degrees Celsius. Its properties are very similar to those of the 300 stainless steel series, especially 316.

It has a density of roughly 4420 kg/m^3, Young's modulus of 110 GPa, and tensile strength of 1000 MPa. By comparison, annealed type 316 stainless steel has a density of 8000 kg/m^3, modulus of 193 GPa, and tensile strength of only 570 MPa. And tempered 6061 aluminium alloy has 2700 kg/m^3, 69 GPa, and 310 MPa, respectively.

HEAT TREATING OF TITANIUM AND TITANIUM ALLOYS

Titanium and titanium alloys are heat treated in order to:
1. Reduce residual stresses developed during fabrication (stress relieving).
2. Produce an optimum combination of ductility, machinability, and dimensional and structural stability (annealing).
3. Increase strength (solution treating and ageing).
4. Optimise special properties such as fracture toughness, fatigue strength, and high-temperature creep strength.

Various types of annealing treatments (single, duplex, (β), and recrystallisation annealing, for example), and solution treating and ageing treatments, are imposed to achieve selected mechanical properties. Stress relieving and annealing may be employed to prevent preferential chemical attack in some corrosive environments, to prevent distortion (a stabilisation treatment) and to condition the metal for subsequent forming and fabricating operations.

Alloy Types and Response to Heat Treatment

The response of titanium and titanium alloys to heat treatment depends on the composition of the metal and the effects of alloying elements on the α-β crystal transformation of titanium. In addition, not all heat treating cycles are applicable to all titanium alloys, because the various alloys are designed for different purposes.
1. Alloys Ti-5Al-2Sn-2Zr-4Mo-4Cr and Ti-6Al-2Sn-4Zr-6Mo are designed for strength in heavy sections.
2. Alloys Ti- 6Al-2Sn-4Zr-2Mo and Ti-6Al-5Zr-0.5Mo-0.2Si for creep resistance.
3. Alloys Ti-6Al-2Nb-1 Ta-1Mo and Ti-6Al-4V, for resistance to stress corrosion in aqueous salt solutions and for high fracture toughness.
4. Alloys Ti-5Al-2.5Sn and Ti-2.5Cu for weldability.
5. Ti-6Al-6V-2Sn, Ti-6Al-4V and Ti-10V-2Fe-3Al for high strength at low-to-moderate temperatures.

Effects of alloying elements on α-β transformation

Unalloyed titanium is allotropic. Its close-packed hexagonal structure (α phase) changes to a body-centered cubic, structure (β-phase) at 885°C (1625°F), and this structure persists at temperatures up to the melting point. With respect to their effects on the allotropic transformation, alloying elements in titanium are classified as a stabilisers or β stabilisers. Alpha stabilisers, such as oxygen and aluminum, raise the α-to-β transformation temperature. Nitrogen and carbon are also stabilisers, but these elements usually are not added intentionally in alloy formulation. Beta stabilisers, such as manganese, chromium, iron, molybdenum, vanadium, and niobium, lower the α- to β-transformation temperature and, depending on the amount added, may result in the retention of some β phase at room temperature.

Alloy types

Based on the types and amounts of alloying elements they contain, titanium alloys are classified as α, near-α, α-β, or β alloys. The response of these alloy types to heat treatment is briefly described below.

Alpha and near-alpha titanium alloys can be stress relieved and annealed, but high strength cannot be developed in these alloys by any type of heat treatment (such as ageing after a solution beta treatment and quenching).

The commercial β alloys are, in reality, metastable β alloys. When these alloys are exposed to selected elevated temperatures, the retained β phase decomposes and strengthening occurs. For β alloys, stress-relieving and ageing treatments can be combined, and annealing and solution treating may be identical operations.

Alpha-beta alloys are two-phase alloys and, as the name suggests, comprise both α and β phases at room temperature. These are the most common and the most versatile of the three types of titanium alloys.

Oxygen and iron levels have significant effects on mechanical properties after heat treatment. It should be realised that:

1. Oxygen and iron must be near specified maximums to meet strength levels in certain commercially pure grades.
2. Oxygen must be near a specified maximum to meet strength levels in solution treated and aged Ti-6Al-4 V.
3. Oxygen levels must be kept as low as possible to optimise fracture toughness. However, the oxygen level must be high enough to meet tensile strength requirements.
4. Iron content must be kept as low as possible to optimise creep and stress-rupture properties. Most creep-resistant alloys require iron levels at or below 0.05wt%.

Stress Relieving

Titanium and titanium alloys can be stress relieved without adversely affecting strength or ductility. Stress-relieving treatments decrease the undesirable residual stresses that result from first, nonuniform hot forging or deformation from cold forming and straightening, second, asymmetric machining of plate or forgings, and, third, welding and cooling of castings. The removal of such stresses helps maintain shape stability and eliminates unfavourable conditions, such as the loss of compressive yield strength commonly known as the Bauschinger effect.

When symmetrical shapes are machined in the annealed condition using moderate cuts and uniform stock removal, stress relieving may not be required. Compressor disks made of Ti-6Al-4V has been machined satisfactorily in this manner, conforming with dimensional requirements. In contrast, thin rings made of the same alloy could be machined at a higher production rate to more stringent dimensions by stress relieving 2 hrs at 540°C (1000°F) between, rough and final machining. Separate stress relieving may be omitted when the manufacturing sequence can be adjusted to use annealing or hardening as the stress-relieving process. For example, forging stresses may be relieved by annealing prior to machining.

Annealing

The annealing of titanium and titanium alloys serves primarily to increase fracture toughness, ductility at room temperature, dimensional and thermal stability, and creep resistance. Many titanium alloys are placed in service in the annealed state. Because improvement in one or more properties is generally obtained at the expense of some other property, the annealing cycle should be selected according to the objective of the treatment.

Common annealing treatments are:
1. Mill annealing.
2. Duplex annealing.
3. Recrystallisation annealing.
4. Beta annealing.

Mill annealing is a general-purpose treatment given to all mill products. It is not a full anneal and may leave traces of cold or warm working in the microstructures of heavily worked products, particularly sheet. Duplex annealing alters the shapes, sizes, and distributions of phases to those required for improved creep resistance or fracture toughness. In the duplex anneal of the Corona 5 alloy, for example, the first anneal is near the β transus to globularise the deformed α and to minimise its volume fraction. This is followed by a second, lower-temperature anneal to precipitate new lenticular (acicular) α between the globular α particles. This formation of acicular α is associated with improvements in creep strength and fracture toughness.

Recrystallisation annealing and β annealing are used to improve fracture toughness. In recrystallisation annealing, the alloy is heated into the upper end of the α-β range, held for a time, and then cooled very slowly. In recent years, recrystallisation annealing has replaced β annealing for fracture critical airframe components.

β (Beta) Annealing: Like recrystallisation annealing, β annealing improves fracture toughness. Beta annealing is done at temperatures above the β transus of the alloy being annealed. To prevent excessive grain growth, the temperature for β annealing should be only slightly higher than the β transus. Annealing times are dependent on section thickness and should be sufficient for complete transformation. Time at temperature after transformation should be held to a minimum to control β grain growth. Larger sections should be fan cooled or water quenched to prevent the formation of α phase at the β grain boundaries.

Straightening, sizing, and flattening of titanium alloys are often necessary in order to meet dimensional requirements. The straightening of bar to close tolerances and the flattening of sheet present major problems for titanium producers and fabricators.

Unlike aluminum alloys, titanium alloys are not easily straightened when cold because the high yield strength and modulus of elasticity of these alloys result in significant springback. Therefore, titanium alloys are straightened primarily by creep straightening and/or hot straightening (hand or die), with the former being considerably more prevalent than the latter.

Straightening, sizing, and flattening may be combined with annealing by the use of appropriate fixtures. The parts, in bulk or in fixtures, may be charged directly into a furnace operating at the annealing temperature. At annealing temperatures many titanium alloys have a creep resistance low enough to permit straightening during annealing.

Creep straightening may be readily accomplished during the annealing and/or ageing processes of most titanium alloys. However, if the annealing/ageing temperature is below about 540° to 650°C (1000° to 1200°F), depending on the alloy, the times required to accomplish the desired creep straightening can be extended. Creep straightening is accomplished with rudimentary or sophisticated fixtures and loading systems, depending on part complexity and the degree of straightening required.

Creep flattening consists of heating titanium sheet between two clean, flat sheets of steel in a furnace containing an oxidising or inert atmosphere. Vacuum creep flattening is used to produce stress-free flat plate for subsequent machining. The plate is placed on a large, flat ceramic bed that has integral electric heating elements. Insulation is placed on top of the plate, and a plastic sheet is sealed to the frame.

Stability: In α-β titanium alloys, thermal stability is a function of β-phase transformations. During cooling from the annealing temperature, β may transform and, under certain conditions and in β alloys, may form a brittle intermediate phase known as ω.

A stabilisation annealing treatment is designed to produce a stable β-phase capable of resisting further transformation when exposed to elevated temperatures in service. Alpha-beta alloys that are lean in β, such as Ti-6Al-4V, can be air cooled from the annealing temperature without impairing their stability. To obtain maximum creep resistance and stability in the near-α alloys Ti-8Al-1 Mo-1 V and Ti-6Al-2Sn-4Zr-2Mo, a duplex annealing treatment is employed. This treatment begins with solution annealing at a temperature high in the α-β range, usually 25° to 55°C (50° to 100°F) below the β transus for Ti-8Al-1Mo-1 V and 15 to 25°C (25° to 50°F) below the α-β transus for Ti-6Al-2Sn-4Zr-2Mo.

Solution Treating and Ageing

A wide range of strength levels can be obtained in α-β or β alloys by solution treating and ageing. With the exception of the unique Ti-2.5Cu alloy (which relies on strengthening from the classic age-hardening reaction of Ti-2Cu precipitation similar to the formation of Guinier-Preston zones in aluminum alloys), the origin of heat-treating responses of titanium alloys lies in the instability of the high-temperature β phase at lower temperatures. Heating an α-β alloy to the solution-treating temperature produces a higher ratio of β phase. This partitioning of phases is maintained by quenching; on subsequent ageing, decomposition of the unstable β phase occurs, providing high strength. Commercial β alloys generally supplied in the solution-treated condition, and need only to be aged.

After being cleaned, titanium components should be loaded into fixtures or racks that will permit free access to the heating and quenching media. Thick and thin components of the same alloy may be solution treated together, but the time at temperature is determined by the thickest section. Time/temperature combinations for solution treating are given in Table 13.1. A load may be charged directly into a furnace operating at the solution-treating temperature. Although preheating is not essential, it may be used to minimise the distortion of complex parts.

Table 13.1. Recommended solution and ageing treatments for titanium alloy.

Alloy	Solution temperature (°C)	Solution time (hr)	Cooling rate	Ageing temperature (°C)	Ageing time (hr)
α or near-α alloys					
Ti-8Al-1Mo-1V	980–1010	1	Oil or water	565–595	
Ti-2.5Cu (IMI 230)	795–815	0.5–1	Air or water	390–410	8–24 (step 1)
				465–485	8 (step 2)
Ti-6Al-2Sn-4Zr-2Mo	955–980	1	Air	595	8
Ti-6Al-5Zr-0.5Mo-0.2Si (IMI 685)	1040–1060	0.5–1	Oil	540–560	24
Ti-5.5Al-3.5Sn-3Zr-1Nb-0.3Mo-0.3Si (IMI 829)	1040–1060	0.5–1	Air or oil	615–635	2
Ti-5.8Al-4Sn-3.5Zr-0.7Nb-0.5Mo-0.3Si (IMI 834)	1020	2	Oil	625	2
α-β alloys					
Ti-6Al-4V	955–970	1	Water	480–595	4–8
	955–970	1	Water	705–760	2–4
Ti-6al-6V-2Sn (Cu+Fe)	885–910	1	Water	480–595	4–8
Ti-6Al-2Sn-4Zr-6Mo	845–890	1	Air	580–605	4–8
Ti-4Al-4Mo-2Sn-0.5Si (IMI 550)	890–910	0.5–1	Air	490–510	24

(Contd ...)

Alloy	Solution temperature (°C)	Solution time (hr)	Cooling rate	Ageing temperature (°C)	Ageing time (hr)
Ti-4Al-4Mo-4Sn-0.5Si (IMI 551)	890–910	0.5–1	Air	490–510	24
Ti-5Al-2Sn-2Zr-4Mo-4Cr	845–870	1	Air	580–605	4–8
Ti-6Al-2Sn-2Zr-2Mo-2Cr-0.25Si	870–925	1	Water	480–595	4–8
β or near-β alloys					
Ti-13V-11Cr-3Al	775–800	1/4–1	Air or water	425–480	4–100
Ti-11.5Mo-6Zr-4.5Sn (Beta III)	690–790	1/8–1	Air or water	480–595	8–32
Ti-3Al-8V-6Cr-4Mo-4Zr (Beta C)	815–925	1	Water	455–540	8–24
Ti-10V-2Fe-3Al	760–780	1	Water	495–525	8
Ti-15V-3Al-3Cr-3Sn	790–815	1/4	Air	510–595	8–24

Solution treating: Solution treating of titanium alloys generally involves heating to temperatures either slightly above or slightly below the β transus temperature. The solution-treating temperature selected depends on the alloy type and practical considerations briefly described below.

β (Beta) alloys: β (Beta) alloys are normally obtained from producers in the solution-treated condition. If reheating is required, soak times should be only as long as necessary to obtain complete solutioning. Solution-treating temperatures for β alloys are above the β transus; because no second phase is present, grain growth can proceed rapidly.

α-β (Alpha-beta) alloys: Selection of a solution-treatment temperature for α-β alloys is based on the combination of mechanical properties desired after ageing. A change in the solution-treating temperature of α-β alloys alters the amounts of β phase and consequently changes the response to ageing.

To obtain high strength with adequate ductility, it is necessary to solution treat at a temperature high in the α-β field, normally 25° to 85°C (50° to 150°F) below the β transus of the alloy. If high fracture toughness or improved resistance to stress corrosion is required, β annealing or β solution treating may be desirable. However, heat treating α-β alloys in the β range causes a significant loss in ductility. These alloys are usually solution heat treated below the β transus to obtain an optimum balance of ductility, fracture toughness, creep, and stress rupture properties.

Chapter 14
Die Casting Alloys

INTRODUCTION

Die casting alloys are normally non-ferrous and there is a large number available with a wide range of physical and mechanical properties covering almost every conceivable application a designer might require. Aluminum and zinc alloys are the most widely used. Followed by magnesium, zinc-aluminum (ZA) alloys, copper, tin and lead. Zinc, lead and tin based alloys are classified as low melting point metals because they turn melt at less than 725° (385°C). Zinc-aluminum (ZA) alloys have a slightly higher melting range of 800° to 900°F (426° to 482°C). Aluminum and magnesium alloys are considered to be moderate melting point alloys, being cast in the 1150° to 1300°F (621° to 704°C) range. Copper alloys are considered to be high melting point alloys, over 1650°F (899°C). Low melting point alloys are cast in hot chamber machines. Intermediate and high melting point alloys are cast in cold chamber machines.

ALUMINUM ALLOYS

Aluminum die casting alloys (Table 14.1) are lightweight, offer good corrosion resistance, ease of casting, good mechanical properties and dimensional stability. Although a variety of aluminum alloys can be die cast from primary or recycled metal, most designers select a standard alloy listed below. Special alloys for special applications are available but their use usually involves significant cost premiums:

1. A360—Selected for best corrosion resistance and pressure tightness.
2. A380—The most common and cost effective of all die casting alloys. Provides the best combination of utility and cost.
3. A383 and A384—These alloys are a modification of 380. Both provide better die filling but with a moderate sacrifice in mechanical properties such as toughness.
4. A390—Selected for special applications where high strength, fluidity and wear-resistance/bearing properties are required.
5. A413 (A13)—Used for maximum pressure tightness and fluidity.

ZINC ALLOYS

Various types of zinc alloy parts are usually made using the zinc die casting process. All types of zinc alloy parts can be relied on for their strength and durability. Zinc alloy parts also come in a broader range of shapes and sizes since zinc alloy is more capable of producing multi-cavity complex shapes than most other metal alloys.

Table 14.1. Aluminum die casting alloys.

Alloy composition	A360	A380	A383	A384	A390	A413 (A13)
Composition (% max or range)						
Silicon	9–10	7.5–9.5	9.5–11.5	10.5–12	16–18	11–13
Iron	1.3	1.3	1.3	1.3	1.3	1.3
Copper	0.6	3–4	2–3	3–4.5	4–5	1.0
Manganese	0.35	0.50	0.50	0.50	0.50	0.35
Magnesium	0.4-0.6	0.10	0.10	0.10	0.45–0.65	0.10
Nickel	0.50	0.50	0.30	0.50	0.10	0.50
Zinc	0.50	3.0	3.0	3.0	1.5	0.50
Tin	0.15	0.35	0.15	0.35	0.20	0.15
Titanium	–	–	–	–	0.20	–
Total others	0.25	0.50	0.50	0.50	0.20	0.25
Aluminium	Bal.	Bal.	Bal.	Bal.	Bal.	Bal.
Properties						
Ultimate tensile strength (ksi)	46	47	45	48	40.5	42
Tensile yield strength (ksi)	24	23	22	24	35	19
Elongation (% in 2″ G.L.)	3.5	3.5	3.5	1–2.5		3.5
Hardness (HB)	75	80	80		85	120
Shear strength (ksi)	26	27	25			29
Charpy impact strength (ft. lb.—unnotched)	4.2	3.5				2.0
Fatigue strength (ksi) (limit @500 million cycles)	18	20	19	20		20
Density (lb./in.^{3})	0.095	0.098	0.097	0.098	0.099	0.096
Melting range (°F) approx.	1035–1105	1000–1100	960–1080	960–1080	945–1200	1065–1080
Specific heat (Btu/lb.°F)	0.23	0.23				
Coefficient of thermal expansion (in./in./°F)	11.8	11.7	11.5	11.3	11.7	10.3
Thermal conductivity (Btu/fthr°F)	65.3	55.6	55.6	56	78.6	67.7
Electrical conductivity (% IACS)	29	31	23	23	25	31
Modulus of elasticity (10^6 psi)	10.3	10.3	10.3	10.3	11.9	10.3
Characteristics (1-most desirable; 4–least desirable)						
Resistance to hot cracking	2	2	–	2	–	1
Pressure tightness	1	2	2	2	–	1
Polishing	3	3	–	3	–	4
Fluidity	2	2	1	1	–	1
Corrosion resistance	3	4	3	4	–	2
Machine-ability	2	2	2	3	–	4
Strength at elev. temp.	3	2	2	1	–	2
Anti-die soldering tend.	3	1	2	2	–	2
Electroplating	1	1	–	2	–	3
Anodising appearance	4	4	–	4	–	4

Zinc-based alloys are the easiest to die cast. Ductility is high and impact strength is excellent, making these alloys suitable for a wide range of products. Zinc alloys can be cast with thin walls and excellent surface smoothness making preparation for plating and painting relatively easy. It is essential that only high purity (99.99+ %) zinc metal be used in the formulation of alloys. Low limits on lead, tin and cadmium ensure the long-term integrity of the alloy's strength and dimensional stability.

Zinc alloy's characteristic low melting point makes it flexible enough to be used for both hot-chamber die casting machines and cold-chamber die casting machines. As a result, there are more types of zinc alloy parts manufactured and sold in the market today, with the automotive industry enjoying the largest share in the output of zinc die castings.

The zinc die casting process involves the injection of molten zinc metal alloy into dies made of hardened tool steel. Over a century ago, molten metal was squeesed into die cast dies or die cast moulds to manufacture axe heads. From simple shapes, zinc alloy die casting technology has improved the process to be able to manufacture more complex shapes.

There are two processes for zinc alloy die casting:
1. The hot-chamber method and the cold-chamber method. In the hot-chamber method, a pool of molten metal is used to fill the steel die while maintaining pressure until the metal hardens in the die.
2. The cold-chamber method, on the other hand, uses separate chambers to melt and then hold the melted metal before pouring the zinc alloy into a shot cylinder and injecting them into the die casting dies.

Various metal alloys are used in the production of parts using the die casting process. Tin and lead were the first metal alloys that were used in die casting of metal printer's types. Throughout the years, a number of other metal alloys ensued as medium for die casting parts. Among the most popular metal alloys is zinc alloy.

Zinc-based alloys (Table 14.2) are the easiest to die cast. Ductility is high and impact strength is excellent, making these alloys suitable for a wide range of products. Zinc alloys can be cast with thin walls and excellent surface smoothness making preparation for plating and painting relatively easy. It is essential that only high purity (99.99+%) zinc metal be used in the formulation of alloys. Low limits on lead, tin and cadmium ensure the long-term integrity of the alloy's strength and dimensional stability.

ZINC-ALUMINUM (ZA) ALLOYS

ZA alloys represent a new family of zinc-based die casting materials that contain higher aluminum content than standard zinc alloys. These alloys provide high strength characteristics plus high hardness and good bearing properties (Table 14.2). Thin wall castability characteristics and die life are similar to zinc alloys. ZA-8 is recommended for hot chamber die casting. ZA-12 and ZA-27 must be cast by the cold chamber die casting process. All ZA alloys offer similar creep properties and are superior to standard zinc alloys.

ZA-8: Provides strength, hardness and creep properties.

ZA-12: Provides excellent bearing properties with strength and hardness characteristics between ZA-8 and ZA-27. Good dimensional stability properties and somewhat better castability than ZA-27.

ZA-27: Offers the highest mechanical properties of the ZA family and is therefore recommended when maximum performance is required.

Table 14.2. Zinc die casting alloys.

Alloy composition (% max or range)	Zinc #3	Zinc #5	Zinc #7	ZA-8	ZA-12	ZA-27
Aluminium	3.5–4.3	3.5–4.3	3.5–4.3	8–8.8	10.5–11.5	25–28
Copper	0.25	0.75–1.25	0.25	0.8–1.3	0.5–1.25	2–2.5
Magnesium	0.02–0.05	0.03–0.08	0.005–0.020	0.015–0.030	0.015–0.30	0.010–0.020
Iron	0.100	0.100	0.075	0.10	0.075	0.10
Lead	0.005	0.005	0.0030	0.004	0.004	0.004
Cadmium	0.004	0.004	0.0020	0.003	0.003	0.003
Tin	0.003	0.003	0.0010	0.002	0.002	0.002
Nickel	–	–	0.005–0.020	–	–	–
Zinc	Bal.	Bal.	Bal.	Bal.	Bal.	Bal.
Properties						
Ultimate tensile strength (ksi)	40	48	41	54	58.5	61
Tensile yield strength (ksi)	–	–	–	42	46	53
Elongation [% in 2″ (55 mm)]	10	7	13	6–10	4–7	1–3
Hardness (HB)	82	91	80	95–110	95–115	105–125
Shear strength (ksi)	31	38	–	35	37	42
Charpy impact strength (ft. lb.– unnotched)	43	48	43	31	21	3
Fatigue strength (ksi) (limit @ 500 million cycles)	6.9	8.2	–	7.5	15	25
Density (lb./in.^{3})	0.24	0.24	0.247	0.227	0.218	0.181
Melting range (°F)	718–728	717–727	718–728	707–759	710–810	708–903
Specific heat (Btu/lb.°F)	0.10	0.10	0.10	0.104	0.107	0.125
Coefficient of thermal expansion (in./in./°F)	15.2	15.2	15.2	12.9	13.4	14.4
Thermal conductivity (Btu/fthr.°F)	65.3	62.9	65.3	66.3	67.1	72.5
Electrical conductivity (% IACS)	27.0	26.0	27.0	27.7	28.3	29.7
Modulus of rupture (10^6 psi)	95,000	105,000	–	–	–	–
Modulus of elasticity (10^6 psi)	–	–	–	10.2	10.3	10.3
Die shrinkage (in./in.)	0.007	0.007	0.007	0.007	0.0075	0.008
Characteristics (1–most desirable; 4–least desirable)						
Resistance to hot cracking	1	1	1			
Pressure tightness	1	1	1			
Polishing	1	1	1			
Fluidity	1	2	1			
Corrosion resistance	1	1	1			
Machine-ability	1	1	1			
Strength at elev. temp.	4	4	4			
Anti-die soldering tend.	1	1	1			
Electroplating	1	1	1			
Anodising appearance	–	–	–			

Chapter 15

Grain Refinement of Light Alloys

INTRODUCTION

The use of aluminium and magnesium alloys in the automobile industry is continuously increasing. The driving force is reduced green house gas emissions resulting from light weighting of the vehicles and efficient scrap recycling. The present consumption of aluminium and magnesium in passenger cars is 120–140 kg and ~5 kg per vehicle respectively; these figures are expected to rise further in the next decade. In order to maintain this momentum it is necessary to pay attention to all processing (solidification, mechanical and thermal) aspects of the alloys and optimise the properties. Grain refining plays an important role in this context. Reduction in grain size can be achieved in three different stages—during solidification of the molten metal, thermomechanical treatments involving recovery and recrystallisation of the deformed material and severe plastic deformation using processes such as equichannel angular processing (ECAP), hydrostatic extrusion and roll bonding.

The resulting grain size varies from a few hundred µm (molten metal solidification) to a fraction (severe plastic deformation) of µm. Grain refinement resulting from solidification is the mother of all these treatments and is applicable to both cast and wrought alloys. In view of the increasing applications of the light alloys in the automobile sector many of these studies are revisited in the recent years and fine tuning done to ensure that the process is efficient and environmentally friendly.

Grain refinement offers a number of advantages in foundry operations and in subsequent mechanical and thermal processing and surface finishing stages. Benefits in the foundry operation include improved feeding, reduced chemical segregation, porosity and hot tearing and increased pressure tightness; the advantages during the subsequent processing stages are improved mechanical properties in heavier sections, consistent properties after heat treatment, improved machinability and better appearance in anodised coatings.

Grain refinement during solidification involves the formation of fine equiaxed grains at the expense of dendrites. The methods favouring the formation of fine grains include addition of trace elements in the form of master alloys, inoculation of borides and carbides, use of ultrasonic treatment or electromagnetic field, introduction of fine gas bubbles and applying coatings to the mould surface. Inoculation is the most commonly employed method and is carried out using grain refiners such as Al-Ti, Al-Ti-B, Al-Ti-C, Al-B and Al-Sr-B alloys. Studies on the performance of grain refiners indicate that the grain size attains a minimum value after a certain length of time, followed by an increase (fade). Alloying elements like Si, Zr and V are found to poison the grain refiners, thereby reducing the efficiency of grain refinement. Al-Ti-C alloys are more effective and are not poisoned by Zr or V, but suffer from disadvantages of easy fade and inferiority to Al-Ti-B in the treatment of recycled material. Aluminium-free magnesium alloys are commonly grain refined by the addition of Zr in the form of Mg-Zr master alloy. Introduction of carbon in the aluminium containing alloys leads to grain refinement but there is ample scope for improving the process. The standard method for the manufacture of Al-Ti-B involving the use of K_2TiF_6 and KBF_4 results in considerable fluoride emissions and formation of fluoride salts as slag. Trials are currently in progress to minimise these effects and control pollution. The mechanisms proposed for grain refinement are based on heterogeneous nucleation of the aluminium grains on the inoculants, solute retardation of grain growth and edge-to-edge matching of planes in the substrate and the solidifying grain. The ultimate aim of understanding the mechanism is to predict the grain refiners that would be suitable for a given alloy.

GRAIN REFINEMENT METHODS

Aluminium Alloys

Trace additions of Mn, Cr and Zr (in the form of master alloys) to aluminium refine the grain size, the effect being prominent after thermomechanical treatments. Fine (a few tens to hundred nm size) dispersoids of Al_3Zr, Al_6Mn and Al_7Cr are effective in pinning grain boundaries, thereby restricting their movement. Scandium is an efficient addition to aluminium to achieve grain refinement during solidification of the molten metal and also during subsequent mechanical and thermal processing stages. The extent of addition for efficient grain refinement depends on the nature of the alloy. For example ~0.6–0.7 per cent Sc is necessary for refining pure aluminium while for an Al-Zn-Mg-Zr alloy ~0.2 per cent Sc is sufficient. The lower amount of Sc in the presence of Zr is attributed to the formation of composite Al_3Sc-Al_3Zr particles as well as to the possible lowering of eutectic composition in the ternary system. Similar results are also obtained with AA356.0 alloy. In view of the prohibitively high cost of Al-Sc master alloys, use of reduced amounts is desirable. The addition of carbon and iron also contribute to grain refining although the effect is not prominent. Also iron forms insolubles of the Al_3Fe, AlFeSi type which are detrimental to the mechanical properties.

Salt flux treatment for grain refining and production of Al-Ti and Al-Ti-B master alloys are both based on the interaction between double fluoride salts and aluminium melt in accordance with the following equations:

$$3K_2TiF_6 + 4Al \rightarrow 3Ti + 4AlF_3 + 6KF \qquad \ldots (15.1)$$
$$2KBF_4 + 3Al \rightarrow AlB_2 + 2AlF_3 + 2KF \qquad \ldots (15.2)$$
$$3K_2TiF_6 + 6KBF_4 + 10Al \rightarrow 3TiB_2 + 10AlF_3 + 12KF \qquad \ldots (15.3)$$

Flux treatment leads to *in situ* generation of the nucleants such as AlB_2 and TiB_2; the production of master alloys based on the above chemical equations results in a fine dispersion of the borides in aluminium which can be subsequently added to aluminium alloys. Process control is somewhat difficult in flux treatment as the borides may get entrapped with the slag particles leading to less efficient grain refinement and the introduction of slag inclusions in the solidified aluminium alloy. Other disadvantages of using fluxes include their hygroscopic nature, release of corrosive fumes during melting, possibility of reaction with modifying agents such as Na and Sr (in Al-Si Alloys) and the unpredictable recovery behaviour of Ti and B. Master alloys are usually produced in induction furnaces and are cast-as *in-got*, waffle, sheared rod or shotted product. The main problem encountered in making the alloys is the pronounced tendency for the particles to segregate arising from differences in melting points of the **elements and the density of the phases (molten Al, Al_3Ti and borides).**

Different practice for salt addition introduce marked changes in microstructure and hence the grain refining efficiency of the Al–5Ti–1B master alloys. Mixing the halide salts before addition and a high rate of addition both lead to improved grain refining efficiency. Stirring during addition and reaction temperatures exceeding 850°C are undesirable. The morphology of Al_3Ti particles in the master alloy depends on the temperature of pouring and has considerable influence on grain refining ability. Consequently an optimum procedure for production of efficient grain refiners consists of melting commercial purity aluminium, rapid addition of premixed salts at 800°C, to facilitate spontaneous reaction and gently mixing the salts with the aluminium melt without introducing any stirring.

Al-Ti-C master alloys are produced through several routes—adding C, TiC, $C_2Cl_6 Al_4C_3$ or a mixture of K_2TiF_6 and carbon to the melt, feeding C rod, CCl_4 or TiC through a flux.

Information on commercially available grain refiners is summarised in Table 15.1. The most commonly used alloy is Al-5Ti-1B but recent studies show that some of the dilute alloys can be equally effective. The ratio of Ti to B for the formation of TiB_2 in Al-Ti-B alloys is 2.21:1. The Al-3Ti-1B alloy would, therefore, contain most of the Ti and B in combined form. Since the other compositions have excess Ti, a certain amount of Al_3Ti would coexist with the boride phase. Also in alloys with low B (such as Al-5Ti-0.2B and Al-10Ti-0.4B), the concentration of borides is low; these alloys are preferred for grain refinement operations where the ingot is to be rolled into thin foils. The low carbon concentration of the Al-Ti-C alloys implies small amounts of TiC; the excess Ti would be present as Al_3Ti. The Al-B alloys would contain AlB_2 particles dispersed in aluminium matrix. The Sr-B alloy fulfils the twin objectives of grain refinement (by AlB_2) and modification (by Sr) of the eutectic structure in Al-Si alloys. Typical size of the boride particles is ~ 1 μm in the Al-5Ti-1B alloy, 2–3 μm in Hydloy and 0.05 μm–1 μm in TiBloy.

Table 15.1. Commercially available grain refining alloys.

Alloy type	Composition
Al-Ti	Al-10Ti, Al-6Ti
Al-Ti-B	Al-3Ti-1B, Al-5Ti-1B, Al-5Ti-0.6B, Al-3Ti-0.2B, Al-5Ti-1B, Al-5Ti-0.2B, Al-10Ti-0.4B, Al-1.6Ti-1.4B (TiBloy for hypoeutectic Al-Si alloys), Al-1.2Ti-0.5B (Hydloy), Al-3Ti-3B, Al-1Ti-3B
Al-B	Al-10B, Al-5B, Al-3B, Al-10Sr-2B, Strobloyä, (Al-10Sr-1.6Ti-1.4B)
Al-Ti-C	Al-6Ti-0.02C, Al-3Ti-0.15C
Al-Sc	Al-1Sc, Al-2Sc
Mg-Zr	AM cast (Mg-25Zr), Zirmax (Mg-33.3Zr)

The performance of a grain refiner can be evaluated by withdrawing samples at different times following its addition and determining the grain size of the solidified alloy. A number of standard tests are available for this purpose but the more commonly employed one is the AA TP1 test. This uses a tapering steel (or copper) mould immersed in water up to a certain height, thereby introducing different rates of cooling simulating various cooling conditions encountered in casting processes. The performance characteristics of a set of grain refining additions (flux, Al-Ti and Al-Ti-B) are schematically illustrated in Fig. 15.1(a). The important points to note are the finite time taken by each type of refiner to produce the minimum grain size, the phenomenon of fade where the grain size starts increasing after a certain length of time and the distinct advantage of Al-Ti-B over Al-Ti and flux additions. Macrostructures of aluminium samples grain refined with Al-1.2Ti-0.5B alloy using the AA TP1 test and withdrawn after various time intervals are shown in Fig. 15.1(b). The fading effect is clearly brought out in the macrographs corresponding to long time interval after addition. The phenomenon of fade is associated with agglomeration of the boride particles; large agglomerates present in the grain refiner and their growth by absorption of smaller (and therefore slower settling particles) are responsible for loss of grain refining. These agglomerates lead to a number of quality problems—streaking and porosity in thin foils, scratch-like liner surface defects in litho and bright anodised sheet, internal cracking in extrusion billets, crack initiation in high strength aluminium alloy plate and forgings. A good grain refiner needs to have a short incubation period for reaching the minimum grain size and a sustained time interval before the onset of fade.

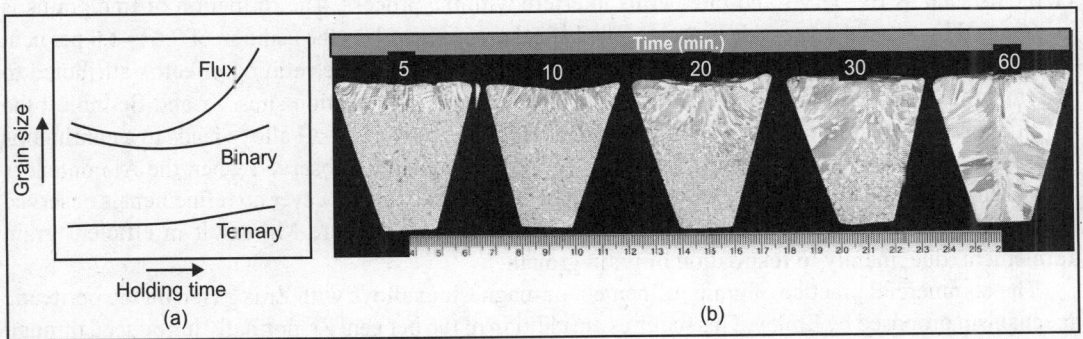

Fig. 15.1. (a) Schematic of grain size variation with holding time for aluminium using flux, binary Al-Ti and ternary Al-Ti-B alloys, and (b) macrographs of commercial aluminium grain refined by Al-1.2Ti-0.5B, 50 ppm Ti addition.

The grain refining behaviour of the Al-Ti-B alloys (particularly the 5Ti-1B alloy) can be adversely affected by solutes such as Si, V and Zr. This poisoning phenomenon is observed in Al-Si alloys when the Si content exceeds ~2 per cent and in the high strength wrought alloys such as those in the 2xxx and 7xxx series. It can be counteracted by excess additions of the grain refiner which adds to the cost of grain refinement. Another possibility is to reduce the Ti content in the master alloys, e.g. Al-3Ti-3B in Table 15.1. The poisoning phenomenon in Al-Si alloys is attributed to the formation of Ti_5Si_3.

Studies on grain refinement of various aluminium alloys by the Al-Ti-B master alloys indicate that the Hydloy (1.2Ti-0.5B) is consistent in producing the lowest grain size at about the same addition level (typically 1.5–2.0 kg/T). The lower titanium content of this alloy implies lower cost and lower concentration of the boride particles and hence less carry over of the inactive nucleants into the solidified product.

Al-Ti-C alloys offer the advantages of higher casting speed, higher yield due to fewer oxide particles, less cracking and agglomeration. However, they are sensitive to casting temperatures and have high fading potential; higher temperatures of pouring reduce grain refining efficiency. The TiC particles are softer than those of TiB_2 and hence there is less die wear during drawing and extrusion operations.

MAGNESIUM ALLOYS

Magnesium alloys can be generally classified into two broad groups; those containing aluminium and the ones free from aluminium. The aluminium-containing alloys are more difficult to refine than those free from aluminium; Zr is effective in the treatment of the latter group of alloys. The subject of grain refinement of magnesium alloys has recently been reviewed by St. John. The methods available include superheating, carbon addition, the Elfinal process, agitation and treatment with Mg-Zr master alloys.

Super heating method of grain refinement involves heating to about 180°–300°C above the liquidus for a short time followed by rapid cooling to the pouring temperature. Presence of at least 1 per cent Al, and smaller amounts of Mn and Fe, adhering to the superheating temperature range strictly and minimum holding time at the pouring temperature, are essential to successful grain refining.

Efficient grain refinement of Mg-Al alloys with more than 2 per cent Al is achieved by the addition of graphite, paraffin wax, lamp black, C_2Cl_6 and carbides such as Al_4C_3, SiC and CaC_2 or bubbling the melt with carbonaceous gases such as CO_2, C_2H_2 and C_2Cl_6. CaC_2 and C_2Cl_6 appear to be more effective; elements such as Be, Ti, Zr and rare earths interfere with the process. The formation of fine grains is encouraged by aluminium carbide particles. The Elfinal process involves the addition of 0.4 to 1.0 per cent anhydrous ferric chloride at temperatures between 740° to 780°C. The refining effect is attributed to intermetallic compounds of Fe and Al acting as heterogeneous nucleation sites. Zr and Be inhibit the refining process. Increasing the aluminium content of hypoeutectic Mg-Al alloys leads to a continuous reduction in grain size up to 5 per cent Al, no further refinement is observed when the Al content is increased. Sr is good for grain refinement of low Al-containing alloys; however no refinement is observed when the Al content is 9 per cent. Additions of Zr, Si and Ca to pure Mg result in efficient grain refinement, due, mainly to retardation of grain growth.

The commercial practice of grain refinement of magnesium alloys with Zr is based on the peritectic mechanism proposed by Emley. This requires an addition of 0.6 per cent Zr, normally introduced through a master alloy (e.g. Zirmax); the low recovery of Zr and the high cost of the master alloy make the grain refining process expensive. Reassessment of the phase compositions in recent years indicate that the peritectic composition is substantially lower, ~ 0.4 per cent. It should, therefore, be possible to add lower amount of Zr for grain refinement which would reduce the cost of the operation. Recent studies on Mg-3.8% Zn-2.2% Ca alloy indicate that the Zr content in the equiaxed grains ahead of the columnar front is between 0.2–0.3 per cent; this is an encouraging result as grain refinement can be obtained with Zr content of <0.3 per cent. There is some evidence that simultaneous addition of Zr and Sc is useful in grain refining the aluminium-containing AZ31 alloy; the effect, brought about by the pinning of the grain boundaries by precipitating phases containing Zr and Sc, is particularly noticeable when the alloy is subjected to severe plastic deformation through ECAP.

Native grain refinement, associated with the purity of magnesium used in alloy making, is reported in Mg-Al alloys; Mg-Al alloys made from high purity magnesium have a finer grain size compared with those made from less pure metal. In contrast Mg-Zn and Mg-Ca alloys exhibit native grain coarsening. Al_4C_3 particles present in the alloys are reported to be responsible for native grain refinement; impurities such as Fe and Mn present in the less pure metal counteract the effect of the carbide nucleants. However, this hypothesis is in conflict with the benefits of Fe introduced by the Elfinal process.

The use of Al-Ti-B type grain refiners in magnesium alloys has not attracted much attention. A recent study indicates that AZ31 and ZA84 alloys can be grain refined by the use of an Al-4Ti-5B master alloy; TiB_2 particles are reported to be the heterogeneous nucleation sites. The use of the standard composition master alloys (Table 15.1) needs a careful study.

While several methods are available for grain refining magnesium alloys, the mechanisms involved are not clear; consequently empirical approaches are often employed and this leads to unsatisfactory results. Attention is now paid to understanding the mechanisms better with a view to developing grain refiners based on theoretical considerations.

ENVIRONMENTAL CONSIDERATIONS

As pointed out earlier, the production of Al-Ti-B grain refiners involves reaction of molten aluminium with KBF_4 and K_2TiF_6. The process is associated with considerable fluoride emissions due to vapourisation of the salts and their reaction with moisture leading to the formation of hydrogen fluoride. Besides the slag formed contains potassium and aluminium fluoride; this presents disposal problems. Consequently several trials have been/are in progress to minimise these effects. The development of the low Ti and B (1.2Ti-0.5B) alloy is a step in this regard. A second approach is to replace KBF_4 by other boron-containing compounds such as borax and boron trioxide and replacing K_2TiF_6 by titanium sponge. Changes in the nature, size and distribution of the boride particles introduced by these processes and the consequent effect on grain refining efficiency and reduced recovery of Ti are problems to be sorted out.

It is recently reported that grain refinement in aluminium can be achieved by using fine argon gas bubbles (introduced through a graphite diffuser) to agitate the melt. This method has great potential for combining grain refinement with melt treatment (an essential prerequisite for producing good quality castings and dealing with minimisation of dissolved hydrogen, Na and Ca and inclusions). The process avoids introduction of borides and their aggregates in the metal and therefore offers longer metal filter life and better mechanical properties.

A recently developed method for grain refinement involves the *in situ* formation of boride nuclei in molten aluminium immediately preceding the casting stage. The process (fy-Gem process) developed under a Department of Energy of the US Government project is carried out by introducing argon—typically 1 per cent BF_3 or BCl_3 mixture into the molten metal in the form of fine bubbles; the trihalide is introduced during the in-line melt treatment stage. Boron dissolving in aluminium combines with Ti, V, Fe, Mn in the metal to form a fine dispersion of borides. BCl_3 can be produced by chlorination of boron carbide at 1000°C. An important step in the process is the design of the rotor head for the introduction of the gas in the form of fine bubbles. The manufacture of the trihalide is considerably simpler than preparing the conventional Al-Ti-B or Al-B grain refiners and has the advantages of environmental, capital and energy savings. Also the process avoids clusters of borides, salt and oxide inclusions that affect adversely the properties of the cast metal. Prolonged experimental trials on the foundry aluminium alloys show that the fy-gem process is as efficient as the best grain refiners currently available; the performance is slightly inferior with the wrought alloys and the Zr-containing alloys pose problems.

THEORIES OF GRAIN REFINEMENT

The mechanisms proposed for grain refinement are based on: (i) heterogeneous nucleation of aluminium grains on inoculant particles (borides and titanium aluminide), (ii) grain growth retardation by solute additions, and (iii) edge-to-edge matching of the planes in the inoculant particle and nucleating aluminium grain. Heterogeneous nucleation on the substrate would depend on compatibility between the crystal structures and lattice parameters of the phases involved. A consideration of these factors indicates that Al_3Ti can be an efficient nucleant. However at the typical levels of addition (a few hundred ppm Ti) for grain refinement, particles of this phase are unstable. Careful high resolution electron optical observations indicate that a thin layer of Al_3Ti formed on TiB_2 facilitates heterogeneous nucleation. Retardation of grain growth is based on the mechanism of constitutional supercooling; the nucleating substrates are mainly the borides with the solute atoms affecting the dendritic growth and building up a constitutionally supercooled zone in front of the solidifying interface which facilitates the nucleation process. The efficiency of the solute atoms in promoting grain refinement is related to the growth restriction factor,

$m(k-1)C_0$ where, C_0 is the solute concentration, m is the slope of the liquidus line at C_0 and k is the equilibrium partition coefficient between the melt and the primary aluminium grains. The higher the value of the growth restriction factor, the smaller will be the grain size.

The value of $m(k-1)$ is the highest for Ti in Al and Zr in Mg. B and Sc, elements of interest in grain refinement of aluminium, have relatively low values of $m(k-1)$. Ta has a high value for $m(k-1)$ in aluminium and is, therefore, of interest; there are very few references in the literature about the use of Ta for grain refinement. The edge-to-edge model is capable of predicting the orientation relationships between the parent and product phases and corresponding habit planes from first principles; it is based on the minimisation of strain energy of the interface. It has been applied to both aluminium and magnesium alloys; studies in aluminium alloys indicate that although TiC, Al_3Ti, TiB_2 and AlB_2 are all effective heterogeneous nucleants, the predicted efficacy of the substrates varies. Al_3Ti is the best grain refiner for Al alloys. The other three are less efficient. Also orientation relationships predicted by the model are in agreement with those from previous observations. It is possible to use the edge-to-edge matching model as a theoretical guide to the discovery of new and more effective grain refiners; this may be of particular relevance to systems that are traditionally difficult to grain refine, such as the Al–Li and Al–Si alloys. This model has been used to identify a new grain refiner, ZnO, for the Mg-Al alloys.

SUMMARY

Al-Ti-B alloys are efficient grain refiners for aluminium alloys but the workhorse Al-5Ti-1B alloy is slowly giving way to the more dilute alloys such as Al-1.2Ti-0.5B. *In situ* formation of the boride nuclei by injection of BCl_3 or BF_3 offers significant advantages in terms of lower amount of nucleants and improved environment.

Injection of fine gas bubbles into the melt satisfies the requirements of both grain refinement and melt treatment; the method requires more elaborate study. Al-free magnesium alloys can be efficiently refined by Zr; the emerging trend is to use lower amount of Zr (typically 0.3 per cent), thereby contributing to economy of the operation. The aluminium-containing alloys are grain refined by the introduction of the carbide nucleants through addition of carbonaceous material. Rapid strides are made in understanding the mechanisms of grain refinement with the ultimate objective of predicting a suitable refiner for a given alloy but more information needs to be collected in this regard.

Chapter 16

Fracture

INTRODUCTION

A fracture is the (local) separation of an object or material into two, or more pieces under the action of stress. Sometimes, in crystalline materials, individual crystals fracture without the body actually separating into two or more pieces. Depending on the substance which is fractured, a fracture reduces strength (most substances) or inhibits transmission of light (optical crystals). A detailed understanding of how fracture occurs in materials may be assisted by the study of fracture mechanics.

FRACTURE STRENGTH

Fracture strength, also known as breaking strength, is the stress at which a specimen fails via fracture. This is usually determined for a given specimen by a tensile test, which charts the stress-strain curve (Fig. 16.1). The final recorded point is the fracture strength.

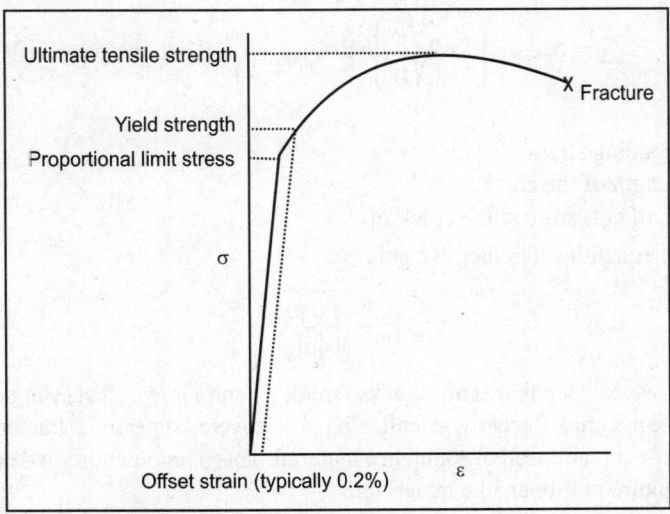

Fig. 16.1. Stress vs. strain curve typical of aluminium.

Ductile materials have a fracture strength lower than the ultimate tensile strength (UTS), whereas in brittle materials the fracture strength is equivalent to the UTS. If a ductile material reaches its ultimate tensile strength in a load-controlled situation, it will continue to deform, with no additional load application, until it ruptures. However, if the loading is displacement-controlled, the deformation of the material may relieve the load, preventing rupture.

If the stress-strain curve is plotted in terms of true stress and true strain the curve will always slope upwards and never reverse, as true stress is corrected for the decrease in cross-sectional area. The true stress on the material at the time of rupture is known as the breaking strength. This is the maximum stress on the true stress-strain curve, given by proportional limit stress.

TYPES OF FRACTURE

Brittle Fracture

In brittle fracture, no apparent plastic deformation takes place before fracture. In brittle crystalline materials, fracture can occur by cleavage as the result of tensile stress acting normal to crystallographic planes with low bonding (cleavage planes). In amorphous solids, by contrast, the lack of a crystalline structure results in a conchoidal fracture, with cracks proceeding normal to the applied tension.

The theoretical strength of a crystalline material is (roughly)

$$\sigma_{theoretical} = \sqrt{\frac{E\gamma}{r_o}}$$

where,
- E is the Young's modulus of the material.
- γ is the surface energy.
- r_o is the equilibrium distance between atomic centers.

On the other hand, a crack introduces a stress concentration modelled by:

$$\sigma_{elliptical\ crack} = \sigma_{applied}\left(1 + 2\sqrt{\frac{a}{\rho}}\right) = 2\sigma_{applied}\sqrt{\frac{a}{\rho}} \quad \text{(For sharp cracks)}$$

where,
- $\sigma_{applied}$ is the loading stress.
- a is half the length of the crack.
- ρ is the radius of curvature at the crack tip.

Putting these two equations together, we get:

$$\sigma_{fracture} = \sqrt{\frac{E\gamma\rho}{4ar_o}}$$

Looking closely, we can see that sharp cracks (small ρ) and large defects (large a) both lower the fracture strength of the material. Recently, scientists have discovered supersonic fracture, the phenomenon of crack motion faster than the speed of sound in a material. This phenomenon was recently also verified by experiment of fracture in rubber-like materials.

Ductile Fracture

In ductile fracture, extensive plastic deformation takes place before fracture. The terms rupture or ductile rupture describe the ultimate failure of tough ductile materials loaded in tension. Rather than cracking, the material 'pulls apart', generally leaving a rough surface. In this case there is slow propagation and an absorption of a large amount energy before fracture (Fig. 16.2).

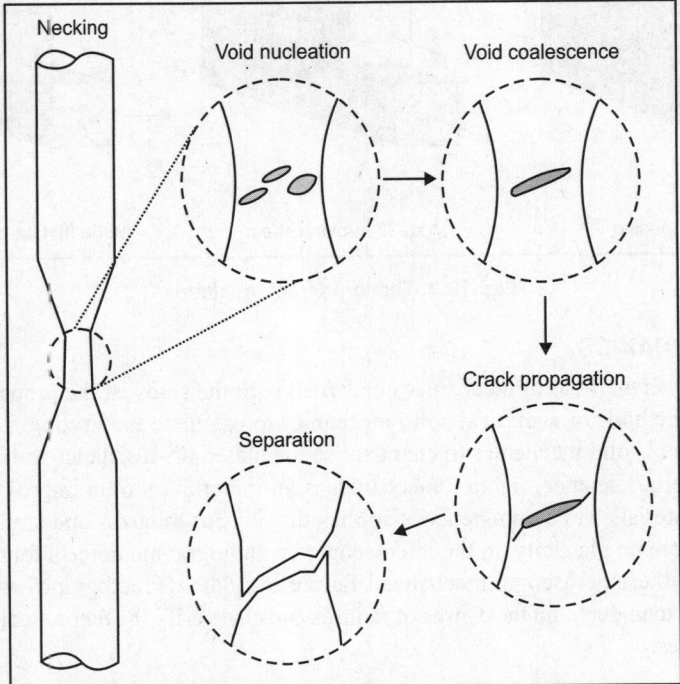

Fig. 16.2. Schematic representation of the steps in ductile fracture (in pure tension).

Many ductile metals, especially materials with high purity, can sustain very large deformation of 50–100 per cent or more strain before fracture under favourable loading condition and environmental condition. The strain at which the fracture happens is controlled by the purity of the materials. At room temperature, pure iron can undergo deformation up to 100 per cent strain before breaking, while cast iron or high-carbon steels can barely sustain 3 per cent of strain.

Because ductile rupture involves a high degree of plastic deformation, the fracture behaviour of a propagating crack as modelled above changes fundamentally. Some of the energy from stress concentrations at the crack tips is dissipated by plastic deformation before the crack actually propagates.

The basic steps sample of smallest cross-sectional area, void formation, void coalescence (also known as crack formation), crack propagation, and failure, often resulting in a cup-and-cone shaped failure surface.

CRACK SEPARATION MODES

There are three ways of applying a force to enable a crack to propagate (Fig. 16.3):
1. Mode I crack—Opening mode (a tensile stress normal to the plane of the crack).
2. Mode II crack—Sliding mode (a shear stress acting parallel to the plane of the crack and perpendicular to the crack front).
3. Mode III crack—Tearing mode (a shear stress acting parallel to the plane of the crack and parallel to the crack front).

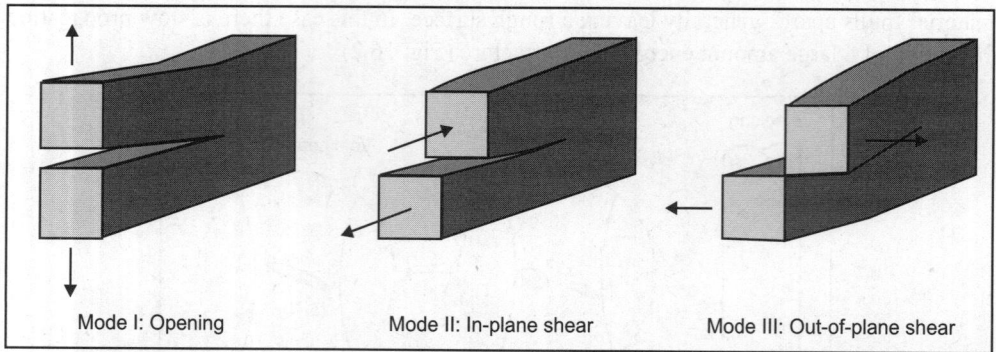

Fig. 16.3. The three fracture modes.

FRACTURE MECHANICS

Fracture mechanics is the field of mechanics concerned with the study of the propagation of cracks in materials. It uses methods of analytical solid mechanics to calculate the driving force on a crack and those of experimental solid mechanics to characterise the material's resistance to fracture.

In modern materials science, fracture mechanics is an important tool in improving the mechanical performance of materials and components. It applies the physics of stress and strain, in particular the theories of elasticity and plasticity, to the microscopic crystallographic defects found in real materials in order to predict the macroscopic mechanical failure of bodies. Fractography is widely used with fracture mechanics to understand the causes of failures and also verify the theoretical failure predictions with real life failures.

Linear Elastic Fracture Mechanics

Griffith's criterion

Fracture mechanics was developed during World War I by English aeronautical engineer, A. A. Griffith, to explain the failure of brittle materials. Griffith's work was motivated by two contradictory facts:
1. The stress needed to fracture bulk glass is around 100 MPa (15,000 psi).
2. The theoretical stress needed for breaking atomic bonds is approximately 10,000 MPa (1,500,000 psi).

A theory was needed to reconcile these conflicting observations. Also, experiments on glass fibres that Griffith himself conducted suggested that the fracture stress increases as the fibre diameter decreases. Hence the uniaxial tensile strength, which had been used extensively to predict material failure before Griffith, could not be a specimen-independent material property. Griffith suggested that the low fracture strength observed in experiments, as well as the size-dependence of strength, was due to the presence of microscopic flaws in the bulk material (Fig. 16.4).

To verify the flaw hypothesis, Griffith introduced an artificial flaw in his experimental specimens. The artificial flaw was in the form of a surface crack which was much larger than other flaws in a specimen. The experiments showed that the product of the square root of the flaw length (a) and the stress at fracture (σ_f) was nearly constant, which is expressed by the equation:

$$\sigma_f = \sqrt{a} \approx C$$

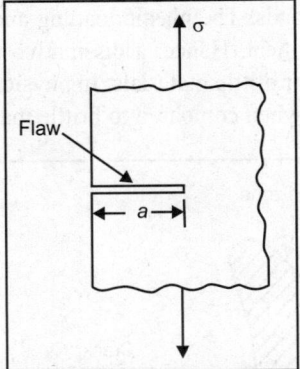

Fig. 16.4. An edge crack (flaw) of length *a* in a material..

An explanation of this relation in terms of linear elasticity theory is problematic. Linear elasticity theory predicts that stress (and hence the strain) at the tip of a sharp flaw in a linear elastic material is infinite. To avoid that problem, Griffith developed a thermodynamic approach to explain the relation that he observed.

The growth of a crack requires the creation of two new surfaces and hence an increase in the surface energy. Griffith found an expression for the constant C in terms of the surface energy of the crack by solving the elasticity problem of a finite crack in an elastic plate. Briefly, the approach was:
1. Compute the potential energy stored in a perfect specimen under an uniaxial tensile load.
2. Fix the boundary so that the applied load does no work and then introduce a crack into the specimen. The crack relaxes the stress and hence reduces the elastic energy near the crack faces. On the other hand, the crack increases the total surface energy of the specimen.
3. Compute the change in the free energy (surface energy—elastic energy) as a function of the crack length. Failure occurs when the free energy attains a peak value at a critical crack length, beyond which the free energy decreases by increasing the crack length, i.e. by causing fracture.

Using this procedure, Griffith found that:

$$C = \sqrt{\frac{2E\gamma}{\pi}}$$

where, E is the Young's modulus of the material and γ is the surface energy density of the material. Assuming $E = 62$ GPa and $\gamma = 1$ J/m^2 gives excellent agreement of Griffith's predicted fracture stress with experimental results for glass.

Irwin's modification

Griffith's theory provides excellent agreement with experimental data for brittle materials such as glass. For ductile materials such as steel, though the relation $\sigma_y \sqrt{a} = C$ still holds, the surface energy (γ) predicted by Griffith's theory is usually unrealistically high. A group working under G. R. Irwin at the US Naval Research Laboratory (NRL) during World War II realised that plasticity must play a significant role in the fracture of ductile materials (Fig. 16.5).

In ductile materials (and even in materials that appear to be brittle), a plastic zone develops at the tip of the crack. As the applied load increases, the plastic zone increases in size until the crack grows and the material behind the crack tip unloads. The plastic loading and unloading cycle near the crack tip leads to the dissipation of energy as heat. Hence, a dissipative term has to be added to the energy balance relation devised by Griffith for brittle materials. In physical terms, additional energy is needed for crack growth in ductile materials when compared to brittle materials.

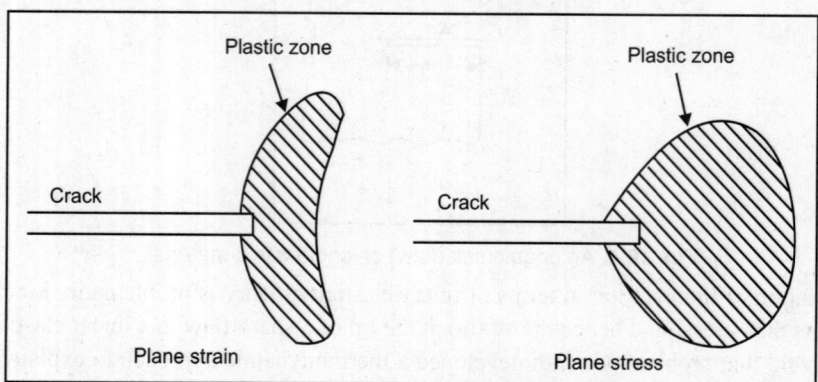

Fig. 16.5. The plastic zone around a crack tip in a ductile material.

Irwin's strategy was to partition the energy into two parts:
1. The stored elastic strain energy which is released as a crack grows. This is the thermodynamic driving force for fracture.
2. The dissipated energy which includes plastic dissipation and the surface energy (and any other dissipative forces that may be at work). The dissipated energy provides the thermodynamic resistance to fracture. Then the total energy dissipated is:
$$G = 2\gamma + G_p$$
where, γ is the surface energy and G_p is the plastic dissipation (and dissipation from other sources) per unit area of crack growth.

The modified version of Griffith's energy criterion can then be written as:
$$\sigma_f \sqrt{a} = \sqrt{\frac{EG}{\pi}}.$$

For brittle materials such as glass, the surface energy term dominates and $G \approx 2\gamma = 2 J/m^2$. For ductile materials such as steel, the plastic dissipation term dominates and $G \approx G_p = 1000 \ J/m^2$. For polymers close to the glass transition temperature, we have intermediate values of $G \approx 2 - 1000 \ J/m^2$.

Stress intensity factor

Another significant achievement of Irwin and his colleagues was to find a method of calculating the amount of energy available for fracture in terms of the asymptotic stress and displacement fields around a crack front in a linear elastic solid. This asymptotic expression for the stress field around a crack tip is:
$$\sigma_{ij} \approx \left(\frac{K}{\sqrt{2\pi r}}\right) f_{ij}(\theta)$$
where, σ_{ij} are the Cauchy stresses, r is the distance from the crack tip, θ is the angle with respect to the plane of the crack, and f_{ij} are functions that are independent of the crack geometry and loading conditions.

Irwin called the quantity K the stress intensity factor. Since the quantity f_{ij} is dimensionless, the stress intensity factor can be expressed in units of $MPa - \sqrt{m}$.

When a rigid line inclusion is considered, a similar asymptotic expression for the stress fields is obtained.

Strain energy release

Irwin was the first to observe that if the size of the plastic zone around a crack is small compared to the size of the crack, the energy required to grow the crack will not be critically dependent on the state of stress at the crack tip. In other words, a purely elastic solution may be used to calculate the amount of energy available for fracture.

The energy release rate for crack growth or strain energy release rate may then be calculated as the change in elastic strain energy per unit area of crack growth, i.e.

$$G = -\left[\frac{\partial U}{\partial a}\right]_P = -\left[\frac{\partial U}{\partial a}\right]_u$$

where, U is the elastic energy of the system and a is the crack length. Either the load P or the displacement u can be kept fixed while evaluating the above expressions.

Irwin showed that for a mode I crack (opening mode) the strain energy release rate and the stress intensity factor are related by:

$$G = G_I = \begin{cases} \dfrac{K_I^2}{E} & \text{plane stress} \\ \dfrac{(1-v^2)K_I^2}{E} & \text{plane strain} \end{cases}$$

where, E is the Young's modulus, v is Poisson's ratio, and K_I is the stress intensity factor in mode I. Irwin also showed that the strain energy release rate of a planar crack in a linear elastic body can be expressed in terms of the mode I, mode II (sliding mode), and mode III (tearing mode) stress intensity factors for the most general loading conditions.

Next, Irwin adopted the additional assumption that the size and shape of the energy dissipation zone remains approximately constant during brittle fracture. This assumption suggests that the energy needed to create a unit fracture surface is a constant that depends only on the material. This new material property was given the name fracture toughness and designated G_{Ic}. Today, it is the critical stress intensity factor K_{Ic} which is accepted as the defining property in linear elastic fracture mechanics.

Limitations

But a problem arose for the NRL researchers because naval materials, e.g. ship-plate steel, are not perfectly elastic but undergo significant plastic deformation at the tip of a crack. One basic assumption in Irwin's linear elastic fracture mechanics is that the size of the plastic zone is small compared to the crack length. However, this assumption is quite restrictive for certain types of failure in structural steels though such steels can be prone to brittle fracture, which has led to a number of catastrophic failures.

Linear-elastic fracture mechanics is of limited practical use for structural steels for another more practical reason. Fracture toughness testing is very expensive and engineers believe that sufficient information for selection of steels can be obtained from the simpler and cheaper Charpy impact test.

Nonlinear Elasticity and Plasticity

Most engineering materials show some nonlinear elastic and inelastic behaviour under operating conditions that involve large loads. In such materials the assumptions of linear elastic fracture mechanics may not hold, that is:
1. The plastic zone at a crack tip may have a size of the same order of magnitude as the crack size.
2. The size and shape of the plastic zone may change as the applied load is increased and also as the crack length increases.

Therefore a more general theory of crack growth is needed for elastic-plastic materials that can account for:
1. The local conditions for initial crack growth which include the nucleation, growth, and coalescence of voids or decohesion at a crack tip.
2. A global energy balance criterion for further crack growth and unstable fracture.

R-curve

An early attempt in the direction of elastic-plastic fracture mechanics was Irwin's crack extension resistance curve or R-curve. This curve acknowledges the fact that the resistance to fracture increases with growing crack size in elastic-plastic materials. The R-curve is a plot of the total energy dissipation rate as a function of the crack size and can be used to examine the processes of slow stable crack growth and unstable fracture. However, the R-curve was not widely used in applications until the early 1970s. The main reasons appear to be that the R-curve depends on the geometry of the specimen and the crack driving force may be difficult to calculate.

J-integral

In the mid-1960s James R. Rice and G. P. Cherepanov independently developed a new toughness measure to describe the case where there is sufficient crack-tip deformation that the part no longer obeys the linear-elastic approximation. Rice's analysis, which assumes non-linear elastic (or monotonic deformation-theory plastic) deformation ahead of the crack tip, is designated the J integral. This analysis is limited to situations where plastic deformation at the crack tip does not extend to the furthest edge of the loaded part. It also demands that the assumed non-linear elastic behaviour of the material is a reasonable approximation in shape and magnitude to the real material's load response. The elastic-plastic failure parameter is designated J_{Ic} and is conventionally converted to K_{Ic} using Eq. 16.9 of the Appendix to this chapter. Also note that the J integral approach reduces to the Griffith theory for linear-elastic behaviour.

Fully plastic failure

If the material is so tough that the yielded region ahead of the crack extends to the far edge of the specimen before fracture, the crack is no longer an effective stress concentrator. Instead, the presence of the crack merely serves to reduce the load-bearing area. In this regime the failure stress is conventionally assumed to be the average of the yield and ultimate strengths of the material.

Engineering Applications

The following information is needed for a fracture mechanics prediction of failure:
1. Applied load.
2. Residual stress.

3. Size and shape of the part.
4. Size, shape, location, and orientation of the crack.

Usually not all of this information is available and conservative assumptions have to be made. Occasionally post-mortem fracture-mechanics analyses are carried out. In the absence of an extreme overload, the causes are either insufficient toughness (K_{Ic}) or an excessively large crack that was not detected during routine inspection.

APPENDIX: MATHEMATICAL RELATIONS

Griffith's Criterion

For the simple case of a thin rectangular plate with a crack perpendicular to the load Griffith's theory becomes:

$$G = \frac{\pi \sigma^2 a}{E} \qquad \ldots (16.1)$$

where, G is the strain energy release rate, σ is the applied stress, a is half the crack length, and E is the Young's modulus. The strain energy release rate can otherwise be understood as: the rate at which energy is absorbed by growth of the crack.

However, we also have that:

$$G_c = \frac{\pi \sigma_f^2 a}{E} \qquad \ldots (16.2)$$

If $G \geq G_c$, this is the criterion for which the crack will begin to propagate.

Irwin's Modifications

Eventually a modification of Griffith's solids theory emerged from this work; a term called stress intensity replaced strain energy release rate and a term called fracture toughness replaced surface weakness energy. Both of these terms are simply related to the energy terms that Griffith used:

$$K_I = \sigma \sqrt{\pi a} \qquad \ldots (16.3)$$

and

$$K_c = \sqrt{E G_c} \quad \text{(for plane stress)} \qquad \ldots (16.4)$$

$$K_c = \sqrt{\frac{E G_c}{1 - v^2}} \quad \text{(for plane strain)} \qquad \ldots (16.5)$$

where, K_I is the stress intensity, K_c the fracture toughness, and v is Poisson's ratio. It is important to recognise the fact that fracture parameter K_c has different values when measured under plane stress and plane strain

Fracture occurs when $K_I \geq K_c$. For the special case of plane strain deformation, K_c becomes K_{Ic} and is considered a material property. The subscript I arises because of the different ways of loading a material to enable a crack to propagate. It refers to so-called 'mode I' loading as opposed to mode II or III. There are three ways of applying a force to enable a crack to propagate:

1. Mode I crack—Opening mode (a tensile stress normal to the plane of the crack).

2. Mode II crack—Sliding mode (a shear stress acting parallel to the plane of the crack and perpendicular to the crack front).
3. Mode III crack—Tearing mode (a shear stress acting parallel to the plane of the crack and parallel to the crack front).

We must note that the expression for K_I in Eq. 16.3 will be different for geometries other than the center-cracked infinite plate, as already discussed in stress intensity. Consequently, it is necessary to introduce a dimensionless correction factor, Y, in order to characterise the geometry. We thus have:

$$K_I = Y\sigma\sqrt{\pi a} \qquad \text{...(16.6)}$$

where, Y is a function of the crack length and width of sheet given by:

$$Y\left(\frac{a}{W}\right) = \sqrt{\sec\left(\frac{\pi a}{W}\right)} \qquad \text{...(16.7)}$$

for a sheet of finite width W containing through-thickness crack of length $2a$, or

$$Y\left(\frac{a}{W}\right) = 1.12 - \frac{0.41}{\sqrt{\pi}}\frac{a}{W} + \frac{18.7}{\sqrt{\pi}}\left(\frac{a}{W}\right)^2 \qquad \text{...(16.8)}$$

for a sheet of finite width W containing a through-thickness edge crack of length a.

Elasticity and Plasticity

Since engineers became accustomed to using K_{Ic} to characterise fracture toughness, a relation has been used to reduce J_{Ic} to it:

$$K_{Ic} = \sqrt{E^* J_{Ic}} \quad \text{where, } E^* = E \text{ for plane stress and } E^* = \frac{E}{1-v^2} \text{ for plane strain} \qquad \text{...(16.9)}$$

The remainder of the mathematics employed in this approach is interesting, but is probably better summarised in external pages due to its complex nature.

FRACTURE TOUGHNESS

In materials science, fracture toughness is a property which describes the ability of a material containing a crack to resist fracture, and is one of the most important properties of any material for virtually all design applications. It is denoted K_{Ic} and has the units of $Pa\sqrt{m}$.

The subscript Ic denotes mode I crack opening under a normal tensile stress perpendicular to the crack, since the material can be made deep enough to stand shear (mode II) or tear (mode III). Fracture toughness is a quantitative way of expressing a material's resistance to brittle fracture when a crack is present. If a material has much fracture toughness it will probably undergo ductile fracture. Brittle fracture is very characteristic of materials with less fracture toughness.

Fracture mechanics, which leads to the concept of fracture toughness, was broadly based on the work of A. A. Griffith who, among other things, studied the behaviour of cracks in brittle materials.

A related concept is the work of fracture (γ_{wof}) which is directly proportional to K_{Ic}^2/E, where, E is the Young's modulus of the material. Note that, in SI units, γ_{wof} is given in J/m².

Some typical values of fracture toughness for various materials are given in Table 16.1.

Table 16.1. Typical values of fracture toughness for various materials.

Material	K_{Ic} (MPa-m$^{1/2}$)
Metals	
Aluminium alloy (7075)	24
Steel alloy (4340)	50
Titanium alloy	44–66
Aluminium	14–28
Ceramics	
Aluminium oxide	3–5
Silicon carbide	3–5
Soda-lime-glass	0.7–0.8
Concrete	0.2–1.4
Polymers	
Polymethyl methacrylate	0.7–1.6
Polystyrene	0.7–1.1
Composites	
Mullite-fibre composite	1.8–3.3
Silica aerogels	0.0008–0.0048

Crack Growth as a Stability Problem

Consider a body with flaws (cracks) that is subject to some loading; the stability of the crack can be assessed as follows. We can assume for simplicity that the loading is of constant displacement or displacement controlled type (such as loading with a screw jack); we can also simplify the discussion by characterising the crack by its area, A. If we consider an adjacent state of the body as being one with a broader crack (area $A + dA$), we can then assess strain energy in the two states and evaluate strain energy release rate.

The rate is reckoned with respect to the change in crack area, so if we use U for strain energy, the strain energy release rate is numerically dU/dA. It may be noted that for a body loaded in constant displacement mode, the displacement is applied and the force level is dictated by stiffness (or compliance) of the body. If the crack grows in size, the stiffness decreases, so the force level will decrease. This decrease in force level under the same displacement (strain) level indicates that the elastic strain energy stored in the body is decreasing—is being released. Hence the term strain energy release rate which is usually denoted with symbol G.

The strain energy release rate is higher for higher loads and broader cracks. If the strain energy so released exceeds a critical value G_c, then the crack will grow spontaneously. For brittle materials, G_c can be equated to the surface energy of the (two) new crack surfaces. In other words, in brittle materials, a crack will grow spontaneously if the strain energy released is equal to or more than the energy required to grow the crack surface(s). The stability condition can be written as:

Elastic energy released = Surface energy created.

If the elastic energy releases is less than the critical value, then the crack will not grow; equality signifies neutral stability and if the strain energy release rate exceeds the critical value, the crack will start growing in an unstable manner. For ductile materials, energy associated with plastic deformation has to be taken into account. When there is plastic deformation at the crack tip (as occurs most often in metals) the energy to propagate the crack may increase by several orders of magnitude as the work related to plastic deformation may be much larger than the surface energy. In such cases, the stability criterion has to restated as:

Elastic energy released = Surface energy + Plastic deformation energy.

Practically, this means a higher value for the critical value G_c. From the definition of G, we can deduce that it has dimensions of work (or energy)/area or force/length. For ductile metals G_{Ic} is around 50–200 kJ/m^2, for brittle metals it is usually 1–5 and for glasses and brittle polymers it is almost always less than 0.5. The problem can also be formulated in terms of stress instead of energy, leading to the terms stress intensity factor K (or KI for mode I) and critical stress intensity factor K_c (and K_{Ic}). These K_c and K_{Ic} (etc.) quantities are commonly referred to as fracture toughness, though it is equivalent to use G_c. Typical values for K_{Ic} are 150 MN/m$^{3/2}$ for ductile (very tough) metals, 25 for brittle ones and 1–10 for glasses and brittle polymers. Notice the different units used by G_{Ic} and K_{Ic}. Engineers tend to use the latter as an indication of toughness.

Transformation Toughening

Composites exhibiting the highest level of fracture toughness are typically made of a pure alumina or some silica-alumina (SiO_2/Al_2O_3) matrix with tiny inclusions of zirconia (ZrO_2) dispersed as uniformly as possible within the solid matrix. (*Note: a wet chemical approach is typically necessary in order to establish the compositional uniformity of the ceramic body before firing).

The process of 'transformation toughening' is based on the assumption that zirconia undergoes several martensitic (displacive, diffusionless) phase transformations (cubic → tetragonal → monoclinic) between room temperature and practical sintering (or firing) temperatures. Thus, due to the volume restrictions induced by the solid matrix, metastable crystalline structures can become frozen in which impart an internal strain field surrounding each zirconia inclusion upon cooling. This enables a zirconia particle (or inclusion) to absorb the energy of an approaching crack tip front in its nearby vicinity.

Thus, the application of large shear stresses during fracture nucleates the transformation of a zirconia inclusion from the metastable phase. The subsequent volume expansion from the inclusion (via an increase in the height of the unit cell) introduces compressive stresses which therefore strengthen the matrix near the approaching crack tip front. Zirconia 'whiskers' may be used expressly for this purpose.

Appropriately referred to by its first discoverers as 'ceramic steel', the stress intensity factor values for window glass (silica), transformation toughened alumina, and a typical iron/carbon steel range from 1 to 20 to 50 respectively.

Conjoint Action

There are number of instances where this picture of a critical crack is modified by corrosion. Thus, fretting corrosion occurs when a corrosive medium is present at the interface between two rubbing surfaces. Fretting (in the absence of corrosion) results from the disruption of very small areas that bond and break as the surfaces undergo friction, often under vibrating conditions. The bonding contact areas deform under the localised pressure and the two surfaces gradually wear away. Fracture mechanics dictates that each minute localised fracture has to satisfy the general rule that the elastic energy released as the bond fractures has to exceed the work done in plastically deforming it and in creating the (very tiny) fracture surfaces. This process is enhanced when corrosion is present, not least because the corrosion products act as an abrasive between the rubbing surfaces.

Fatigue is another instance where cyclical stressing, this time of a bulk lump of metal, causes small flaws to develop. Ultimately one such flaw exceeds the critical condition and fracture propagates across the whole structure. The fatigue life of a component is the time it takes for criticality to be reached, for a given regime of cyclical stress. Corrosion fatigue is what happens when a cyclically stressed structure is subjected to a corrosive environment at the same time. This not only serves to initiate surface cracks but actually modifies the crack growth process. As a result the fatigue life is shortened, often considerably.

Stress–Corrosion Cracking (SCC)

This phenomenon is the unexpected sudden failure of normally ductile metals subjected to a constant tensile stress in a corrosive environment. Certain austenitic stainless steels and aluminium alloys crack in the presence of chlorides, mild steel cracks in the presence of alkali (boiler cracking) and copper alloys crack in ammoniacal solutions (season cracking). Worse still, high-tensile structural steels crack in an unexpectedly brittle manner in a whole variety of aqueous environments, especially chloride. With the possible exception of the latter, which is a special example of hydrogen cracking, all the others display the phenomenon of subcritical crack growth, i.e. small surface flaws propagate (usually smoothly) under conditions where fracture mechanics predicts that failure should not occur. That is, in the presence of a corrodent, cracks develop and propagate well below K_{Ic}. In fact, the subcritical value of the stress intensity, designated as K_{Iscc}, may be less than 1 per cent of K_{Ic}, as the following Table 16.2 shows.

Table 16.2. Stress–corrosion cracking (SCC).

Alloy	K_{Ic} (MN/m$^{3/2}$)	SCC environment	K_{Iscc} (MN/m$^{3/2}$)
13Cr steel		3% NaCl	12
18Cr-8Ni	200	42% MgCl$_2$	10
Cu-30Zn	200	NH$_4$OH, pH7	1
Al-3Mg-7Zn	25	Aqueous halides	5
Ti-6Al-1V	60	0.6M KCl	20

The subcritical nature of propagation may be attributed to the chemical energy released as the crack propagates. That is:

Elastic energy released + Chemical energy = Surface energy + Deformation energy.

The crack initiates at K_{Iscc} and thereafter propagates at a rate governed by the slowest process, which most of the time is the rate at which corrosive ions can diffuse to the crack tip. As the crack advances so K rises (because crack size appears in the calculation of stress intensity). Finally it reaches K_{Ic}, whereupon swift fracture ensues and the component fails. One of the practical difficulties with SCC is its unexpected nature. Stainless steels, for example, are employed because under most conditions they are passive, i.e. effectively inert. Very often one finds a single crack has propagated whiles the left metal surface stays apparently unaffected.

Chapter 17

Fatigue

INTRODUCTION

In materials science, fatigue is the progressive and localised structural damage that occurs when a material is subjected to cyclic loading. The nominal maximum stress values are less than the ultimate tensile stress limit, and may be below the yield stress limit of the material.

Fatigue occurs when a material is subjected to repeated loading and unloading. If the loads are above a certain threshold, microscopic cracks will begin to form at the surface. Eventually a crack will reach a critical size, and the structure will suddenly fracture. The shape of the structure will significantly affect the fatigue life; square holes or sharp corners will lead to elevated local stresses where fatigue cracks can initiate. Round holes and smooth transitions or fillets are therefore important to increase the fatigue strength of the structure.

FATIGUE LIFE

ASTM defines fatigue life, N_f, as the number of stress cycles of a specified character that a specimen sustains before failure of a specified nature occurs.

One method to predict fatigue life of materials is the Uniform Material Law (UML). UML was developed for fatigue life prediction of aluminium and titanium alloys by the end of 20th century and extended to high-strength steels.

Characteristics of Fatigue

1. In metals and alloys, the process starts with dislocation movements, eventually forming persistent slip bands that nucleate short cracks.
2. Fatigue is a stochastic process, often showing considerable scatter even in controlled environments.
3. The greater the applied stress range, the shorter the life.
4. Fatigue life scatter tends to increase for longer fatigue lives.
5. Damage is cumulative. Materials do not recover when rested.
6. Fatigue life is influenced by a variety of factors, such as temperature, surface finish, microstructure, presence of oxidising or inert chemicals, residual stresses, contact (fretting), etc.
7. Some materials (e.g. some steel and titanium alloys) exhibit a theoretical fatigue limit below which continued loading does not lead to structural failure.
8. In recent years, researchers (for example, the work of Bathias, Murakami, and Stanzl-Tschegg) have found that failures occur below the theoretical fatigue limit at very high fatigue lives

(10^9 to 10^{10} cycles). An ultrasonic resonance technique is used in these experiments with frequencies around 10–20 kHz.
9. High cycle fatigue strength (about 10^3 to 10^8 cycles) can be described by stress-based parameters. A load-controlled servo-hydraulic test rig is commonly used in these tests, with frequencies of around 20–50 Hz. Other sorts of machines—like resonant magnetic machines—can also be used, achieving frequencies up to 250 Hz.
10. Low cycle fatigue (typically less than 10^3 cycles) is associated with widespread plasticity in metals; thus, a strain-based parameter should be used for fatigue life prediction in metals and alloys. Testing is conducted with constant strain amplitudes typically at 0.01–5 Hz.

High-Cycle Fatigue

Historically, most attention has focused on situations that require more than 10^4 cycles to failure where stress is low and deformation primarily elastic.

S-N curve

In high-cycle fatigue situations, materials performance is commonly characterised by an *S-N* curve, also known as a Wöhler curve. This is a graph of the magnitude of a cyclic stress (*S*) against the logarithmic scale of cycles to failure (*N*) (Fig. 17.1).

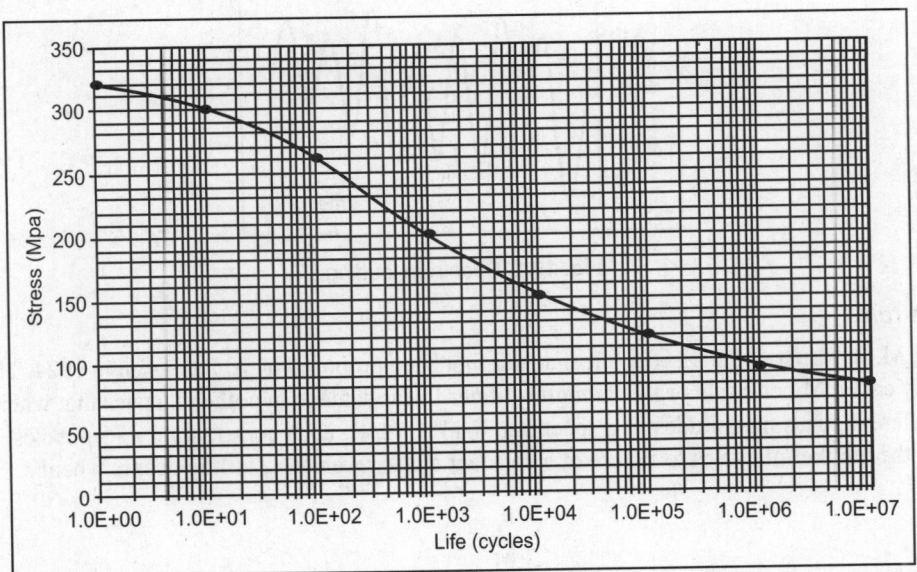

Fig. 17.1. *S-N* curve for brittle aluminium with a UTS of 320 MPa.

S-N curves are derived from tests on samples of the material to be characterised (often called coupons) where a regular sinusoidal stress is applied by a testing machine which also counts the number of cycles to failure. This process is sometimes known as coupon testing. Each coupon test generates a point on the plot though in some cases there is a runout where the time to failure exceeds that available for the test. Analysis of fatigue data requires techniques from statistics, especially survival analysis and linear regression.

Probabilistic nature of fatigue

As coupons sampled from a homogeneous frame will manifest variation in their number of cycles to failure, the S-N curve should more properly be an S-N-P curve capturing the probability of failure after a given number of cycles of a certain stress. Probability distributions that are common in data analysis and in design against fatigue include the lognormal distribution, extreme value distribution, Birnbaum–Saunders distribution, and Weibull distribution.

Complex loadings

In practice, a mechanical part is exposed to a complex, often random, sequence of loads, large and small. In order to assess the safe life of such a part:
1. Reduce the complex loading to a series of simple cyclic loadings using a technique such as rainflow analysis.
2. Create a histogram of cyclic stress from the rainflow analysis to form a fatigue damage spectrum (Fig. 17.2).
3. For each stress level, calculate the degree of cumulative damage incurred from the S-N curve.
4. Combine the individual contributions using an algorithm such as Miner's rule.

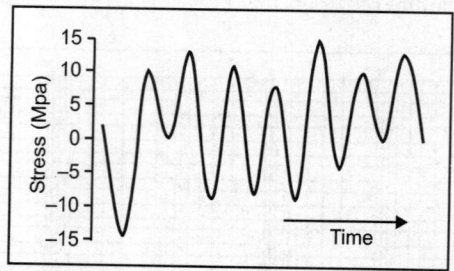

Fig. 17.2. Spectrum loading.

Miner's rule

In 1945, M. A. Miner popularised a rule that had first been proposed by A. Palmgren in 1924. The rule, variously called Miner's rule or the Palmgren-Miner linear damage hypothesis, states that where there are k different stress magnitudes in a spectrum, S_i ($1 \leq i \leq k$), each contributing $n_i(S_i)$ cycles, then if $N_i(S_i)$ is the number of cycles to failure of a constant stress reversal S_i, failure occurs when:

$$\sum_{i=1}^{k} \frac{n_i}{N_i} = C$$

C is experimentally found to be between 0.7 and 2.2. Usually for design purposes, C is assumed to be 1.

This can be thought of as assessing what proportion of life is consumed by stress reversal at each magnitude then forming a linear combination of their aggregate. Though Miner's rule is a useful approximation in many circumstances, it has several major limitations:
1. It fails to recognise the probabilistic nature of fatigue and there is no simple way to relate life predicted by the rule with the characteristics of a probability distribution. Industry analysts often use design curves, adjusted to account for scatter, to calculate $N_i(S_i)$.

2. There is sometimes an effect in the order in which the reversals occur. In some circumstances, cycles of low stress followed by high stress cause more damage than would be predicted by the rule. It does not consider the effect of overload or high stress which may result in a compressive residual stress. High stress followed by low stress may have less damage due to the presence of compressive residual stress.

Paris' relationship

In Fracture mechanics, Anderson, Gomez and Paris derived relationships for the stage II crack growth with cycles N, in terms of the cyclical component ΔK of the stress intensity factor K:

$$\frac{da}{dN} = C(\Delta K)^m$$

where, a is the crack length and m is typically in the range 3 to 5 (for metals) (Fig. 17.3).

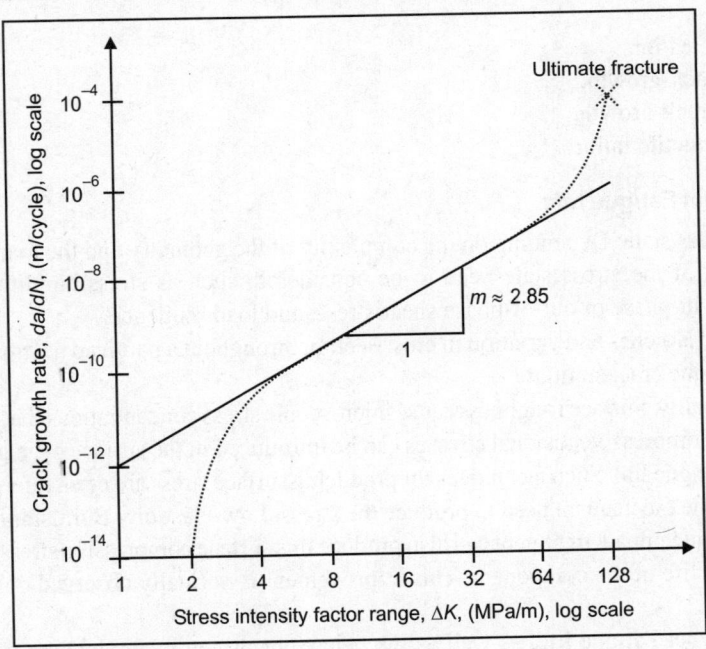

Fig. 17.3. Typical fatigue crack growth rate graph.

This relationship was later modified to make better allowance for the mean stress, by introducing a factor depending on $(1-R)$ where, R = min. stress/max stress, in the denominator.

Low-Cycle Fatigue

Where the stress is high enough for plastic deformation to occur, the account in terms of stress is less useful and the strain in the material offers a simpler description. Low-cycle fatigue is usually characterised by the Coffin-Manson relation:

$$\frac{\Delta \varepsilon_p}{2} = \varepsilon'_f (2N)^c$$

where,

$\Delta\varepsilon_p/2$ is the plastic strain amplitude.

ε_f' is an empirical constant known as the fatigue ductility coefficient, the failure strain for a single reversal.

$2N$ is the number of reversals to failure (N cycles).

c is an empirical constant known as the fatigue ductility exponent, commonly ranging from −0.5 to −0.7 for metals in time independent fatigue. Slopes can be considerably steeper in the presence of creep or environmental interactions.

A similar relationship for materials such as zirconium, used in the nuclear industry.

Fatigue and Fracture Mechanics

The account above is purely empirical and, though it allows life prediction and design assurance, life improvement or design optimisation can be enhanced using fracture mechanics. It can be developed in four stages.

1. Crack nucleation.
2. Stage I crack-growth.
3. Stage II crack-growth.
4. Ultimate ductile failure.

Factors that Affect Fatigue Life

1. Cyclic stress state: Depending on the complexity of the geometry and the loading, one or more properties of the stress state need to be considered, such as stress amplitude, mean stress, biaxiality, in-phase or out-of-phase shear stress, and load sequence,
2. Geometry: Notches and variation in cross section throughout a part lead to stress concentrations where fatigue cracks initiate.
3. Surface quality. Surface roughness cause microscopic stress concentrations that lower the fatigue strength. Compressive residual stresses can be introduced in the surface by, e.g. shot peening to increase fatigue life. Such techniques for producing surface stress are often referred to as peening, whatever the mechanism used to produce the stress. Low Plasticity Burnishing, Laser peening, and ultrasonic impact treatment can also produce this surface compressive stress and can increase the fatigue life of the component. This improvement is normally observed only for high-cycle fatigue.
4. Material type: Fatigue life, as well as the behaviour during cyclic loading, varies widely for different materials, e.g. composites and polymers differ markedly from metals.
5. Residual stresses: Welding, cutting, casting, and other manufacturing processes involving heat or deformation can produce high levels of tensile residual stress, which decreases the fatigue strength.
6. Size and distribution of internal defects: Casting defects such as gas porosity, nonmetallic inclusions and shrinkage voids can significantly reduce fatigue strength.
7. Direction of loading: For non-isotropic materials, fatigue strength depends on the direction of the principal stress.
8. Grain size: For most metals, smaller grains yield longer fatigue lives, however, the presence of surface defects or scratches will have a greater influence than in a coarse grained alloy.

9. Environment: Environmental conditions can cause erosion, corrosion, or gas-phase embrittlement, which all affect fatigue life. Corrosion fatigue is a problem encountered in many aggressive environments.
10. Temperature: Extreme high or low temperatures can decrease fatigue strength.

Design Against Fatigue

Dependable design against fatigue-failure requires thorough education and supervised experience in structural engineering, mechanical engineering, or materials science. There are three principal approaches to life assurance for mechanical parts that display increasing degrees of sophistication:

1. Design to keep stress below threshold of fatigue limit (infinite lifetime concept).
2. Design (conservatively) for a fixed life after which the user is instructed to replace the part with a new one (a so-called lifed part, finite lifetime concept or 'safe-life' design practice).
3. Instruct the user to inspect the part periodically for cracks and to replace the part once a crack exceeds a critical length. This approach usually uses the technologies of nondestructive testing and requires an accurate prediction of the rate of crack-growth between inspections. This is often referred to as damage tolerant design or 'retirement-for-cause'.

Stopping fatigue

Fatigue cracks that have begun to propagate can sometimes be stopped by drilling holes, called drill stops, in the path of the fatigue crack. This is not recommended as a general practice because the hole represents a stress concentration factor which depends on the size of the hole and geometry. There is thus the possibility of a new crack starting in the side of the hole. It is always far better to replace the cracked part entirely.

Material change

Changes in the materials used in parts can also improve fatigue life. For example, parts can be made from better fatigue rated metals. Complete replacement and redesign of parts can also reduce if not eliminate fatigue problems. Thus helicopter rotor blades and propellers in metal are being replaced by composite equivalents. They are not only lighter, but also much more resistant to fatigue. They are more expensive, but the extra cost is amply repaid by their greater integrity, since loss of a rotor blade usually leads to total loss of the aircraft. A similar argument has been made for replacement of metal fuselages, wings and tails of aircraft.

FATIGUE FAILURE

In service many components undergo thousands, often millions, of changes of stress. Some are repeatedly stressed and unstressed, while some undergo alternating stresses of compression and tension. For others the stress may just fluctuate about some value. Many materials subject to such conditions fail, even though the maximum stress in anyone stress change is less than the fracture stress as determined by a simple tensile test. Such a failure, as a result of repeated stressing, is called a fatigue failure.

The source of the alternating stresses can be due to the conditions of use of a component. Thus, in the case of an aircraft, the changes of pressure between the cabin and the outside of the aircraft every time it flies subject the cabin skin to repeated stressing. Components such as a crown wheel and pinion are subject to repeated stressing by the very way in which they are used, while others receive their stressing 'accidentally'. Vibration of thee component can occur as a result of the transmission of vibration from some machine nearby. Turbine blades may vibrate in use in such a way that they fail by fatigue. It has been said that fatigue causes at least 80 per cent of the failures in modern engineering components.

A fatigue crack often starts at some point of stress concentration. This point of origin of the failure can be seen on the failed material as a smooth, flat, semicircular or elliptical region, often referred to as the nucleus. Surrounding the nucleus is a burnished zone with ribbed markings. This smooth zone is produced by the crack propagating relatively slowly through the material and the resulting fractured surfaces rubbing together during the alternating stressing of the component. When the component has become so weakened by the crack that it is no longer able to carry the load, the final, abrupt fracture occurs, which shows a typically crystalline appearance. Figure 17.4 shows the various stages in the growth of a fatigue crack failure.

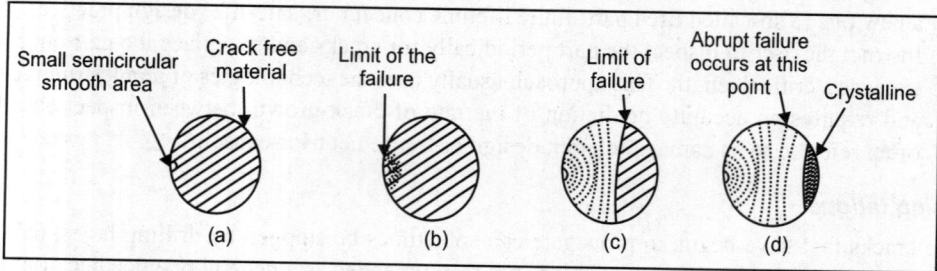

Fig. 17.4. Fatigue failure with a metal: (a) the nucleus, limit of the failure, (b) the crack grows slowly, (c) the crack continuing to grow slowly, and (d) complete failure.

Stages in Fatigue Failure

A metal progressing to fatigue failure can be considered to pass through three stages.

Stage 1—The nucleus and initial crack

This is the initiation zone of the fatigue crack. Under repeated stressing slip occurs as a result of the movement of dislocations. Slip may occur one way on one slip plane and the reverse way on an adjacent slip plane during the reverse stress cycle. The reverse direction of slip on the first slip plane is inhibited by local work hardening, i.e. an increase in dislocation density in this slip plane as a result of its plastic deformation. The result of such behaviour is a number of slip bands, essentially a series of grooves and extended tongues of metal from the metal surface (Fig. 17.5). From this discontinuity the fatigue cracks start. The initial crack growth is in a plane which is about 45° to the direction of the applied stress. This is a consequence of the slip occurring as a result of spear. After a few grains the direction of the crack changes to be at right-angles to the applied stress direction. This change in direction is the beginning of Stage 2.

Stage 2—Crack propagation

The mode of failure of the material in Stage 1 is a shear mode, in Stage 2 the mode is a tensile mode with the crack being forced open (Fig. 17.6). The Stage 2 crack surfaces show a series of fine striations. The striations are a series of ridges and result from the alternating stresses applied to the material, each stress cycle producing a striation. The striations are concentric on the nucleus and the spacing between successive striations increases as the crack propagates out from the nucleus.

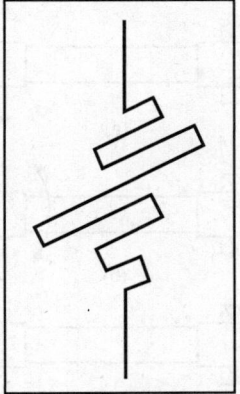

Fig. 17.5. Slip bands at the nucleus of fatigue failure.

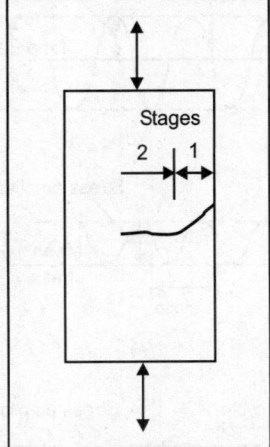

Fig. 17.6. Stages 1 and 2 crack propagation.

Stage 3—Failure

The Stage 2 crack continues growing until point is reached when there is a sudden complete failure of the material. This final fracture zone is likely to show a crystalline surface appearance, quite different from the striations of Stage 2.

Fatigue Tests

Fatigue tests can be carried out in a number of ways, the way used being the one needed to simulate the type of stress changes that will occur to the material of a component when in service. There are thus bending-stress machines which bend a test piece of the material alternately one way and then the other [Fig. 17.7(a)], and torsional-fatigue machines which twist the test piece alternately one way and then the other [Fig. 17.7(b)]. Another type of machine can be used to produce alternating tension and compression by direct stressing [Fig. 17.7(c)].

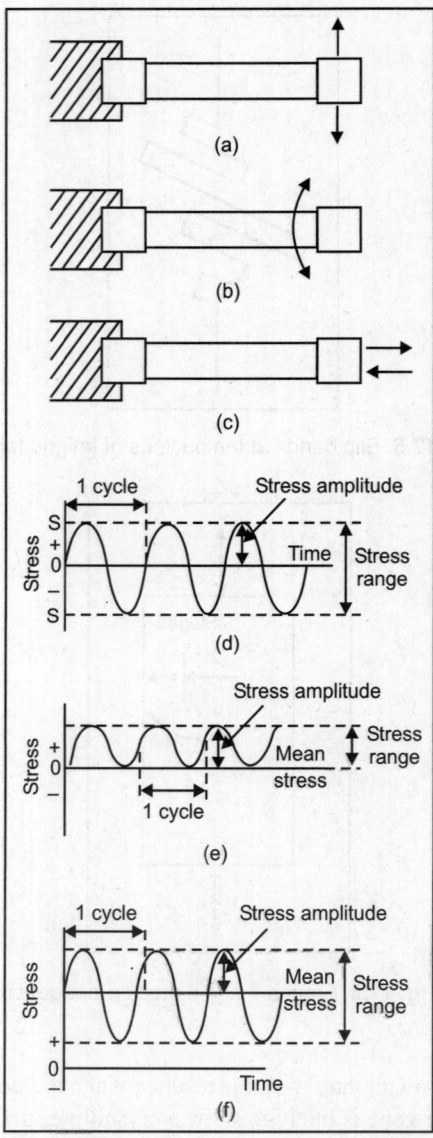

Fig. 17.7. Fatigue testing: (a) bending, (b) torsion, (c) direct stress, (d) alternating stress, (e) repeated stress, and (f) fluctuating stress.

The tests can be carried out with stresses which alternate about zero stress [Fig. 17.7(d)], apply a repeated stress which varies from zero to some maximum stress [Fig. 17.7(e)] or apply a stress which varies about some stress value and does not reach zero at all [Fig. 17.7(f)]. In the case of the alternating stress [Fig. 17.7(d)], the stress varies between $+S$ and $-S$. The tensile stress is denoted by a positive sign, the compressive stress by a negative sign; the stress range is thus $2S$. The mean stress is zero as the stress alternates equally about the zero stress. With the repeated stress [Fig. 17.7(e)], the mean stress is half the stress range. With the fluctuating stress [Fig. 17.7(f)] the mean stress is more than half the stress range. During the fatigue tests, the machine is kept running, alternating the stress, until the specimen fails, the number of cycles of stressing up to failure being recorded by the machine. The test is repeated for the specimen subject to different stress ranges. Such tests enable graphs similar to those in Fig. 17.8 to be plotted. The vertical axis is the stress amplitude, half the stress range. For a stress amplitude greater than the value given by the graph line, failure occurs for the number of cycles concerned. These graphs are known as S/N graphs, the S denoting the stress amplitude and the N the number of cycles.

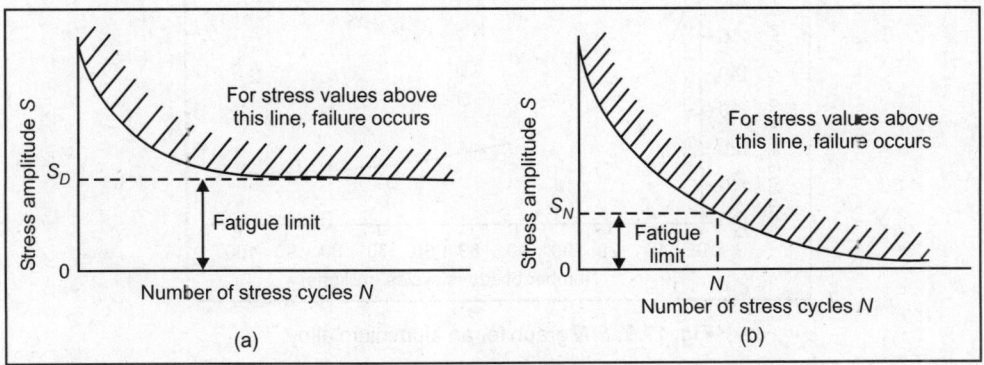

Fig. 17.8. Typical S/N graphs for (a) a steel, and (b) a nonferrous alloy.

For the S/N graph in Fig. 17.8(a) there is a stress amplitude for which the material will endure an indefinite number of stress cycles. The maximum value, S_D, being called the fatigue limit. For any stress amplitude greater than the fatigue limit, failure will occur if the material undergoes a sufficient number of stress cycles. With the S/N graph shown in Fig. 17.8(b) there is no stress amplitude at which failure cannot occur; for such materials a fatigue limit S_N is quoted for N cycles. The term endurance limit is sometimes used where the material will endure an infinite number of cycles.

The number of reversals that a specimen can sustain before failure occurs depends on the stress amplitude, the bigger the stress amplitude the smaller the number of cycles of stress and reversals that can be sustained. Some typical results for an aluminium alloy specimen are given in Table 17.1.

Table 17.1. S/N values for an aluminium alloy specimen.

Stress amplitude/MN m^{-2}	Number of cycles before failure ($\times 10^6$)
185	1
155	5
145	10
120	50
115	100

With a stress amplitude of 185 MN m^{-2}, e.g. a stress alternating from +185 MN m^{-2} to −185 MN m^{-2}, one million cycles are needed before failure occurs. With a smaller stress amplitude of 115 MN m^{-2} one hundred million cycles are needed before failure occurs. Figure 17.9 shows the S/N graph for the above data. Extrapolation of the graph seems to indicate that for a greater number of cycles, failure will occur at even smaller stress amplitudes. There seems to be no stress amplitude for which failure will not occur; the material has no fatigue limit. If a component made of that material had a service life of 100 million stress cycles then we could specify that during the lifetime, failure should not occur for stress amplitudes less than 115 MN m^{-2}. The endurance limit for 100 million cycles is thus 115 MN m^{-2}.

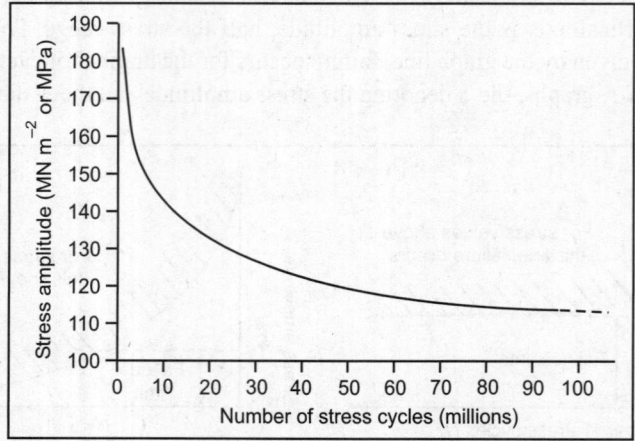

Fig. 17.9. *S/N* graph for an aluminium alloy.

Table 17.2 gives some typical results for a steel, the fatigue tests being bending stress (Fig. 17.10).

Table 17.2. *S/N* values for a steel specimen.

Stress amplitude/MN m^{-2}	Number of cycles before failure ($\times 10^6$)
750	0.01
550	0.1
450	1
450	10
450	100

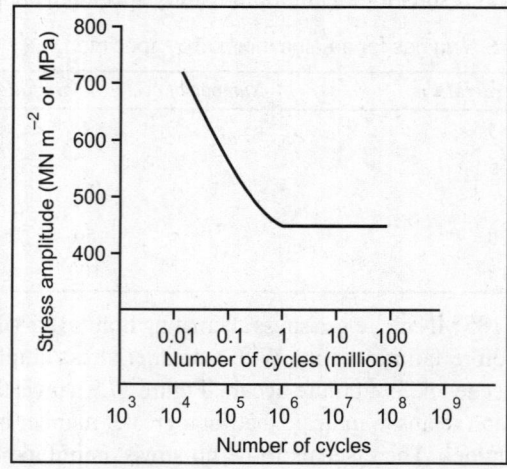

Fig. 17.10. *S/N* graph for a steel. Note: number of cycles shown on logarithmic scale.

With a stress amplitude of 750 MN m^{-2}, e.g. a stress alternating from +750 MN m^{-2} to –750 MN m^{-2}, 0.01 million cycles or ten thousand cycles are needed before failure occurs. For one million, ten million and one hundred million cycles the stress amplitude for failure is the same, 450 MN m^{-2}. For stress amplitudes below this value the material should not fail, however long the test continues. The fatigue limit is thus 450 MN m^{-2}.

The fatigue limit, or the endurance limit at about 500 million cycles, for metals tends to lie between about a third and a half of the static tensile strength. This applies to most steels, aluminium alloys, brass, nickel and magnesium alloys. For example, a steel with a tensile strength of 420 MN m^{-2} has a fatigue limit of 180 MN m^{-2}, just under half the tensile strength.

If used in a situation where it were subject to alternating stresses, such a steel would need to be limited to stress amplitudes below 180 MN m^{-2} if it were not to fail at some time. A magnesium alloy with a tensile strength of 290 MN m^{-2} has an endurance limit of 120 MN m^{-2}, just under half the tensile strength. Such an alloy would need to be limited to stress amplitudes below 120 MN m^{-2} if it were to last to 500 million cycles. It must be recognised that there is a relatively large scatter of results in any fatigue test. Thus an S/N graph is essentially drawn through data points which represent the mean value of the life at each stress range. This variation in life must be considered in interpreting S/N graphs.

Effect of Mean Stress

For any particular value of the mean stress it is possible to determine an S/N graph. When the mean stress is zero the fatigue limit that is given is that which occurs in the absence of any stress, however when the mean stress is tensile strength for the material, then the fatigue limit is zero since the material fails without any cycles being undertaken. Between these two limits of mean stress, increasing the mean stress decreases the fatigue limit. A number of empirical relationships have been devised to describe the relationship between fatigue limit and the mean stress. Figure 17.11 shows the relationship proposed by Goodman. The graph between stress amplitude and mean stress is a straight line drawn between two points, the stress amplitude being the fatigue limit in the absence of mean stress at the zero value of mean stress and the stress amplitude being zero when the mean stress equals the tensile strength.

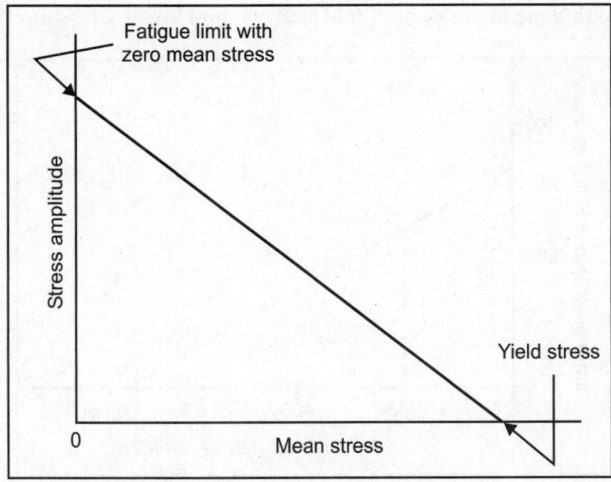

Fig. 17.11. The Goodman relationship.

If, for given conditions, the point representing the value of mean stress and stress amplitude lies below the straight line in the graph then the Goodman relationship considers it will not fail by fatigue.

Another relationship is that pur forward by Soderberg. He proposed that the graph of stress amplitude against mean stress should be drawn between the points of the stress amplitude being the fatigue limit in the absence of mean stress—at the zero value of mean stress and the stress amplitude being zero when the mean stress equals the yield stress (Fig. 17.12).

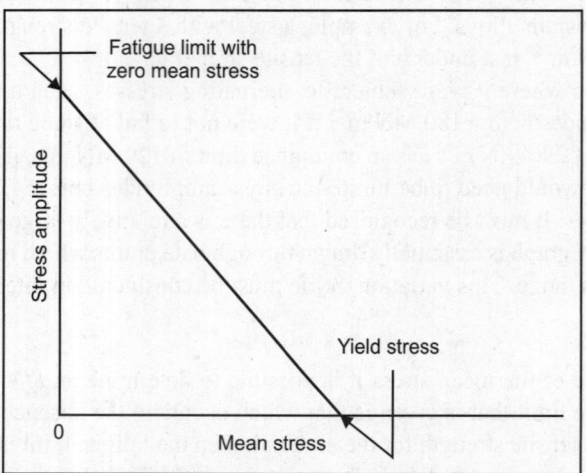

Fig. 17.12. The Soderberg relationship.

An important consequence of the above is that an S/N graph or values for fatigue or endurance limits should not be used without a consideration of the mean stress.

As an illustration of the use of a Goodman diagram, consider a 0.6 per cent carbon steel with a fatigue limit of 320 MN m^{-2} and a tensile strength of 740 MN m^{-2}. Figure 17.13 shows the resulting Goodman diagram. Thus on the basis of this diagram we can predict that a stress amplitude of 240 MN m^{-2} will cause failure with a mean stress of 200 MN m^{-2}—any lower stress amplitude would be safe.

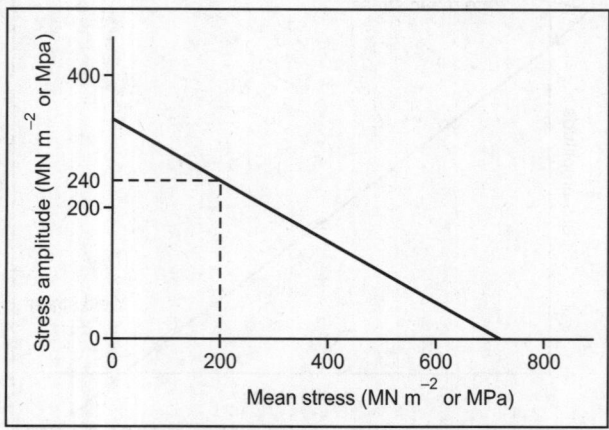

Fig. 17.13. Goodman diagram for a 0.6 per cent carbon steel.

Cumulative Damage

During service many components are subject to cyclic loading but not necessarily regularly repeated loading at the same stress amplitude. A simple relationship that is used to assess the effects of cycles at different stress amplitudes is that of Miner, the relationship being known as Miner's law. If the component is subject to n_1 cycles at a stress amplitude for which fatigue failure would occur at N_1 cycles, and n_2 cycles at a stress amplitude for which fatigue failure would occur at N_2 cycles, and n_3 cycles at a stress amplitude for which failure would occur at N_3 cycles, etc. then the component will fail if the sum of n/N ratios equals 1.

$$\frac{n_1}{N_1} + \frac{n_2}{N_2} + \frac{n_3}{N_3} + \text{etc.} = 1$$

The relationship must only be regarded as a useful approximation. The condition for failure is, for instance, affected by the sequence of the different load cycles.

FACTORS AFFECTING THE FATIGUE PROPERTIES OF METALS

The main factors affecting the fatigue properties of a component are:
1. Stress concentrations caused by component design.
2. Corrosion.
3. Residual stresses.
4. Surface finish/treatment.
5. Temperature.
6. Microstructure of alloy.
7. Heat treatment.

Fatigue of a component depends on the stress amplitude attained, the bigger the stress amplitude the fewer the stress cycles needed for failure. Stress concentrations caused by sudden changes in cross-section, keyways, holes or sharp corners can thus more easily lead to a fatigue failure. The presence of a countersunk hole was considered in one case to have led to a stress concentration which could have led to a fatigue failure. Figure 17.14 shows the effect on the fatigue properties of a steel of a small hole acting as a stress raiser. With the hole, at every stress amplitude value less cycles are needed to reach failure. There is also a lower fatigue limit with the hole present, 700 MN m^{-2} instead of over 1000 MN m^{-2}.

Figure 17.15 shows the effect on the fatigue properties of a steel of exposure to salt solution. The effect of the corrosion resulting from the salt solution attack on the steel is to reduce the number of stress cycles needed to reach failure for every stress amplitude. The non-corroded steel has a fatigue limit of 450 MN^{-2}, the corroded steel has no fatigue limit. There is thus no stress amplitude below which failure will not occur. The steel can be protected against the corrosion by plating; for example, chromium or zinc plating of the steel can result in the same S/N graph as the non-corroded steel even though it is subject to a corrosive atmosphere.

Residual stresses can be produced by many fabrication and finishing processes. If the stresses produced are such that the surfaces have compressive residual stresses then the fatigue properties are improved, but if tensile residual stresses are produced at the surfaces then poorer fatigue properties result. The case-hardening of steels by carburising results in compressive residual stresses at the surface, hence carburising improves the fatigue properties. Figure 17.16 shows the effect of carburising a hardened steel. Many, machining processes result in the production of surface tensile residual stresses and so result in poorer fatigue properties.

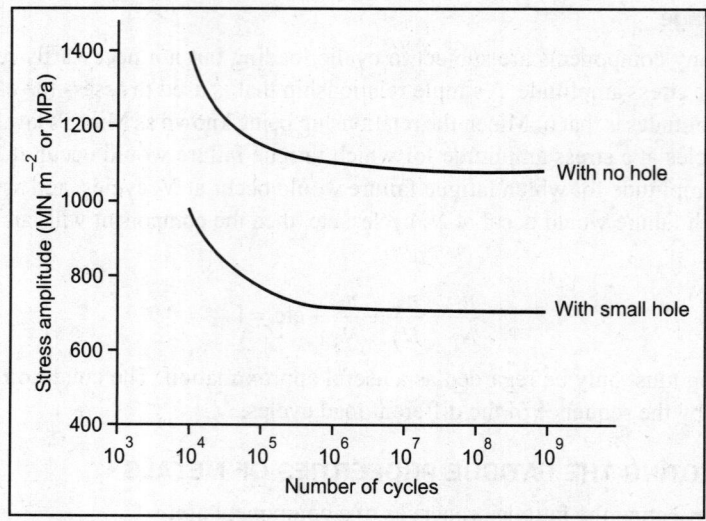

Fig. 17.14. S/N graphs for a steel both with and without a small hole by acting as a stress raiser.

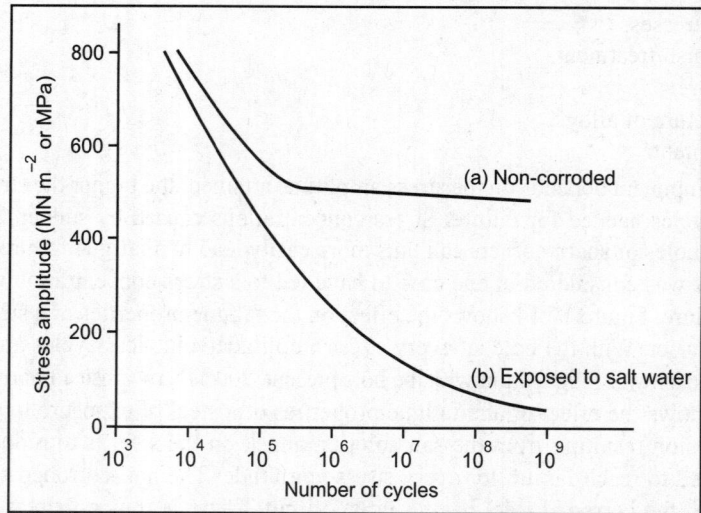

Fig. 17.15. S/N graphs for a steel: (a) with no corrosion, and (b) corroded to exposure to salt solution.

The effect of surface finish on the fatigue properties of a component is very significant. Scratches, dents or even surface identification markings can act as stress raisers and so reduce the fatigue properties. Shot peening a surface produces surface compressive residual stresses and improves the fatigue performance. Some surface treatments, e.g. conventional electroplating can, however, have a detrimental effect on the fatigue properties. This is because the surfaces end up with tensile residual stresses.

An increase in temperature can lead to a reduction in fatigue properties as a consequence of oxidation or corrosion of the metal surface. For example, the nickel-chromium alloy Nimonic 90 undergoes surface degradation at temperatures around 700° to 800°C and there is a poorer fatigue performance as a result. In many instances an increase in temperature does result in a poorer fatigue performance.

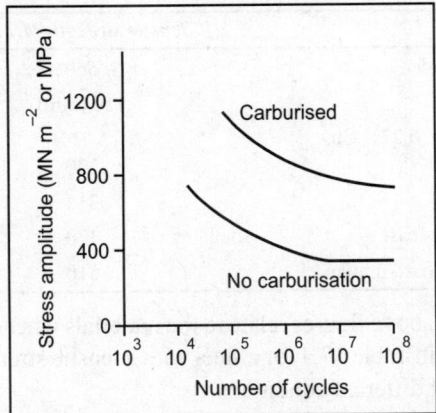

Fig. 17.16. *S/N* graph for a steel, showing effect of carburisation.

The microstructure of an alloy is a factor in determining the fatigue properties. This is because the origins of fatigue failure are extremely localised, involving slip at crystal planes. Because of this, the composition of an alloy and its grain size can affect its fatigue properties. Inclusions, such as lead in steel, can act as nuclei for fatigue failure and so impair fatigue properties.

Heat treatment can change or produce residual stresses within a metal. As mentioned earlier, case hardening improves fatigue properties as a result of producing compressive residual stresses in surfaces. However, some heat treatments can reduce surface compressive stresses and so adversely affect fatigue properties. Some hardening and tempering treatments fall into this category.

Materials and Fatigue Resistance

Steels typically have a fatigue limit which is generally about 0.4 to 0.5 times the tensile strength of the material. Inclusions in steels can impair the fatigue properties, thus steels with lead or sulphur present to enhance machanability are to avoided if good fatigue properties are required. The optimum structure for steels is tempered martensite for good fatigue resistance. Cast steels and cast irons tend to have relatively low endurance limits.

With steels there is generally a fatigue limit below which fatigue failure will not occur regardless of how many load cycles occur. However, with nonferrous alloys this is generally not the case and a fatigue limit is quoted for a specific number of load cycles, usually 10^7 or 10^8 cycles.

The fatigue limit for aluminium alloys is generally about 0.3 to 0.4 times the tensile strength of the material. Copper alloys tend to have fatigue limits about 0.4 to 0.5 times the tensile strength of the material.

Table 17.3 gives some typical values of tensile strength and fatigue limit, to about 10^7 or 10^8 cycles.

Table 17.3. Tensile strength and fatigue limit data.

Material	Tensile strength/MN m^{-2}	Fatigue limit/MN m^{-2}
0.10% carbon steel, normalised	360	190
0.60% carbon steel, normalised	740	320
Alloy steel, 3.5% Ni, 1.55% Cr oil quenched and tempered 550°C	850	470

(Contd...)

Material	Tensile strength/MN m^{-2}	Fatigue limit/MN m^{-2}
Stainless steel, 18% Cr, 8% Ni annealed	560	240
Grey cast iron	150 (min)	70
Aluminium, wrought alloy, 1.0% Mg, 0.27% Cu, 0.60% Si, 0.20% Cr, annealed	130	60
Solution treated and aged	315	100
Aluminium, casting alloy, 5% Mg, as cast	170	50
Copper alloy, cupro-nickel, 30% Ni hard drawn	510	230

It should be realised that the above figures relate to the materials when used in perfect conditions. To illustrate this, consider the data in Table 17.4 for a steel with a tensile strength of about 800 MN m^{-2} and the effect on the fatigue limit of different conditions.

Table 17.4. Effect of conditions on fatigue limit.

Condition	Fatigue limit/MN m^{-2}
Mirror polished surface, no flaws	470
Machined surface	420
Surface with a 0.1 mm notch	310
Hot worked surface	220
Under fresh water	170
Under sea water	120

Chapter 18

Forming Processes with Metals

INTRODUCTION

The range of forming processes can be divided broadly into four categories:
1. Casting, shaping a material by pouring the liquid material into a mould.
2. Manipulative process, shaping a material by plastic deformation processes.
3. Powder techniques, producing a shape by compacting a powder.
4. Cutting and grinding, producing a shape by metal removal.

The choice of forming process will depend on a number of factors:
1. The quantity of items required.
2. The dimensional accuracy required.
3. The surface finish required.
4. The size of the items, both overall size and section thicknesses.
5. The requirement for holes, inserts and undercuts.

Another factor to be considered is whether a joining process would be more economic or more suitable for the form of the item concerned. Linked with the choice of process is the choice of material, one cannot be considered without the other.

CASTING

Most metal products have at some stage in their manufacture been cast. Casting is the shaping of an object by pouring the liquid metal into a mould and then allowing it to solidify. The resulting shape may be that of the final manufactured object or one that requires some machining, or an ingot which is then further processed by manipulative processes.

The mould used to form the shape into which the liquid metal is poured has to be designed in such a way that, however complicated the shape, the liquid metal flows easily and quickly to all parts. This has implications for the finished casting in that sharp corners and re-entrant sections have to be avoided and gradually tapered changes in sections used. Account has also to be taken of the fact that the dimensions of the finished casting will be less than those of the mould due to shrinkage occurring when the metal cools from the liquid state to room temperature. Moulds are generally made in two or more parts, which are clamped together while the liquid metal is poured into them, then separated, when the metal has solidified; to enable the finished casting to be extracted. Complex castings can be achieved by the use of moulds having a number of parts. Hollow castings or holes or cavities can be achieved by incorporating separate loose pieces inside the mould, known as cores.

There are a number of casting methods possible and the factors determining the choice of a particular method are:
1. Size of casting required.
2. The number of castings required.
3. The cost per casting.
4. Complexity of casting.
5. The mechanical properties required for the casting.
6. The surface finish required.
7. Dimensional accuracy required.
8. The metal to be used.

Casting is a manufacturing process by which a liquid material is usually poured into a mould, which contains a hollow cavity of the desired shape, and then allowed to solidify. The solidified part is also known as a casting, which is ejected or broken out of the mould to complete the process. Casting materials are usually metals or various cold setting materials that cure after mixing two or more components together; examples are epoxy, concrete, plaster and clay. Casting is most often used for making complex shapes that would be otherwise difficult or uneconomical to make by other methods.

Sand Casting

Sand casting, also known as sand moulded casting, is a metal casting process characterised by using sand as the mould material. It is relatively cheap and sufficiently refractory even for steel foundry use. A suitable bonding agent (usually clay) is mixed or occurs with the sand. The mixture is moistened with water to develop strength and plasticity of the clay and to make the aggregate suitable for moulding. The term 'sand casting' can also refer to a casting produced via the sand casting process. Sand castings are produced in specialised factories called foundries. Over 70 per cent of all metal castings are produced via a sand casting process. There are six steps in this process:
1. Place a pattern in sand to create a mould.
2. Incorporate the pattern and sand in a gating system.
3. Remove the pattern.
4. Fill the mould cavity with molten metal.
5. Allow the metal to cool.
6. Break away the sand mould and remove the casting.

Main types of sand casting

In general, we can distinguish between two methods of sand casting; the first one using green sand and the second being the air set method.

Green sand method

These expendable moulds are made of wet sands that are used to make the mould's shape. The name comes from the fact that wet sands are used in the moulding process. Green sand is not green in colour, but 'green' in the sense that it is used in a wet state (akin to green wood). Unlike the name suggests, 'green sand' is not a type of sand on its own, but is rather a mixture of:
1. Silica sand (SiO_2), or chromite sand ($FeCr_2O$), or zircon sand ($ZrSiO_4$), 75 to 85 per cent.
2. Bentonite (clay), 5 to 11 per cent.
3. Water, 2 to 4 per cent.

4. Inert sludge 3 to 5 per cent.
5. Anthracite (0 to 1 per cent).

There are many recipes for the proportion of clay, but they all strike different balances between mouldability, surface finish, and ability of the hot molten metal to degas. The coal, typically referred to in foundries as sea-coal, which is present at a ratio of less than 5 per cent, partially combusts in the presence of the molten metal leading to offgassing of organic vapors.

Air set method

The air set method uses dry sand bonded with materials other than clay, using a fast curing adhesive. The latter may also be referred to as no bake mould casting. When these are used, they are collectively called 'air set' sand castings to distinguish them from 'green sand' castings. Two types of moulding sand are natural bonded (bank sand) and synthetic (lake sand); the latter is generally preferred due to its more consistent composition.

With both methods, the sand mixture is packed around a master pattern, forming a mould cavity. If necessary, a temporary plug is placed in the sand and touching the pattern in order to later form a channel into which the casting fluid can be poured. Air-set moulds are often formed with the help of a two-part mould having a top and bottom part, termed the cope and drag. The sand mixture is tamped down as it is added around the pattern, and the final mould assembly is sometimes vibrated to compact the sand and fill any unwanted voids in the mould. Then the pattern is removed along with the channel plug, leaving the mould cavity. The casting liquid (typically molten metal) is then poured into the mould cavity. After the metal has solidified and cooled, the casting is separated from the sand mould. There is typically no mould release agent, and the mould is generally destroyed in the removal process.

The accuracy of the casting is limited by the type of sand and the moulding process. Sand castings made from coarse green sand impart a rough texture to the surface, and this makes them easy to identify. Air-set moulds can produce castings with much smoother surfaces. Surfaces can also be later ground and polished, for example when making a large bell. After moulding, the casting is covered with a residue of oxides, silicates and other compounds. This residue can be removed by various means, such as grinding, or shot blasting.

During casting, some of the components of the sand mixture are lost in the thermal casting process. Green sand can be reused after adjusting its composition to replenish the lost moisture and additives. The pattern itself can be reused indefinitely to produce new sand moulds. The sand moulding process has been used for many centuries to produce castings manually.

Sand casting involves the making of a mould using a mixture of sand with clay, for the traditional moulding material. This is packed around a pattern of the casting, generally of a hard wood and larger than the required casting to allow for shrinkage. The mould is made in two or more parts so that the pattern can be extracted after the sand has been packed round it (Fig. 18.1). Sand casting can be used for a wide range of casting sizes and for small- or large-number production. It is the cheapest process for small-number production and a reasonably priced process for large-number production. Complex castings can be produced by this method. The mechanical properties, surface finish and dimensional accuracy of the casting are however limited. A wide range of alloys can be cast by this process.

Die Casting

Die casting is a metal casting process that is characterised by forcing molten metal under high pressure into a mould cavity. The mould cavity is created using two hardened tool steel dies which have been machined into shape and work similarly to moulds during the process. Most die castings are made from non-ferrous metals, specifically zinc, copper, aluminium, magnesium, lead, and tin based alloys. Depending on the type of metal being cast, a hot- or cold-chamber machine is used.

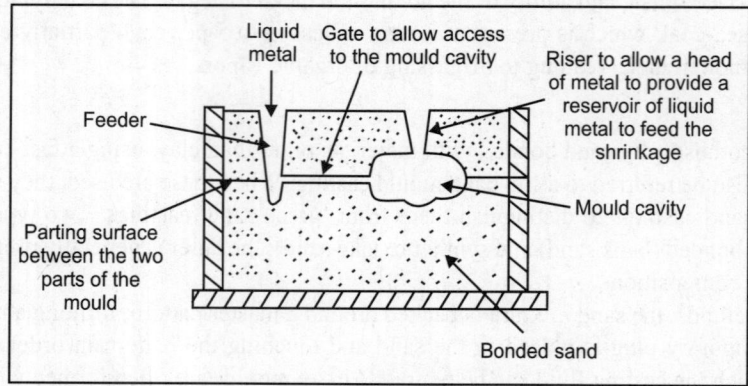

Fig. 18.1. Sand casting.

The casting equipment and the metal dies represent large capital costs and this tends to limit the process to high volume production. Manufacture of parts using die casting is relatively simple, involving only four main steps, which keeps the incremental cost per item low. It is especially suited for a large quantity of small to medium sized castings, which is why die casting produces more castings than any other casting process. Die castings are characterised by a very good surface finish (by casting standards) and dimensional consistency.

Two variants are pore-free die casting, which is used to eliminate gas porosity defects; and direct injection die casting, which is used with zinc castings to reduce scrap and increase yield.

Die casting involves the use of a metal mould. Two types of die casting are used. Gravity die casting is similar to sand casting in that the metal mould has the liquid metal poured into it in a similar way to that adopted with a sand casting. The head of liquid metal in the feeder forces the metal into the various parts of the mould. With pressure die casting the liquid metal is injected into the mould under pressure. This has the advantage that the metal can be forced into all parts of the mould cavity and thus very complex shapes with high dimensional accuracy can be produced. There are limitations to the size of the casting that can be produced by die casting, that for pressure die casting being smaller than that for gravity die casting. The cost of the mould is high and thus the process is relatively uneconomic for small-number production. Large-number production is necessary to spread the cost of the mould. These initial high costs may, however, be more than compensated for with large-number production by the reduction or complete elimination of machining or finishing costs. The mechanical properties, surface finish and dimensional accuracy of the casting are very good. The metals that can be used for this process are, however, restricted to the lower melting point metals and alloys, e.g. aluminium, copper, magnesium and zinc and their alloys.

Another method which is used to force the liquid metal into the various parts of the mould is known as centrifugal casting. The mould is rotated (Fig. 18.2) and the forces resulting from this rotation force the metal against the sides of the mould. This method is used for simple geometrical shapes, e.g. large diameter pipes. The method is not suitable for complex castings.

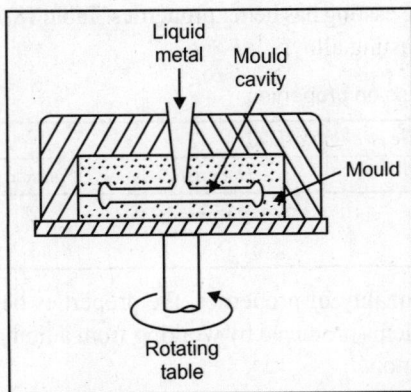

Fig. 18.2. Centrifugal casting.

Investment or lost wax casting is a process that can be used for metals that have to withsand very high temperatures, and so have high melting points, and for which high dimensional accuracy is required; areo engine blades are a typical product. The process is not restricted to high-melting-point metals but can also be used with low-melting-point metals. It is, however, the only casting method that can be used for the high-melting-point metals. Such metals cause rapid die failures when used with die casting. Modern investment casting uses metal moulds to produce wax patterns. The wax patterns are then coated with a ceramic paste. When this coated wax pattern is heated the ceramic hardens and the wax melts to give a ceramic mould.

The liquid metal is then injected into this ceramic mould by pressure or the centrifugal process. After the mould has cooled the ceramic broken away to release the casting. The size of castings that can be produced in this way is limited and it is an expensive process for large-number production. It is, however, relatively cheap for small-number products, particularly where high dimensional accuracy and good surface finish are required. It is suitable for complex castings.

Casting and Grain Structure

Casting involves the shaping of a product by the pouring of liquid metal into a mould. The grain structure within the product is determined by the rate of cooling. Thus, the metal in contact with the moulds cools faster than that in the centre of the casting. This gives rise to small crystals, termed chill crystals, near the surfaces. These are smaller because the metal has cooled too rapidly for the crystals to grow to any size. The cooling rate nearer the centre is, however, much less, and so some chill crystals can develop in an inward direction. This results in large elongated crystals perpendicular to the mould walls called columnar crystals. In the centre of the mould the cooling rate is the lowest. While growth of the columnar crystals is taking place small crystals are growing in this central region. These grow in the liquid metal which is constantly on the move due to convection currents. The final result is a central region of medium-sized, almost spherical, crystals called equiaxed crystals.

In general a casting structure having entirely small equiaxed crystals is preferred. This type of structure can be promoted by a more rapid rate of cooling for the casting. Castings in which the mould is made of sand tend to have a slow cooling rate as sand has low thermal conductivity. Thus, sand castings tend to have large columnar grains and hence relatively low strength. Die casting involving metal moulds has a much faster rate of cooling and so gives castings having a bigger zone of equiaxed crystals. As these are smaller than columnar crystals the casting has better properties. Table 18.1 shows the types of differences that can occur with aluminium casting alloys.

Table 18.1. Effect of casting process on properties.

Material	Tensile strength (MPa)		Percentage elongation	
	Sand cast	Die cast	Sand cast	Die cast
5% Si, 3% Cu	140	150	2	2
12% Si	160	185	5	7

Castings do not show directionality of properties, the properties being the same in all directions. They do, however, have the problems produced by working from a liquid metal of blowholes and other voids occurring during solidification.

MANIPULATIVE PROCESSES

Manipulative processes involve the shaping of a material by plastic deformation processes. Where the deformation is carried out at a temperature in excess of the recrystallisation temperature of the metal, the process is said to involve hot working. Plastic deformation at temperatures below the recrystallisation temperature is called cold working. The main hot working processes are rolling, forging and extrusion. Cold working processes are cold rolling, drawing, pressing, spinning and impact extrusion.

An increase in temperature at which a metal is worked means less energy is required to work the metal, i.e. the metal is more malleable. High temperatures can mean, however, surface scaling or damage occurring. The initial cast metal has coarse grains; hot working breaks the grains down to give a finer structure and thus better mechanical properties.

In addition to the alloying elements present in a metal there are impurities derived from the fluxes and slags used in the melting operation. With the cast ingot these impurities are reasonably randomly distributed but with hot working they tend to become oriented as fibres in the direction of the working. Thus with rolled products the fibre lines tend to be in a direction parallel to the direction of rolling [Fig. 18.3(a)]. With a forging the work pattern, shown in Fig. 18.3(b) is more complex and so the fibre direction is more complex.

The effect of the fibres having a specific direction is to give a corresponding directionality of mechanical properties. Thus although hot working improves the mechanical properties it does lead to the properties varying in different directions. The fibres can act as lines along which cracks can be propagated, so the design of a product should, as far as is possible, be such as to have the fibre direction, parallel to the tensile stresses and not at right angles to them.

Cold working involves the use of a greater amount of energy than a hot working process to obtain a particular amount of deformation. During cold working the crystal structure becomes broken up and distorted, leading to an increase in mechanical strength and hardness. Unlike hot working, cold working can give a clean, smooth surface finish.

Cold Working

The term cold working is applied to any process which results in plastic deformation at a temperature which does not alter the structural changes produced by the working. Table 18.2 shows some of the changes that take place when a sheet of annealed aluminium is rolled and its thickness reduced.

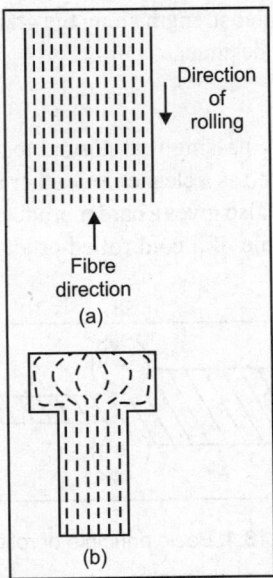

Fig. 18.3. Fibre directions with (a) rolling, and (b) forging.

Table 18.2. Effect of work hardening on properties.

Reduction in sheet thickness %	Tensile strength (MV m^{-2} or MPa)	Elongation %	Hardness HV
0	92	40	20
15	107	15	28
30	125	8	33
40	140	5	38
60	155	3	43

As the amount of plastic deformation is increased so the tensile strength increases, the hardness increases and the elongation decreases. The material is becoming harder as a result of the cold working, hence the term sometimes applied to cold working of work hardening. The more the material is worked the harder it becomes.

Also, as the percentage elongation results above indicate the more a material is worked the more brittle it becomes. A stage can, however, be reached when the strength and hardness are a maximum and the elongation a minimum and further plastic deformation is not possible, the material is too brittle. With the rolled aluminium sheet referred to in the Table 18.2, this condition has been reached with about a 60 per cent reduction in sheet thickness. The material is then said to be fully work hardened.

Structure of cold worked metals

When stress is applied to a metal grain, deformation starts along the slip planes most suitably orientated. The effect of this is to cause the grains to become elongated and distorted. The grains have become elongated into fibre-like structures, which has the effect of giving the material different mechanical properties in different directions; a greater strength along the grain than at right angles to the grain. This effect can be used to advantage by the designer.

Cold working processes

Cold rolling is the shaping of metal by passing it at normal temperature, between rollers (Fig. 18.4). Sheet and strip metal are often cold rolled as a cleaner, smoother finish to the metal surfaces is produced than if hot working is used. The process also gives a harder product, the aluminium foil used for wrapping sweets, such as chocolate, is an example of a cold rolled product. Cold rolling requires more energy than hot rolling.

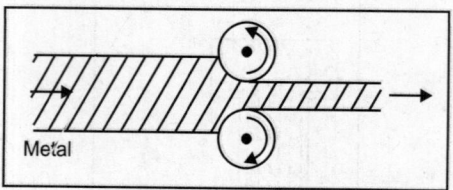

Fig. 18.4. Basic principle of rolling.

Drawing involves the pulling of metal through a die (Fig. 18.5). Wire manufacture can involve a number of drawing stages in order that the initial material can be brought down to the required size. As cold working hardens a metal there may have to be annealing operations between the various drawing stages to soften the material for further drawing to take place.

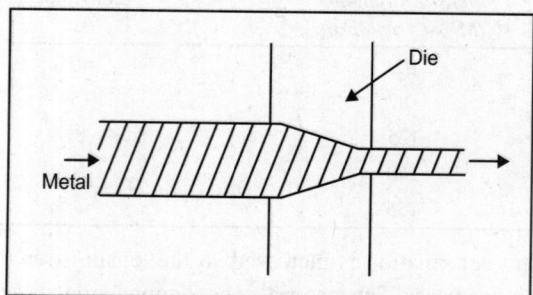

Fig. 18.5. Drawing a wire.

With deep drawing, sheet metal is pushed through an aperture by a punch (Fig. 18.6). The more ductile materials such as aluminium, brass and mild steel are used and the products are deep cup-shaped articles such as cartridge cases. With deep drawing the sheet metal is not clamped round the edges and so is drawn into the die by the pressure from the punch. If the material is clamped round the edges then the process is known as pressing (Fig. 18.7). Car body panels, kitchen pans and other cooking utensils are typical examples of the products obtained by pressing. Ductile materials are used.

Spinning is a process that can be used for the production of circular section objects. A circular blank of metal is rotated in a lathe type of machine and then pressure applied to deflect the blank into the required shape (Fig. 18.8). Aluminium, brass and mild steel are examples of materials used for forming by this process. Spinning is an economic method for producing products required in small numbers and can be used also for large products where other forms of forming would be too expensive.

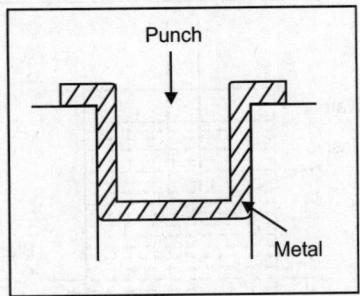

Fig. 18.6. Deep drawing.

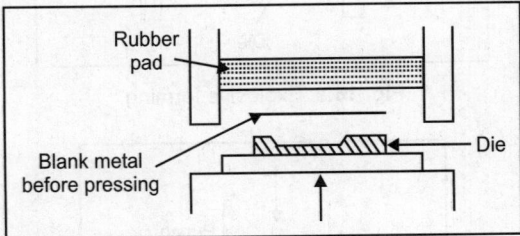

Fig. 18.7. Pressing.

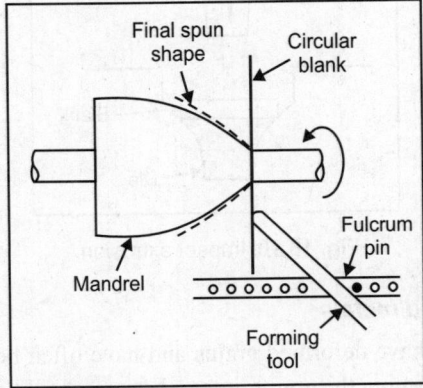

Fig. 18.8. Spinning with a hand-held tool.

    Explosive forming is used mainly for the forming of sheets of relatively large surface area on a comparatively small number production basis. An explosive charge is detonated under water and the resulting pressure wave used to press a metal blank against a die (Fig. 18.9). Communication reflectors and contoured panels are examples of the products of this process.

    Impact extrusion is the process used for the production of rigid or collapsible tubes or cans, e.g. zinc dry battery cases and toothpaste tubes, in softer materials such as zinc, lead and aluminium. Figure 18.10 shows the essential features of the process, a punch forcing a blank to flow into the die. The punch descends very rapidly and hence the term 'impact' for this form of extrusion.

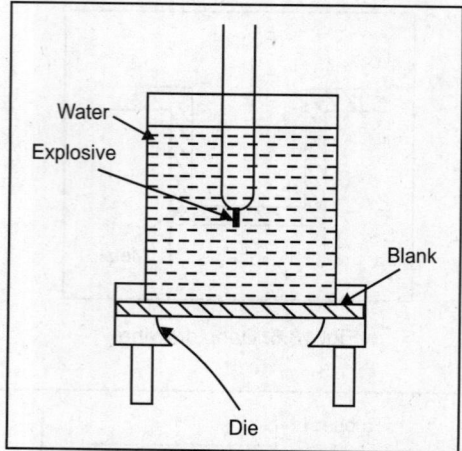

Fig. 18.9. Explosive forming.

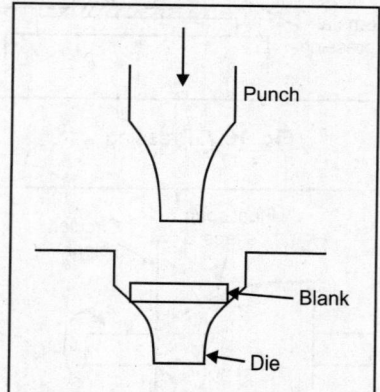

Fig. 18.10. Impact extrusion.

Effect of heat on cold-worked metals

Cold-worked metals generally have deformed grains and have often become rather brittle due to the working. In this process of deforming the grains, internal stresses build-up. When a cold-worked metal is heated to temperatures up to about $0.3\,T_m$ where, T_m is the melting point of the metal concerned on the Kelvin scale of temperature, then the internal stresses start to become relieved. There are no changes in grain structure during this but just some slight rearrangement of atoms in order that the stresses become relieved.

This process is known as recovery. Copper has a melting point of 1083°C or 1356 K. Hence stress relief with copper requires heating to above about 407 K, i.e. 134°C.

If the heating is contained to a temperature of about 0.3 to 0.5 T_m there is a very large change in hardness. The strength and also the structure of the metal change. Table 18.3 shows how the hardness of copper changes, the copper having been subject to a 30 per cent cold working.

Table 18.3. Effect of temperature on hardness.

Temperature			Hardness HV
/°C	/K		
Initially			86
150	423	$(0.3\ T_m)$	85
200	473		80
250	523	$(0.4\ T_m)$	74
300	573		61
350	623	$(0.5\ T_m)$	46
450	723		24
600	873	$(0.6\ T_m)$	15

Figure 18.11 shows the results of Table 18.3 graphically. Between $0.3\ T_m$ and $0.5\ T_m$ there is a very large change in hardness. The strength also decreases while the elongation increases. What is happening is that the metal is recrystallising.

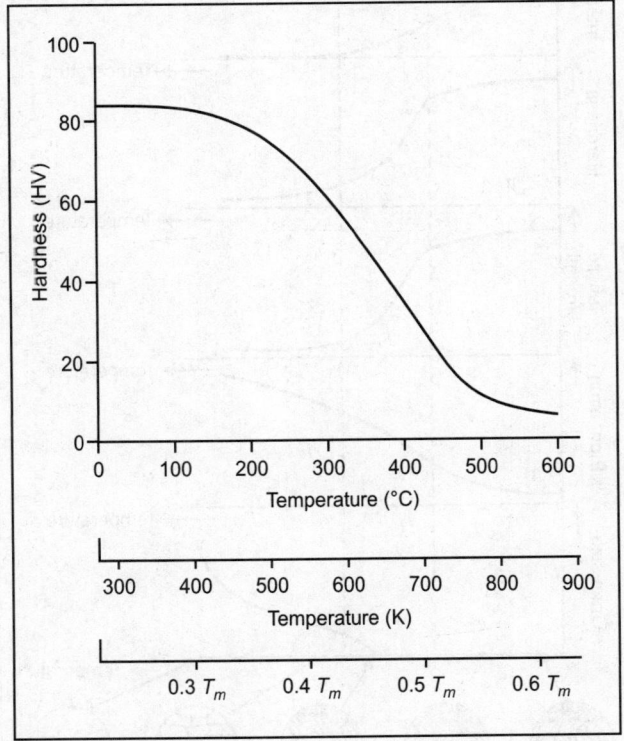

Fig. 18.11. The effect of heat treatment on cold-worked copper.

With recrystallisation crystals begin to grow from nuclei in the most heavily deformed parts of the metal. The temperature at which recrystallisation just starts is called the recrystallisation temperature. This is, for pure metals, about 0.3 to $0.5\ T_m$ (Table 18.4).

Table 18.4. Recrystallisation temperatures.

Material	Melting point		Recrystallisation temperature		
	/°C	/K	/°C	/K	
Aluminium	660	933	150	423	0.05 T_m
Copper	1083	1356	200	473	0.3 T_m
Iron	1535	1808	450	723	0.4 T_m
Nickel	1452	1725	620	893	0.5 T_m

As the temperature is increased from the recrystallisation temperature so the crystals grow until they have completely replaced the original distorted cold worked structure. Figure 18.12 illustrates this sequence and its relationship to the changes in physical properties.

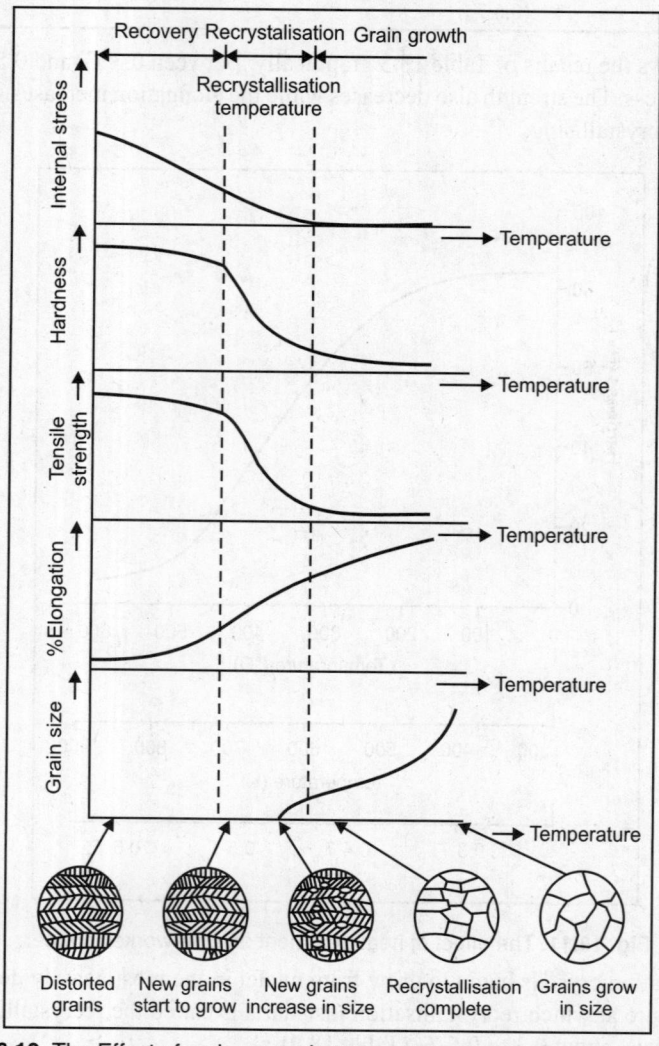

Fig. 18.12. The Effect of an increase in temperature on cold-worked materials.

The sequence of events that occurs when a cold-worked metal is heated can be broken down into three phases:
1. Recovery—the only significant change during this phase is the relief of internal stresses.
2. Recrystallisation—the hardness, tensile strength and percentage elongation all change noticeably during this phase.
3. Grain growth—the hardness, tensile strength and percentage elongation change little during this phase. The only change is that the grains grow and the material becomes large-grained.

During the grain-growth phase the newly-formed grains grow by absorbing other neighbouring grains. The amount of grain growth depends on the temperature and the time for which the material is at that temperature (Fig. 18.13).

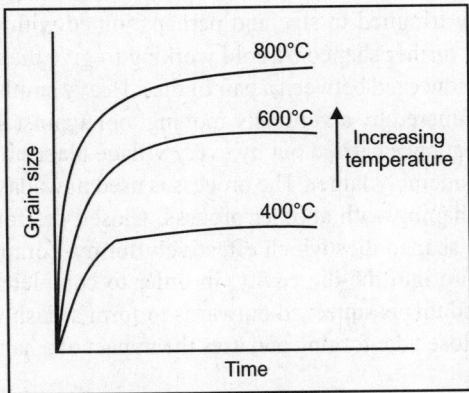

Fig. 18.13. The effect of time and temperature on grain growth.

The term annealing is used for the heating process used to change the properties of a material. Thus, in the case of aluminium that has been cold worked and has become too brittle to work further, heating to above the recrystallisation temperature of 150°C enables new grains to grow and the material to become more ductile. The aluminium can then be worked further. This sequence of events, cold working followed by annealing and then further cold working, is used in many manufacturing processes.

Factors affecting recrystallisation

1. A minimum amount of deformation is necessary before recrystallisation can occur. The permanent deformation necessary depends on the metal concerned.
2. The greater the amount of cold work the lower the crystallisation temperature for a particular metal.
3. Alloying increases the recrystallisation temperature.
4. No recrystallisation takes place below the recrystallisation temperature. The higher the temperature above the recrystallisation temperature the shorter the time needed at that temperature for a given crystal condition to be attained.
5. The resulting grain size depends on the annealing temperature. The higher the temperature the larger the grain size.
6. The amount of cold work prior to the annealing affects the size of the grains. The greater the amount of cold work the smaller the resulting grain size. The greater the amount of cold work the more centres are produced for crystal growth.

Hot Working

Hot working processes

The main hot working processes are rolling, forging and extrusion. Rolling is the shaping of metal by the passing of the hot metal between rollers. Forging is the shaping of metal by a succession of hammer blows or application of pressure. Extrusion shapes metal by a hot ingot being forced, under pressure, through a die.

Rolling is a continuous process in which the metal is passed through the gap between a pair of rotating rollers. When cylindrical rollers are used, the product is in the form of a bar or sheet, but profiled rollers can be used to produce contoured surfaces, e.g. structural beam sections. A wide variety of cross-sections can be produced. These are often used as the basis for structures, e.g. window frames, the rolled product being only trimmed to size and perhaps joined with other rolled shapes. In some instances the product may be further shaped by cold working to give the final product.

With forging, the metal is squeezed between a pair of dies. Heavy smith's forging or open die forging involves the metal being hammered by a vertically moving tool against a stationary tool (Fig. 18.14). This type of forging is like that once carried out by every village blacksmith, only now the ingot being hammered is likely to be considerably larger. The process is used nowadays, mainly for an initial rough shaping of an ingot before shaping with another process. Closed die forging involves the hot metal being squeezed between two shaped dies which effectively form a complete mould (Fig. 18.15). The metal flows under the pressure into the die cavity. In order to completely fill the die cavity a small excess of metal is allowed and this is squeezed outwards to form a flash which is later trimmed away. Drop forging is one form of closed die forging and uses the impact of a hammer to cause the metal billet to flow and fill the die cavity.

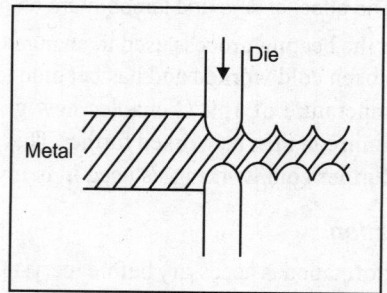

Fig. 18.14. Open die forging.

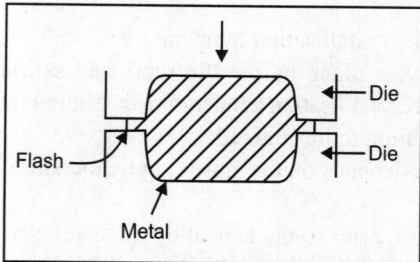

Fig. 18.15. Closed die forging.

Closed die forging can be used to produce large numbers of components with high dimensional accuracy and better mechanical properties would be produced by casting or machining. This is because the fibre direction can be arranged to give the greatest strength.

With hot extrusion the hot metal is forced, under pressure, to flow through a die, i.e. a shaped orifice (Fig. 18.16). It is rather like squeezing toothpaste out of its tube. Quite complex sections can be extruded.

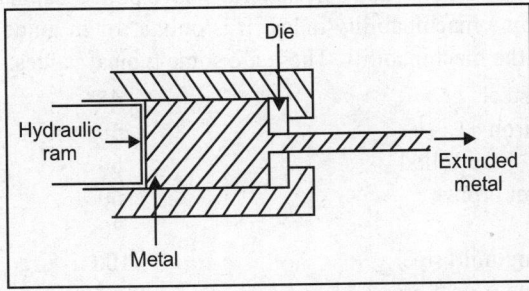

Fig. 18.16. Extrusion.

MACHINING

Machining is the removal of material from the workpiece, the block of material being machined, by the action of a tool. The tool moves relative to the workpiece and detaches thin layers of the unwanted material, known as 'chips'. Figure 18.17 shows some of the main machining methods.

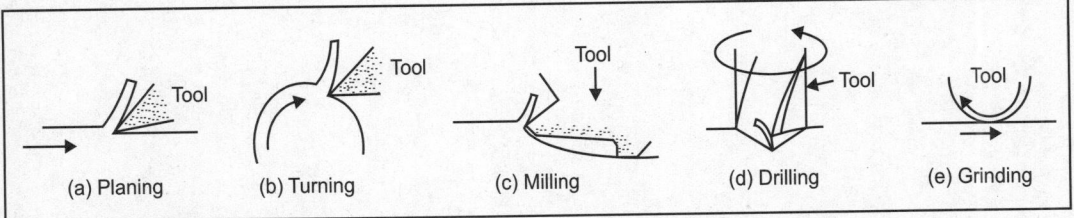

Fig. 18.17. Machining methods (a) planing, (b) turning, (c) milling, (d) drilling, and (e) grinding.

Machining is generally a secondary process, following a primary process such as casting or forging, and is used to produce the final shape to the required accuracy and surface finish. Machining results invariably in waste material being produced and thus any costing of a machining process has to allow for this. To keep the waste to a aluminium the primary process should give a product as near the final required dimensions as possible, bearing in mind any need to remove material to give a good surface finish.

Machining involves using a tool that is of a harder material than that of the workpiece. Tools may be made of high speed steels, metal carbides or ceramics. Metal carbide and ceramic tools are made by sintering appropriate mixtures of powders.

In machining, the cutting tool causes the workpiece material at the cutting edge to become highly stressed and subject to plastic deformation. The more ductile the material the greater the amount of plastic deformation and the more the material of the workpiece spreads along the tool face. The more this happens the greater the force needed to machine the material and so the greater the expenditure of energy in the machining process. A ductile material on machining gives rise to a continuous chip while a more brittle material leads to small discontinuous chips being produced. Less energy is needed for machining in this case.

The term machinability is used to describe the ease of machining. A material with good machinability will produce small chips, need low cutting forces and energy expenditure, be capable of being machined quickly and give long tool life. Ductile and soft materials have poor machinability. A relative measure of machinability is given by a machinability index. It is only a rough guide to machinability, but the higher the index the better the machinability, These are some typical values:

Material	Index
Stainless steel	45
Wrought iron	50
Copper, ¼ hard rolled	60
Aluminium bronze	60
Cast steel	70
Free cutting mild steel	100
Free cutting α or β brass	200–400

The machinability of a metal can be improved if its ductility is decreased. Work hardening can make an improvement. Some multiphase alloys have good machinability as the insoluble phase can provide discontinuities within the material and assist in breaking up a continuous chip to give small chips. The addition of small amount of lead to a mild steel improves its machinability. For optimum machinability, the workpiece material must have low ductility and also low hardness.

Chapter 19
Joining Materials

INTRODUCTION
The main joining processing can be summarised as—adhesive bonding, soldering and brazing, welding and fastening systems. The factors that determine the joining process to be chosen are:
1. The material involved.
2. The shape of the components being joined.
3. Whether a permanent or temporary joint is required.
4. Limitations imposed by the environment.
5. Cost.

ADHESIVE
An adhesive or glue, is a mixture in a liquid or semi-liquid state that adheres or bonds items together. Adhesives may come from either natural or synthetic sources. The types of materials that can be bonded are vast but they are especially useful for bonding thin materials. Adhesives cure (harden) by either evaporating a solvent or by chemical reactions that occur between two or more constituents.

Adhesives are advantageous for joining thin or dissimilar materials, minimising weight, when a vibration dampening joint is needed. A disadvantage to adhesives is that they do not form an instantaneous joint, unlike most other joining processes, because the adhesive needs time to cure.

Types of Adhesives
Adhesives are typically organised by the method of adhesion. These are then organised into reactive and non-reactive adhesives, which refers to if the adhesive chemically reacts to harden. Alternatively they can be organised by whether the raw stock is of natural or synthetic origin, or by their starting physical phase.

Nonreactive adhesives

Drying adhesives
There are two types of adhesives that harden by drying: solvent based adhesives and polymer dispersion adhesives, also known as emulsion adhesives. Solvent based adhesives are a mixture of ingredients (typically polymers) dissolved in a solvent. White glue, contact adhesives and rubber cements are members of the drying adhesive family. As the solvent evaporates, the adhesive hardens. Depending on the chemical composition of the adhesive, they will adhere to different materials to greater or lesser

degrees. Polymer dispersion adhesives are milky-white dispersions often based on polyvinyl acetate (PVAc). Used extensively in the woodworking and packaging industries. Also used with fabrics and fabric-based components, and in engineered products such as loudspeaker cones.

Pressure sensitive adhesives

Pressure sensitive adhesives (PSA) form a bond by the application of light pressure to marry the adhesive with the adherend. They are designed with a balance between flow and resistance to flow. The bond forms because the adhesive is soft enough to flow (i.e. wet) the adherend. The bond has strength because the adhesive is hard enough to resist flow when stress is applied to the bond. Once the adhesive and the adherend are in close proximity, molecular interactions, such as Van der Waals forces, become involved in the bond, contributing significantly to its ultimate strength.

Contact adhesives

Contact adhesives are used in strong bonds with high shear-resistance like laminates, such as bonding formica to a wooden counter, and in footwear, as in attaching outsoles to uppers. Natural rubber and polychloroprene (Neoprene) are commonly used contact adhesives. Both of these elastomers undergo strain crystallisation. Contact adhesives must be applied to both surfaces and allowed some time to dry before the two surfaces are pushed together. Some contact adhesives require as long as 24 hours to dry before the surfaces are to be held together. Once the surfaces are pushed together, the bond forms very quickly. It is usually not necessary to apply pressure for a long time, so there is less need for clamps.

Hot adhesives

Hot adhesives, also known as hot melt adhesives, are simply thermoplastics applied in molten form (in the 65°–180°C range) which solidify on cooling to form strong bonds between a wide range of materials. Ethylene-vinyl acetate based hot-melts are particularly popular for crafts because of their ease of use and the wide range of common materials they can join. A glue gun is one method of applying hot adhesives. The glue gun melts the solid adhesive then allows the liquid to pass through its barrel onto the material, where it solidifies.

Reactive adhesives

Multi-part adhesives

Multi-part adhesives harden by mixing two or more components which chemically react. This reaction causes polymers to cross-link into acrylics, urethanes, and epoxies. There are several commercial combinations of multi-component adhesives in use in industry. Some of these combinations are:
1. Polyester resin—polyurethane resin.
2. Polyols—polyurethane resin.
3. Acrylic polymers—polyurethane resins.

The individual components of a multi-component adhesive are not adhesive by nature. The individual components react with each other after being mixed and show full adhesion only on curing. The multi-component resins can be either solvent-based or solvent-less. The solvents present in the adhesives are a medium for the polyester or the polyurethane resin. The solvent is dried during the curing process.

One-part adhesives

One-part adhesives harden via a chemical reaction with an external energy source, such as radiation, heat, and moisture. Ultraviolet (UV) light curing adhesives, also known as light curing materials (LCM), have become popular within the manufacturing sector due to their rapid curing time and strong bond strength. Light curing adhesives can cure in as little as a second and many formulations can bond dissimilar substrates (materials) and withstand harsh temperatures. These qualities make UV curing adhesives essential to the manufacturing of items in many industrial markets such as electronics, telecommunications, medical, aerospace, glass, and optical. Unlike traditional adhesives, UV light curing adhesives not only bond materials together but they can also be used to seal and coat products. They are generally acrylic based.

Heat curing adhesives consist of a pre-made mixture of two or more components. When heat is applied the components react and cross-link. This type of adhesive includes epoxies, urethanes, and polyimides.

Moisture curing adhesives cure when they react with moisture present on the substrate surface or in the air. This type of adhesive includes cyanoacrylates and urethanes.

Natural adhesives

Natural adhesives are made from organic sources such as vegetable matter, starch (dextrin), natural resins or from animals, e.g. casein or animal glue. They are often referred to as bioadhesives. One example is a simple paste made by cooking flour in water.

Synthetic adhesives

Synthetic adhesives are based on elastomers, thermoplastics, emulsions, and thermosets. Examples of thermosetting adhesives are: epoxy, polyurethane, cyanoacrylate and acrylic polymers.

Application of Adhesion

Applicators of different adhesives are designed according to the adhesive being used and the size of the area to which the adhesive will be applied. The adhesive is applied to either one or both of the materials being bonded. The pieces are aligned and pressure is added to aid in adhesion and rid the bond of air bubbles. Common ways of applying an adhesive include brushes, rollers, using films or pellets, spray guns and applicator guns (e.g. caulk gun). All of these can be done manually or can be automated into a machine.

Mechanisms of Adhesion

Adhesion, the attachment between adhesive and substrate may occur either by mechanical means, in which the adhesive works its way into small pores of the substrate, or by one of several chemical mechanisms. The strength of adhesion depends on many factors, including the means by which it occurs.

In some cases, an actual chemical bond occurs between adhesive and substrate. In others, electrostatic forces, as in static electricity, hold the substances together. A third mechanism involves the Van der Waals forces that develop between molecules. A fourth means involves the moisture-aided diffusion of the glue into the substrate, followed by hardening.

Failure of the Adhesive Joint

There are several factors that could contribute to the failure of two adhered surfaces. Sunlight and heat may weaken the adhesive. Solvents can deteriorate or dissolve adhesive. Physical stresses may also cause the separation of surfaces. When subjected to loading, debonding may occur at different locations in the adhesive joint.

The major fracture types are the following.

Cohesive fracture

Cohesive fracture is obtained if a crack propagates in the bulk polymer which constitutes the adhesive. In this case the surfaces of both adherents after debonding will be covered by fractured adhesive. The crack may propagate in the centre of the layer or near an interface. For this last case, the cohesive fracture can be said to be 'cohesive near the interface'. Most quality control standards consider a good adhesive bond to be cohesive.

Interfacial fracture

The fracture is adhesive or interfacial when debonding occurs between the adhesive and the adherent. In most cases, the occurrence of interfacial fracture for a given adhesive goes along with a smaller fracture toughness. The interfacial character of a fracture surface is usually to identify the precise location of the crack path in the interphase.

Design of Adhesive Joints

As a general design rule, the material properties of the object need to be greater than the forces anticipated during its use (i.e. geometry, loads, etc.). The engineering work will consist of having a good model to evaluate the function. For most adhesive joints, this can be achieved using fracture mechanics. Concepts such as the stress concentration factor and the strain energy release rate can be used to predict failure. In such models, the behaviour of the adhesive layer itself is neglected and only the adherents are considered.

As the loads are usually fixed, an acceptable design will result from combination of a material selection procedure and geometry modifications, if possible. In adhesively bonded structures, the global geometry and loads are fixed by structural considerations and the design procedure focuses on the material properties of the adhesive and on local changes on the geometry.

Testing the Resistance of the Adhesive

A wide range of testing devices have been devised to evaluate the fracture resistance of bonded structures. Most of these devices are beam type specimens.

1. Double cantilever beam tests (DCB) measure the fracture resistance of adhesives in a fracture mechanics framework. These tests consist in opening an assembly of two beams by applying a force at the ends of the two beams. The test is unstable (i.e. the crack propagates along the entire specimen once a critical load is attained) and a modified version of this test characterised by a non constant inertia was proposed called the tapered double cantilever beam (TDCB) specimen.
2. Peel tests measure the fracture resistance of a thin layer bonded on a thick substrate or of two layers bonded together. They consist in measuring the force needed for tearing an adherent layer from a substrate or for tearing two adherent layers one from another. Whereas the structure is not symmetrical, various mode mixities can be introduced in these tests. This is one of the more common methods of evaluating paper strength in library and archival preservation.
3. Wedge tests consist in inserting a wedge in between two bonded plates. A critical energy release rate can be derived from the crack length during testing.
4. End notch flexure tests consist in two bonded beams built-in on one side and loaded by a force on the other.
6. Crack lap shear tests (CLS) are application-oriented fracture resistance tests. They consist in two plates bonded on a limited length and loaded in tension on both ends. The test can be either

symmetrical or dis-symmetrical. In the first case two cracks can be initiated and in the second only one crack can propagate.

SOLDERING

Soldering is a process in which two or more metal items are joined together by melting and flowing a filler metal into the joint, the filler metal having a relatively low melting point. Soft soldering is characterised by the melting point of the filler metal, which is below 400°C (752°F). The filler metal used in the process is called solder.

Soldering is distinguished from brazing by use of a lower melting-temperature filler metal. The filler metals are typically alloys that have liquidus temperatures below 350°C. It is distinguished from welding by the base metals not being melted during the joining process which may or may not include the addition of a filler metal.

In a soldering process, heat is applied to the parts to be joined, causing the solder to melt and be drawn into the joint by capillary action and to bond to the materials to be joined by wetting action. After the metal cools, the resulting joints are not as strong as the base metal, but have adequate strength, electrical conductivity, and watertightness for many uses.

Applications

One of the most frequent applications of soldering is assembling electronic components to printed circuit boards (PCBs). Another common application is making permanent but reversible connections between copper pipes in plumbing systems. Joints in sheet metal objects such as food cans, roof flashing, rain gutters and automobile radiators have also historically been soldered, and occasionally still are. Jewellery components are assembled and repaired by soldering. Small mechanical parts are often soldered as well. Soldering is also used to join lead and copper foil in stained glass work. Soldering can also be used as a semipermanent patch for a leak in a container or cooking vessel.

One guideline to consider when soldering is that, since soldering temperatures are so low, a soldered joint has limited service at elevated temperatures. Solders generally do not have much strength, so the process should not be used for load-bearing members.

Some examples of solder types and their applications include tin–lead (general purpose), tin–zinc for joining aluminium, lead-silver for strength at higher than room temperature, cadmium–silver for strength at high temperatures, zinc–aluminium for aluminium and corrosion resistance, and tin–silver and tin–bismuth for electronics.

Solders

Soldering filler materials are available in many different alloys for differing applications. In electronics assembly, the eutectic alloy of 63 per cent tin and 37 per cent lead (or 60/40, which is almost identical in performance to the eutectic) has been the alloy of choice. Other alloys are used for plumbing, mechanical assembly, and other applications.

An eutectic formulation has several advantages for soldering; chief among these is the coincidence of the liquidus and solidus temperatures, i.e. the absence of a plastic phase. This allows for quicker wetting as the solder heats up, and quicker setup as the solder cools. A non-eutectic formulation must remain still as the temperature drops through the liquidus and solidus temperatures. Any differential movement during the plastic phase may result in cracks, giving an unreliable joint. Additionally, a

eutectic formulation has the lowest possible melting point, which minimises heat stress on electronic components during soldering. Common solder alloys are mixtures of tin and lead, respectively:
1. 63/37: melts at 183°C (361°F) (eutectic: the only mixture that melts at a point, instead of over a range).
2. 60/40: melts between 183°–190°C (361°–374°F).
3. 50/50: melts between 185°–215°C (365°–419°F).

Lead-free solders are suggested anywhere young children may come into contact with (since young children are likely to place things into their mouths), or for outdoor use where rain and other precipitation may wash the lead into the groundwater. Lead-free solder alloys melt around 250°C (482°F), depending on their composition.

For environmental reasons, 'no-lead' solders are becoming more widely used. Unfortunately most 'no-lead' solders are not eutectic formulations, making it more difficult to create reliable joints with them. Other common solders include low-temperature formulations (often containing bismuth), which are often used to join previously-soldered assemblies without unsoldering earlier connections, and high-temperature formulations (usually containing silver) which are used for high-temperature operation or for first assembly of items which must not become unsoldered during subsequent operations.

Alloying silver with other metals changes the melting point, adhesion and wetting characteristics, and tensile strength. Of all the brazing alloys, the silver solders have the greatest strength and the broadest applications.

Speciality alloys are available with properties such as higher strength, better electrical conductivity and higher corrosion resistance.

Flux

In high-temperature metal joining processes (welding, brazing and soldering), the primary purpose of flux is to prevent oxidation of the base and filler materials. Tin-lead solder, for example, attaches very well to copper, but poorly to copper oxides (which form quickly at soldering temperatures). Flux is nearly inert at room temperature, yet becomes strongly reductive when heated. This helps remove oxidation from the metals to be joined, and inhibits oxidation of the base and filler materials. Secondarily, flux acts as a wetting agent in the soldering process, reducing the surface tension of the molten solder and causing it to better wet out the parts to be joined.

Fluxes currently available in three basic formulations:
1. Water-soluble fluxes (no VOC's required for removal) are higher activity fluxes designed to be removed with water after soldering.
2. No-clean fluxes which are mild enough to not require removal at all due to the non-conductive and non-corrosive residue. Performance of the flux needs to be carefully evaluated; a very mild 'no-clean' flux might be perfectly acceptable for production equipment, but not give adequate performance for a poorly-controlled hand-soldering operation.
3. Traditional rosin fluxes are available in non-activated (R), mildly activated (RMA) and activated (RA) formulations. RA and RMA fluxes contain rosin combined with an activating agent, typically an acid, which increases the wettability of metals to which it is applied by removing existing oxides. The residue resulting from the use of RA flux is corrosive and must be cleaned off the piece being soldered. RMA flux is formulated to result in a residue which is not significantly corrosive, with cleaning being preferred but optional.

Basic Soldering Techniques

Soldering operations can be performed with hand tools, one joint at a time, or *en masse* on a production line. Hand soldering is typically performed with a soldering iron, soldering gun, or a torch, or occasionally a hot-air pencil. Sheetmetal work was traditionally done with 'soldering coppers' directly heated by a flame, with sufficient stored heat in the mass of the soldering copper to complete a joint; torches or electrically-heated soldering irons are more convenient. All soldered joints require the same elements of cleaning of the metal parts to be joined, fitting up the joint, heating the parts, applying flux, applying the filler, removing heat and holding the assembly still until the filler metal has completely solidified. Depending on the nature of flux material used, cleaning of the joints may be required after they have cooled.

The distinction between soldering and brazing is arbitrary, based on the melting temperature of the filler material. A temperature of 450°C is usually used as a practical cutoff. Different equipment and/or fixturing is usually required since (for instance) a soldering iron generally cannot achieve high enough temperatures for brazing. Practically speaking there is a significant difference between the two processes —brazing fillers have far more structural strength than solders, and are formulated for this as opposed to maximum electrical conductivity. Brazed connections are often as strong or nearly as strong as the parts they connect, even at elevated temperatures.

'Hard soldering' or 'silver soldering' (performed with high-temperature solder containing up to 40 per cent silver) is also often a form of brazing, since it involves filler materials with melting points in the vicinity of, or in excess of, 450°C. Although the term 'silver soldering' is used much more often than 'silver brazing', it may be technically incorrect depending on the exact melting point of the filler in use. In silver soldering (hard soldering), the goal is generally to give a beautiful, structurally sound joint, especially in the field of jewelry. Thus, the temperatures involved, and the usual use of a torch rather than an iron, would seem to indicate that the process should be referred to as 'brazing' rather than 'soldering', but the endurance of the 'soldering' appellation serves to indicate the arbitrary nature of the distinction (and the level of confusion) between the two processes.

Induction soldering is a process which is similar to brazing. The source of heat in induction soldering is induction heating by high-frequency AC current in a surrounding copper coil. This induces currents in the part being soldered, heat then being generated by resistive heating. The copper rings can be made to fit the part needed to be soldered for precision in the work piece. Induction soldering is a process in which a filler metal (solder) is placed between the facing surfaces of (to be joined) metals. The filler metal in this process is melted at a fairly low temperature. Fluxes are commonly used in induction soldering. This is a process which is particularly suitable for soldering continuously. The process is usually done with coils that wrap around a cylinder/pipe that needs to be soldered.

Some metals are easier to solder than others. Copper, silver, and gold are easy. Iron, mild steel and nickel are found to be more difficult. Because of their thin, strong oxide films, stainless steel and aluminium are even more difficult. Titanium, magnesium, cast irons, some high-carbon steels, ceramics, and graphite can be soldered but it involves a process similar to joining carbides. They are first plated with a suitable metallic element that induces interfacial bonding.

To simplify soldering, beginners are usually advised to apply the soldering iron and the solder separately to the joint, rather than the solder being applied direct to the iron. When sufficient solder is applied, the solder wire is removed. When the surfaces are adequately heated, the solder will flow around the joint. The iron is then removed from the joint.

Since non-eutectic solder alloys have a small plastic range, the joint must not be moved until the solder has cooled down through both the liquidus and solidus temperatures. Visually, a good solder joint will appear smooth and shiny, with the outline of the soldered wire clearly visible. A matte grey surface is a good indicator of a joint that was moved during soldering. Too little solder will result in a dry and unreliable joint; too much solder (the 'solder blob' very familiar to beginners) is not necessarily unsound, but tends to mean poor wetting. With some fluxes, flux residue remaining on the joint may need to be removed, using water, alcohol or other solvents compatible with the process. Excess solder and unconsumed flux and residue is sometimes wiped from the soldering iron tip between joints. The tip of the iron is kept wetted with solder (tinned) when hot to minimise oxidation and corrosion of the tip itself.

Hot-bar reflow

Hot-bar reflow is a selective soldering process where two prefluxed, solder coated parts are heated with heating element (called a thermode) to a sufficient temperature to melt the solder.

Pressure is applied through the whole process (usually 15 s) to ensure that components stay in place during cooling. The heating element is heated and cooled for each connection. Up to 4000 W can be used in the heating element allowing fast soldering, good results with connections requiring high energy.

Laser

Laser soldering is a technique where a ~30–50 W laser is used to melt and solder an electrical connection joint. Diode laser systems based on semiconductor junctions are used for this purpose. Wavelengths are typically 808 nm through 980 nm. The beam is delivered via an optical fibre to the workpiece, with fibre diameters 800 µm and smaller. Since the beam out of the end of the fibre diverges rapidly, lenses are used to create a suitable spot size on the workpiece at a suitable working distance. A wire feeder is used to supply solder.

Both lead-tin and silver-tin material can be soldered. Process recipes will differ depending on the alloy composition. For soldering 44-pin chip carriers to a board using soldering preforms, power levels were on the order of 10 Watts and solder times approximately 1 second. Low power levels can lead to incomplete wetting and the formation of voids, both of which can weaken the joint.

Pipe soldering

Copper pipe or tube, is commonly joined by soldering. Copper conducts heat away faster than a soldering iron or gun can provide, so a propane torch is most commonly used. Solder fittings, which are short sections of smooth pipe designed to slide over the outside of the mating tube, are usually used for copper joints. There are two types of fittings: end feed fittings which contain no solder, and solder ring fittings, in which there is a ring of solder in a small circular recess inside the fitting. As with all solder joints, all parts to be joined must be clean and oxide free.

Internal and external wire brushes are available for the common pipe and fitting sizes; emery cloth and wire-wool are frequently used as well, although metal wool products are discouraged, as they can contain oil, which would contaminate the joint.

Solder connections are usually considered the most difficult of the three methods of connecting copper tubing, but soldering copper is a very simple process, provided some basic conditions are provided:

1. The tubing and fittings must be cleaned to bare metal with no tarnish.
2. Any pressure which is formed by heating of the tubing must have an outlet.

Copper is only one material that is joined in this manner. Brass fittings are often used for valves or as a connection fitting between copper and other metals. Brass piping is soldered in this manner in the making of brass and some woodwind (saxophone and flute) musical instruments

Mechanical and aluminium soldering

A number of solder materials, primarily zinc alloys, are used for soldering aluminium metal and alloys and to some lesser extent steel and zinc. This mechanical soldering is similar to a low temperature brazing operation, in that the mechanical characteristics of the joint are reasonably good and it can be used for structural repairs of those materials.

The American welding society defines brazing as using filler metals with melting points over 450°C (842°F) or, by the traditional definition in the United States, above 800°F (427°C). Aluminium soldering alloys generally have melting temperatures around 730°F (388°C). This soldering/brazing operation can use a propane torch heat source.

These materials are often advertised as 'aluminium welding', but the process does not involve melting the base metal, and therefore is not properly a weld.

Stained glass soldering

Historically, stained glass soldering tips were copper, heated by being placed in a charcoal-burning brazier. Multiple tips were used; when one tip cooled down from use, it was placed back in the brazier of charcoal and the next tip was used.

More recently, electrically heated soldering irons are used. These are heated by a coil or ceramic heating element inside the tip of the iron. Different power ratings are available, and temperature can be controlled electronically. These characteristics allow longer beads to be run without interrupting the work to change tips. Soldering irons designed for electronic use are often effective though they are sometimes underpowered for the heavy copper and lead came used in stained glass work.

Tiffany type stainglass is made by gluing copper foil around the edges of the pieces of glass and then soldering them together. This method makes it possible to create three dimensional stainglass pieces.

Solderability

The solderability of a substrate is a measure of the ease with which a soldered joint can be made to that material.

Desoldering and Resoldering

Used solder contains some of the dissolved base metals and is unsuitable for reuse in making new joints. Once the solder's capacity for the base metal has been achieved it will no longer properly bond with the base metal, usually resulting in a brittle cold solder joint with a crystalline appearance.

It is good practice to remove solder from a joint prior to resoldering—desoldering braids or vacuum desoldering equipment (solder suckers) can be used. Desoldering wicks contain plenty of flux that will lift the contamination from the copper trace and any device leads that are present. This will leave a bright, shiny, clean junction to be resoldered.

The lower melting point of solder means it can be melted away from the base metal, leaving it mostly intact, though the outer layer will be 'tinned' with solder. Flux will remain which can easily be removed by abrasive or chemical processes. This tinned layer will allow solder to flow into a new joint, resulting in a new joint, as well as making the new solder flow very quickly and easily.

Lead-free Electronic Soldering

It is a common misconception that lead free soldering requires higher soldering temperatures than lead/tin solder; the wetting temperature in lead/tin solder is higher than the melting point and is the controlling factor. Wave soldering can proceed at the same temperature as previous lead/tin soldering. Nevertheless many new technical challenges have arisen with this endeavour; to reduce the melting point of tin based solder alloys various new alloys have had to be researched, with additives of copper, silver, bismuth as typical minor additives to reduce melting point and control other properties, additionally tin is a more corrosive metal, and can eventually lead to the failure of solder baths, etc.

Soldering Defects

Various problems may arise in the soldering process which lead to joints which are non functional either immediately or after a period of use. The most common defect when hand-soldering results from the parts being joined not exceeding the solder's liquidus temperature, resulting in a 'cold solder' joint. This is usually the result of the soldering iron being used to heat the solder directly, rather than the parts themselves. Properly done, the iron heats the parts to be connected, which in turn melt the solder, guaranteeing adequate heat in the joined parts for thorough wetting. In 'electronic' hand soldering solder the flux is embedded in the solder. Therefore heating the solder first may cause the flux to evaporate before it cleans the surfaces (pcb pad and component connection) being soldered.

An improperly selected or applied flux can cause joint failure, or if not properly cleaned off the joint, may corrode the metals in the joint over time and cause eventual joint failure. Without flux the joint may not be clean, or may be oxidised, resulting in an unsound joint.

Movement of metals being soldered before the solder has cooled will cause a highly unreliable cracked joint. In electronics' soldering terminology this is known as a 'dry' joint. It has a characteristically dull or grainy appearance immediately after the joint is made, rather than being smooth, bright and shiny. This appearance is caused by crystallisation of the liquid solder. A dry joint is weak mechanically and a poor conductor electrically.

Tools

Hand-soldering tools include the electric soldering iron, which has a variety of tips available ranging from blunt to very fine to chisel heads for hot-cutting plastics, and the soldering gun, which typically provides more power, giving faster heat-up and allowing larger parts to be soldered. Hot-air guns and pencils allow rework of component packages which cannot easily be performed with electric irons and guns. A soldering copper is a tool with a large copper head and a long handle which is heated in a blacksmith's forge fire and used to apply heat to sheet metal for soldering. Typical soldering coppers have heads weighing between one and four pounds. The head provides a thermal mass, which can store enough heat for soldering large areas between reheating the copper in the fire. The larger the head, the longer the working time it affords. Historically, soldering coppers were a standard tool used in auto bodywork, although body solder has been mostly superseded by spot welding for mechanical connection and nonmetallic fillers for contouring.

BRAZING

Brazing is a metal-joining process whereby a filler metal is heated above and distributed between two or more close-fitting parts by capillary action. The filler metal is brought slightly above its melting (liquidus) temperature while protected by a suitable atmosphere, usually a flux. It then flows over the base metal (known as wetting) and is then cooled to join the workpieces together. It is similar to soldering, except the temperatures used to melt the filler metal is above 450°C (842°F), or as traditionally defined in the United States, above 800°F (427°C).

In order to obtain high-quality brazed joints, parts must be closely fitted, and the base metals must be exceptionally clean and free of oxides. In most cases, joint clearances of 0.03 to 0.08 mm (0.0012 to 0.0031 inch) are recommended for the best capillary action and joint strength. However, in some brazing operations it is not uncommon to have joint clearances around 0.6 mm (0.024 inch). Cleanliness of the brazing surfaces is also of vital importance, as any contamination can cause poor wetting. The two main methods for cleaning parts, prior to brazing are chemical cleaning, and abrasive or mechanical cleaning. In the case of mechanical cleaning, it is of vital importance to maintain the proper surface roughness as wetting on a rough surface occurs much more readily than on a smooth surface of the same geometry.

Another consideration that cannot be overlooked is the effect of temperature and time on the quality of brazed joints. As the temperature of the braze alloy is increased, the alloying and wetting action of the filler metal increases as well. In general, the brazing temperature selected must be above the melting point of the filler metal. However, there are several factors that influence the joint designer's temperature selection. The best temperature is usually selected so as to: (i) be the lowest possible braze temperature, (ii) minimise any heat effects on the assembly, (iii) keep filler metal/base metal interactions to a minimum, and (iv) maximise the life of any fixtures or jigs used. In some cases, a higher temperature may be selected to allow for other factors in the design (e.g. to allow use of a different filler metal, or to control metallurgical effects, or to sufficiently remove surface contamination). The effect of time on the brazed joint primarily affects the extent to which the aforementioned effects are present; however, in general most production processes are selected to minimise brazing time and the associated costs. This is not always the case, however, since in some non-production settings, time and cost are secondary to other joint attributes (e.g. strength, appearance).

Flux: In the case of brazing operations not contained within an inert or reducing atmosphere environment (i.e. a furnace), flux is required to prevent oxides from forming while the metal is heated. The flux also serves the purpose of cleaning any contamination left on the brazing surfaces. Flux can be applied in any number of forms including flux paste, liquid, powder or pre-made brazing pastes that combine flux with filler metal powder. Flux can also be applied using brazing rods with a coating of flux, or a flux core. In either case, the flux flows into the joint when applied to the heated joint and is displaced by the molten filler metal entering the joint. Excess flux should be removed when the cycle is completed because flux left in the joint can lead to corrosion, impede joint inspection, and prevent further surface finishing operations. Phosphorus-containing brazing alloys can be self-fluxing when joining copper to copper. Fluxes are generally selected based on their performance on particular base metals. To be effective, the flux must be chemically compatible with both the base metal and the filler metal being used. Self-fluxing phosphorus filler alloys produce brittle phosphides if used on iron or nickel. As a general rule, longer brazing cycles should use less active fluxes than short brazing operations.

Filler materials: A variety of alloys are used as filler metals for brazing depending on the intended use or application method. In general, braze alloys are made up of 3 or more metals to form an alloy with the desired properties. The filler metal for a particular application is chosen based on its ability to wet the base metals, withstand the service conditions required, and melt at a lower temperature than the base metals or at a very specific temperature.

Braze alloy is generally available as rod, ribbon, powder, paste, cream, wire and preforms (such as stamped washers). Depending on the application, the filler material can be pre-placed at the desired location or applied during the heating cycle. For manual brazing, wire and rod forms are generally used as they are the easiest to apply while heating. In the case of furnace brazing, alloy is usually placed beforehand since the process is usually highly automated.

Common Techniques

Torch brazing

Torch brazing is by far the most common method of mechanised brazing in use. It is best used in small production volumes or in specialised operations, and in some countries, it accounts for a majority of the brazing taking place. There are three main categories of torch brazing in use: manual, machine, and automatic torch brazing.

1. Manual torch brazing: Manual torch brazing is a procedure where the heat is applied using a gas flame placed on or near the joint being brazed. The torch can either be hand held or held in a fixed position depending on if the operation is completely manual or has some level of automation. Manual brazing is most commonly used on small production volumes or in applications where the part size or configuration makes other brazing methods impossible. The main drawback is the high labour cost associated with the method as well as the operator skill required to obtain quality brazed joints. The use of flux or self-fluxing material is required to prevent oxidation.
2. Machine torch brazing: Machine torch brazing is commonly used where a repetitive braze operation is being carried out. This method is a mix of both automated and manual operations with an operator often placing brazes material, flux and jigging parts while the machine mechanism carries out the actual braze. The advantage of this method is that it reduces the high labour and skill requirement of manual brazing. The use of flux is also required for this method as there is no protective atmosphere, and it is best suited to small to medium production volumes.
3. Automatic torch brazing: Automatic torch brazing is a method that almost eliminates the need for manual labour in the brazing operation, except for loading and unloading of the machine. The main advantages of this method are: a high production rate, uniform braze quality, and reduced operating cost. The equipment used is essentially the same as that used for machine torch brazing, with the main difference being that the machinery replaces the operator in the part preparation.

Furnace brazing

Furnace brazing is a semiautomatic process used widely in industrial brazing operations due to its adaptability to mass production and use of unskilled labour. There are many advantages of furnace brazing over other heating methods that make it ideal for mass production. One main advantage is the ease with which it can produce large numbers of small parts that are easily jigged or self-locating. The process also offers the benefits of a controlled heat cycle (allowing use of parts that might distort under localised heating) and no need for post braze cleaning. Common atmospheres used include: inert, reducing or vacuum atmospheres all of which protect the part from oxidation. Some other advantages include: low unit cost when used in mass production, close temperature control, and the ability to braze multiple joints at once. Furnaces are typically heated using either electric, gas or oil depending on the type of furnace and application. However, some of the disadvantages of this method include: high capital equipment cost, more difficult design considerations and high power consumption (Fig. 19.1).

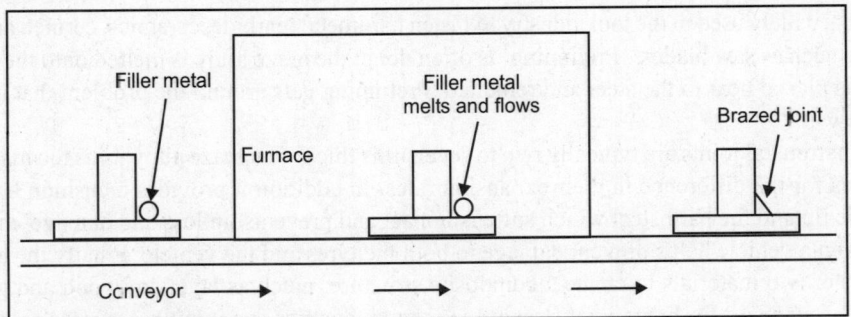

Fig. 19.1. Furnace brazing schematic.

There are four main types of furnaces used in brazing operations: batch type; continuous; retort with controlled atmosphere; and vacuum.

1. Batch type: Batch type furnaces have relatively low initial equipment costs and heat each part load separately. It is capable of being turned on and off at will which reduces operating expenses when not in use. These furnaces are well suited to medium to large volume production and offer a large degree of flexibility in type of parts that can be brazed. Either controlled atmospheres or flux can be used to control oxidation and cleanliness of parts.
2. Continuous type: Continuous type furnaces are best suited to a steady flow of similar-sized parts through the furnace. These furnaces are often conveyor fed, allowing parts to be moved through the hot zone at a controlled speed. It is common to use either controlled atmosphere or pre-applied flux in continuous furnaces. In particular, these furnaces offer the benefit of very low manual labour requirements and so are best suited to large scale production operations.
3. Retort-type: Retort-type furnaces differ from other batch-type furnaces in that they make use of a sealed lining called a 'retort'. The retort is generally sealed with either a gasket or is welded shut and filled completely with the desired atmosphere and then heated externally by conventional heating elements. Due to the high temperatures involved, the retort usually made of heat resistant alloys that resist oxidation. Retort furnaces are often either used in a batch or semi-continuous versions.
4. Vacuum furnaces: Vacuum furnaces is a relatively economical method of oxide prevention and is most often used to braze materials with very stable oxides (aluminium, titanium and zirconium) that cannot be brazed in atmosphere furnaces. Vacuum brazing is also used heavily with refractory materials and other exotic alloy combinations unsuited to atmosphere furnaces. Due to the absence of flux or a reducing atmosphere, the part cleanliness is critical when brazing in a vacuum. The three main types of vacuum furnace are: single-wall hot retort, double-walled hot retort, and cold-wall retort. Typical vacuum levels for brazing range from pressures of 1.3 to 0.13 pascals (10^{-2} to 10^{-3} Torr) to 0.00013 Pa (10^{-6} Torr) or lower. Vacuum furnaces are most commonly batch-type, and they are suited to medium and high production volumes.

Silver brazing

Silver brazing, colloquially (however, incorrectly) known as a silver soldering or hard soldering, is brazing using a silver alloy based filler. These silver alloys consist of many different percentages of silver and other metals, such as copper, zinc and cadmium.

Brazing is widely used in the tool industry to fasten hardmetal (carbide, ceramics, cermet, and similar) tips to tools such as saw blades. 'Pretinning' is often done: the braze alloy is melted onto the hardmetal tip, which is placed next to the steel and remelted. Pretinning gets around the problem that hardmetals are hard to wet.

Brazed hardmetal joints are typically two to seven mils thick. The braze alloy joins the materials and compensates for the difference in their expansion rates. In addition it provides a cushion between the hard carbide tip and the hard steel which softens impact and prevents tip loss and damage, much as the suspension on a vehicle helps prevent damage to both the tyres and the vehicle. Finally the braze alloy joins the other two materials to create a composite structure, much as layers of wood and glue create plywood. The standard for braze joint strength in many industries is a joint that is stronger than either base material, so that when under stress, one or other of the base materials fails before the joint.

One special silver brazing method is called pinbrazing or pin brazing. It has been developed especially for connecting cables to railway track or for cathodic protection installations. The method uses a silver- and flux-containing brazing pin which is melted down in the eye of a cable lug. The equipment is normally powered from batteries.

Braze welding

Braze welding, also known as fillet brazing, is the use of a bronze or brass filler rod coated with flux to join steel workpieces. The equipment needed for braze welding is basically identical to the equipment used in brazing. Since braze welding usually requires more heat than brazing, acetylene or methylacetylene-propadiene (MPS) gas fuel is commonly used. The American Welding Society states that the name comes from the fact that no capillary action is used.

Braze welding has many advantages over fusion welding. It allows the joining of dissimilar metals, minimisation of heat distortion, and can reduce the need for extensive pre-heating. Additionally, since the metals joined are not melted in the process, the components retain their original shape; edges and contours are not eroded or changed by the formation of a fillet. Another side effect of braze welding is the elimination of stored-up stresses that are often present in fusion welding. This is extremely important in the repair of large castings. The disadvantages are the loss of strength when subjected to high temperatures and the inability to withstand high stresses.

Carbide, cermet and ceramic tips are plated and then joined to steel to make tipped band saws. The plating acts as a braze alloy.

Cast iron 'welding'

The 'welding' of cast iron is usually a brazing operation, with a filler rod made chiefly of nickel being used although true welding with cast iron rods is also available. Ductile cast iron pipe may be also 'cadwelded', a process which connects joints by means of a small copper wire fused into the iron when previously ground down to the bare metal, parallel to the iron joints being formed as per hub pipe with neoprene gasket seals. The purpose behind this operation is to use electricity along the copper for keeping underground pipes warm in cold climates.

Vacuum brazing

Vacuum brazing is a materials joining technique that offers significant advantages: extremely clean, superior, flux-free braze joints of high integrity and strength. The process can be expensive because it must be performed inside a vacuum chamber vessel. Temperature uniformity is maintained on the work piece when heating in a vacuum, greatly reducing residual stresses due to slow heating and cooling cycles. This, in turn, can significantly improve the thermal and mechanical properties of the material, thus providing unique heat treatment capabilities. One such capability is heat-treating or age-hardening the workpiece while performing a metal-joining process, all in a single furnace thermal cycle.

Vacuum brazing is often conducted in a furnace; this means that several joints can be made at once because the whole workpiece reaches the brazing temperature. The heat is transferred using radiation, as many other methods cannot be used in a vacuum.

Dip brazing

Dip brazing is especially suited for brazing aluminium because air is excluded, thus preventing the formation of oxides. The parts to be joined are fixtured and the brazing compound applied to the mating surfaces, typically in slurry form. Then the assemblies are dipped into a bath of molten salt (typically NaCl, KCl and other compounds) which functions both as heat transfer medium and flux.

Heating methods

There are many heating methods available to accomplish brazing operations. The most important factor in choosing a heating method is achieving efficient transfer of heat throughout the joint and doing so within the heat capacity of the individual base metals used. The geometry of the braze joint is also a crucial factor to consider, as is the rate and volume of production required. The easiest way to categorise brazing methods is to group them by heating method, which are given below:

1. Torch brazing.
2. Furnace brazing.
3. Induction brazing.
4. Dip brazing.
5. Resistance brazing.
6. Infrared brazing.
7. Blanket brazing.
8. Electron beam and laser brazing.
9. Braze welding.

Advantages and disadvantages

Brazing has many advantages over other metal-joining techniques, such as welding. Since brazing does not melt the base metal of the joint, it allows much tighter control over tolerances and produces a clean joint without the need for secondary finishing. Additionally, dissimilar metals and nonmetals (i.e. metalised ceramics) can be brazed. In general, brazing also produces less thermal distortion than welding due to the uniform heating of a brazed piece. Complex and multi-part assemblies can be brazed cost-effectively. Another advantage is that the brazing can be coated or clad for protective purposes. Finally, brazing is easily adapted to mass production and it is easy to automate because the individual process parameters are less sensitive to variation.

One of the main disadvantages is: the lack of joint strength as compared to a welded joint due to the softer filler metals used. The strength of the brazed joint is likely to be less than that of the base metal(s) but greater than the filler metal. Another disadvantage is that brazed joints can be damaged under high service temperatures. Brazed joints require a high degree of base-metal cleanliness when done in an industrial setting. Some brazing applications require the use of adequate fluxing agents to control cleanliness. The joint colour is often different than that of the base metal, creating an aesthetic disadvantage.

WELDING

Welding is a fabrication or sculptural process that joins materials, usually metals or thermoplastics, by causing coalescence. This is often done by melting the workpieces and adding a filler material to form a pool of molten material (the weld pool) that cools to become a strong joint, with pressure sometimes used in conjunction with heat, or by itself, to produce the weld. This is in contrast with soldering and brazing, which involve melting a lower-melting-point material between the workpieces to form a bond between them, without melting the workpieces.

Many different energy sources can be used for welding, including a gas flame, an electric arc, a laser, an electron beam, friction, and ultrasound. While often an industrial process, welding can be done in many different environments, including open air, under water and in outer space. Regardless of location, welding remains dangerous, and precautions are taken to avoid burns, electric shock, eye damage, poisonous fumes, and overexposure to ultraviolet light.

Processes Involved in Welding

Arc welding

These processes use a welding power supply to create and maintain an electric arc between an electrode and the base material to melt metals at the welding point. They can use either direct (DC) or alternating (AC) current, and consumable or non-consumable electrodes. The welding region is sometimes protected by some type of inert or semi-inert gas, known as a shielding gas, and filler material is sometimes used as well. To supply the electrical energy necessary for arc welding processes, a number of different power supplies can be used. The most common welding power supplies are constant current power supplies and constant voltage power supplies. In arc welding, the length of the arc is directly related to the voltage, and the amount of heat input is related to the current. Constant current power supplies are most often used for manual welding processes such as gas tungsten arc welding and shielded metal arc welding, because they maintain a relatively constant current even as the voltage varies. This is important because in manual welding, it can be difficult to hold the electrode perfectly steady, and as a result, the arc length and thus voltage tend to fluctuate.

Processes

One of the most common types of arc welding is shielded metal arc welding (SMAW); it is also known as manual metal arc welding (MMA) or stick welding. Electric current is used to strike an arc between the base material and consumable electrode rod, which is made of steel and is covered with a flux that protects the weld area from oxidation and contamination by producing carbon dioxide (CO_2) gas during the welding process. The electrode core itself acts as filler material, making a separate filler unnecessary.

The process is versatile and can be performed with relatively inexpensive equipment, making it well suited to shop jobs and field work. An operator can become reasonably proficient with a modest amount of training and can achieve mastery with experience. Weld times are rather slow, since the consumable electrodes must be frequently replaced and because slag, the residue from the flux, must be chipped away after welding. Furthermore, the process is generally limited to welding ferrous materials, though special electrodes have made possible the welding of cast iron, nickel, aluminium, copper, and other metals. Gas metal arc welding (GMAW), also known as metal inert gas or MIG welding, is a semiautomatic or automatic process that uses a continuous wire feed as an electrode and an inert or semi-inert gas mixture to protect the weld from contamination. Since the electrode is continuous, welding speeds are greater for GMAW than for SMAW.

A related process, flux-cored arc welding (FCAW), uses similar equipment but uses wire consisting of a steel electrode surrounding a powder fill material. This cored wire is more expensive than the standard solid wire and can generate fumes and/or slag, but it permits even higher welding speed and greater metal penetration. Gas tungsten arc welding (GTAW), or tungsten inert gas (TIG) welding, is a manual welding process that uses a nonconsumable tungsten electrode, an inert or semi-inert gas mixture, and a separate filler material. Especially useful for welding thin materials, this method is characterised by a stable arc and high quality welds, but it requires significant operator skill and can only be accomplished at relatively low speeds.

GTAW can be used on nearly all weldable metals, though it is most often applied to stainless steel and light metals. It is often used when quality welds are extremely important, such as in bicycle, aircraft and naval applications. A related process, plasma arc welding, also uses a tungsten electrode but uses plasma gas to make the arc. The arc is more concentrated than the GTAW arc, making transverse control more critical and thus generally restricting the technique to a mechanised process.

Submerged arc welding (SAW) is a high-productivity welding method in which the arc is struck beneath a covering layer of flux. This increases arc quality, since contaminants in the atmosphere are blocked by the flux. The slag that forms on the weld generally comes off by itself, and combined with the use of a continuous wire feed, the weld deposition rate is high. Working conditions are much improved over other arc welding processes, since the flux hides the arc and almost no smoke is produced. The process is commonly used in industry, especially for large products and in the manufacture of welded pressure vessels. Other arc welding processes include atomic hydrogen welding, electroslag welding, electrogas welding, and stud arc welding.

Gas welding

The most common gas welding process is oxyfuel welding, also known as oxyacetylene welding. It is one of the oldest and most versatile welding processes, but in recent years it has become less popular in industrial applications. It is still widely used for welding pipes and tubes, as well as repair work.

The equipment is relatively inexpensive and simple, generally employing the combustion of acetylene in oxygen to produce a welding flame temperature of about 3100°C. The flame, since it is less concentrated than an electric arc, causes slower weld cooling, which can lead to greater residual stresses and weld distortion, though it eases the welding of high alloy steels. A similar process, generally called oxyfuel cutting, is used to cut metals.

Resistance welding

Resistance welding involves the generation of heat by passing current through the resistance caused by the contact between two or more metal surfaces. Small pools of molten metal are formed at the weld area as high current (1000–1,00,000 A) is passed through the metal. In general, resistance welding methods are efficient and cause little pollution, but their applications are somewhat limited and the equipment cost can be high.

Spot welding is a popular resistance welding method used to join overlapping metal sheets of up to 3 mm thick. Two electrodes are simultaneously used to clamp the metal sheets together and to pass current through the sheets. The advantages of the method include efficient energy use, limited workpiece deformation, high production rates, easy automation, and no required filler materials. Weld strength is significantly lower than with other welding methods, making the process suitable for only certain applications. It is used extensively in the automotive industry—ordinary cars can have several thousand spot welds made by industrial robots. A specialised process, called shot welding, can be used to spot weld stainless steel. Like spot welding, seam welding relies on two electrodes to apply pressure and current to join metal sheets.

However, instead of pointed electrodes, wheel-shaped electrodes roll along and often feed the workpiece, making it possible to make long continuous welds. In the past, this process was used in the manufacture of beverage cans, but now its uses are more limited. Other resistance welding methods include butt welding, flash welding, projection welding, and upset welding.

Energy beam

Energy beam welding methods, namely laser beam welding and electron beam welding, are relatively new processes that have become quite popular in high production applications. The two processes are quite similar, differing most notably in their source of power. Laser beam welding employs a highly focused laser beam, while electron beam welding is done in a vacuum and uses an electron beam. Both have a very high energy density, making deep weld penetration possible and minimising the size of the weld area. Both processes are extremely fast, and are easily automated, making them highly productive. The primary disadvantages are their very high equipment costs (though these are decreasing) and a susceptibility to thermal cracking. Developments in this area include laser-hybrid welding, which uses principles from both laser beam welding and arc welding for even better weld properties, and X-ray welding.

Solid-state

Like the first welding process, forge welding, some modern welding methods do not involve the melting of the materials being joined. One of the most popular, ultrasonic welding, is used to connect thin sheets or wires made of metal or thermoplastic by vibrating them at high frequency and under high pressure. The equipment and methods involved are similar to that of resistance welding, but instead of electric current, vibration provides energy input. Welding metals with this process does not involve melting the materials; instead, the weld is formed by introducing mechanical vibrations horizontally under pressure. When welding plastics, the materials should have similar melting temperatures, and the vibrations are introduced vertically. Ultrasonic welding is commonly used for making electrical connections out of aluminium or copper, and it is also a very common polymer welding process.

Another common process, explosion welding, involves the joining of materials by pushing them together under extremely high pressure. The energy from the impact plasticises the materials, forming a weld, even though only a limited amount of heat is generated. The process is commonly used for welding dissimilar materials, such as the welding of aluminium with steel in ship hulls or compound plates. Other solid-state welding processes include friction welding (including friction stir welding), electromagnetic pulse welding, coextrusion welding, cold welding, diffusion welding, exothermic welding, high frequency welding, hot pressure welding, induction welding, and roll welding.

Welds in Steel

Figure 19.2 shows a cross-section of a weld between two plates. Molten steel is produced between the two plates in the welding process and during this melting and then solidification heat is conducted into the plates on either side of the weld. The term heat-affected zone is used to describe those parts of the plates which have their temperatures raised to above the critical point A_1.

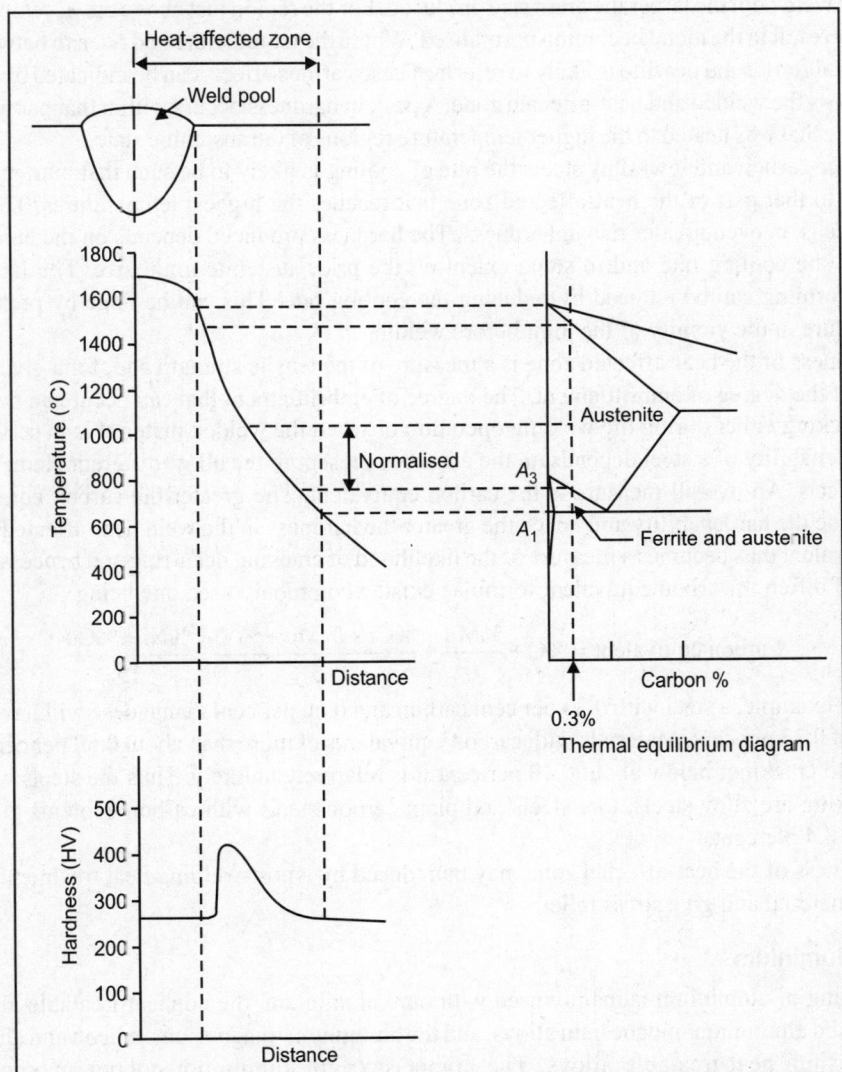

Fig. 19.2. The effect of welding heat on the hardness of a 0.3 per cent carbon steel.

In the weld pool the metal shows the typical cast-metal structure of columnar grains. In the case of a multi-pass weld deposit each pass forms a heat-affected zone in the weld metal immediately below it. The result is a more complex microstructure.

In the heat-affected zone there will be a wide variation in temperature as illustrated in Fig. 19.2. For a 0.3 per cent carbon steel, close to the weld pool the temperature will rise to well above the A_3 temperature, while at the edge of the heat-affected zone it will be just A_1. Thus, close to the weld pool the metal will have been heated into the austenitic state while near the edge of the heat-affected zone it will be ferrite plus austenite. With the low-carbon steel where the temperature rises to above A_3 grain growth occurs—the closer to the weld pool the larger the grain size produced. For the region just above the A_3 temperature the cooling may result in the metal becoming normalised. Where the temperature had risen to between A_1 and A_3 the original ferrite and pearlite is likely to reform. These various effects can be indicated by a hardness traverse across the welded and heat-affected zone. A peak in hardness occurs within that part of the heat-affected zone that was heated to the higher temperature regions of the austenitic state.

For higher-carbon and low-alloy steels the rate of cooling is likely to be such that martensite forms, particularly in that part of the heat-affected zone that reaches the highest temperatures. The result of such changes is an even greater rise in hardness. The hardness produced depends on the harden ability of the steel, the cooling rate and to some extent on the prior austenite grain size. The likelihood of martensite forming can be reduced by reducing the cooling rate. This can be done by preheating the whole structure in the vicinity of the joint before welding.

The hardness of the heat-affected zone is a measure of the tensile strength and, for a given alloy, an indication of the degree of embrittlement. The degree of embrittlement that can occur can be sufficient to cause cracking either during the welding operation or when the welded material is in service.

The hardenability of a steel depends on the elements present in the alloy, different elements having different effects. An overall measure is the carbon equivalent. The greater the carbon equivalent the greater will be the hardenability and hence the greater the hardness in the weld heat-affected zone. The carbon equivalent thus becomes a measure of the likelihood of cracking occurring and hence weldability. A number of different carbon equivalent formulae exist, a commonly used one being:

$$\text{Carbon equivalent} = \%C + \frac{\%Mn}{6} + \frac{\%Cr + \%Mo + \%V}{5} + \frac{\%Ni + \%Cu}{15}$$

Thus, for example, a steel with 0.23 per cent carbon and 0.60 per cent manganese will have a carbon equivalent of 0.33 per cent. Materials with carbon equivalents of more than about 0.50 per cent are very susceptible to cracking; below about 0.40 per cent it is relatively unlikely. Thus the steels with a high risk of cracking are alloy steels, tool steels and plain carbon steels with carbon contents greater than about 0.3 to 0.4 per cent.

The hardness of the heat-affected zone may be reduced by a post-welding heat treatment. This can temper the material and give stress relief.

Welds in Aluminium

Fusion welding of aluminium is mainly used with pure aluminium, the nonheat-treatable aluminium–manganese and aluminium–magnesium alloys, and the aluminium–magnesium–silicon and aluminium–zinc–magnesium heat-treatable alloys. The higher strength aluminium–copper–magnesium and duraluminium alloys cannot be effectively fusion-welded and such alloys, which are mainly used for aircraft structures, are normally joined by riveting.

Figure 19.3 shows the results of a hardness traverse of a weld between two plates of a nonheat-treatable aluminium alloy. Within the heat-affected zone the alloy is fully or partially annealed by the temperatures produced during the welding. The result is that the work-hardened material is much softer in the weld region than in the unaffected material. Since the tensile strength is related to the hardness this means there is a drop in strength. This effect is in the main irreversible, although the strength of the weld pool area can be improved by rolling or hammering.

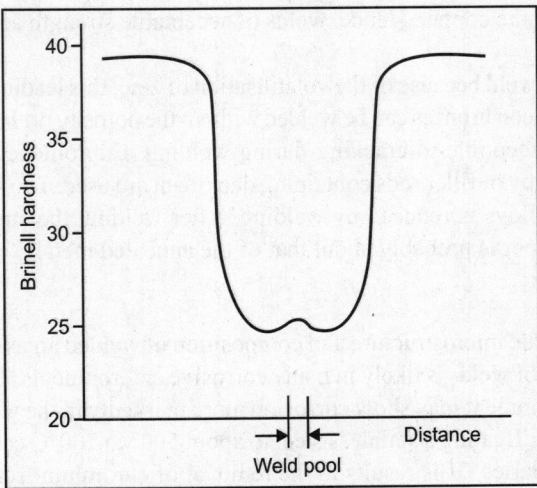

Fig. 19.3. Hardness of weld zone in a nonheat-treatable aluminium alloy.

Figure 19.4 shows the results of a hardness traverse of a weld between two plates of a heat-treatable aluminium alloy. Softening and a reduction in tensile strength occur within the heat-affected zone. However, the strength may be almost completely recoverable by solution treatment and ageing of the component.

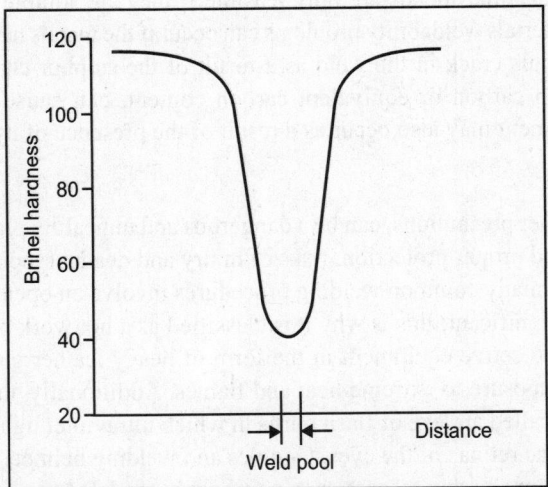

Fig. 19.4. Hardness of weld zone in a heat-treatable aluminium alloy.

Welds in Copper

Copper oxide reacts with hydrogen, at temperatures above about 500°C, to give copper and steam. A consequence of this is that the steam gives rise to porosity in the weld pool, as well as causing fissures to develop and embrittlement to occur in the heat-affected zone close to the weld pool. To reduce this effect the copper has to be deoxidised prior to welding. This can be achieved by the presence of small amounts of phosphorus in the copper. Hence, welds of acceptable strength are possible in phosphorus-deoxidised copper.

Brasses are difficult to weld because of the volatilisation of zinc, this leading to porosity. Tin bronzes, aluminium bronzes and silicon bronzes can be welded without the porosity problem occurring. Aluminium bronzes, however, are susceptible to cracking during welding. Cupronickels can be welded without porosity if a deoxidised alloy or filler rods containing deoxidant are used. The strength of work hardened or age-hardened copper alloys is reduced by welding. After welding the strength of a fusion welded joint in a hard temper copper is probably about that of the annealed metal.

Corrosion of Welds

Because of differences in the microstructure and composition of welded areas compared with the parent metal, selective corrosion of welds is likely in many corrosive environments. Thus welded carbon steels exposed to a marine environment may show corrosion more markedly in the weld metal or heat-affected zone than the parent metal. Heating a stainless steel to about 500° to 700°C can lead to the precipitation of carbides at grain boundaries. This results in the removal of chromium from grains to the boundary and hence a reduction in corrosion resistance. The effect is known as weld decay since such effects occur during the welding of stainless steels. The defect can be overcome by heat treating the steel or using a stabilised stainless steel, i.e. one which includes niobium or titanium.

Weldability

The term weldability is used to describe the ease with which a sound weld can be made between materials. Sound welds between dissimilar metals are only feasible if they are soluble in each other. With both similar and dissimilar materials weldability problems can occur if the metals have a high sulphur content. This is because such metals crack in the weld as a result of the sulphur causing low strength in the solidifying metal. A high carbon or equivalent carbon content, can cause problems as a result of embrittlement. Embrittlement may also occur as a result of the presence of hydrogen.

Safety Issues

Welding, without the proper precautions, can be a dangerous and unhealthy practice. However, with the use of new technology and proper protection, risks of injury and death associated with welding can be greatly reduced. Because many common welding procedures involve an open electric arc or flame, the risk of burns and fire is significant; this is why it is classified as a hot work process. To prevent them, welders wear personal protective equipment in the form of heavy leather gloves and protective long sleeve jackets to avoid exposure to extreme heat and flames. Additionally, the brightness of the weld area leads to a condition called arc eye or flash burns in which ultraviolet light causes inflammation of the cornea and can burn the retinas of the eyes. Goggles and welding helmets with dark face plates are worn to prevent this exposure, and in recent years, new helmet models have been produced that feature a face plate that self-darkens upon exposure to high amounts of UV light. To protect bystanders, translucent welding curtains often surround the welding area. These curtains, made of a polyvinyl chloride plastic film, shield nearby workers from exposure to the UV light from the electric arc, but should not be used to replace the filter glass used in helmets.

Welders are also often exposed to dangerous gases and particulate matter. Processes like flux-cored arc welding and shielded metal arc welding produce smoke containing particles of various types of oxides. The size of the particles in question tends to influence the toxicity of the fumes, with smaller particles presenting a greater danger. This is due to the fact that smaller particles have the ability to cross the blood brain barrier. Additionally, many processes produce fumes and various gases, most commonly carbon dioxide, ozone and heavy metals, that can prove dangerous without proper ventilation and training.

Exposure to manganese welding fumes, for example, even at low levels (<0.2 mg/m^3), may lead to neurological problems or to damage to the lungs, liver, kidneys, or central nervous system. Furthermore, because the use of compressed gases and flames in many welding processes poses an explosion and fire risk, some common precautions include limiting the amount of oxygen in the air and keeping combustible materials away from the workplace.

FASTENER

A fastener is a hardware device that mechanically joins or affixes two or more objects together. Fasteners can also be used to close a container such as a bag, a box or an envelope; or they may involve keeping together the sides of an opening of flexible material, attaching a lid to a container, etc. There are also special-purpose closing devices, e.g. a bread clip. Fasteners used in these manners are often temporary, in that they may be fastened and unfastened repeatedly.

Some types of woodworking joints make use of separate internal reinforcements, such as dowels or biscuits, which in a sense can be considered fasteners within the scope of the joint system, although on their own they are not general purpose fasteners. Furniture supplied in flat-pack form often uses cam dowels locked by cam locks, also known as conformat fasteners.

Items like a rope, string, wire (e.g. metal wire, possibly coated with plastic, or multiple parallel wires kept together by a plastic strip coating), cable, chain, or plastic wrap may be used to mechanically join objects; but are not generally categorised as fasteners because they have additional common uses. Likewise, hinges and springs may join objects together, but are ordinarily not considered fasteners because their primary purpose is to allow articulation rather than rigid affixment.

Other alternative methods of joining materials include crimping, welding, soldering, brazing, taping, gluing, cementing, or the use of other adhesives. The use of force may also be used, such as with magnets, vacuum (like suction cups) or even friction.

Fastening Systems

The choice of fastener will depend on a number of factors:
1. Environmental, e.g. temperature, corrosive conditions.
2. Nature of the external loading on the fastener, e.g. tension, compression, shear, cyclic, impact, and its magnitude.
3. Life and service requirements, e.g. frequent assembly and disassembly.
4. Design of the components being joined and types of material involved.
5. Quantity of fasteners required and their cost.

Fasteners provide a clamping force between two pieces of material. A wide variation exists in types of fastener and the materials used for making them. The types of fastener available can be classified as threaded, non-threaded and special-purpose. Steel is probably the most common material used, although aluminium alloys, brass and nickel are among other metals used. Aluminium alloy fasteners have the advantage over steel of being much lighter, nonmagnetic and more corrosion resistant. Nickel has the particular advantage of strength at high temperatures.

With a threaded fastener, the clamping force holding the two pieces of material together is produced by a torque being applied to the fastener and being maintained during the service life of the fastener. Bolts mated with nuts, and screws with threads in the material, are examples of threaded fasteners.

Nails, rivets and pins are examples of non-threaded fasteners. Nails are used extensively for making joints between pieces of wood. Rivets, however, are used for joining dissimilar or similar materials, both metallic and nonmetallic. Both nails and rivets are low-cost fasteners designed for making joints which are intended to be permanent and non demounted.

Fatigue properties of fastened joints

The use, for example, of bolts or rivets as fasteners for joints can introduce fretting damage. Fretting is the wear process that occurs at the areas of contact of two metals undergoing small amplitude cyclic slip. On steels this damage may be visible as the red oxide of iron, on aluminium as black oxides. The damage is referred to as galling or scuffing. Such damage can lower the fatigue by factors as high as three for aluminium alloys. One form of anti-fret treatment is to separate the metal surfaces by using polytetrafluoroethylene (PTFE) shims or a coating of a paint containing the solid lubricant molybdenum disulphide.

Rail Fastening System

A rail fastening system is a means of fixing rails to railroad ties (United States) or sleepers (international). The terms rail anchors, tie plates, chairs and track fasteners are used to refer to parts or all of a rail fastening system. Various types of fastening have been used over the years.

Spikes and screws

Rail spikes

A rail spike (also known as a cut spike or crampon) is a large nail with an offset head that is used to secure rails and base plates to railroad ties in the track.

A rail spike is roughly chisel shaped and with a flat edged point; the spike is driven with the edge against the grain, which gives greater resistance to loosening. The main function is to keep the rail in gauge. When attaching tie plates the attachment is made as strong as possible, whereas when attaching a rail to tie or tie plate the spike is not normally required to provide a strong vertical force, allowing the rail some freedom of movement.

Screw spikes

A screw spike, rail screw (or lag bolt) is a large (~6″ length, slightly under 1″ diameter) metal screw used to fix a tie plate or fasten rail. Screw spikes are fixed into a hole bored in the sleeper. The screw spike has a higher cost to manufacture that the rail spike but has the advantage of greater fixing power; approximately twice that of a rail spike, and can be used in combination with spring washers.

Fang bolts

Fang bolts have also been used for fixing rails or chairs to sleepers; the fang bolt is a bolt inserted through a hole in the sleeper with a fanged nut that bites into the lower surface of the sleeper. For fastening flat bottomed rails an upper lipped washer can be used to grip the edge of the rail. They are more resistant to loosening by vibrations and movement of the rail. They are thought more effective than spikes and screws and so are used in positions such as switch (point) tieplates, and on sharp curves.

Spring spikes

Spring spikes, (or elastic rail spikes) are used with flat bottomed rail, baseplates and wooden sleepers; the spring spike holds the rail down and prevents tipping, and also secures the baseplate to the sleeper. The Macbeth spike (tradename) is a two pronged U shaped staple like spike bent at the bend so that it appears M shaped when viewed side on. Inverted J shaped single pointed spikes have also been used.

Chairs

Chairs have been fixed to the sleeper using wooden spikes (trenails), screws, fang-bolts or spikes.

Tie plates

A tie plate, baseplate or sole plate is a steel plate used on rail tracks between flanged T rail and the crossties. The tie plate increases bearing area and holds the rail to correct gauge. They are fastened to wooden ties by means of spikes or bolts through holes in the plate.

The part of the plate under the rail base is tapered, setting the cant of the rail, an inward rotation from the vertical. The usual slope is one in forty (1.4 degrees). The top surface of the plate has one or two shoulders that fit against the edges of the base of the rail. The double-shoulder type is currently used. Older single-shoulder types were adaptable for various rail widths, with the single shoulder positioned on the outside (field side) of the rails. Most plates are slightly wider on the field side, without which the plates tend to cut more into the outsides of the tie, reducing cant angle.

Clips

A variety of different types of heavy-duty clips are used to fasten the rails to the underlying baseplate, one common one being the Pandrol fastener (Pandrol clip), named after its maker, which is shaped like a stubby paperclip. Another one is the Vossloh Tension Clamp. The newer Pandrol fastclip is applied at right angles to the rail. Because the clip is captive, it has to be installed at the time of manufacture of the concrete sleeper.

Chapter 20
Mechanical and Nondestructive Tests

INTRODUCTION

The subject of mechanical testing of metals is an important one to both the engineer and the metallurgist. During the seventeenth century Robert Hooke established the famous law named after him, which forms the basis of many mechanical tests, but it was the industrial revolution that provided the impetus to the study of mechanical testing. The development of modern transport, particularly the aeroplane, is associated with a vast increase in varieties of alloys and the necessity for making full use of their properties. More recently, the development of nuclear energy has stimulated the need for entirely new metals and alloys. Today, more attention is being given to the interpretation of the test results in terms of service, performance, but this is hampered by the fact that some of the tests are of a purely empirical nature. Nevertheless, many of these have been proved to give reliable indications of the ability of the material to perform certain types of duty.

Mechanical tests are employed, too, in investigational work in order to obtain data for use in design; also for acceptance work, the main purpose of which is to check whether the material meets the specification. For this latter purpose the tests should yield the information accurately, rapidly and economically.

Mechanical properties indicate the response of a metal or alloy to elastic and plastic deformations under the applied forces. The success of metal forming operations is related to the mechanical properties of the metals being formed, and many finished products are accepted or rejected on the basis of their mechanical properties. Evaluation of these properties is essential for proper selection of materials for the given service requirements. There are many tests to determine mechanical properties. However, some of the important tests such as tensile test (tension), compression test, hardness test, impact test, fatigue test and creep test are described in this chapter.

In the UK the British Standards Institution (BSI) provides facilities for the drafting and publication of specifications, which frequently contain clauses relating to method of manufacture, chemical composition, heat-treatment, the selection of test pieces and mechanical tests. The Air Ministry also issues DTD specifications of aircraft materials not dealt with by the BSI. In America the American Society for Testing Materials (ASTM) publish yearly proceedings which contain research papers and tentative standards. The ASTM standards are published every three years and contain standard specifications and methods of testing adopted by the Society. The New International Association for Testing Materials provides means for discussing tests and issuing papers in English, French and German, but it does not put out definite specifications.

HARDNESS

The property of hardness largely determines the resistance to scratching, wear, penetration, machinability and the ability to cut. Some thirty methods have been used for measuring hardness, but only four important tests can be considered here.

Brinell Test

The Brinell test consists of indenting the surface of the metal by a hardened steel ball under a load, and measuring the average diameter of the impression with a low-power portable microscope fitted with a scale. The spherical area is calculated from the diameter of the impression. The Brinell number, H, is:

$$H = \frac{Load}{Area} = \frac{P}{\frac{\pi D}{2}[D - \sqrt{(D^2 - d^2)}]} \text{ kg/mm}^2$$

where,
- P = load (kilogrammes).
- D = diameter of ball (millimetres).
- d = diameter of impression (millimetres).

To obviate calculation, the Brinell numbers are usually obtained from tables giving values of impression diameters and corresponding Brinell numbers. Typical Brinell numbers are given for a few materials in Table 20.1 compared with hardness values obtained by other tests.

Table 20.1. Comparison of hardness values.

Material	Brinell		Vickers pyramid number	Rockwell scale		Shore
	Impression dia mm	Number		C	B	
Soft brass	–	60	61	–	–	–
Mild steel	5.20	131	131	–	74	20
Soft chisel steel	3.95	235	235	22	99	34
White cast iron	3.00	415	437	44	114	57
Nitrided surface	2.25	745	1050	68	–	100

The diameter of the ball is usually 10 mm and the load 3000 kg for steel, 1000 kg for copper and 500 kg for aluminium. If other sizes of ball are used the load is varied according to the relation: P/D^2 = constant. The constant is 30 for steel, 10 for copper and 5 for aluminium. The time of loading is 15 seconds and the thickness of the specimen should not be less than 10 times the depth of the impression. The piling up of metal round the edge of the impression indicates a low rate of hardening by deformation; sinking denotes the ability for work-hardening (Fig. 20.1). The approximate tensile strength (N/mm^2) of steels can be obtained by multiplying the Brinell number by 3.54 for annealed condition and by 3.24 for quenched and tempered steels. Errors arise when the Brinell test is used on very hard materials, resulting in low values owing to: (i) the spherical shape of indentor, and (ii) flattening of the ball.

Vickers Machine

The errors mentioned above are eliminated in this machine by using a diamond square-based pyramid which does not readily deform and which gives geometrically similar impressions under different loads.

The angularity of the pyramid is 136° and loads ranging from 5 to 120 kg can be used. The rate and duration of loading are controlled by a piston and a dash pot of oil.

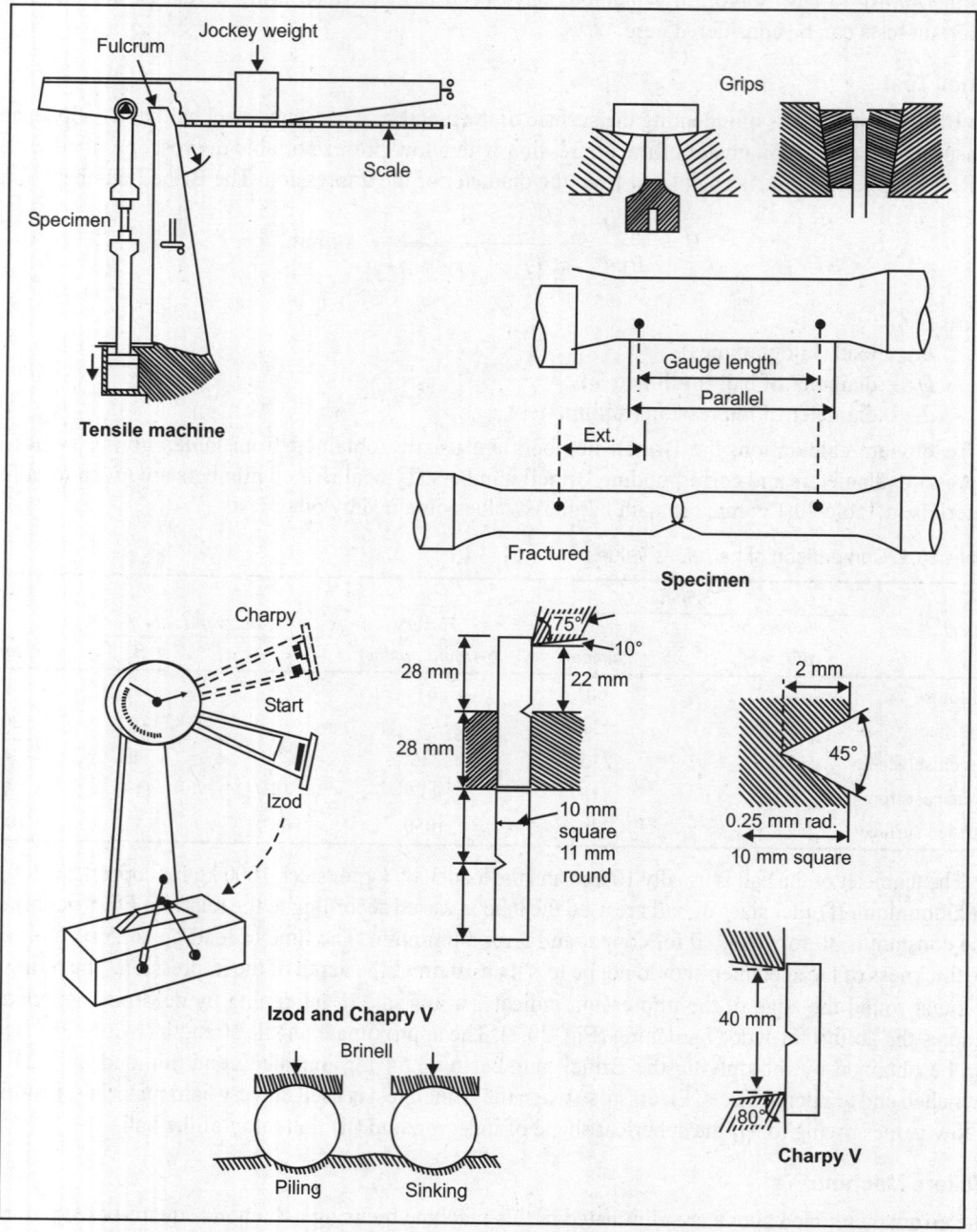

Fig. 20.1. Tensile and Izod Charpy V machines.

A microscope can be swung over the square impression, the diagonals of which are measured between knife edges instead of hair wires or scale, and the reading is taken from a digit counter. The load divided by the contact area of the impression gives the Vickers pyramid number (VPN).

Since the impressions are small, the machine is very suitable for testing polished and hardened material. The Brinell and Vickers hardness values are practically identical up to a hardness of 300. The Brinell number is not reliable above 600 as shown in Table 24.1.

Rockwell Test

This uses either a steel ball 1.58 mm diameter loaded with 100 kg (scale B) or 150 kg on a diamond cone having a 120° angle (scale C). The penetrator is first loaded with a minor load of 10 kg to take out any slack in the machine and the indicator, for measuring the depths of the impression, set to zero. The above major load is applied and after its removal the dial gauge records the depth of the impression in terms of Rockwell numbers. The Rockwell test is particularly useful for rapid routine tests on finished products.

Shore Scleroscope

Shore scleroscope consists of a small diamond-pointed hammer weighing 2.5 g, which is allowed to fall freely from a height of 250 mm down a glass tube graduated into 140 equal parts. The height of the first rebound is taken as the index of hardness. This test is used for testing rolls, dies and gears and leaves no visible impression.

Ductility

Ductility is a mechanical property that describes the extent in which solid materials can be plastically deformed without fracture.

In materials science, ductility is a solid material's ability to deform under tensile stress; this is often characterised by the material's ability to be stretched into a wire. Malleability, a similar property, is a material's ability to deform under compressive stress; this is often characterised by the material's ability to form a thin sheet by hammering or rolling. Both of these mechanical properties are aspects of plasticity, the extent to which a solid material can be plastically deformed without fracture. Also, these material properties are dependent on temperature.

A material's ductility and malleability are not always coextensive. For instance, while gold is both ductile and malleable, lead is only malleable. The word ductility is sometimes used to embrace both types of plasticity.

Ductility is especially important in metalworking, as materials that crack or break under stress cannot be manipulated using metal forming processes, such as hammering, rolling, and drawing. Malleable materials can be formed using stamping or pressing, whereas brittle metals and plastics must be moulded.

High degrees of ductility occur due to metallic bonds, which are found predominantly in metals and leads to the common perception that metals are ductile in general. In metallic bonds valence shell electrons are delocalised and shared between many atoms. The delocalised electrons allow metal atoms to slide past one another without being subjected to strong repulsive forces that would cause other materials to shatter.

The ductile-brittle transition temperature (DBTT), nil ductility temperature (NDT), or nil ductility transition temperature of a metal represents the point at which the fracture energy passes below a predetermined point (for steels typically 40 J for a standard Charpy impact test). DBTT is important since, once a material is cooled below the DBTT, it has a much greater tendency to shatter on impact instead of bending or deforming.

TENSILE TEST

The tensile testing machine consists of two essential parts: (i) the straining device, such as a screw and nut, driven electrically, or a plunger subjected to oil pressure, and (ii) the measurement of the load on the specimen, determined from the oil pressure, care having been taken to obviate errors due to friction, or from the position of a jockey-weight on a beam balanced upon a knife edge and also attached to one end of the specimen. During a test the weight is slid along the beam in order to keep it floating as the load on the specimen increases (Fig. 20.1).

The specimen may be round or rectangular in cross-section, depending on the nature of the product being tested. The centre is usually reduced in section to form the gauge length. A sharp change in section from the parallel portion to the shoulders should be avoided, otherwise concentrations of stress occur and a brittle material would fracture at an apparently low stress. With ductile materials deformation occurs at such places, distributing the concentration of stress over a wider area. A similar effect occurs when the line of action of the force is eccentric to the axis of the specimen. This effect can be obviated by the use of self-aligning grips fitted with spherical seats in the testing machine. The specimen may be held by flanges, pins, screw thread or serrated wedges (Fig. 20.1). Before placing the specimen in the machine its diameter is measured with a micrometer, and two small 'pop' marks are made at a distance apart corresponding to the gauge length on which the extension is to be measured.

Stress–Strain Curve

The relation of extension to the applied stress is shown in Fig. 20.2(a) for mild steel. Up to E the extension of the specimen is very small and necessitates the use of magnifying devices—called extensometers—for its measurement. On removing the load the specimen returns to its previous dimensions and exhibits elasticity. The stress at E is called the elastic limit and in some metals point E does not coincide with P, which denotes the point at which the curve deviates from a straight line; the stress corresponding to P is called the limit of proportionality. Up to P, therefore, the stress is proportional to the strain and can be calculated:

$$\text{Stress} = \frac{\text{Load}}{\text{Cross-sectional area}}, \text{ e.g. N/mm}^2$$

$$\text{Strain} = \frac{\text{Extension of gauge length}}{\text{Original gauge length}}$$

Therefore, by Hooke's Law

$$\frac{\text{Stress}}{\text{Strain}} = \frac{\dfrac{\text{Load}}{\text{Cross-sectional area}}}{\dfrac{\text{Extension of gauge length}}{\text{Original gauge length}}}$$

$$= E, \text{ a constant known as Young's Modulus.}$$

Young's Modulus is fixed by the nature of the material and for ordinary steel the value of about 200 kN/mm^2 is not much affected by composition or heat-treatment, but decreases with temperature.

The value for steels decreases 25 per cent between 15° and 600°C. The springiness of a material is indicated by its Young's Modulus and when stiffness is required by design, the Modulus has to be considered when changing from mild steel to high tensile steels with similar values or to nonferrous metals with low values of Young's Modulus.

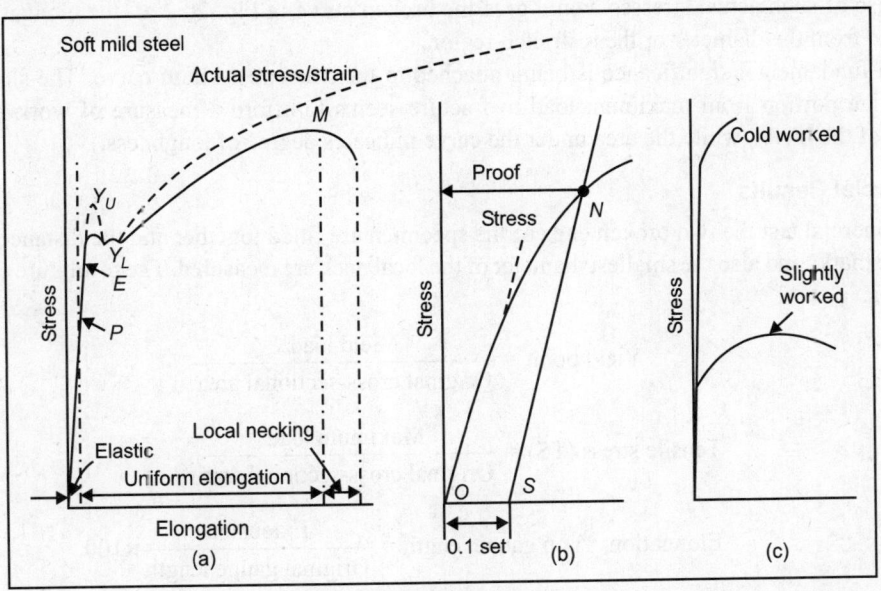

Fig. 20.2. Stress-elongation curves.

Recent investigations have shown, however, that the limit of proportionality becomes lower as more sensitive instruments are used to measure the extension. Some of the high values now in use are due to the inability of the extensometer to detect small amounts of permanent extension.

As the load on the test piece is increased beyond the elastic limit there comes a point at which there is a sudden extension, indicated by the drop of the beam and continued extension with a lower load. If the load is removed, the specimen does not recover its original dimensions and it is said to have undergone plastic deformation or plastic flow. A coating of brittle lacquer is useful for indicating plastic yielding.

In Fig. 20.2(a) the upper yield point is denoted by Y_U, the highest stress before sudden extension occurs, and its value is affected by surface finish, shape of test piece and rate of loading. The lower yield point, which is normally measured in commercial testing, is denoted by Y_L, the lowest stress producing the large elongation. This large elongation of the metal only occurs in a very few materials such as wrought iron and mild steels. 'Stretcher strains' occur in the latter owing to this pronounced yield point, but can be prevented by temper rolling the steel, with the result that the stress-strain curve is smoothed out [Fig. 20.2(c)]. Heavy cold working raises the ultimate tensile stress, yield point and limit of proportionality but reduces the elongation.

Much engineering design has been based on tensile strength rather than yield strength, which is the primary criterion of load-carrying ability. With the older materials of engineering the ratio of yield to tensile strength is fairly constant, but the newer materials, especially alloy steels, have much higher ratios and design should be based on yield strength or proof stress, unless fatigue is an important criterion. As the load is increased the specimen continues to extend (i.e. plastic deformation) until a constriction occurs in the gauge length and the beam drops. This corresponds to the maximum load [M, Fig. 20.2(a)] on the specimen. The load now acts on a diminishing area and produces a stress sufficient to break the specimen. The actual breaking stress, which is never used in practice, is obtained by dividing the breaking load by the actual sectional area of the fracture.

The use of such actual stresses would give the broken curve in Fig. 20.2(a), the elongation being calculated from the diameter or the restricted region.

Much fundamental significance is being attached to the true stress-strain curve. The slope of the straight-line portion from maximum load to fracture seems to afford a measure of work-hardening capacity of the metal; while the area under the curve indicates degree of toughness.

Commercial Results

In a commercial test the two broken ends of the specimen are fitted together and the distance between the gauge marks and also the smallest diameter of the local neck are measured. The results are calculated as follows:

$$\text{Yield point} = \frac{\text{Yield load}}{\text{Original cross-sectional area}}$$

$$\text{Tensile stress (TS)} = \frac{\text{Maximum load}}{\text{Original cross-sectional area}}$$

$$\text{Elongation, \% on gauge length} = \frac{\text{Extension}}{\text{Original gauge length}} \times 100$$

$$\text{Reduction of area, \%} = \left(\frac{\text{Original area} - \text{Final area}}{\text{Original area}}\right) \times 100$$

Proof Stress

For the harder steels and nonferrous metals there is no sharply defined yielding of the material, and a curve is obtained as shown in Fig. 20.2(b). For aircraft materials it has become essential to specify a stress which corresponds to a definite amount of permanent extension, and it is called proof stress, commonly obtained as illustrated in Fig. 20.2(b). A line, SN, is drawn from S, so that OS represents 0.1 per cent, or some other permanent set. SN is drawn parallel to the rectilinear portion of the curve and cutting it at N. The stress corresponding to N is the 0.1 per cent proof stress. The material fulfils the specification if, after the proof stress is applied for 15 seconds and removed, the specimen has not permanently extended more than 0.1 per cent of the gauge length.

Elongation

The total elongation of a test piece is made up of two separate parts:
1. Uniform extension, which occurs up to the maximum load (M) and is proportional to the gauge length.
2. Local extension, due to the necking. This is independent of the gauge length, but varies with the cross-sectional area of the specimen. As the gauge length is increased, the effect of the necking on the value of the total elongation decreases, as shown in Fig. 20.3. It is essential, therefore,

that the gauge length should be stated when an elongation figure is mentioned. In practice, it is found that geometrically similar test bars of a given material deform similarly (Barba's Law), giving the same percentage elongation if:

$$\frac{\text{Guage length}}{\sqrt{(\text{Cross-sectional area})}} = \text{Constant}$$

which allows for variation of the gauge length with the cross-sectional area of a specimen. Unfortunately the same constant is not used in various parts of the world and consequently values of elongation cannot be directly compared with each other without the use of formulae. The gauge length used in England was 4 √(area), but has now been changed to 5.65 √(area), i.e. 5 dia for round specimens (ISO) in Germany, 11.3 √(area); and in America, 4.47 √(area).

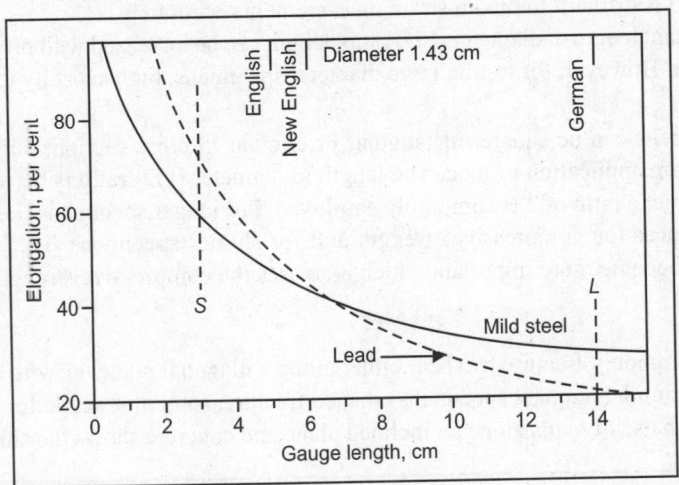

Fig. 20.3. Effect of gauge length on percentage elongation.

Values of elongation obtained on such arbitrary gauge lengths do not afford a guide as to the relative manner in which two different materials will behave in service. From Fig. 20.3 it will be seen that if measurement is made on the gauge length S, the steel appears to be better, while if the gauge length L is used the reverse is the case. For steel plates a fixed gauge length of 200 mm is used with a width varying with the thickness of the plate. The values of elongation and of reduction of area indicate the ductility of a metal. A high reduction of area indicates that the material has a low rate of hardening by deformation. 18/8 stainless steel has a high elongation but a low reduction of area, and this indicates that the alloy is tough but hardens extremely rapidly when deformed.

COMPRESSION TEST

Theoretically, compression test is merely the opposite of the tension test with respect to the direction of applied stress. The compression test can be done on the same machine on which the tension test is done like universal testing machine or some other machine which is designed specifically for the purpose. In general, brittle materials are good in compression than in tension and therefore, they are used for compressive loads. Due to this, compression test is mainly used to test brittle materials such as cast irons, concrete stone, bricks and ceramic products. During testing, fracture occurs in brittle materials and therefore, the ultimate strength is determined corresponding to the fracture point; but no fracture occurs for ductile materials and hence ultimate strength is found out for some arbitrary amount of deformation. It has been observed that some errors are always bound to come in the compression test due to the following practical difficulties.

1. Since the top and bottom faces of the specimen are seldom perfectly parallel to each other and there is always a tendency for bending of the specimen during testing, it is very difficult to apply truly axial loads.
2. The friction between the ends of the specimen and heads of the testing machine prevent the deformation of the specimen uniformly throughout the length. This results in more lateral expansion in the central region than the other regions giving a barrel like shape to specimen.
3. Since the length of specimen is kept short enough (not more than twice its diameter) to avoid its buckling, it is difficult to obtain strain measurements accurately.
4. For a constant length to diameter (l/D) ratio, length can be increased with proportionate increase in diameter. However, for testing large diameter specimens, high capacity testing machines are required.

The test specimens can be square, rectangular or circular in cross section; but circular section is preferred for uniform application of load. The length to diameter (l/D) ratio is between 1.5 and 10 for different materials but a ratio of 2 is commonly employed. For longer specimens (i.e. l/D >10) bending is more which reduces the compressive strength and for shorter specimens (i.e. l/D <1.5) frictional effects at the ends become more important which increases the compressive strength.

Type of Fracture

Brittle materials commonly fracture by shear either along a diagonal plane, or with a cone (cylindrical specimens) or a pyramidal- (square specimens) shaped fracture, sometimes called as hourglass fracture (Fig. 20.4). Cast iron usually fails along an inclined plane and concrete shows the cone type of fracture.

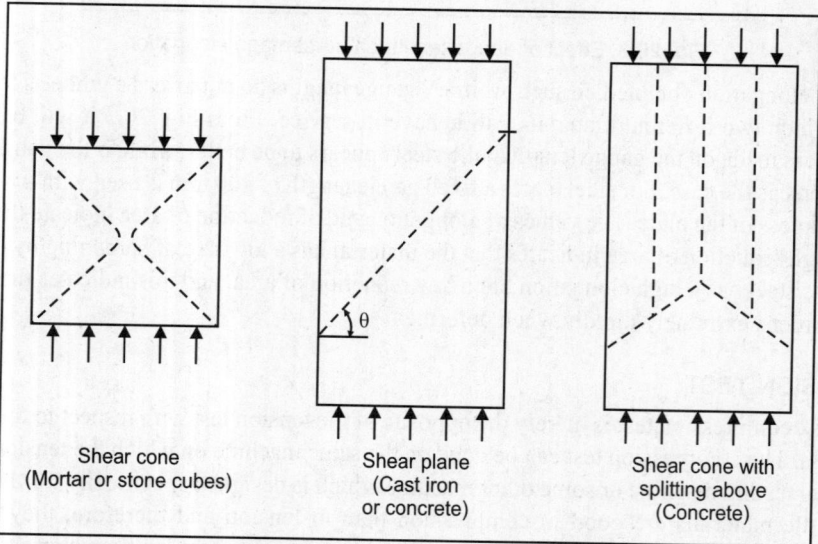

Fig. 20.4. Types of fractures of brittle materials under compressive loads.

The resolved shear stress is maximum at 45° to the load axis and therefore, the fracture should occur on a plane at 45° to the load axis. However, due to internal friction, non-homogeneous composition and structure, and friction at the ends of the specimen, the fracture plane is between 50° and 60° to the load axis. If the specimen is so short that a normal failure plane cannot develop within its length, then the strength is appreciably increased and other types of failures such as crushing may occur.

Ductile and plastic materials bulge laterally and take a barrel shape as they are compressed, provided the specimen does not bend or buckle. Due to this, the compressive stress continues to increase almost without any limit as there is no failure of the material.

Effect of size and shape of specimens on the compressive strength

In the majority of cases, compression test specimens are either square or circular in cross-section and hence the important variable is length-to-width (or length-to-diameter) ratio. As the length-to-diameter (l/D) ratio increases, compressive strength decreases (Fig. 20.5). This is due to increased amount of bending stresses.

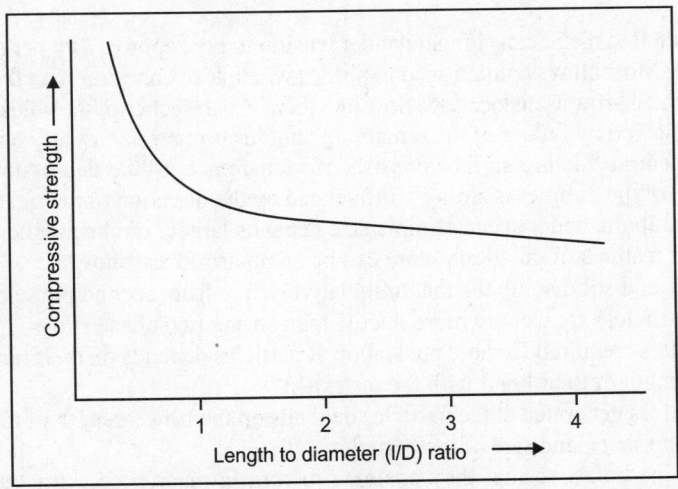

Fig. 20.5. Schematic illustration of the effect of length-to-diameter ratio on compressive strength of brittle materials.

Speed of Loading

It is necessary to take into account the wide variation of actual strain rates in a tensile test which may affect the results obtained. For measurement of yield stresses a rate of strain and of stress not exceeding 0.15 min. and 0.3 N/mm^2/s respectively is recommended. Speed is particularly important in the case of soft metals and also of hard metals tested at high temperatures. At high testing speeds the tensile stress increases and the elongation decreases. At sufficiently high speeds there may not be time to conduct away the heat produced by plastic working and the temperature may rise sufficiently to soften the deforming material. Plastic flow may thus be concentrated in zones which eventually rupture. Outside the zone of failure little deformation is evident and an apparent brittle failure is indicated.

On the other hand, the embrittling effect of hydrogen on high tensile steel becomes more effective on slow or sustained dead loading.

Effect of Previous Deformation

With steels deformation only slightly in excess of the yield point has the effect of lowering the limit of proportionality. After a rest at room temperature or a short time at 100°–300°C, the proportional limit for tension stresses is raised, accompanied by a reduction in the corresponding value for compression stresses.

	Yield point N/mm^2	Proportional limit N/mm^2
First loading	256	238
Overstrained	266	164
Strained and rested	357	337

Heavy deformation affects the stress-strain curve as shown in Fig. 20.2(c).

Fracture

Ductile fracture

A pure and inclusion free metal can elongate under tension to give approx. 100 per cent RA and a point fracture (Fig. 20.6). Most alloys contain second phases which lose cohesion with the matrix or fracture and the voids so formed grow as dislocations flow into them. Coalescence of the voids forms a continuous fracture surface followed by failure of the remaining annulus of material usually on plane at 45° to the tension axis. The central fracture surface consists of numerous cup-like depressions generally called dimples. The shape of the dimples is strongly influenced by the direction of major stresses—circular in pure tension and parabolic under shear. Dimple size depends largely on the number of inclusion sites.

Some important features of ductile fracture can be summarised as follows:
1. Pure metals and solid solutions that are relatively free from second phase particles (including impurity particles) are usually more ductile than strong two phase alloys.
2. The local stress required for hole nucleation at particles depends on their resistance to cracking and the strength of their bond with the matrix.
3. The local stress generated at the particles depends on the flow strength of the alloy, the applied strain and the shape and size of the particles.
4. Growth of the holes, so that they coalesce to form a macroscopic fracture, depends on the applied stresses being tensile. Much higher ductilities are achieved in compressive straining.

In cleavage fracture the material fails along well defined crystallographic planes within the grain but the crack path is affected by grain boundaries and inclusions. Basically a cleavage fracture surface contains large smooth areas separated by cleavage steps and feathers, river markings and cleavage tongues which are the direct result of crack path disturbances.

Intercrystalline

Intercrystalline fracture is characterised by separation of the grains to reveal a surface composed of grain boundary facets. This type of fracture is found in stress-corrosion creep hot tearing and hydrogen embrittlement.

Fatigue fractures

Fatigue fractures are characterised by striations representing the extent of crack propagation under each cycle of loading.

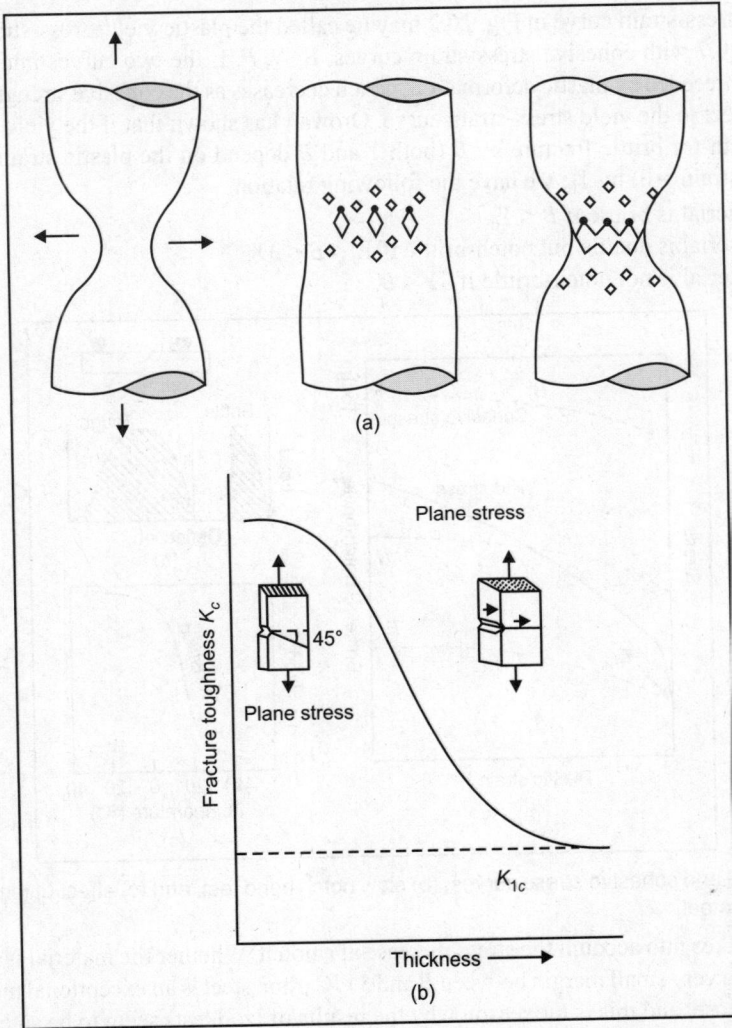

Fig. 20.6. (a) Stages in ductile fracture from inclusions, and (b) fracture toughness v thickness.

Compound stresses and brittle fracture

The failure of some American all-welded ships during the Second World War has stimulated much work on the causes of brittle fracture in steel. In the tensile test plastic deformation involves shearing slip along crystal planes within the crystals, but in the presence of tension of equal magnitude in each principal direction, shearing stresses are absent, plastic deformation is prevented and a brittle fracture occurs as soon as the cohesive strength of the material is exceeded. Equal triaxial tension stresses do not arise frequently in practice, but it is common to find a triaxial tension superimposed on a unidirectional tension, and if the margin between cohesive strength and plastic yield strength is small, a brittle fracture may occur in a material ordinarily considered highly ductile. Compound stresses arise in a weld in very thick plate and in a tube under internal pressure and an axial tension.

The actual stress-strain curve in Fig. 20.2 may be called the plastic yield stress-strain curve. This is shown in Fig. 20.7 with cohesive stress-strain curves, B, N, F. If the two curves intersect at Y, brittle fracture occurs preceded by plastic deformation, which decreases as the cohesive strength curve becomes lower with respect to the yield stress-strain curve. Orowan has shown that if the yield stress is denoted by Y, the strength for brittle fracture by B (both Y and B depend on the plastic strain), and the initial value of Y (for strain = 0) by Y_0, we have the following relation:

1. The material is brittle if $B < Y_0$.
2. The material is ductile but notch-brittle if $Y_0 < B < 3Y$.
3. The material is not notch-brittle if $3Y < B$.

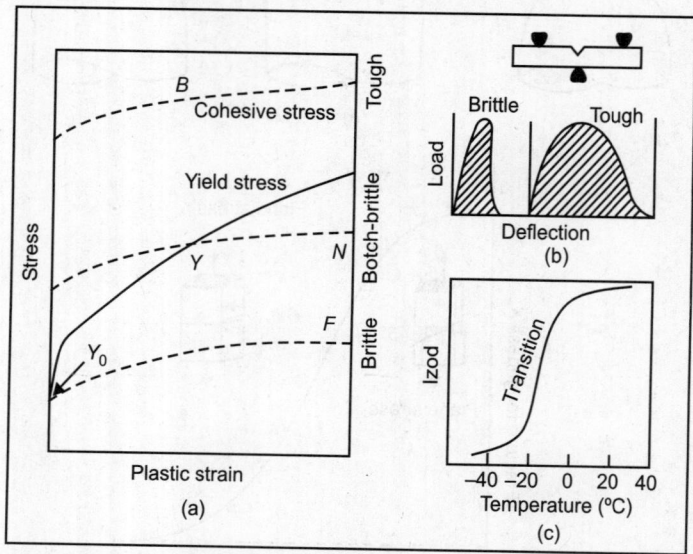

Fig. 20.7. (a) Yield and cohesive stress curves, (b) slow notch bend test, and (c) effect of temperature on the Izod value of mild steel.

The factor 3 takes into account the stress increase at a notch. Whether the material is notch-brittle or not depends on the very small margin between B and $3Y$. Carbon steel is an exceptional material, because $3Y$ and B are so close, and this is the reason why the results of Izod tests seem to be so erratic, and why notch brittleness is so sensitive to slight variations of composition, previous treatment and temperature.

Brittle fracture is characterised by the very small amount of work absorbed and by a crystalline appearance of the surfaces of fracture, often with a chevron pattern pointing to the origin of fracture, due to the formation of discontinuous cleavage cracks which join up. It can occur at a low stress of 75–120 N/mm² with great suddenness; the velocity of crack propagation is probably not far from that of sound in the material. In this type of fracture plastic deformation is very small, and the crack need not open up considerably in order to propagate, as is necessary with a ductile failure.

The work required to propagate a crack is given by Griffith's formula:

$$\sigma \approx \sqrt{E\gamma/c}$$

where, σ = tensile stress required to propagate a crack of length c.
γ = surface energy of fracture faces.
E = Young's modulus.

Orowan modified the Griffith theory to include a plastic strain energy factor, p, since some plastic flow is always found near the fracture surface.:

$$\sigma = \sqrt{E(\gamma + p)/c}$$

When the temperature is above the brittle-ductile transition temperature, p is large and the stress, σ, required to make the crack grow will also be large. Below the transition temperature the metal is brittle and p will be smaller. The stress necessary to cause crack growth, therefore, will be reduced. The reason for the increasing speed of crack propagation, once a crack has started, is clear from both Griffith's and Orowan's equations: as the crack grows in length, the stress required for propagation continually decreases.

Notched Bar Tests

Notches produce triaxial tension stresses which increase the ratio of tensile to shear stresses and the use of an Izod test is an attempt to subject metals to a controllable triaxial tension, and not to measure the resistance of the material to impact, since the velocity of testing is too low. Test pieces, either 10 mm^2 section or 11 mm diameter (Fig. 20.1), are gripped in a vice, with the root of the notch level with the top of the vice. A weighted pendulum, swinging on ball bearings, is raised to a standard height and allowed to strike the specimen on the same side as the notch. The striking energy of 163 J is partially absorbed in fracturing the specimen, and this amount is indicated by the pointer. The sharpness of the notch largely controls the test, but geometrically similar notches do not produce the same results on large parts as they do on small test pieces.

Consequently true behaviour of a material under the unmeasurable triaxial tension in service can only be obtained by testing full-sized parts as they will be stressed in service. The Izod figures, therefore, have no design value. A material of 40 J is not 'twice as strong as one of 20 J' and with equal room temperature Izod values, two materials may respond quite differently to temperature, size of specimen and dimensions of notch.

The Izod test is accurate for its particular geometry and stress conditions and is useful to the metallurgist in detecting differences due to casting, mechanical and heat treatment, not indicated by the tensile test. For material susceptible to notch-brittle fracture it gives a guide to the resistance against failure at a discontinuity or change in section and also indicates the resistance of a material to the spread of a crack after it has formed. Notched-bar test results form no basis for approval or condemnation of a metal for services under conditions of notch-fatigue.

In assessing the notch ductility of steel the important factors are state of stress (notch effect), speed of deformation and temperature. Earlier, the effect of temperature was ignored and steels were classified as tough or brittle by the results of an Izod test at room temperature. Because it is so much easier to test specimens over a range of temperature the Charpy V-notch test has displaced the Izod test in recent years. In the Charpy machine the specimen, 10 mm^2 section is supported as a beam, 40 mm span using the standard Izod notch instead of the Charpy keyhole notch. The Charpy machine has a lighter tup but a higher striking velocity, giving a striking energy of 280 J.

In spite of the same notch geometry the results of the two tests differ; in general the Izod test gives higher energy values and lower crystalline areas of fracture than the Charpy V-notch test. Some authorities consider that the area of brittle fracture is a better criterion than an energy value and this is easier to estimate on large specimens. Many tests employing the full plate thickness have been introduced. A slow V-notch bend test 70 × 225 mm is used by Van der Veen, while the Tipper test employs a notched tensile specimen. These various tests do not indicate the same transition temperature for a steel but they usually rate steels in the same order of merit. Of much more use to the engineer is the Robertson test. In this a specimen is subjected to a uniform applied stress and also to a temperature gradient. At the cold end is a sharp defect—a saw cut—and a crack is initiated from this defect by means of a blow. The crack propagates under these conditions and the temperature at the point where the failure changes from brittle to ductile is known as the crack arrest temperature. From a series of such tests carried out over a range of applied stresses, Robertson finds a temperature at which the stress required to propagate a brittle fracture increases rapidly.

Fracture Mechanics and Fracture Toughness

Although the Charpy test has been used as a guide and a quality control test for toughness in the past its limitations, from the design point of view, are becoming increasingly apparent especially with the development of new materials, for which previous experience is lacking. The use of linear fracture mechanics is now being applied to many design problems to give a fracture-safe structure containing a given defect size. Essentially, the technique involves a study of the stresses and strains at the tips of sharp cracks or defects and relates them to the applied loading.

Chapter 21

Metallography

INTRODUCTION

Metallography is the general study of metals and their behaviour, with particular reference to their microstructure and macrostructure. Microstructure is the characteristic appearance and physical arrangement of a metal as observed with a microscope. The macrostructure is the appearance and physical arrangement as observed with the naked eye or with a low power magnification. Naturally, these two groups of characteristics are closely interrelated with each other and a knowledge of both is essential for a full understanding of any metal. Since this branch of metallurgy is probably the widest in scope it is natural that precise techniques have been developed for much of the work and that new techniques are continually being developed and old ones modified.

Crystallographic are obviously important to the metallographer by giving him a submicroscopic picture together with a better understanding of the microscopic picture and it is sometimes difficult to see where one field ends and the other begins. Perhaps the easiest way of looking at it is to consider it from the aspect of the type of the field of observation. Crystallography covers atomic arrangement and distribution as obtained by inference and deduction, electron microscopy looks into the interplay of atomic groupings by electronically-assisted direct observation using an electron beam, while micrography concerns itself with the smallest characteristics directly observable with optical assistance; macrography deals with conditions in the massive range within the scope of unaided or only slightly aided observation.

PREPARING METALLOGRAPHIC SPECIMENS

The surface of a metallographic specimen is prepared by various methods of grinding, polishing, and etching. After preparation, it is often analysed using optical or electron microscopy. Using only metallographic techniques, a skilled technician can identify alloys and predict material properties.

Mechanical preparation is the most common preparation method. In a series of steps, successively finer abrasive particles are used to remove material from the sample surface until the desired surface quality is achieved. Many different machines are available for doing this grinding and polishing, able to meet different demands for quality, capacity, and reproducibility.

A systematic preparation method is the easiest way to achieve the true structure. Sample preparation must therefore pursue rules which are suitable for most materials. Different materials with similar properties (hardness and ductility) will respond alike and thus require the same consumables during preparation. Metallographic specimens are typically 'mounted' using a hot compression thermosetting resin. In the past, phenolic thermosetting resins have been used, but modern epoxy is becoming more popular because reduced shrinkage during curing results in a better mount with superior edge retention. A typical mounting cycle will compress the specimen and mounting media to 4000 psi (28 MPa) and heat to a temperature of 350°F (177°C). When specimens are very sensitive to temperature, 'cold mounts' may be made with a two-part epoxy resin. Mounting a specimen provides a safe, standardised, and ergonomic way by which to hold a sample during the grinding and polishing operations.

After mounting, the specimen is wet ground to reveal the surface of the metal. The specimen is successively ground with finer and finer abrasive media. Silicon carbide abrasive paper was the first method of grinding and is still used today. Many metallographers, however, prefer to use a diamond grit suspension which is dosed onto a reusable fabric pad throughout the polishing process. Diamond grit in suspension might start at 9 micrometers and finish at one micrometer. Generally, polishing with diamond suspension gives finer results than using silicon carbide papers (SiC papers), especially with revealing porosity, which silicon carbide paper sometimes 'smear' over. After grinding the specimen, polishing is performed. Typically, a specimen is polished with a slurry of alumina, silica, or diamond on a napless cloth to produce a scratch-free mirror finish, free from smear, drag, or pull-outs and with minimal deformation remaining from the preparation process.

After polishing, certain microstructural constituents can be seen with the microscope, e.g. inclusions and nitrides. If the crystal structure is non-cubic (e.g. a metal with a hexagonal-closed packed crystal structure, such as Ti or Zr) the microstructure can be revealed without etching using crossed polarised light (light microscopy). Otherwise, the microstructural constituents of the specimen are revealed by using a suitable chemical or electrolytic etchant. A great many etchants have been developed to reveal the structure of metals and alloys, ceramics, carbides, nitrides, and so forth. While a number of etchants may work for a given metal or alloy, they generally produce different results, in that some etchants may reveal the general structure, while others may be selective to certain phases or constituents.

ANALYSIS TECHNIQUES

Prepared specimens should be examined after etching with the unaided eye to detect any visible areas that respond differently to the etchant as a guide to where the microscopical examination should be employed. Light optical microscopy (LOM) examination should always be performed prior to any electron metallographic (EM) technique, as these are more time-consuming to perform and the instruments are much more expensive.

Further, certain features can be best observed with the LOM, e.g. the natural colour of a constituent can be seen with the LOM but not with EM systems. Also, image contrast of microstructures at relatively low magnifications, e.g. <500X, is far better with the LOM than with the scanning electron microscope (SEM), while transmission electron microscopes (TEM) generally cannot be utilised at magnifications below about 2000 to 3000X. LOM examination is fast and can cover a large area. Thus, the analysis can determine if the more expensive, more time-consuming examination techniques using the SEM or the TEM are required and where on the specimen the work should be concentrated.

Design, Resolution and Image Contrast

Light microscopes are designed for placement of the specimen's polished surface on the specimen stage either upright or inverted. Each type has advantages and disadvantages. Most LOM work is done at magnifications between 50 and 1000X. However, with a good microscope, it is possible to perform examination at higher magnifications, e.g. 2000X, and even higher, as long as diffraction fringes are not present to distort the image. However, the resolution limit of the LOM will not be better than about 0.2

to 0.3 micrometers. Special methods are be used at magnifications below 50X, which can be very helpful when examining the microstructure of cast specimens where greater spatial coverage in the field of view may be required to observe features such as dendrites.

Besides considering the resolution of the optics, one must also maximise visibility by maximising image contrast. A microscope with excellent resolution may not be able to image a structure, that is there is no visibility, if image contrast is poor. Image contrast depends upon the quality of the optics, coatings on the lenses, and reduction of flare and glare; but, it also requires proper specimen preparation and good etching techniques. So, obtaining good images requires maximum resolution and image contrast. Bright field illumination, where sample contrast comes from absorbance of light in the sample.

Bright and Dark Field Microscopy

Most LOM observations are conducted using bright field (BF) illumination, where the image of any flat feature perpendicular to the incident light path is bright, or appears to be white. But, other illumination methods can be used and, in some cases, may provide superior images with greater detail. Dark field microscopy (DF), although not used much today, provides high contrast images and actually greater resolution than bright field. In dark field, the light from features perpendicular to the optical axis is blocked and appears dark while the light from features inclined to the surface, which look dark in BF, appear bright, or 'self luminous' in DF grain boundaries, for example, are more vivid in DF than BF.

Polarised Light Microscopy

Polarised light (PL) is very useful when studying the structure of metals with non-cubic crystal structures (mainly metals with hexagonal close-packed (hcp) crystal structures). If the specimen is prepared with minimal damage to the surface, the structure can be seen vividly in crossed polarised light (the optic axis of the polariser and analyser are 90 degrees to each other, i.e. crossed). In some cases, an hcp metal can be chemically etched and then examined more effectively with PL.

Tint etched surfaces, where a thin film (such as a sulphide, molybdate, chromate or elemental selenium film) is grown epitaxially on the surface to a depth where interference effects are created when examined with BF producing colour images, can be improved with PL. If it is difficult to get a good interference film with good colouration, the colours can be improved by examination in PL using a sensitive tint (ST) filter.

Differential Interference Contrast Microscopy

Another useful imaging mode is differential interference contrast (DIC), which is usually obtained with a system designed by the Polish physicist Georges Nomarski. This system gives the best detail. DIC converts minor height differences on the plane-of-polish, invisible in BF, into visible detail. The detail in some cases can be quite striking and very useful. If an ST filter is used along with a Wollaston prism, colour is introduced. The colours are controlled by the adjustment of the Wollaston prism, and have no specific physical meaning, *per se*. But, visibility may be better.

Oblique Illumination

DIC has largely replaced the older oblique illumination (OI) technique, which was available on reflected light microscopes prior to about 1975. In OI, the vertical illuminator is offset from perpendicular, producing shading effects that reveal height differences. This procedure reduces resolution and yields uneven illumination across the field of view. Nevertheless, OI was useful when people needed to know if a second phase particle was standing above or was recessed below the plane-of-polish, and is still available on a few microscopes. OI can be created on any microscope by placing a piece of paper under one corner of the mount so that the plane-of-polish is no longer perpendicular to the optical axis.

Scanning Electron and Transmission Electron Microscopes

If a specimen must be observed at higher magnification, it can be examined with a scanning electron microscope (SEM), or a transmission electron microscope (TEM). When equipped with an energy dispersive spectrometer (EDS), the chemical composition of the microstructural features can be determined. The ability to detect low-atomic number elements, such as carbon, oxygen, and nitrogen, depends upon the nature of the detector used. But, quantification of these elements by EDS is difficult and their minimum detectable limits are higher than when a wavelength-dispersive spectrometer (WDS) is used. But quantification of composition by EDS has improved greatly over time. The WDS system has historically had better sensitivity (ability to detect low amounts of an element) and ability to detect low-atomic weight elements, as well as better quantification of compositions, compared to EDS, but it was slower to use. Again, in recent years, the speed required to perform WDS analysis has improved substantially. Historically, EDS was used with the SEM while WDS was used with the electron microprobe analyser (EMPA). Today, EDS and WDS is used with both the SEM and the EMPA. However, a dedicated EMPA is not as common as an SEM.

X-ray Diffraction Techniques

Characterisation of microstructures has also been performed using X-ray diffraction (XRD) techniques for many years. XRD can be used to determine the percentages of various phases present in a specimen if they have different crystal structures. For example, the amount of retained austenite in a hardened steel is best measured using XRD (ASTM E 975). If a particular phase can be chemically extracted from a bulk specimen, it can be identified using XRD based on the crystal structure and lattice dimensions. This work can be complemented by EDS and/or WDS analysis where the chemical composition is quantified. But EDS and WDS are difficult to apply to particles less than 2-3 micrometers in diameter. For smaller particles, diffraction techniques can be performed using the TEM for identification and EDS can be performed on small particles if they are extracted from the matrix using replication methods to avoid detection of the matrix along with the precipitate.

QUANTITATIVE METALLOGRAPHY

A number of techniques exist to quantitatively analyse metallographic specimens. These techniques are valuable in the research and production of all metals and alloys and nonmetallic or composite materials.

Microstructural quantification is performed on a prepared, two-dimensional plane through the three-dimensional part or component. Measurements may involve simple metrology techniques, e.g. the measurement of the thickness of a surface coating, or the apparent diameter of a discrete second-phase particle, (for example, spheroidal graphite in ductile iron). Measurement may also require application of stereology to assess matrix and second-phase structures. Stereology is the field of taking 0-, 1- or 2-dimensional measurements on the two-dimensional sectioning plane and estimating the amount, size, shape or distribution of the microstructure in three dimensions. These measurements may be made using manual procedures with the aid of templates overlaying the microstructure, or with automated image analysers. In all cases, adequate sampling must be made to obtain a proper statistical basis for the measurement. Efforts to eliminate bias are required.

Some of the most basic measurements include determination of the volume fraction of a phase or constituent, measurement of the grain size in polycrystalline metals and alloys, measurement of the size and size distribution of particles, assessment of the shape of particles, and spacing between particles.

Standards organisations, including ASTM International's Committee E-4 on Metallography and some other national and international organisations, have developed standard test methods describing how to characterise microstructures quantitatively.

For example, the amount of a phase or constituent, that is, its volume fraction, is defined in ASTM E 562; manual grain size measurements are described in ASTM E 112 (equiaxed grain structures with a single size distribution) and E 1182 (specimens with a bimodal grain size distribution); while ASTM E 1382 describes how any grain size type or condition can be measured using image analysis methods. Characterisation of nonmetallic inclusions using standard charts is described in ASTM E 45 (historically, E 45 covered only manual chart methods and an image analysis method for making such chart measurements was described in ASTM E 1122. The image analysis methods are currently being incorporated into E 45). A stereological method for characterising discrete second-phase particles, such as nonmetallic inclusions, carbides, graphite, etc. is presented in ASTM E 1245.

METALLOGRAPHIC EXAMINATION

Metallography requires the removal of small samples, which are then mounted in a resin or bakelite block, polished and etched in dilute acid, before examination under a metallurgical microscope. This reveals the crystal structure of the metal, from which an assessment of the type of alloy and its mechanical and heat treatment history can be made. Metallography thus provides a good measure of the quality of the metal and its suitability for a particular application. Scott provides a good introduction to the structure of metals, metallography and the phase diagrams which help explain the microstructures it reveals.

The structure of many ancient alloys is, typically, heterogeneous. Ferrous alloys were never heated to melting temperature and therefore retain quantities of slag as well as an uneven distribution of alloying elements, particularly carbon and phosphorus. Nonferrous alloys may show segregation of certain elements towards the centre or surface of the artefact. All alloys can show depletion of elements at the surface following oxidation, either during manufacture or after post-depositional corrosion

Because of this heterogeneity, bulk chemical analyses, especially of the surface, may be misleading. Metallography, especially when combined with micro-analysis, investigates rather than ignores the microstructure of the metal and provides a greater insight into the technological and post depositional history of the artefact.

Ferrous alloys: It is with iron alloys that metallography can extract the most detailed information. The following notes show the sort of features which can be determined.

Slag Content

Examination of the unetched sample allows the slag inclusions to be measured, both by volume, and by shape. The shape of the inclusions show the way the artefact has been wrought.

Alloy Identification

Prior to the introduction of the blast furnace three main ferrous alloys were in use.

Ferritic iron

The grains of ferrite appear white and contain no impurity elements; it is a soft, ductile metal.

Phosphoric iron

Indicated by grain enlargement and 'ghosting'. Phosphorus contents in the region of 0.1–0.2 per cent are sufficient to give a significantly harder, tougher alloy. Steel: The dark etching regions, are known as pearlite (and contain 0.8 per cent carbon). Steel is not only harder and tougher than iron but allows further hardening by heating and quenching.

Heat Treatment

An acicular structure, martensite, results from the rapid cooling (quenching) of steel without subsequent tempering. This is a very hard material but with a tendency to brittleness. Tempered martensite appears less distinct and although not as hard provides a much tougher metal. Metals worked at low or ambient temperatures and not subsequently annealed show deformed, elongated grains. This cold working increases the hardness of both iron and steel.

Composite Artefacts

To capitalise on the hardness of steel and the ductility (and cheapness) of iron the two alloys were welded together to form composite artefacts. Such structures are frequently found in edged tools and weapons. A weld is generally seen as a sharp division between two metal types (although carbon may diffuse across a boundary). Scale and silicate inclusions may also be trapped at the interface. Techniques for combining different alloys may have important cultural implications. For example, in many Saxon knife blades a steel edge was butt welded to an iron back, whilst Anglo-Scandinavian smiths favoured 'sandwiching' the steel between two low carbon sides. Carburisation was an alternative means of creating a hardenable surface. The iron was heated with a carbon-rich material in a reducing atmosphere so carbon diffused into the surface. Unfortunately this thin layer may be lost to corrosion in all but the best preserved artefacts.

Nonferrous Alloys

Identification of phases present allows the nature of the alloy to be determined. For instance, in leaded copper alloys the lead is immiscible and will be visible as dark grey areas at the grain (crystal) boundaries.

The shape of the metal crystals will show how the object was produced. Cast alloys generally have the characteristic dendritic structure, but this is broken down by subsequent annealing which produces equiaxed crystals. Cold working is indicated by deformation of these crystals and subsequent annealing produces a twinned crystal structure.

Fabrication Techniques

Whilst ancient iron could be fire welded by heating and hammering, most nonferrous alloys required additional liquid metal to bond the parts together. This may be of similar composition to the object's parts or an alloy chosen because is has a lower melting point (or melting range) than the material to be joined. Surface treatments such as gilding, silvering and tinning were all used in antiquity. Metallography can identify the method used to apply the coating by examination of compounds formed between the two dissimilar metals.

Alternative Approaches

Occasionally it is possible to polish a small area of the surface of a well preserved artefact, and examine it without the removal of a specimen. This will be of more limited value, because it does not allow the examination of a complete section, however it may be the only method considered acceptable.

Associated methods

Both microhardness and analysis in the SEM or microprobe are extremely useful in extending studies of metallographic sections because they operate on a scale that allows individual phases to be examined. A microhardness tester measures the indentation produced by a diamond under a set load and provides a direct measure of the hardness of the metal.

Justification

Most opposition to metallography arises because of the need to 'destructively' remove samples. This must always be balanced against the potential evidence which could be obtained by the technique. Metallography can be a very informative investigative technique but programs need to be well thought out to ensure that valid conclusions can be reached.

Associated with metallography there is, in addition to micrography and macrography, a range of techniques covering control of physical treatment of metals by which it is possible to correlate external influences with the observed state of a metal. This range includes systems of temperature measurement and control, methods for controlled heating and cooling, hardness testing and assessment of mechanical properties. There are also the techniques concerned with the recording of observed results including such systems as equilibrium diagrams and time-temperature-transformation diagrams.

It is difficult to give a consecutive account of metallographic work but the sequence followed is first to describe the means and methods of examination, then to consider measurement and control and finally, to discuss methods of recording and interpreting the results of observation.

METHODS OF EXAMINATION

Methods of examination will be covered by starting with the ordinary light microscope, since most people are familiar with elementary optical principles, then going on to the electron microscope and finally to macrography.

Micrography

The ordinary, biological, optical microscope is probably familiar to most people and its principles are fairly well understood. A light beam passes through the object to be observed and is refracted through a system of lenses in such a way that the beam is widely diverged to make the object seem larger. Two methods of examination can be used, namely, direct visual observation of a virtual image, formed as shown in Fig. 21.1(a), and photographic record of a real image focused on a light-sensitive film, as shown in Fig. 21.1(b), the latter method being called 'photomicrography'. Recording in the first method has to be by diagram and written description, whereas the photographic record, once made, is always directly available and if colour film is used, may need no written description. Both systems are used extensively in accordance with the purpose of the examination.

An immediate difficulty encountered in trying to use the ordinary microscope on metals is that the light cannot be transmitted through the object, so a different system of illumination using reflected light has to be employed, the metallurgical microscope being particularly adapted to this system. Two methods are available: (i) oblique illumination [Fig. 21.2(a)] in which the light comes in at an angle between the microscope objective lens and the surface of the opaque object, and (ii) direct illumination [Fig. 21.2(b)] in which the illuminating system is incorporated into the microscope system in such a way that the illuminating beam goes down axially on to the object surface and reflects back along the same axis, but through the glass slip into eyepiece.

418 Physical Metallurgy

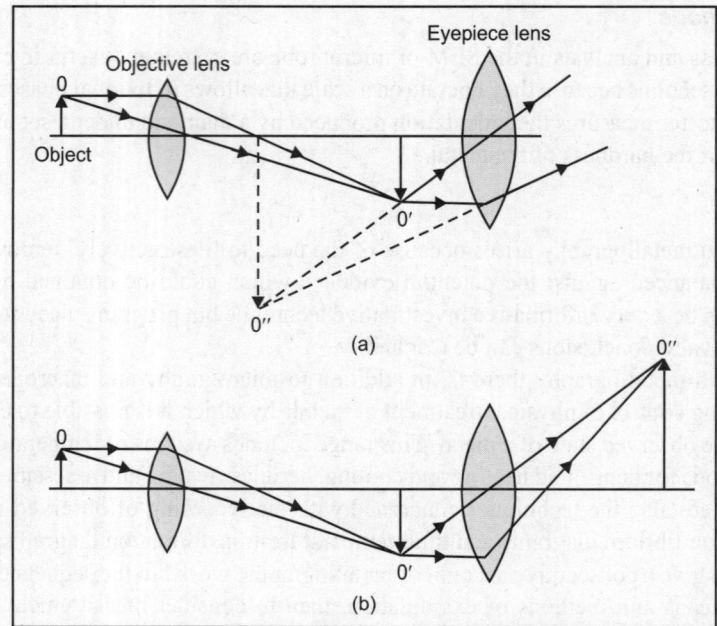

Fig. 21.1. Image formation in a microscope. (a) For visual work, inverted virtual image 0″ is formed and (b) for photography, real image 0″ is projected all a screen.

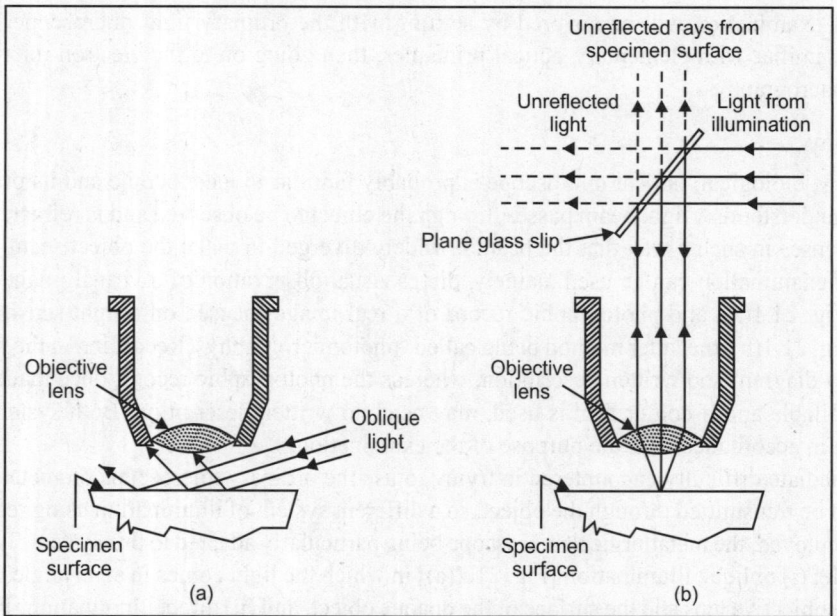

Fig. 21.2. Metallurgical microscope illumination systems. (a) Oblique illuminations. Much light is lost by random reflection, and (b) direct illumination. Some light is lost by poor reflection by the glass slip and by random reflection of rays from the specimen surface.

With oblique illumination, surface irregularities will look bright against a dark background because only irregularities will reflect light into the microscope. On the other hand, direct illumination shows irregularities as darker than the normal plane surfaces because the former do not reflect all the light back into the lens system. Each system has its own application but most use is made of direct illumination.

A diagrammatic illustration of a metallurgical microscope is given in Fig. 21.3 but it must be borne in mind that there are many varieties and types of microscopes, including those using reflecting lens systems and those types specially adapted to photomicrographic work.

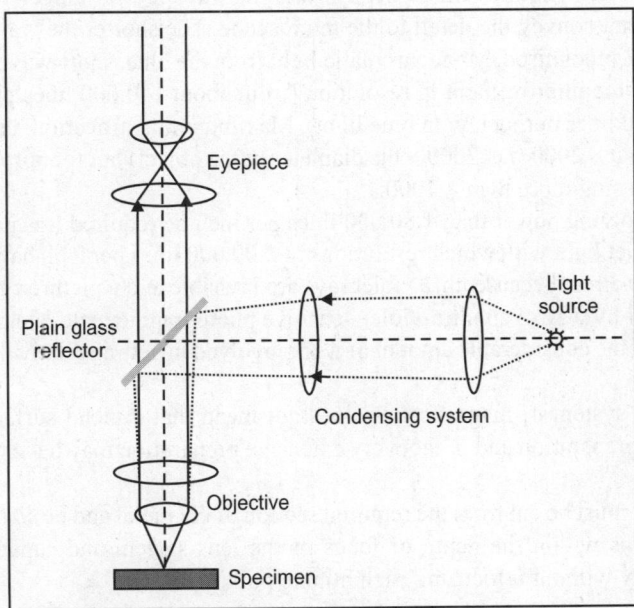

Fig. 21.3. Optical system of metallurgical microscope.

Magnification is not the only purpose in microscopy-resolving power is of greater importance. The resolving power or resolution is the capacity of the microscope for distinguishing detail and is measured by finding the maximum number of parallel lines scribed within the distance of one inch which can be clearly distinguished with its aid. Indeed, the quality of a microscope is better determined by its resolving power than by its nominal magnification. Unaided, the human eye cannot usually distinguish anything measuring much less than 0.1 mm across, so any smaller detail must be clearly magnified to at least this dimension before it becomes recognisable. Illumination intensity is very important in this connection and every effort must be made to make it as uniform as possible over the field of vision.

High-magnification objective lenses have very short focal lengths and are of small diameter; therefore much of the reflected light tends to get lost by divergence from the objective area as it is refracted in the air gap. If the refractive index of the transmitting medium, between the work and the lens, can be raised to a value near to that of the glass of the lens then the numerical aperture or equivalent light-collecting capacity of the lens can also be raised and the resolution improved. Not many media are adaptable to this purpose but cedar oil is one and high magnification lenses are specially made to use with it. A drop of the oil is placed on the surface at the place to be examined, and the lens dipped right into it, giving a so-called 'immersion' lens.

There are severe limitations to the use of optical microscopes because of the nature of light. White light is not monochromatic as it is made up of a combination of frequencies of radiation, each type of wave tending to diffract by a different amount in each lens, so clarity is lost. Some of this trouble can be offset by using compound lenses but these are much more costly to make. Alternatively monochromatic light, produced by interposing a colour filter into the path of the illuminating beam, may be used although this is not an ideal solution to the problem as colour distinction may be lost. Another difficulty is the limitation of magnifying power set by the wave nature of light rays. If the size of a detail is very small and approaching the wavelength of the light rays then the rays are no longer reflected in a simple uniform way and cannot convey the detail to the microscope. The shorter the wavelength, the smaller the detail which can be recognised. Monochromatic light from the blue, short-wave end of the spectrum can be used to give some improvement in resolution (from about 140,000 lines per inch with yellow-green light to 1,80,000 lines per inch with blue light). Maximum magnification, under best conditions, with white light is about × 2000 (i.e. 2000 × the diameter of the object) but for normal visual work there is rarely any point in using more than × 1000.

Should greater resolving power than 1,80,000 lines per inch be required it is possible (with special lenses) to use ultraviolet light with which resolutions of 2,00,000 lines per inch have been obtained, but the vision is no longer direct because ultra violet rays are invisible and a picture can be formed only on a fluorescent screen or by way of an ultra-violet-sensitive photographic plate. Not much use is made of this system because of the considerable amount of work involved in getting relatively little improvement in result.

Having an optical system of magnification does not mean that a metal surface can be examined immediately without preparation and in fact very extensive preparation may have to be made and three conditions satisfied.

1. The specimen must be cut from the required section of the metal and be so flat that all of a given field of view is within the depth of focus of the lens system and capable of being viewed simultaneously without refocusing each minute point.
2. The preparation system must not modify the structure in any way. Nothing should be added, either in the nature of scratches or modification of the state of the metal, due either to plastic deformation or heat modification. Most metals are very liable to scratch and deform and many will change their structures under the influence of frictional heat. Likewise, nothing which is present should be removed from the surface. This may not be as easy to ensure as it sounds because it is very easy to disturb hard particles or phases embedded in a soft matrix or to lose brittle phases out of a hard matrix.
3. Surface details of the structure must be clear. Treatment may be required to achieve this.

Preparation of a specimen for examination can be done in a number of ways. Machining, grinding or abrasive wheel cutting to a reasonable standard of machine finish is the first essential. Properly sharpened tools and unglazed grinding wheels must be used to avoid deep surface smearing. Hand abrasion follows to remove the marks and other effects which inevitably arise from the machining process. Starting with relatively coarse grinding paper, used either wet or dry (wet gives better results), this stage progresses through successively finer grades of paper until a flat surface is produced with a uniform finish corresponding to the last grade of abrasive to be used. Subsequently one or more final polishing operations are required. The most common methods use cloth-covered polishing wheels to which the polishing agent (usually alumina or diamond dust) is applied in combination with a suitable liquid lubricant. Those operations are continued until a bright mirror finish is obtained. With all mechanical abrasion treatments, even the final stage of polishing may not entirely remove the effects of previous treatment so it is often necessary to remove this surface film by a chemical attack (or etch) in some suitable chemical reagent, such as an acid, followed by a further very light polish.

An alternative method of finishing, which is widely used, is electrolytic polishing by immersing the metal specimen in a suitable electrolyte and passing an electric current, using an appropriate metal for the cathode and the specimen as anode. If the conditions are right and the metal structure is not too heterogeneous, a good, uniform polished surface is obtained free of any scratches or plastic deformation effects.

After such treatment the specimen is ready for its first examination under the microscope. Sometimes, if the different phases have not polished equally uniformly and a relief effect has resulted, a polished finish will reveal structural features but certainly any cracks, fissures, porosity, or nonmetallic inclusions which are present, or phases of differing colours will be revealed, The best magnification to use will depend on circumstances but it is usually worth while using a low magnification first, to get a general picture, before more detailed examination with higher magnification.

Often the polished surface of a specimen does not show all that the metallurgist would like to see and therefore the surface has to be etched, usually by immersion in a suitable etchant, to bring out the desired features. An etchant may be used to pick out grain boundaries and to reveal grain size and form; to reveal lack of uniformity in a structure (such as the 'coring'); or to reveal grain orientation and to expose and identify differing phases. Considerable skill is required in selecting etchants and interpreting their effects but, once this skill is acquired, a metallographer can gain a surprising amount of information by alternate polishing, etching and examination using different etchants. Other means are also available for etching. A similar process to electrolytic polishing can give an electrolytic etch. Sometimes the structural condition can also be revealed by 'thermal' etching or tinting. In thermal etching the specimen is heated in a vacuum to a sufficiently high temperature to cause thermally assisted adjustments at grain boundaries and sometimes in other areas which assist examination under the microscope by producing relief effects on the surface. In thermal tinting the specimen is kept in air and the temperature raised sufficiently to form a thin oxide skin which reveals itself as a tinting effect due to interference between the thin oxide film and the wavelengths of the incident light. Different phases oxidise at different rates and so the tints for a given time and temperature will differ because the oxide film thickness differs. This latter method is not used much because it can be unreliable.

Examination is usually restricted to room temperature, so in those metals in which an elevated temperature structure cannot be retained at room temperature after rapid quenching of the specimen, little information can be obtained about their structural behaviour at elevated temperature. In these cases much can be done by using a 'hot stage' microscope. This is a microscope which carries on its stage a miniature furnace (usually electrically heated) with a transparent, heat-resisting window through which the microscope can focus on the polished surface of the specimen as it lies inside. Provision is made for keeping the specimen under vacuum or in an inert atmosphere so that the polished surface will not oxidise or tarnish. Very high magnifications cannot be used because of the difficulty in getting the lens close to the surface

Electron Microscope

Many attempts have been made to overcome the limitations which the wave nature of light rays imposes on resolution and magnification. The most successful of these is the use of an electron beam in an electron microscope. The principle of magnification is similar to that for light rays except that the lenses are magnetic or electrostatic fields. Electrons are invisible to the naked eye so visibility is obtained by focusing the beam on a fluorescent screen, as in television, giving an image which may be studied or photographed. The electron beam has its source in a heated tungsten filament which is also the cathode of the system, emission being controlled and directed towards the anode. In the latter there is a circular, axial hole through which a stream of electrons may pass to the specimen. The stream passes through the specimen, then through the 'lenses' to the fluorescent screen, as shown in Fig. 21.4.

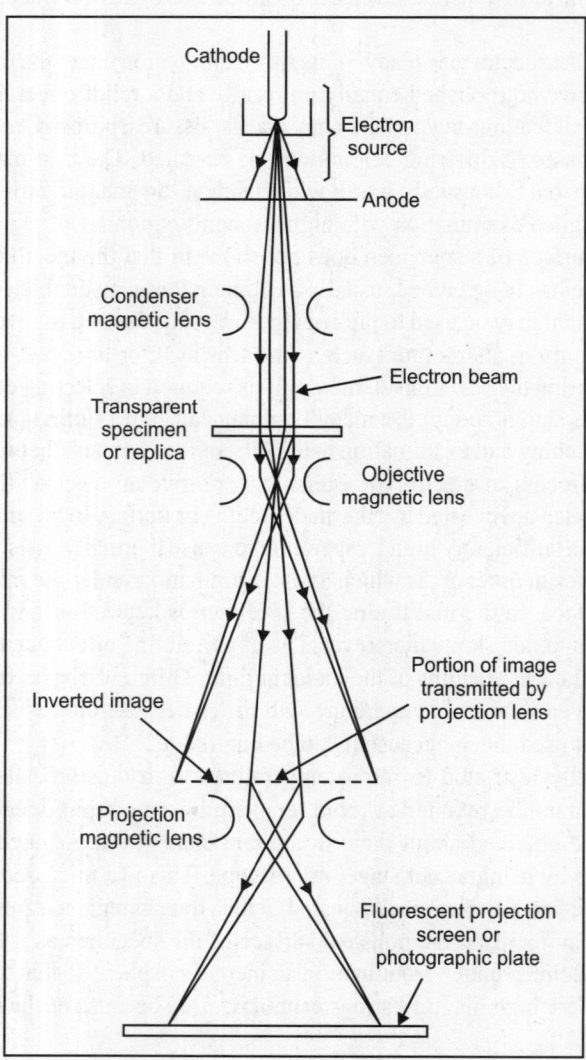

Fig. 21.4. The principle of the electron microscope.

Electrons do not travel well or far in air, so the whole source and lens system has to be evacuated. The wavelength of the electron beam can be varied by varying the potential between the cathode and the anode, 10,000 volts giving a wavelength of 0.1227 Å. (1 Ångström unit = 10^{-8} cm) and 70,000 volts giving 0.0447 Å. Magnification up to 100,000 times or more is possible, with resolutions down to the order of 20 A (equivalent to about 13 million lines per inch). Focusing is performed by adjusting the current or potential to the lenses, while resolution and penetration are adjusted by varying the potential at the source (to change the wavelength).

Many difficulties beset the use of the electron microscope in addition to those such as spherical and chromatic aberration which are analogous to ocular microscope difficulties. Examination by reflection methods is exceptionally difficult, if not impossible, so transmission systems have to be used. Metals are a real problem under transmission conditions because of their dense nature. Two methods of approach have been used: (i) the replica method, and (ii) the preparation of films of the metal so thin that they become transparent to the electron beam.

Replicas can be prepared in two ways: either by taking an impression of the surface of the metal with some externally applied skin, such as collodion or, alternatively, by forming an oxide film on the surface and then dissolving the metal away to leave the oxide film which will be accurately shaped to the contours of the metal surface. This method gives a shadow picture approximating to the contour of the metal surface but there is always uncertainty as to whether or not the replica is undistorted (it is extremely fragile to handle, especially if mechanically removed from the parent surface, and is liable to distort and twist) and as to whether or not it has taken a true representation by penetrating into all crevices, etc. Not surprisingly, the results are hard to interpret.

Thin film preparation is begun by rolling the metal down to a foil and then is continued by electrolytic 'machining' or corrosive attack to dissolve down to the required thinness. Obtaining and interpreting the results requires great skill and patience and it is unlikely that electron microscopy will become a routine tool except for research work.

Macrography

Macrography is another branch of metallography which requires consideration in relation to the study of topography of sectioned surfaces. Its use is intended to give a broad picture of the interior of a metal by studying relatively large sectioned areas either with the unaided eye or at magnification up to about ×15. By its means the incidence of grosser defects can readily be seen, the grain size of cast metal can be studied, some idea can be obtained concerning distribution of constituents and a clear picture obtained of the way in which the metal may have been caused to 'flow' in the course of forming. The last of these is particularly important to those industrial metallurgists and engineers who are concerned with the mechanical working processes, such as forging and rolling.

Preparation follows similar lines to those for micro-examination but need not be taken to such a high degree of surface finish and so the final stages of polishing can be omitted.

A hardness survey is usually made on a macro-surface to give some idea of its uniformity in regard to properties or treatment. Such hardness tests are made in a regular pattern according to the shape of the section and in a sufficient number to give a reasonably accurate picture.

Etching of the prepared surface can be used to show grain size and distribution, nonmetallic inclusions (e.g. slag and oxides), defects resulting from manufacturing processes, such as casting and mechanical working, and other structural features. For instance, some idea of the influence of casting and working processes on uniformity of a metal can be obtained by locating and plotting the distribution of some low-melting-point, solid, insoluble constituent. Such a constituent will be the last to solidify and so will tend to outline crystals which have formed in the metal. A constituent of this type will also tend to concentrate more in the liquid metal which freezes last and thus a greater proportion will be present in such areas after solidification. These facts, taken together, can give a very useful indication of the mode of solidification when the distribution of the constituent is traced. Should a cast structure be broken down by forging or some other mechanical working process, the distribution of the low-melting-point insoluble constituent being known for the cast condition, then tracing its distribution after mechanical working will help towards an understanding of the mode of deformation of the metal as a whole. Probably the most useful method of this type is the use of 'sulphur printing' on sections of low-alloy steel components.

Sulphur is almost invariably present in low-alloy steel, although the amount is kept to a minimum, and exists in the form of various sulphides, notably manganese sulphide which will evolve hydrogen sulphide gas if attacked by dilute acid. Bromide printing paper stains in the presence of hydrogen sulphide, so if bromide paper is soaked in dilute sulphuric acid (3 per cent aqueous solution) just long enough to give saturation (under 2 minutes) and the paper is placed, sensitised side down, in close contact with the prepared, unetched surface then hydrogen sulphide will be evolved. Through reaction of the acid with the sulphides, staining will be caused in the vicinity of the evolution. Time of exposure decides the intensity of the stain but excessive time also causes spreading and blurring, so a compromise is adopted on the basis of experience. The staining of the paper can be 'fixed' in the usual way after the print has been made. Often deeply etched surfaces can be 'printed' by smearing them with printer's ink, carefully removing excess, and then pressing white paper into contact with the surface or, alternatively, a photograph can be taken. In neither case should such prints be confused with sulphur prints although, with a cast structure, both may give the same appearance. Each has its own purpose, the latter giving a good idea of the chemical distribution in the metal, whereas the former gives a more accurate picture of the state of the structure. It should be remembered that a part must be destroyed if it is to be sectioned and subjected to macro-examination and, furthermore, that more than one section may have to be so examined if a true estimate is to be made of the state and history of the metal forming the component; thus the process is not speedy or economic to apply on a large scale. Probably, the main use of macroexamination is in two fields:

1. Examining a part which has failed in service, to find the cause of failure.
2. Doing preliminary research to plan a manufacturing process or sequence such as casting or forging.

Measurement and Control

Much of the work of the metallographer is experimental, so he has to have standards by which he can measure and control the processes which he employs, temperature has to be measured and controlled, cooling and testing rates determined, testing conditions specified and so on. It is intended now to give some attention to the more important of these aspects.

Heating

Nearly all metallurgical treatments involve the use of heat in one way or another; therefore heat application and control form a very important part of the work and probably the most important part in industrial practice. Laboratory-type heating is mainly confined to electrical heating, usually by a resistance heating method, although gas is used to a limited extent. The great advantage of electrical heating lies in the ease of control and in its cleanliness and convenience.

Control is not the simple matter it might seem at first sight. The inherent heating and cooling rates of the furnace must be taken into account as well as the speed of response between the heating system and the control. In fact, for many applications the critical factor is not the accuracy of the control medium but rather its positioning in relation to the heat source. It is not much use having a control medium with a response of ±1/10°C if it takes ten minutes for the effect of a change in heating conditions to penetrate to the control position.

Furthermore, the conditions in a furnace are not necessarily uniform and they can vary considerably between furnaces of apparently identical construction and control. Each case has to be considered on its merits in relation both to the arrangement of the equipment and to the degree of accuracy which is required. Manual control may be good enough, or it may be necessary to combine some automatic control with manual control, or it may be necessary to employ fully automatic control and, simultaneously, circulate the furnace atmosphere to keep it uniform.

The technique of measuring temperature is normally called thermometry but in metallurgy, where concern lies mainly with elevated temperature, the term 'pyrometry' is more frequently employed. Temperatures can be measured in a number of ways against standard scales. The scale which is most commonly used in Britain is based on the Centigrade scale which arbitrarily divides the difference in temperature between that of melting ice and boiling water, under normal atmospheric pressure, into 100 equal divisions or degrees. Alternatively, the Kelvin absolute scale is sometimes employed. This scale uses the same mode of division in the same range but starts at absolute zero (273°K = 0°C).

Various means for measuring temperature are available. Mercury and alcohol thermometers are used in the lower temperature range, up to 350°C, although a bi-metal strip instrument may be used as an alternative, up to 400°C. A bi-metal strip made from two dissimilar metals bonded together side by side will deflect with changing temperature and can be used to indicate temperature by moving a needle on a calibrated scale.

Beyond this range other methods must be adopted. Two methods are in common use; one for temperatures up to 700°C and the other for temperatures up to 1500°C. The former is the resistance pyrometer which measures temperature by making use of the fact that the electrical resistance of a metal changes in a known relationship with temperature. Platinum, because of its stable characteristics and resistance to oxidation, is most commonly used for this application. It's use is not widespread but there are some applications for which it is particularly suited.

The alternative and most common method is to use a thermocouple which depends for its operation on the fact that if two dissimilar metals are in contact there will be a potential difference between them, the magnitude of which will depend on the temperature. Thus, if two wires of dissimilar metals are joined by welding together one pair of ends, as shown at Fig. 21.5(a), and the other two ends are joined to a sensitive galvanometer, then a deflection will be shown on the galvanometer, the magnitude of deflection depending on the temperature difference between the welded and unwelded ends. If the unwelded ends are maintained at a constant temperature, say 0°C in melting ice, then the deflection indicated by the galvanometer will have a definite relationship to the temperature at the welded end. The unwelded ends, connected together by way of the galvanometer, are called the 'cold junction' and the welded ends the 'hot junction'.

If it is not possible or practical to maintain a cold junction at a fixed temperature then 'cold junction compensation' may be used. This takes the form of a piece of equipment which, when incorporated in the system, produces a change in the zero setting of the galvanometer needle to compensate for fluctuation in the reference temperature (room temperature). The compensation may take the form of a varying resistance in the circuit or it may be a tension adjustment to the galvanometer suspension.

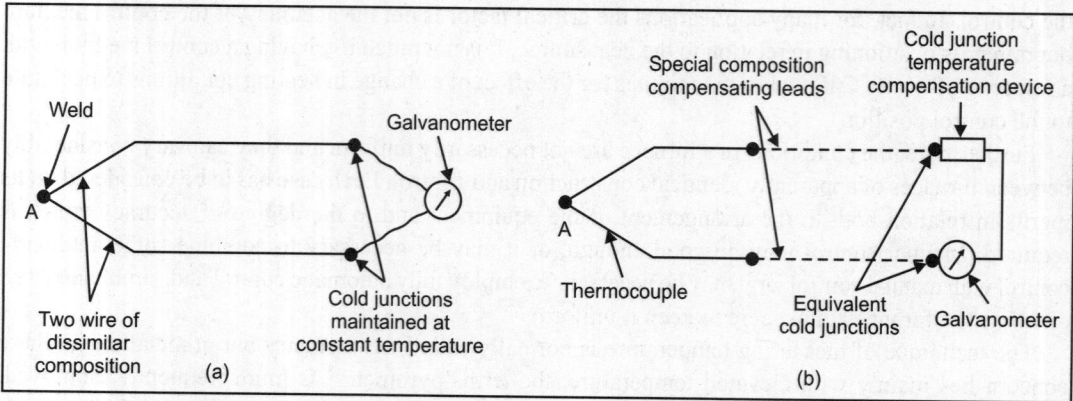

Fig. 21.5. Thermocouples. (a) Basic thermocouple circuit, and (b) thermocouple with leads for extending cold junctions away from heat source and a device to compensate automatically for temperature changes at these cold junctions.

It may not be convenient to have the galvanometer connected directly to the thermocouple wires, so the connection may be made by an extension system using 'compensating' leads composed of metals which will not add to or subtract from the main potential if temperature varies between the cold junction and the galvanometer connections. The cold junction is transferred, in effect, to the outer ends of the compensating leads. The circuit might be as shown in Fig. 21.5(b) which is typical of many industrial applications. Many combinations of metals do not form good thermocouples, either because their potential differences are not great enough or because the relationship between potential difference and temperature is not sufficiently uniform.

The three most common combinations are: (i) iron and constantan (constantan is an alloy containing 60 per cent Cu 40 per cent Ni), used for temperatures up to 300°C, (ii) Chromel (90 per cent Ni 10 per cent Cr) and Alumel (98 per cent Ni_2 per cent Al), used up to 1100°C, and (iii) platinum and a platinum-13 per cent rhodium alloy, for temperatures up to 1500°C. Of the three, the last is the one with the most uniform temperature-potential relationship, but the potential differences are low. Typical potential curves are shown in Fig. 21.6. It is possible to measure temperatures up to 1800°C by a similar system, using a silicon-carbide rod in a carbon tube as the thermocouple, but this application is not common.

For temperatures between 700° and 1500°C thermocouples have an almost exclusive field but are superseded at higher temperature ranges by optical or radiation pyrometers. Any heated body radiates thermal energy which begins to become visible when the temperature rises to 600°C. As temperature rises further, the radiation increases in intensity and changes wavelength, the variation being mainly dependent on the temperature but also on the nature of the radiating substance.

This dependence can be used for measuring temperature within certain limits of accuracy. Trouble arises from two main sources:

1. The full effect of the radiation may not be under observation. (Ideal conditions are approached only if the radiation is observed as it comes from the bottom of a deep narrow hole in the heated body, giving what are called 'black body' conditions of full radiation.)
2. Other adjacent heat sources are liable to give reflections from the surface under observation which cause anomalies in the readings. (This is very likely to happen in a furnace where the heating source must almost inevitably be hotter than the heated object.)

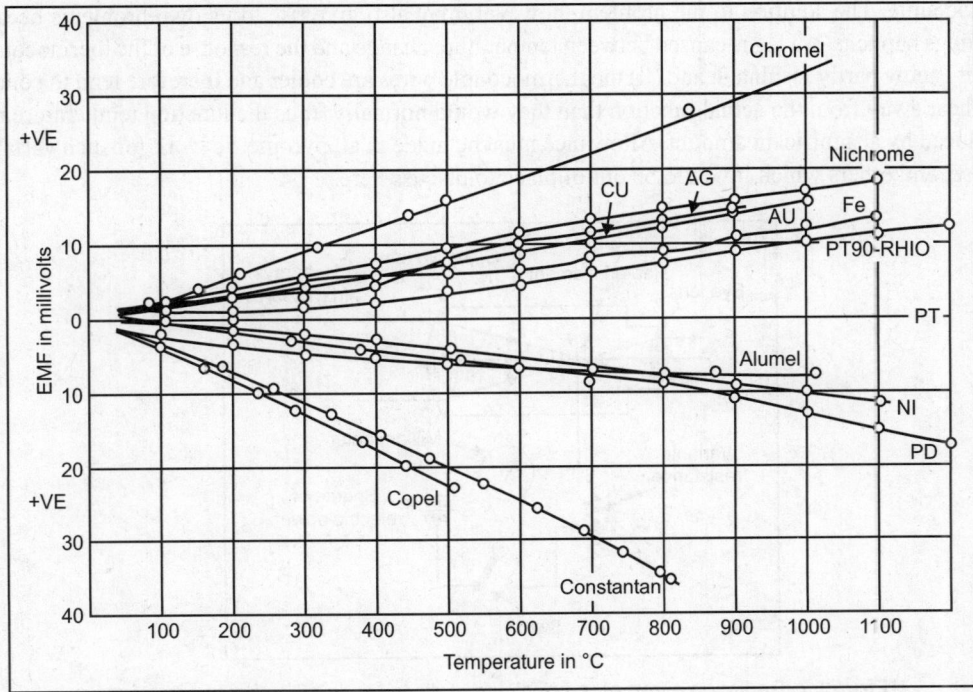

Fig. 21.6. Thermoelectric potentials for various metals and alloys against platinum. Cold junction temperature 0°C.

Altogether, radiation pyrometry cannot attain the accuracy of other methods but, on the other hand, there is a range of temperatures in which only radiation methods can be employed.

Two systems are used: the optical system and the total radiation system. Human judgment is used in the optical system, either to match the radiation intensity with a tinted glass slip or to heat a lamp filament to such intensity that it disappears against the radiating background, as suggested in Fig. 21.7. The colour intensity method gives a rather poor measure of temperature but the current required to produce invisibility in a properly calibrated lamp filament gives reasonably accurate results. Many portable radiation pyrometers are of the disappearing filament type.

Total radiation systems do not rely on human judgment, except to ensure accurate siting and setting of the instrument, so that a true full-radiation beam from the source is focused on a thermocouple, thermopile or photosensitive cell contained inside the instrument. Knowing the characteristics of the instrument and its position, the readings from the potential source in the instrument can be interpreted in terms of the temperature of the heated body.

Although, within its range, a thermocouple is the most convenient means of temperature measurement, there are also some snags. For one thing, the thermocouple is in the same atmosphere and condition as the body whose temperature is being measured. Consequently, if any corrosive gas or vapour is present, the thermocouple is open to attack (e.g. oxidation or corrosion) which may alter its characteristics or cause it to fracture. Moreover, it may be used to measure the temperature of a liquid metal and direct contact can mean diffusion between the liquid metal and the solid thermocouple wires. In either case the problem may be solved by enclosing the thermocouple in a protecting sheath made of a suitably refractory material, such as fused silica, which will give sufficient protection to ensure a reasonable life to the thermocouple. The solution to the problem, however, may also give rise to its own problems because two things happen: (i) a lag is caused between temperature change and the response of the thermocouple, since it is now partly insulated, and (ii) the thermocouple wires are cooler and therefore tend to conduct more heat away from the actual junction than they would normally; thus the junction temperature may be reduced by a significant amount. Allowance must be made in all pyrometric work for such variables as these, and others which it would be out of place to discuss here.

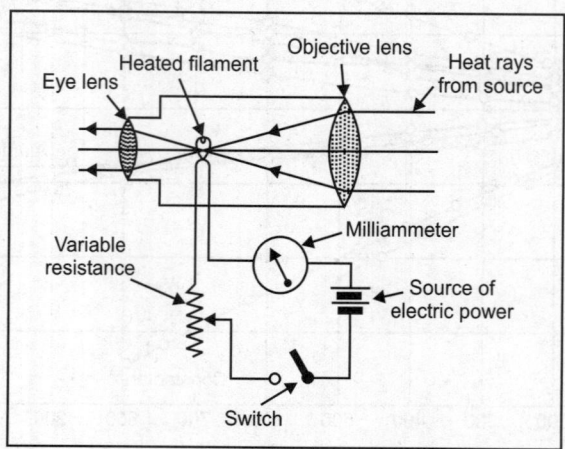

Fig. 21.7. Radiation pyrometer: principles of disappearing filament pyrometer.

Nearly all the instruments which have been mentioned for pyrometric work give indication of temperature by means of a galvanometer in one form or another. Many use the direct indication of the galvanometer, given by means of a needle on a calibrated scale, but this suffers from serious disadvantages due to the limited angle of needle deflection permissible with such instruments. Without making the needle so long that it becomes unstable or mechanically weak the maximum range of needle point deflection which may be attained with a stationary galvanometer is 8–10 inches which must be further reduced if the instrument is to be portable. If a record is to be kept by making the needle of the inking type, a further burden is placed upon the instrument, so both accuracy and efficiency suffer.

For these and other reasons it is often preferred that the potentiometric system of potential measurement or the Wheatstone Bridge method of resistance measurement (according to the type of detecting instrument) be incorporated into an automatically operated instrument. Such instruments are electronically or mechanically powered and may be of indicating, or indicating and recording, or indicating, recording and controlling type according to requirements. Both these measuring methods use a 'null deflection' galvanometer system, that is, the galvanometer is constantly being balanced back to zero deflection, with no current flowing. The balance is achieved either by opposing the potential from the detecting system by an external potential or by balancing the resistance ratios in the bridge, if the latter is used. The balancing has to be done by some servo mechanism, such as an electrically driven mechanical clutch and cam system or an electrically operated servomotor. On such an instrument the indicator or recorder is not direct reading but simply indicates the value of the opposed potential or balance resistance. Power for switch changing and relay operation is available from the servomechanism and so these instruments can readily be made multi-point temperature-indicating (taking a reading from each point over a period of time equal to the response time of the instrument multiplied by the number of points) and/or control operating. Mechanical operation is slower and less accurate than electronic operation; the time of response required to permit an instrument to balance itself is about 20 seconds with the former and 2 or 3 seconds with the latter. Both systems are expensive in first cost.

Direct control of heating from the temperature measuring source is common practice and an essential for all operations requiring accurate temperature maintenance.

Operation of a mechanical or electrical relay system is simple with the servomechanism of the more expensive instruments but not so simple with the direct type of instrument. However, very effective electronic methods are being developed and are in use with many direct reading instruments. One employs a simple electronic circuit tuned in series with a photosensitive transistor which is carried on the control setting arm. The control setting arm is mounted below the galvanometer needle, which carries a little opaque vane of foil. As the temperature rises, the vane swings into the range of the transistor according to where the control arm is set, and upsets the balance of the circuit by shutting off light to the transistor, thus causing a relay system to operate and influence the furnace control to lower the temperature. Falling temperature removes the vane and restores the former conditions and so on, the temperature attaining a stabilised position relative to the control setting.

Instruments are available which perform as indicating-controllers or indicating-controller-recorders in one or other of the ways already described; in addition they will also meter the heating agency (through mechanical or electrical devices) in such a way that the energy input is reduced when the control temperature is approached, so achieving very stable temperature control with the minimum of manual interference. Adjustment of the energy input may be done in several ways, from cutting down the maximum energy to using periods of full heating alternately with the heating energy completely cut off over a short time cycle. The proportioning of the latter type of cycle determines the average heat input. Atmosphere control in a furnace may be important either to protect the charge from oxidation or other attack, or to produce some desirable surface reaction. Control of a gaseous atmosphere may be the most convenient means, or it may be necessary to use a liquid medium, such as a salt bath, in which the charge can be immersed. The latter method has the advantage of very rapid heating, because of the close contact between the salt and the charge and easier control of uniformity of temperature as a result of natural convective circulation.

Cooling

Cooling is a very important factor in many applications but it is difficult to define or standardise in precise terms because no method gives a uniform rate throughout an operation and even the same method will give different rates with differing sizes and shapes of charge. The best that can be done, for general purposes, is to give an order of cooling severity ranging from quenching rapidly in chilled brine (with which the cooling rate is most rapid) to slow cooling in a closed furnace after the heat has been turned off.

Chapter 22

Pyrometry

INTRODUCTION

Pyrometry measures the temperature of objects without touching them. It is standard procedure in many industries today. Due to its accuracy, speed, economy and specific advantages, pyrometry is steadily gaining acceptance in new fields. But how is it possible to measure temperatures without physical contact? Every object whose temperature is above absolute zero (−273.15°C) emits radiation. This emission is heat radiation and is dependent upon temperature. The term infrared radiation is also in use because the wavelengths of the majority of this radiation lie in the electromagnetic spectrum above the visible red light, in the infrared domain.

Temperature is the determining factor of radiation and energy. Infrared radiation transports energy. This radiated energy is used to help determine the temperature of a body being measured (Fig. 22.1).

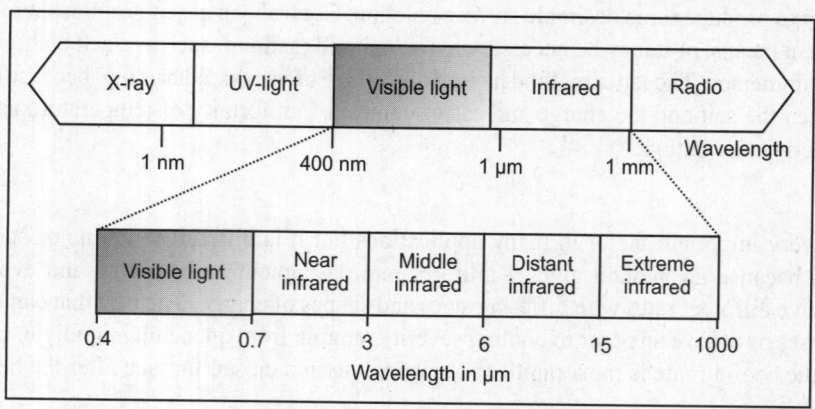

Fig. 22.1. Electromagnetic spectrum.

Similar to radio broadcasting where emitted energy from a transmitter is captured by a receiver via an antenna and then transformed into sound waves, the emitted heat radiation of an object is received by a detecting device and transformed into electric signals.

Thus, the energy emitted by an object is utilised by remote (i.e. non-contact) temperature measuring devices. The instruments which determine an object's temperature in this fashion are called radiation thermometers, radiation pyrometers or simply pyrometers.

Originally, pyrometry was a strictly visual measuring method. Experienced blacksmiths and steel workers could with surprising accuracy gauge the metal's temperature by its brightness and colouration. The first pyrometers could only utilise the visible radiation from an object. Since radiation is visible only when the object is made red hot, early Pyrometry could only be successful when measuring high temperatures. But technical advances have made it possible today to measure temperatures far below freezing point from a distance and without making contact with the object to be measured. In industrial manufacturing and in engineering processes, pyrometry is standard procedure and can no longer be ignored. Be it in glass manufacture, metal working, or food production, accurate temperature measurement remains one of the most important factors to consider during processing.

PRINCIPLE OF OPERATION

A pyrometer has an optical system and detector. The optical system focuses the thermal radiation onto the detector. The output signal of the detector (Temperature T) is related to the thermal radiation or irradiance j^* of the target object through the Stefan–Boltzmann law, the constant of proportionality σ, called the Stefan-Boltzmann constant and the emissivity ε of the object.

$$j^* = \varepsilon \sigma T^4$$

This output is used to infer the object's temperature. Thus, there is no need for direct contact between the pyrometer and the object, as there is with thermocouple and Resistance temperature detector (RTDs).

Modern pyrometers became available when the first disappearing filament pyrometer was built by L. Holborn and F. Kurlbaum in 1901. This device superimposed a thin, heated filament over the object to be measured and relied on the operator's eye to detect when the filament vanished. The object temperature was then read from a scale on the pyrometer.

The temperature returned by the vanishing filament pyrometer and others of its kind, called Brightness Pyrometers, is dependent on the emissivity of the object. With greater use of brightness pyrometers, it became obvious that problems existed with relying on knowledge of the value of emissivity. Emissivity was found to change, often drastically, with surface roughness, bulk and surface composition, and even the temperature itself. To get around these difficulties, the ratio or two-colour pyrometer was developed. They rely on the fact that Planck's Law, which relates temperature to the intensity of radiation emitted at individual wavelengths, can be solved for temperature if Planck's statement of the intensities at two different wavelengths is divided. This solution assumes that the emissivity is the same at both wavelengths and cancels out in the division. This is known as the grey body assumption. Ratio pyrometers are essentially two brightness pyrometers in a single instrument. The operational principles of the ratio pyrometers were developed in the 1920s and 1930s, and they were commercially available in 1939.

As the ratio pyrometer came into popular use, it was determined that many materials, of which metals are an example, do not have the same emissivity at two wavelengths. For these materials, the emissivity does not cancel out and the temperature measurement is in error. The amount of error depends on the emissivities and the wavelengths where the measurements are taken. Two-colour ratio pyrometers cannot measure whether a material's emissivity is wavelength dependent.

To more accurately measure the temperature of real objects with unknown or changing emissivities, multiwavelength pyrometers were envisioned at the US National Institute of Standards and Technology and described in 1992. Multiwavelength pyrometers use three or more wavelengths and mathematical manipulation of the results to attempt to achieve accurate temperature measurement even when the emissivity is unknown, changing, and different at all wavelengths.

Applications

Pyrometers are suited especially to the measurement of moving objects or any surfaces that cannot be reached or cannot be touched.

Smelter industry

Temperature is a fundamental parameter in metallurgical furnace operations. Reliable and continuous measurement of the melt temperature is essential for effective control of the operation. Smelting rates can be maximised, slag can be produced at the optimum temperature, fuel consumption is minimised and refractory life may also be lengthened. Thermocouples were the traditional devices used for this purpose, but they are unsuitable for continuous measurement because they rapidly dissolve.

Over-the-bath pyrometer

Salt bath furnaces operate at temperatures up to 1300°C and are used for heat treatment. At very high working temperatures with intense heat transfer between the molten salt and the steel being treated, precision is maintained by measuring the temperature of the molten salt. Most errors are caused by slag on the surface which is cooler than the salt bath.

Tuyère Pyrometer

The Tuyère pyrometer is an optical instrument for temperature measurement through the tuyeres which are normally used for feeding air or reactants into the bath of the furnace.

Steam boilers

A steam boiler may be fitted with a pyrometer to measure the steam temperature in the superheater.

Hot air balloons

A hot air balloon is equipped with a pyrometer for measuring the temperature at the top of the envelope in order to prevent overheating of the fabric.

Pyrometry of Gases

Pyrometry of gases presents difficulties. These are most commonly overcome by using thin filament pyrometry or soot pyrometry. Both techniques involve small solids in contact with hot gases.

ADVANTAGES OF PYROMETERS

The advantages of pyrometers are:
1. Fast response.
2. No adverse effects on temperatures and materials.
3. Measuring moving objects.
4. Measuring objects which are difficult to access.

Fast Response

Pyrometers have a very short response time. With contact measuring, a probe records the temperature at its tip which is in contact with the object. The probe must first reach the same temperature of the object and this takes time due to thermal conduction. The pyrometer, however, measures the radiation and shows the correct temperature in fractions of a second (Fig. 22.2).

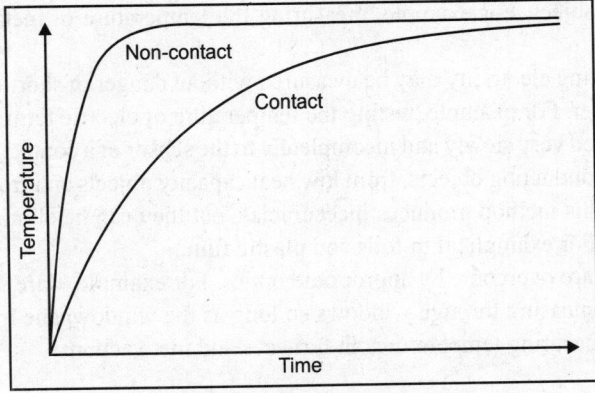

Fig. 22.2. Response time.

No Adverse Effects

1. To measure temperature, a radiation pyrometer uses a portion of the energy that is being emitted from the object anyway. Therefore, the act of measuring itself does not influence the temperature of the object. A contact thermometer must first reach the temperature of the object at the point of contact in order to measure. This process causes heat loss of the object which in turn may change the temperature at the contact point.
2. Using non-contact measuring, sensors cannot be damaged or destroyed in the same way that can happen when using thermocouples and other contact devices. Clearly, the life of contact-free measuring units is considerably longer than that of thermo-elements which are subject to more wear and tear.

Measuring Moving Objects

1. Because of the pyrometer's quick response time, temperatures of moving objects can be determined accurately.
2. Contact thermometers can influence temperature readings because of friction of the sliding temperature probe.
3. Measuring by physical contact can also cause scratching on the measured object's surface.
4. Pyrometers do not damage or destroy the measured object. Neither drilling nor special fastening to the object is needed.

Measuring Objects which are Difficult to Access by Contact Measuring Devices

1. The optics of pyrometers can be adjusted to measure temperatures of small objects. Today it is possible to accurately measure objects with a diameter of 0.2 mm. The measuring error mentioned above (at the contact point) is especially great with small objects. For example, thin wires.
2. High temperatures can be captured easily as there is no direct contact with the heat source. NiCr-Ni thermocouples, for example, change physically at 1300°C and then can no longer achieve repeatable readings. For example, forging steel.
3. Highly aggressive materials can be measured without contact and thus without damage to the sensor. For example, acids in chemical processes.
4. Objects can be measured with pyrometers even though they cannot be physically reached. Pyrometers are compact units that can be installed nearly anywhere. All they need is a clear line

of sight to the object. For example, measuring the temperature of metals during the heating process.
5. Objects conducting electricity may be measured without danger of short-circuiting and without danger to the user. For example, testing the temperature of electric terminals in switch boxes.
6. Heat is transferred very slowly and incompletely to the sensor of a contact measuring instrument from poor heatconducting objects, from low heat capacity objects and from objects which have a small mass. This method produces inaccuracies, but they can be eliminated by using a non-contact device. For example, thin foils and plastic film.
7. Great distances are overcome by appropriate optics. For example, flare stack monitors.
8. It is possible to measure through windows so long as the windowpane material is compatible. For example, measuring temperatures in furnaces and in a vacuum.

PHYSICAL PRINCIPLES

Spectral Intensity

Visible light with all its colours, infrared radiation, X-rays or γ-rays (gamma), are similar in nature. Their differences lie in wavelength, or frequency. The wavelength is expressed as the 'colour' of the light (Fig. 22.3). One should consider the energy or the intensity of the radiation coming from the black body. Figure 22.3 shows the relative distribution of heat radiation (spectral intensity) across the wavelengths. The exponential correlation of intensity and wavelength requires double logarithmic scaling for graphic representation. Figure 22.3 demonstrates that the intensity curve moves left toward the shorter wavelength as the temperature rises. At temperatures over 550°C the curve reaches the area of visible light. The object to be measured begins to glow. At higher temperatures the intensity rises in the visible area. Steel glows red hot at first, then, as the temperature rises, one speaks of white hot which means all spectral colours are represented.

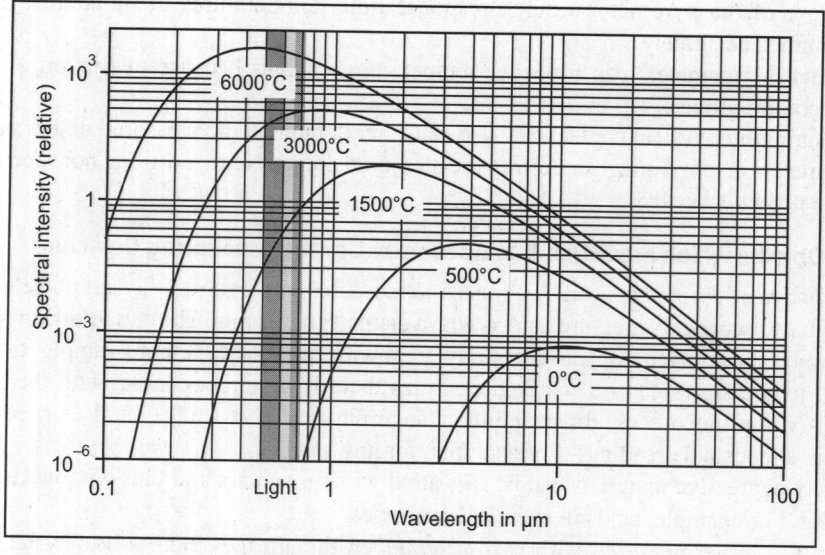

Fig. 22.3. Distribution of intensity.

Wavelength of Maximum Intensity

The curves in Fig. 22.3 indicate that the maximum spectral intensity shifts towards shorter wavelengths as the temperature rises. This correlation is demonstrated in Fig. 22.4 and is called Wien's Law. The wavelength of the maximum intensity of the sun's spectrum lies at 550 nm, in the area of green light. The sun's surface temperature is about 6000°C.

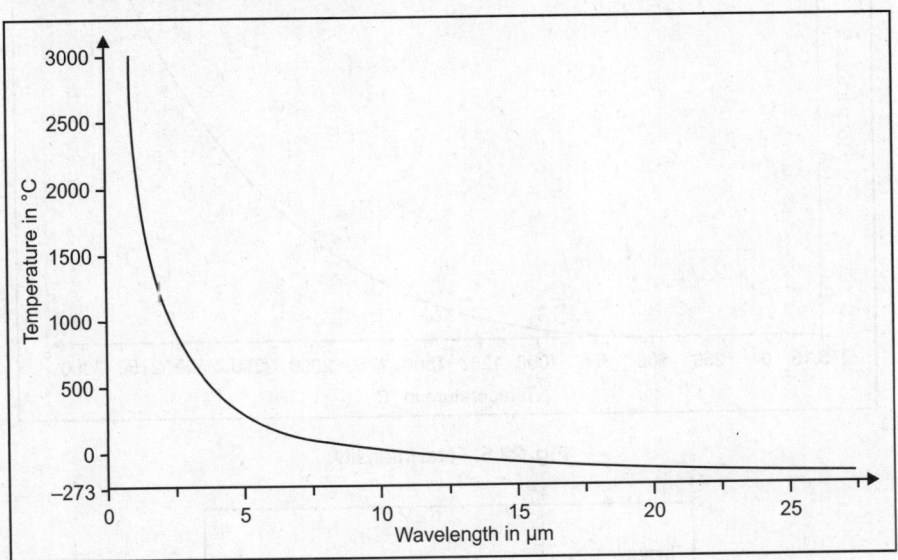

Fig. 22.4. Wien's law.

Total Intensity

When measuring with pyrometers the intensity of radiation is changed into an electric signal. The intensity of radiation across the whole band of all wavelengths is formed by the integral of spectral intensity between 0 µm and infinity, at a given temperature. The total intensity is shown in Fig. 22.3 by the area under the curves.

Total intensity rises to the power of 4 of the absolute temperature. That means that a doubling of the temperature causes a 16-fold rise in intensity. It follows that the intensity at low temperatures is very small. By narrowing the spectral area, as is the case with true pyrometers, a complex relationship between temperature and the intensity reaching the detector results (Fig. 22.5).

PROPERTIES OF REAL OBJECTS

The connections and relationships discussed so far concern black bodies. Real objects, however, have different properties. To clarify this we will look at conditions in the area of visible light, which can also be applied to the infrared region. Real objects have properties called reflection, absorption, and transmission (permeability). A large part of incoming rays are reflected off bright, smooth surfaces. On the one hand we find focused reflection, such as off a mirror or a lacquered surface. On the other hand we have diffuse reflection such as in objects with rough surfaces. Paper, for instance, reflects light in all directions (Fig. 22.6).

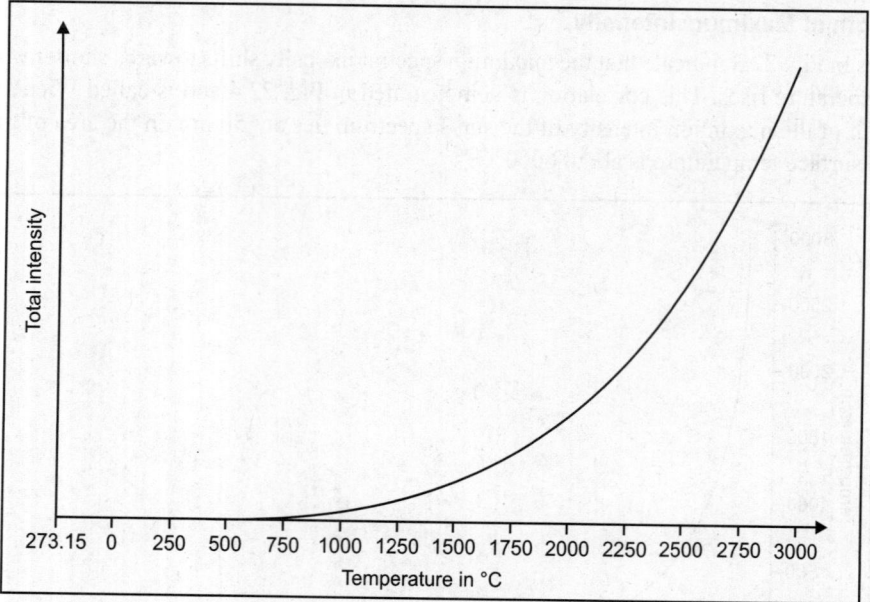

Fig. 22.5. Total intensity.

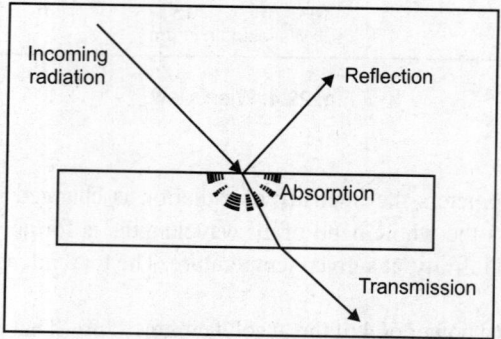

Fig. 22.6. Reflection, absorption, transmission.

Another part of incoming rays is absorbed by dark, rough surfaces. This may happen across a wide or narrow band of the spectrum. In cinemas, much light has to be absorbed by the side walls of the room (often fitted out with dark coloured curtains) so that clear viewing is not impaired by reflections. These dark wall hangings absorb nearly all incoming light. Colours and lacquer, on the other hand, only absorb light selectively. A red car appears red because all other colours are absorbed. The remaining part of incoming rays penetrate the object and are transmitted through it. We speak of transparent materials. This process too may be selective. While normal window glass lets all of the spectrum of visible light pass through, tinted sunglasses let only a certain part of the spectrum through.

Every object has the above mentioned properties, but they are represented in different percentages according to the material under observation. They are described mathematically as reflection rate ρ, absorption rate α, and transmission rate τ. They refer to the ratio of reflected, absorbed, or transmitted intensity to the intensity of the incoming light. The values for ρ, α and τ lie between 0 and 1. Their sum is always 1. With these values a black body's behaviour may be theoretically described as one which absorbs all incoming rays. Its absorption coefficient, α, is 1 (one). It follows then that ρ = 0 (zero), and τ = 0 (zero). In thermal equilibrium, a body which absorbs well, emits well. This means that its absorption coefficient α equals its emission coefficient ε. At a given temperature maximum flow of radiation come from black bodies. Therefore, this object is also called a black body radiation source. In practical terms this condition is evident in soot or in flat black colour.

The emission coefficient ε is the relationship of the emission output of an object to the emission output of a black body radiation source at the same temperature. ε is influenced by the object's material and changes with the wavelength, the temperature or other physical values. In real life, objects match the properties of the black body radiation source only partially or not at all. A body whose emissivity remains constant within a certain spectral area is called a grey body. In visible light it reflects all colours of the light evenly and therefore appears grey. Objects which do not match the properties of a black or a grey body radiation source are called real or coloured radiation bodies (Fig. 22.7).

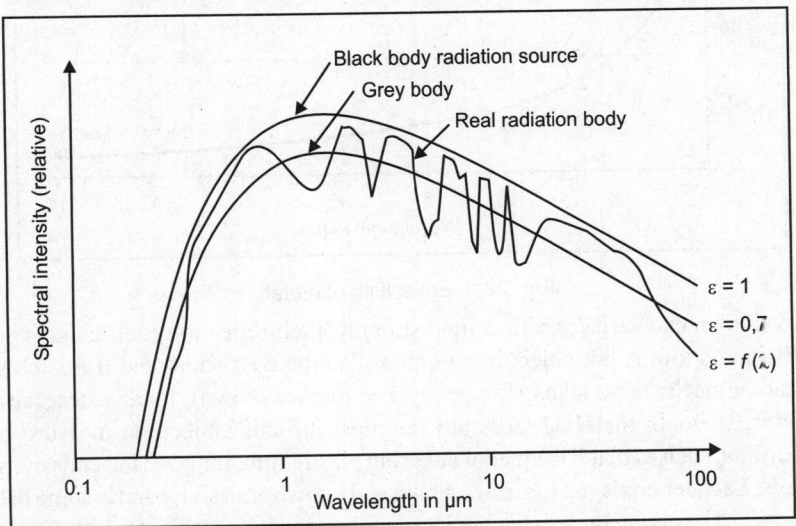

Fig. 22.7. Black body radiation source grey body real radiation body.

EMISSIVITY OF VARIOUS MATERIALS

As already described, the emission coefficient ε of an object is the most important value when determining its temperature with a pyrometer. If one wants to measure the true surface temperature of an object with a pyrometer one must know the emission coefficient, or emissivity, of the object and enter its value in the pyrometric measuring system. To adjust for the material being measured, pyrometers therefore have an emissivity setting. The values for the various materials may be taken from tables. In principle, the emissivity of a material is influenced by wavelength, temperature, etc. Because the emissivity is dependent upon wavelength most materials can be grouped as follows:

1. Metals.
2. Nonmetals.
3. Transparent materials (opaque).

The emissivity of smooth metal surfaces is high at short wavelengths and decreases with lengthening wavelengths. With oxidised and soiled metal surfaces results are not consistent; emissivity may be strongly influenced by temperature and/or wavelength. The emissivity of metals also changes with time due to wear and tear, oxidation or soiling. Pieces of metal are often smooth after processing and their surfaces are changed by heat. Discolouration occurs and can be followed by rust and scale. All this can change the emissivity and must be considered to avoid errors. However, so long as surfaces are not shiny, metals can be measured well in most cases (Fig. 22.8).

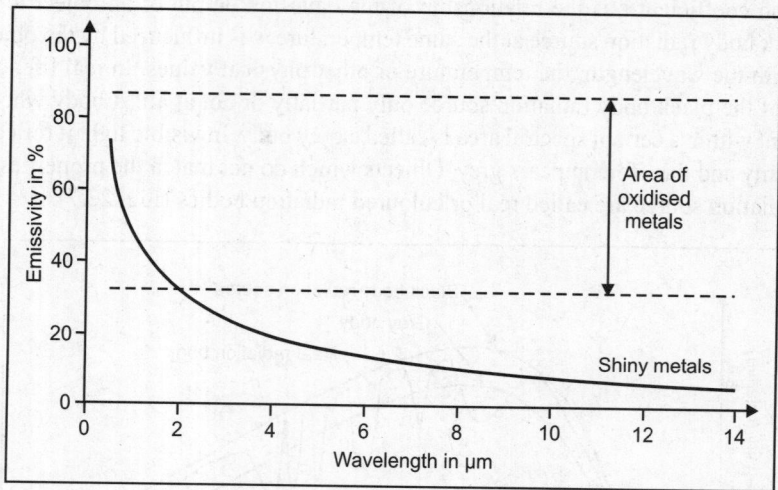

Fig. 22.8. Emissivity of metals.

Smooth and shiny metal surfaces reflect light strongly, their reflection coefficient is high, and their emission coefficient is low. A hot object has a high reflection coefficient and if it is close to where a temperature reading needs to be taken (for example, a furnace crown), it can affect the value of that reading. Therefore, smooth metal surfaces are the most difficult objects to measure in pyrometry. Emissivity modifiers, such as black lacquer or adhering plastic film, improve the emissivity of metals at low temperatures. Lacquer or plastic film have a high and known emissivity and assume the temperature of the metal surface. The nonmetal group includes organic materials, such as food stuffs, wood or paper, as well as ceramics or fire clay. The emissivity of nonmetals rises with increasing wavelength. Generally speaking, from a certain wavelength, the emissivity is nearly constant. With dark materials this begins in the visible spectrum, but with light coloured materials it is above 4 μm (Fig. 22.9).

Penetrable materials like glass, quartz, water, plastics, gases and flames show their own unique emissivity (Fig. 22.10). On the one hand, the emissivity is characterised by transparency in certain areas, on the other hand by absorption. In the absorption band these materials are impenetrable by radiation and therefore are excellent objects for measuring temperatures.

Glass is transparent in visible light and in the near infrared area (to about 3 μm), its transmission coefficient τ is high, and therefore its ε is low. Figure 22.10 shows its emission coefficient is very high in the area of 4.5 to 8.5 μm. The absorption band of glass falls within this area. To measure the glass surface temperature one uses the wavelength of around 5.14 μm, because the values there are not influenced by the absorption band of water vapour or carbon dioxide. Above 7 μm the reflection of glass increases.

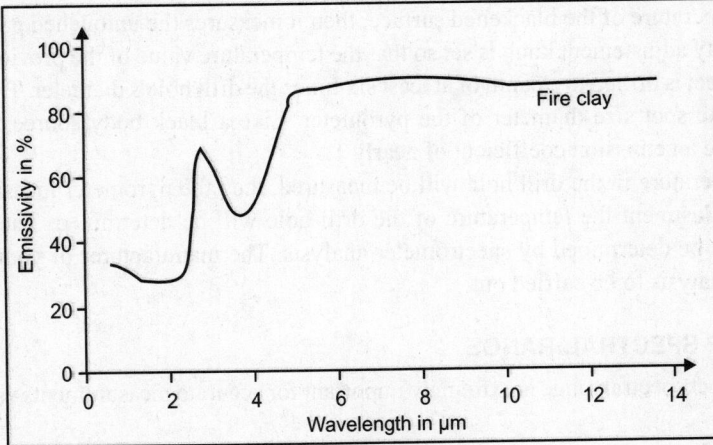

Fig. 22.9. Emissivity of nonmetals.

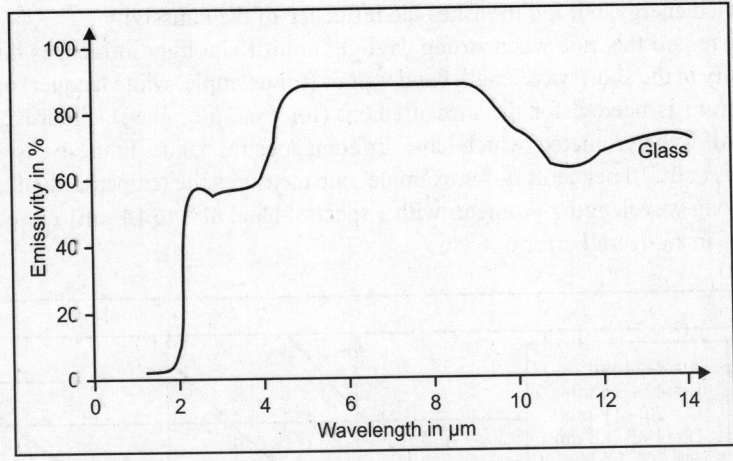

Fig. 22.10. Emissivity of glass (qualitatively).

DETERMINING THE EMISSIVITY OF AN OBJECT

Because the emissivity factor is so important in the calculations that determine temperature, it is essential to establish its value accurately for a given material. There are several ways that this can be done. Tables may be consulted to look up the values of the emission coefficient for many different materials (Table 22.1). For metals, however, the values are mostly qualitative. The temperature of the object is first determined by measuring with a contact thermometer. Then the pyrometer is aimed at the object. Finally, the emissivity adjustment knob is turned until both devices indicate the same temperature. In order to use this method the object must be sufficiently large and accessible.

Part of the object's surface is blackened with special lacquer or soot whose emission coefficient is close to 1, is accurately known and is stable up to the temperature to be measured. The pyrometer measures the temperature of the blackened surface, then it measures the untouched part of the surface. Then the emissivity adjustement knob is set so that the temperature value of the previous measurement is shown. The object is drilled to a depth of at least six times the drill hole's diameter. The diameter must be greater than the spot size diameter of the pyrometer. Like a black body source, the drill hole is considered to have an emission coefficient of nearly 1.

First, the temperature in the drill hole will be measured, then the pyrometer measures the surface, and by correct adjustment the temperature of the drill hole will be determined. The emissivity of a sample object can be determined by spectrometer analysis. The manufacturer of your pyrometer will arrange for this analysis to be carried out.

CHOOSING THE SPECTRAL RANGE

Choosing the correct spectral range is extremely important for accurate measurements using pyrometers.

Emissivity Errors

Here are some rules to observe to avoid emissivity errors. The most important rule is to choose a pyrometer that measures in the shortest wavelength band. This rule may be a disadvantage by not fully utilising the radiated energy, but it diminishes the influence of the emissivity.

It is best to disregard this rule when strong daylight or artificial light influences the measurement, when the emissivity in the short wavelength band is poor (for example, white lacquer) or when a certain area of the spectrum is needed for the measurement (for example, glass). Figure 22.11 shows the measuring errors of five pyrometers which have different spectral bands. In these cases the emissivity had been wrongly set by 10 per cent. If, for example, one measures the temperature of an object heated to 750°C with a long wavelength pyrometer with a spectral band of 8 to 14 µm, a ε setting mistake of 10 per cent results in an overall error of 60°C.

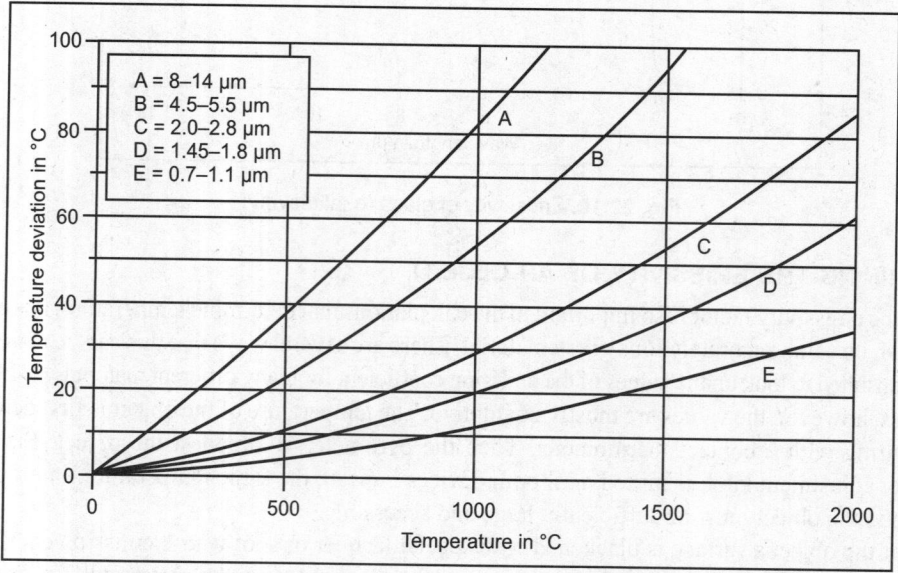

Fig. 22.11. Errors when emissivity setting was out by 10 per cent.

If, however, one uses a pyrometer with a short wavelength spectral band of 0.7 to 1.1 μm the measurement error is reduced to 7°C assuming similar conditions. Just by choosing the right band of the spectrum, errors can be reduced nine fold. This rule is very important when measuring metal objects. With metals the emissivity rises in the short wavelength band which helps prevent errors. In addition, the variation of the emission coefficient that is dependent upon the composition of the material and on the condition of the surface, is diminished when dealing with metals.

For example, the emissivity of pure steel in the spectral area of 0.85 to 1.15 μm shows a value of 0.4 to 0.45. The value for emissivity in the spectral area of 8 to 14 μm, however is 0.1 to 0.3. A potentially false setting of the emission coefficient is reduced to about 6 per cent in the short wavelength band, but can reach 50 per cent in the long wavelength band. Because of their emissivity, measuring the temperature of nonmetals by means of a pyrometer is less complicated.

In this case one must choose pyrometers which the manufacturer has designated for certain materials (for instance, glass, plastics, ceramics, textiles, etc.). The spectral areas in quality pyrometers are chosen so that they are in the wavelengths which have a high and constant emissivity. At those wavelengths, the material is impenetrable and absorption bands of water vapour and carbon dioxide are not found here. In cases where the emission coefficient varies strongly, such as in metalworking processes, it is advisable to use pyrometers which can measure in more than one spectral range. Two colour pyrometers have proven especially successful.

ATMOSPHERIC WINDOWS

The atmosphere is normally the medium through which radiation must pass to reach the pyrometer. Quality pyrometers have been built with spectral ranges which will not allow measurements to be influenced by the atmosphere. These areas are called atmospheric windows. In these windows there are no absorption bands of water vapour and carbon dioxide in the air, so that measuring errors due to moisture in the air or due to a change in measuring distance are eliminated. Figure 22.12 shows where the atmospheric window is located within the spectrum in comparison to the transmission of air and its dependency on wavelength.

Silicon: In the spectral area '1' in Fig. 22.12, temperatures of over 550°C can be measured. Pyrometers with silicon detectors measure the radiation in this window. This spectral area is usually used when measuring metals.

InGaAs and Germanium: In window '2' temperatures of over 250°C are measured. Here Germanium or Indium-Gallium-Arsenide detectors (InGaAs) are used together with optic filters. Metals are mostly measured in this window.

Lead sulphide: In window '3' temperatures of over 75°C are measured. Here lead sulphide detectors (PbS) are used together with optical filters. Metals with low temperatures are measured in this spectral area.

Lead selenide, thermopile, and pyroelectric: In window '4' temperatures of over 50°C are measured. It is especially useful to measure objects behind flames or glass with a penetration depth of 20 mm. Pyrometers are used that have lead selenide (PbSe) detectors, thermopiles, or pyroelectric detectors, together with an optical filter.

Thermopile, and pyroelectric: In window '5' temperatures of over 100°C are measured. This works extremely well with glass surfaces with a penetration depth of 0.7 mm. Pyrometers are used here that have thermopiles and pyroelectric detectors together with an optical filter.

Thermophile and pyroelectric: In window '6' temperatures of over −50°C are measured. Pyrometers are used that have Thermopiles and pyroelectric detectors together with an optical filter. It is used primarily to measure organic substances.

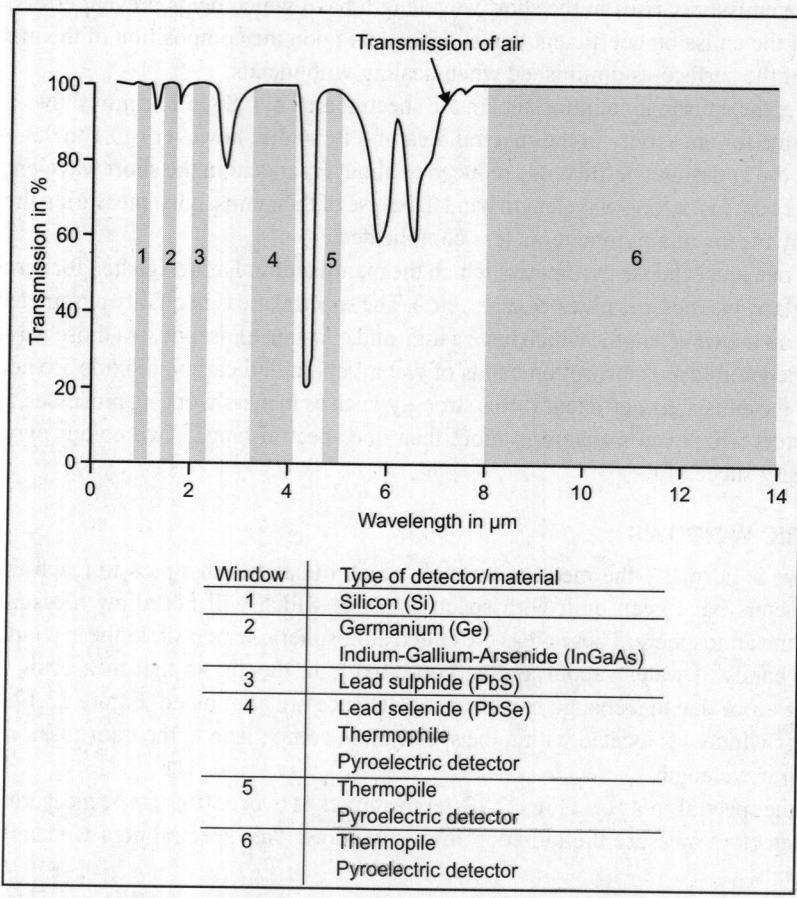

Fig. 22.12. Atmospheric windows and transmission of air.

SPOT SIZE AND MEASURING DISTANCE

The optics of a pyrometer transmit the image of a section of the target area of the measured surface to the detector. This section is called the spot size. By using differently shaped apertures in the pyrometer the spot size may be round or rectangular. The laws of optics mean that the image enlarges as the distance from the lens increases. This is common knowledge in photography. It is possible to measure small objects with pyrometers which are designed for use over short distances. The larger the distance between pyrometer and object, the larger the spot size diameter.

Pyrometers are available with two types of optics:
1. Fixed optics.
2. Optics with variable focus.

Fixed Optics

With fixed optics the minimum diameter of the spot size requires a fixed distance for measuring; the nominal measuring distance. A sharp image on the detector is the result. A different optical variant, with different measuring distances and spot sizes, enables the operator to use the instrument correctly for various applications.

Optics with Variable Focus

These optics allow the pyrometer to be focused on the target from various distances. This kind of equipment is preferred for portable pyrometers. The diameter of the spot size can be calculated by using the distance to target ratio, for example, 100:1. The resulting value expresses the distance to diameter ratio. But there are also tables and spot size diagrams which can be used to determine the spot size diameter. Figure 22.14 shows the correlation between the spot size diameter and the measuring distance. The calculations apply equally to fixed optics and optics with variable focus. The Focus point (M_1) in the diagram represents the distance from the pyrometer at which the lens focuses the measured object sharply, and consequently produces the smallest spot size diameter. If this distance changes, the spot size diameter becomes larger, irrespective of the direction of the change. So long as the object to be measured can fill the predetermined spot size, a fuzzy image on the detector will not cause a measuring error by changing the measuring distance. The manufacturer either supplies the technical explanations for the spot size diagrams as they relate to various optics, or shows the measuring distances with the appropriate spot size diameters. With the help of the formulae for closer or farther distances the spot size diameter for the changes in distance can be calculated (Fig. 22.13). In order to obtain exact results, the measured object must at least fill the spot size (Fig. 22.14).

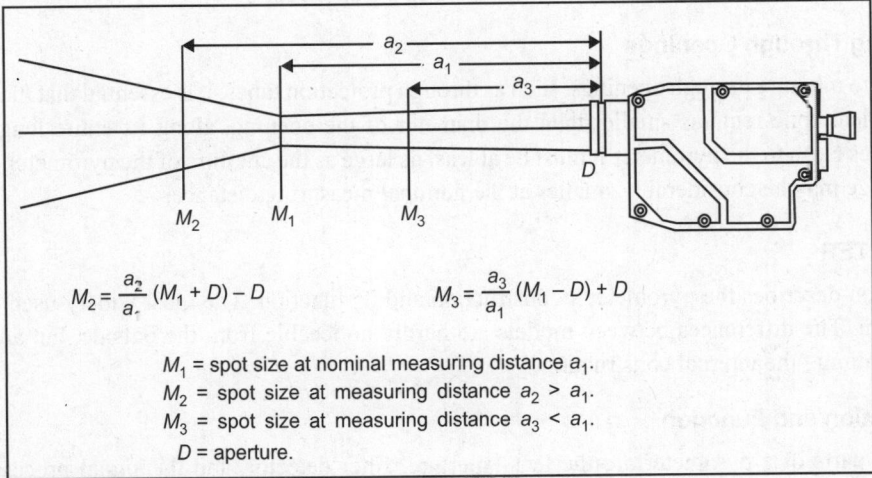

Fig. 22.13. Spot size diagram.

Filling Up the Spot Size

To avoid errors that could arise from adjustments made during operation, it is advisable to use an object size slightly larger than the spot size. When the object does not fill the spot size completely, measuring errors occur.

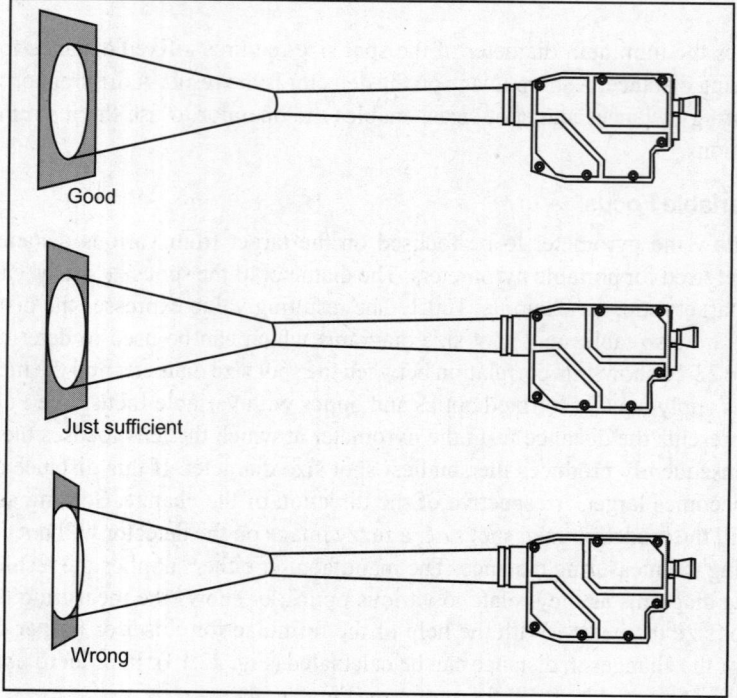

Fig. 22.14. Filling up the spot size.

Measuring Through Openings

If one has to measure through openings, such as through protection tubes, it is essential that the diameter of the optical cone remains smaller than the diameter of the opening, along its entire length. If the opening lies close to the pyrometer it must be at least as large as the aperture of the pyrometer, although the spot size may be considerably smaller at the nominal measuring distance.

PYROMETER

This section describes the pyrometer's construction and its function. The most widely-used types are also shown. The differences between models are hardly noticeable from the outside, but are evident when examining the internal construction.

Construction and Function

The basic parts of a pyrometer are the lens, aperture, filter detector, and the signal processing unit (Fig. 22.15). The infrared radiation coming in from the object to be measured is gathered by the lens. The aperture blocks unwanted rays at the edges.

The filter permits only the desired spectral range to enter. The rays then pass through to the detector which transforms the infrared radiation into electric signals. These signals are then linearised in the signal processing unit and changed into a standard output signal which can then be read in the display, and be used for process control.

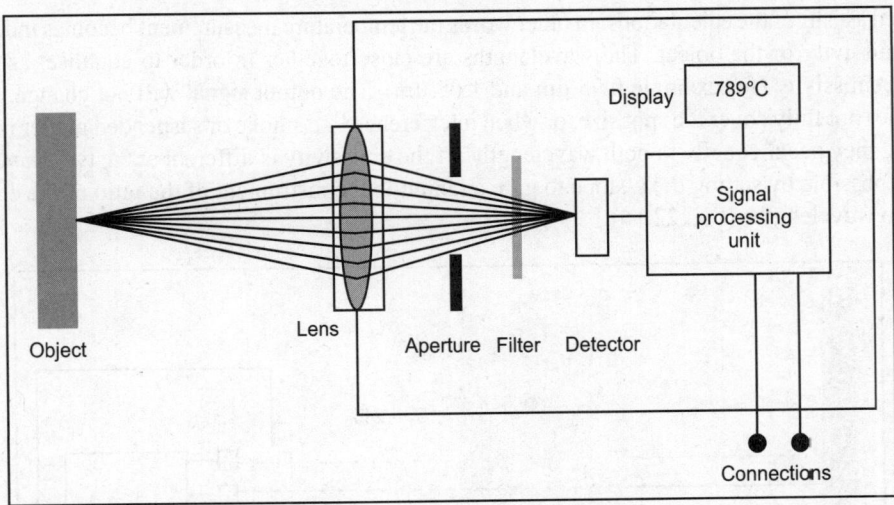

Fig. 22.15. Construction of a pyrometer.

PYROMETER TYPES

The differences between spectral band pyrometers, total band pyrometers, and 2-colour pyrometers are described below. In this category are narrow band pyrometers and broad band pyrometers.

Narrow Band Pyrometers

These pyrometers measure the radiation from a narrow wavelength band, usually just around one wavelength. By using interference filters and appropriate detectors a certain wavelength or a certain wavelength band is chosen.

They are frequently used when measuring glass at 5.14 μm. Metals are also measured with them since their rate of emissivity is high only in a narrow band.

Broad Band Pyrometers

These have a similar construction to that of the narrow band pyrometer. By using other filters and detectors the radiation from a wider wavelength band is measured (for example, 8 to 14 μm). These pyrometers are used for measuring organic materials because they have, in general, a high and constant emissivity at longer wavelengths.

Total Band Pyrometers

These pyrometers are built to detect more than 90 per cent of the emitted radiation of an object. This requires special detectors, lenses and filters which are sensitive to almost the whole spectrum. Today, total band pyrometers are rarely used due to the major errors experienced (atmospheric window, emissivity).

Two-Colour Pyrometer

Two-colour pyrometers measure the radiation using two different wavelengths, then calculate the ratio from the signals, and finally determine the temperature. When forming the ratio, the emissivity is eliminated as part of the calculations; in other words the temperature measurement becomes independent of the emissivity of the object. The wavelengths are close together in order to equalise, as much as possible, emissivity (for example 0.95 µm and 1.05 µm). The output signal will not change when the object does not fully cover the spot size, or when interference like smoke or suspended matter is present, providing they occur equally in both wavelengths. If the emissivity is different at the two wavelengths, then it is possible by setting the ε-slope to give an input to the instrument of the ratio of the emissivity at the two wavelengths (Fig. 22.16).

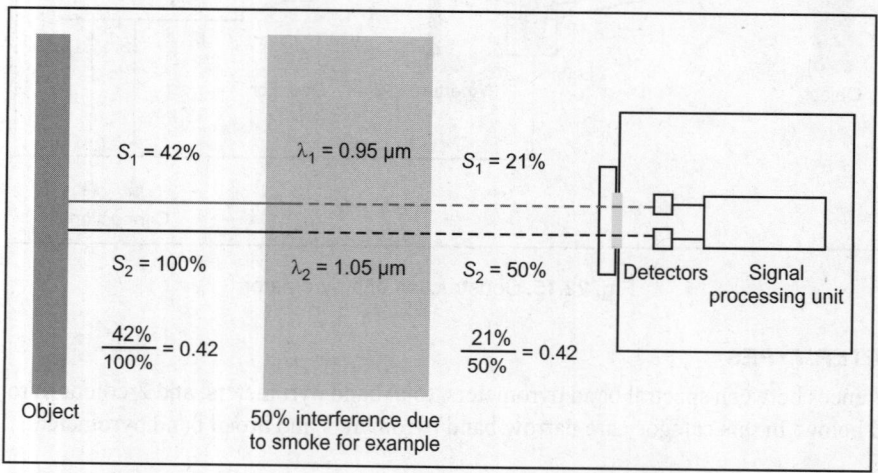

Fig. 22.16. Structure of a two-colour pyrometer.

Two-colour pyrometers are used for difficult measuring tasks.
1. High temperatures.
2. Blocked views or interference in the atmosphere (for example, smoke, suspended matter).
3. The object is smaller than the spot size (down to 10 per cent of the spot size).
4. Changing, low, or unknown emissivity (for example, molten metal).

In order to measure both signals various constructions are used:
1. Sandwich detector.
2. Two separate detectors with different filters.
3. One detector with a rotating filter wheel.

The disadvantage of a pyrometer with a rotating filter wheel is that the signals do not arrive simultaneously. The calculation of the ratio in the pyrometer increases the sensitivity toward changing signals in one of the two detectors. If there are quickly changing temperatures or moving objects a 2-colour pyrometer with rotating filter may record an inaccurate temperature.

Bright Flames Flame Pyrometers

To measure temperatures of bright flames (the most common type of flame) flame pyrometers have been found to work well. The radiation coming to the pyrometer stems from glowing soot or other burning particles. In this case, the soot factor 'n' must be set on the pyrometer in order to record the correct measurement.

Non-Luminous Flames

For the measurement of temperatures of flames that are non-luminous, such as gas burners, spectral pyrometers which measure the radiation of hot carbon dioxide in a very narrow spectral area, are required. That area lies between 4.5 and 4.65 μm.

Four-Colour Pyrometer

Four-colour pyrometers were developed for uses where the emissivity is very low and not stable during processing. Four-colour pyrometers measure the radiation intensity simultaneously in four different spectral areas and they are able to adapt and make a correction of the emissivity setting. These are very special pyrometers because the instrument collects data and effectively goes through a 'learning' process which enables it to adapt to changing emissivities. Two temperature measurements are taken: a spectral radiation measurement and a contact measurement. The corresponding emissivity for each spectral band can then be calculated and stored.

Infrared Radiation Thermometers/Pyrometers

A radiation thermometer, in very simple terms, consists of an optical system and detector. The optical system focuses the energy emitted by an object onto the detector, which is sensitive to the radiation. The output of the detector is proportional to the amount of energy radiated by the target object (less the amount absorbed by the optical system), and the response of the detector to the specific radiation wavelengths. This output can be used to infer the objects temperature. The emitivity or emittance, of the object is an important variable in converting the detector output into an accurate temperature signal.

Infrared radiation thermometers/pyrometers, by specifically measuring the energy being radiated from an object in the 0.7 to 20 micron wavelength range, are a subset of radiation thermometers. These devices can measure this radiation from a distance. There is no need for direct contact between the radiation thermometer and the object, as there is with thermocouples and resistance temperature detectors (RTDs). Radiation thermometers are suited especially to the measurement of moving objects or any surfaces that cannot be reached or can not be touched.

But the benefits of radiation thermometry have a price. Even the simplest of devices is more expensive than a standard thermocouple or resistance temperature detector (RTD) assembly, and installation cost can exceed that of a standard thermowell. The devices are rugged, but do require routine maintenance to keep the sighting path clear, and to keep the optical elements clean. Radiation thermometers used for more difficult applications may have more complicated optics, possibly rotating or moving parts, and microprocessor-based electronics. There are no industry accepted calibration curves for radiation thermometers, as there are for thermocouples and RTDs. In addition, the user may need to seriously investigate the application, to select the optimum technology, method of installation, and compensation needed for the measured signal, to achieve the performance desired.

Emittance, emissivity and the N-factor

Emittance can be identified as a critical parameter in accurately converting the output of the detector used in a radiation thermometer into a value representing object temperature. The terms emittance and emissivity are often used interchangeably. There is, however, a technical distinction. Emissivity refers to the properties of a material; emittance to the properties of a particular object. In this latter sense, emissivity is only one component in determining emittance. Other factors, including shape of the object, oxidation and surface finish must be taken into account (Fig. 22.17).

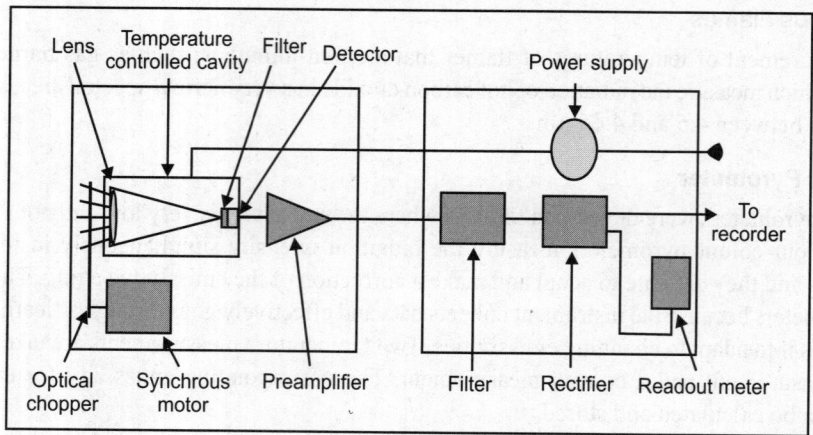

Fig. 22.17. Traditional infrared thermometer.

The apparent emittance of a material also depends on the temperature at which it is determined, and the wavelength at which the measurement is taken. Surface condition affects the value of an object's emittance, with lower values for polished surfaces, and higher values for rough or matte surfaces. In addition, as materials oxidise, emittance tends to increase, and the surface condition dependence decreases.

The basic equation used to describe the output of a radiation thermometer is:

$$V(T) = eKTN$$

where, e = Emitivity.
$V(T)$ = Thermometer output with temperature.
K = Constant.
T = Object temperature.
N = N factor [= 14388/(lT)].

A radiation thermometer with the highest value of N (shortest possible equivalent wavelength) should be selected to obtain the least dependence on target emittance changes. The benefits of a device with a high value of N extends to any parameter that effects the output V. A dirty optical system, or absorption of energy by gases in the sighting path, has less effect on an indicated temperature if N has a high value.

The values for the emissivities of almost all substances are known and published in reference literature. However, the emissivity determined under laboratory conditions seldom agrees with actual emittance of an object under real operating conditions. For this reason, one is likely to use published emissivity data when the values are high. As a rule of thumb, most opaque nonmetallic materials have a high and stable emissivity (0.85 to 0.90). Most unoxidised, metallic materials have a low to medium emissivity value (0.2 to 0.5). Gold, silver and aluminium are exceptions, with emissivity values in the 0.02 to 0.04 range. The temperature of these metals is very difficult to measure with a radiation thermometer. One way to determine emissivity experimentally is by comparing the radiation thermometer measurement of a target with the simultaneous measurement obtained using a thermocouple or RTD. The difference in readings is due to the emissivity, which is, of course, less than one.

For temperatures up to 500°F (260°C) emissivity values can be determined experimentally by putting a piece of black masking tape on the target surface. Using a radiation pyrometer set for an emissivity of 0.95, measure the temperature of the tape surface (allowing time for it to gain thermal equilibrium). Then measure the temperature of the target surface without the tape. The difference in readings determines the actual value for the target emissivity. Many instruments now have calibrated emissivity adjustments. The adjustment may be set to a value of emissivity, or experimentally, as described in the preceding paragraph. For highest accuracy, independent determination of emissivity in a lab at the wavelength at which the thermometer measures, and possibly at the expected temperature of the target, may be necessary (Fig. 22.18).

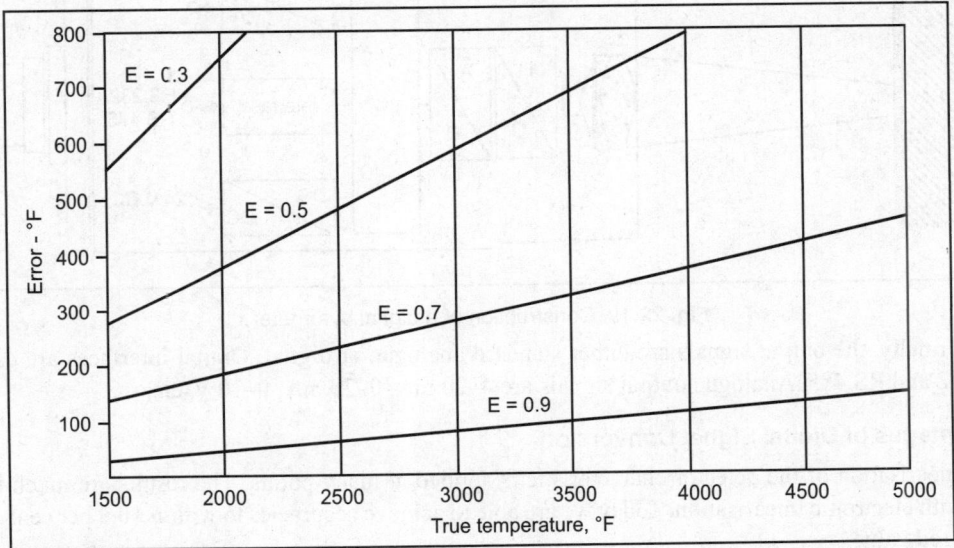

Fig. 22.18. Effect of non-blackbody emissivity on IR thermometer error.

Emissivity values in tables have been determined by a pyrometer sighted perpendicular to the target. If the actual sighting angle is more than 30 or 40 degrees from the normal to the target, lab measurement of emissivity may be required.

In addition, if the radiation pyrometer sights through a window, emissivity correction must be provided for energy lost by reflection from the two surfaces of the window, as well as absorption in the window. For example, about 4 per cent of radiation is reflected from glass surfaces in the infrared ranges, so the effective transmittance is 0.92. The loss through other materials can be determined from the index of refraction of the material at the wavelength of measurement.

The uncertainties concerning emittance can be reduced using short wavelength or ratio radiation thermometers. Short wavelengths, around 0.7 microns, are useful because the signal gain is high in this region. The higher response output at short wavelengths tends to swamp the effects of emittance variations. The high gain of the radiated energy also tends to swamp the absorption effects of steam, dust or water vapour in the sight path to the target. For example, setting the wavelength at such a band will cause the sensor to read within +/–5 to +/–10 degrees of absolute temperature when the material has an emissivity of 0.9 (+/–0.05). This represents about 1 to 2 per cent accuracy.

DIGITAL PYROMETERS: STATE-OF-THE-ART-TECHNOLOGY

With advancing miniaturisation and integration, today's pyrometers are digital. This means that a microprocessor is built into the pyrometer. It does all the calculations and controls the memory functions. Figure 22.19 shows the basic construction. The detector signal is either directly digitised or digitised after an analogue preamplifier (A/D converter). The digital signal is then processed further by the microprocessor.

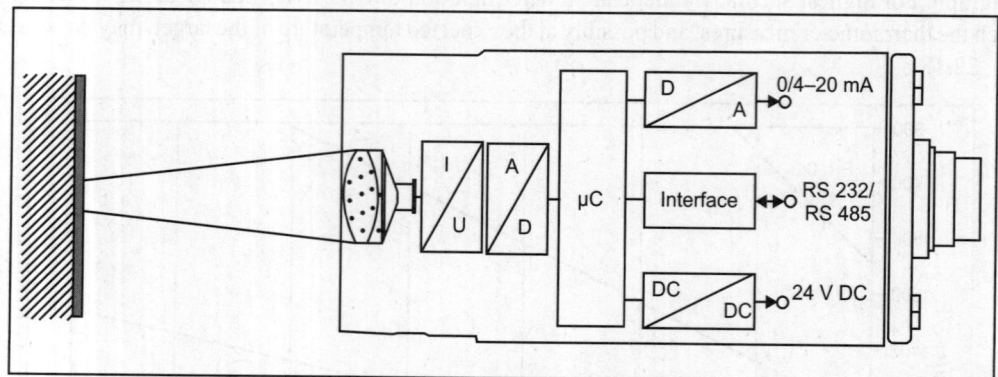

Fig. 22.19. Construction of a digital pyrometer.

Normally, the output signals are either standard analogue or digital. Digital interfaces are usually RS 232 and RS 485. Analogue output signals are 4–20 mA, 0–20 mA, 0–10 V, etc.

Advantages of Digital Signal Conversion

The linearisation of the detector characteristic is applied at many points. The results are much better than with electronic linearisation. Today we are able to achieve accuracies to within ±0.3 per cent of the measured value.

1. Confined spaces: The optical head is small and can fit through narrow openings until it is nearer the object.

In the analogue system, mathematical functions required additional equipment. However, with the digital system, these functions are now integrated into the pyrometer which eliminates the need for peripheral equipment. An example of these functions is the 'maximum value storage'. Communication with the pyrometer is also possible. A PC connected with the appropriate software is usually sufficient. All relevant data can be entered into the pyrometer, such as emissivity, response time, measuring range, maximum value storage, etc. Within the determined basic temperature measuring range, any sub-range can be set via the PC. Accuracy is not affected by changing the measuring range. The advantages are:

1. When replacing old equipment the existing measuring range can be entered. Other equipment and the cables can all be reused.
2. Stores stock levels can be reduced as one range of digital pyrometer can be programmed to cover several different ranges of analogue instruments.
3. The new equipment is easier to use and reduces complications.
4. Optimum adoption to a specific application.

By using an appropriate black body source and software, digital pyrometers can be quickly recalibrated and checked. With the appropriate software all settings are simple to do. On-line graphics are standard today.

FIBRE OPTICS PYROMETER

A fibre optics pyrometer consists of three parts: an optical head, a glass fibre and a signal processing unit. The optical head contains only the optics and no electronics. In the converter is the detector and the signal processing unit. The radiation, coming in through the optical head, is transported via the lens system into the fibre where it can be transmitted along for up to 30 metres to the converter. The glass fibre of the optical fibre is no longer transparent at higher wavelengths. Consequently, the measurement of temperatures with glass fibres is limited to 150°C and above.

Fibre optics pyrometers have proven themselves in difficult situations. Splitting the two components has advantages in these instances:
1. High temperatures: The optical head and the fibre have no electronic components and can easily withstand temperatures of up to 250°C. The pyrometer unit itself, however, is installed at a cooler location and will not be damaged.
2. Strong electromagnetic fields: These have no effect on the measurements because the optical head and the optical fibre contain no electronics and consist of material that cannot be magnetised.
3. Measuring in a vacuum: Access windows and vacuum tight flanges allow an installation of the optical head near the object inside a vacuum chamber.

Radiation transmission in an optical fibre is based on the total reflection of the rays at the interface between the core and the outer shielding (also called cladding). Thus, the transmission is practically without loss (Fig. 22.20).

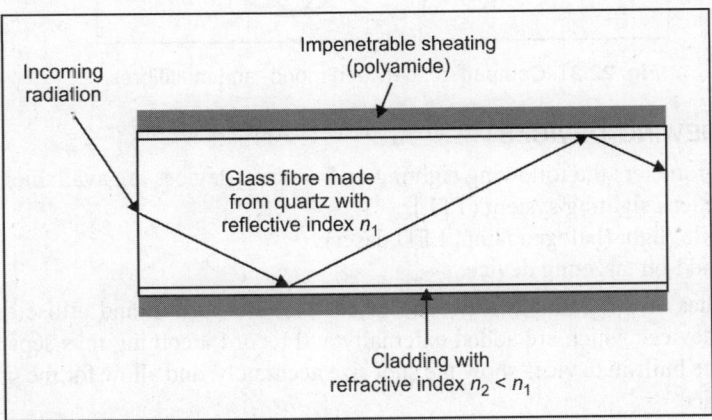

Fig. 22.20. Longitudinal section of a glass fibre.

Optical fibres consist either of a single fibre called monofibre or a fibre bundle called multifibre. Using a monofibre has certain advantages over a multifibre version:
1. Smaller external diameter whilst having the same cross sectional area. There can be losses due to pinching in a multifibre bundle. The diameter of a monofibre is smaller and therefore so is the diameter of the spot size, while the optical area dimension remains the same [Fig. 22.21(a)].
2. Fibre breakage is detected immediately: The break in a monofibre is recognised instantly by the lack of a signal. Breakage of a few fibres in a bundle is not immediately apparent which means that the signal being received by the pyrometer is less than the true signal [Fig. 22.21(b)].
3. There will be no wear and tear due to friction between the individual fibres. With fibre bundles the cladding may be damaged due to friction between fibres and the filler material in between [Fig. 22.21(c)]. The advantages of multifibre bundles lie in their smaller minimal curving radius (ability to bend), and in their lower cost compared with monofibre optical fibres.

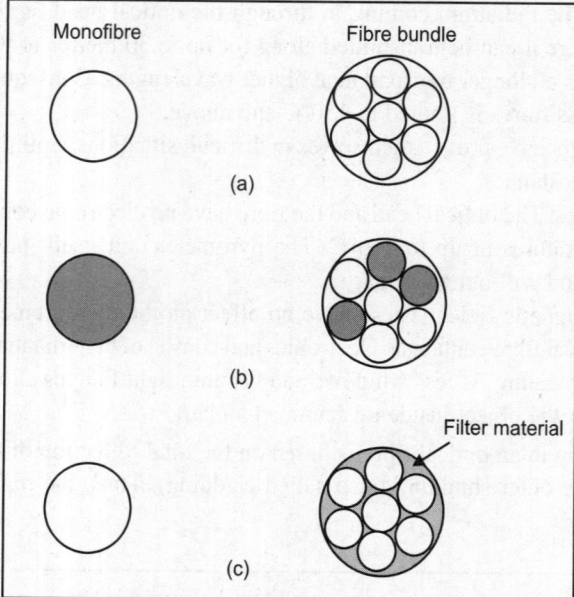

Fig. 22.21. Comparison between mono- and multifibres.

SIGHTING AND VIEWING DEVICES

In order to adjust pyrometers the following sighting and viewing devices are available:
1. Through the lens sighting system (TTL).
2. Integrated pilot light (halogen lamp, LED, laser).
3. Temporary add-on targeting device.

In general, one has to differentiate between devices that are built-in and utilise the pyrometer's optics, and add-on devices which are added externally and record incoming rays separately from the pyrometer optics. The built-in devices show the spot size accurately, and allow for the proper setting of the measuring distance.
1. The user looks at the object as though he were looking through a camera. In the centre of the viewing area are marks which indicate the target area. To protect the eye, filters eliminate UV and infrared radiation, and brightness at high temperatures can be reduced by using polarising filters. Through the lens sighting systems are built-in, but they may be purchased as add-on equipment.
2. The pilot light is built into the pyrometer and indicates by its point of light the size and the location of the target area. It is only usable if the measured object is not too bright. Generally, it is visible on an object up to a temperature of 1000°C. Pilot lights can be a halogen lamp, LED, or laser.
3. The laser pointer indicates with its ray the centre of the target area, or the target area itself. It is very useful when measuring in darkness and for precision measurements. Because of the easily visible pointer light, small and moving objects may be accurately targeted.
4. This device is placed at the front of the pyrometer. It is available with a laser that lies in the lens axis or with two lasers crossing at a defined distance from the lens.

LINEARISATION

The relationship between the incoming radiation intensity and the output of the detector (for example, a change in voltage or resistance), is not linear. However, the output signal of a quality pyrometer must be linear with respect to the temperature, because it is meant to control the peripheral equipment. Depending upon how it is made, the signal processing unit of the pyrometer gives off a standard signal of 0 to 20 mA or 4 to 20 mA. The lower value refers to the beginning of the measuring range, the higher value to the full scale of the measuring range. The linear relationship with respect to temperature is accomplished by linearisation of the input signal. The linearisation of a pyrometer takes place by means of an electronic circuit in analogue equipment, or by means of mathematical calculations in digital equipment (Fig. 22.22).

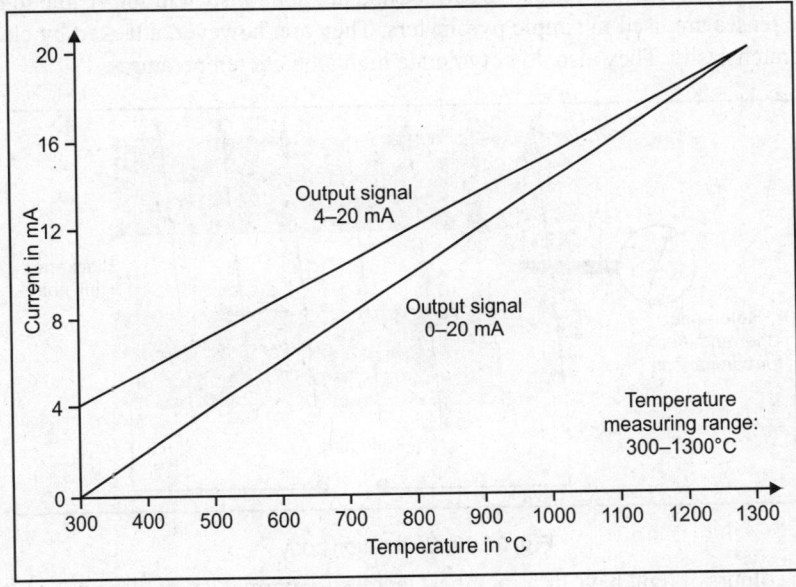

Fig. 22.22. Output signal.

CALIBRATION

Every pyrometer is properly calibrated by the manufacturer before despatch. A certificate accompanies the equipment. To ensure long-term reliability, pyrometers must be regularly checked and, if necessary, recalibrated. A black body furnace is required for this. The depth of the cavity should be at least six times as long as its diameter because the emission coefficient of nearly 1 is reached by multiple reflections in the cavity. The inner surface of the cavity is heated evenly, and the pyrometer is set to the value of the reference thermometer used for comparisons (Fig. 22.23). Recalibration is also necessary when the equipment is being repaired or modified. Calibrations are done by the manufacturer or by an approved calibration laboratory.

OPTICS, LENSES AND WINDOW MATERIAL

One of the most important components of a pyrometer is the optics. If lenses are used the material must be adapted to the spectral properties of the detector.

The material must be permeable to the pyrometer's spectral range, which is determined by the measuring range and the object to be measured.
1. Crown glass (BK7) is used in pyrometers which measure in the short wavelength band (up to 2.7 µm). Crown glass is very stable, resistant to chemicals and easy to clean.
2. Water-free quartz glass (Infrasil) is also used in pyrometers which measure in the short wavelength band (up to 3 µm).
3. Calcium fluoride (CaF_2, Fluorspar) is used especially when glass is measured. It can be used up to 10 µm and has a high transmission coefficient.
4. Germanium lenses are useful for pyrometers which measure in the long wavelength band (up to 18 µm). They have a non-reflective surface and are nontransparent for visible light.
5. Plastic lenses are used in simple pyrometers. They are, however, attacked by cleaning agents and scratch easily. They also do not tolerate high ambient temperatures.

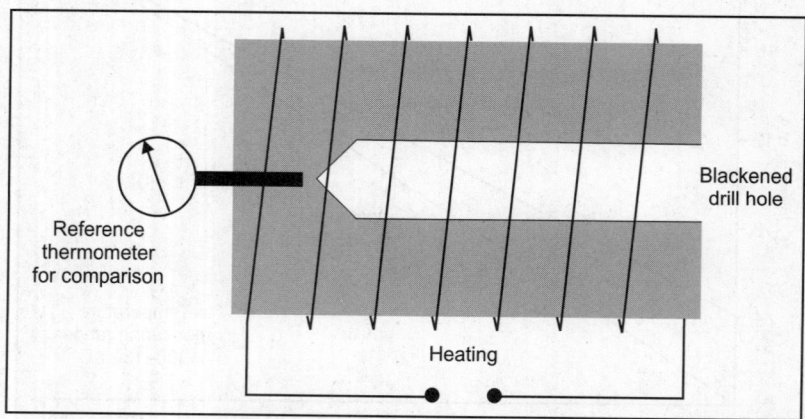

Fig. 22.23. Calibration body.

The various colours of light have different focal lengths for normal lenses. This divergence of colour is called dispersion, and the resulting effect is called chromatic error. To eliminate this error an achromat is used. This is a combination of a convex lens and a diverging lens each with a different refractive index. They are precisely designed so that in the observed wavelength range, the chromatic error is fully compensated for. An achromat also diminishes the spherical error, i.e. the shorter focal distance of peripheral rays. Achromats are used in 2-colour pyrometers because they measure in two different colours. Simple lenses would lead to incorrect measurements. In order to further reduce chromatic and spherical errors, an airgap achromat has been developed.

Unlike more basic achromats, there is a small airgap between the lenses instead of adhesive. This is more suitable where there are high ambient temperatures. Airgap achromats are often used in the optical head of fibre optic pyrometers (Fig. 22.24).

WINDOW MATERIALS

Pyrometers permit non-contact measurement of temperatures of materials in furnaces, vacuum chambers or other enclosed areas. Of course, one needs a special opening through which the pyrometer can 'see' the surface of the object to be measured. In many cases these openings must be closed off by windows (for instance, in a vacuum, when under pressure, when dealing with gases, liquids or viscous masses).

Depending on the temperature range and the spectral range of the pyrometer, the correct choice of window material is essential. The transmission range must be chosen so that it will not conflict with the pyrometer's spectral range, which is determined by temperature and the material of the object to be measured. Among other necessary properties are mechanical strength, moisture and chemical resistance, and the ability to withstand thermal shocks.

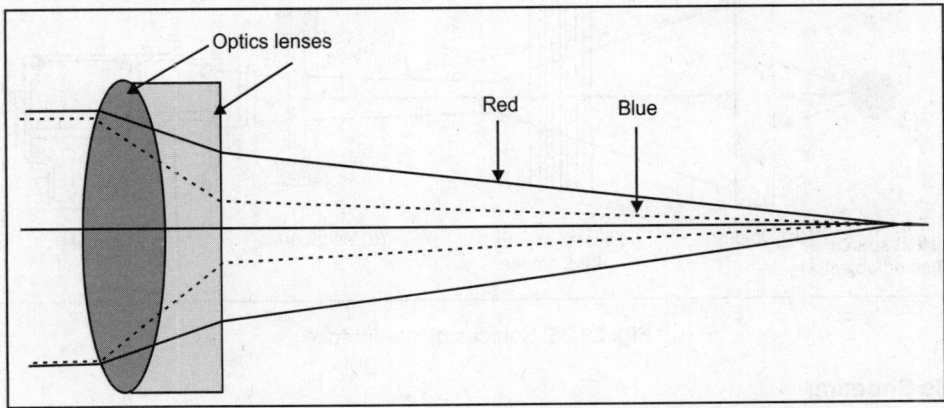

Fig. 22.24. Basic construction of an achromat.

The minimum thickness of the window (d min) to ensure stability under pressure is calculated with the formula:

$$d_{\min} = r \cdot \sqrt{\frac{S \cdot c \cdot \Delta p}{M_r}}$$

where,
- r = radius of the window.
- S = safety factor (≥ 4).
- c = method of window attachment (for instance $c = 1.1$ for loose attachment).
- Δp = Differential pressure
- M_r = Break modulus.

Glass and quartz windows (used for high temperatures) are cost efficient, as are silicon and fluorspar windows (to measure lower temperatures).

SOURCES OF INTERFERENCE

Under most conditions, errors may occur when measuring temperatures due to outside influences. However, once the most commonly occurring sources of these are known, they can be easily avoided. The following list shows the different sources of interference and a troubleshooting guide. Additional infrared radiation from nearby hot objects may be reflected off the surface of the object to be measured [Fig. 22.25(a)].

If there is a heat source behind the object that is to be measured and the object lets radiation pass through, the measurement will be affected [Fig. 22.25(b)]. Infrared radiation can be reduced by dust, water vapour, smoke, or windows [Fig. 22.25 (c/d)].

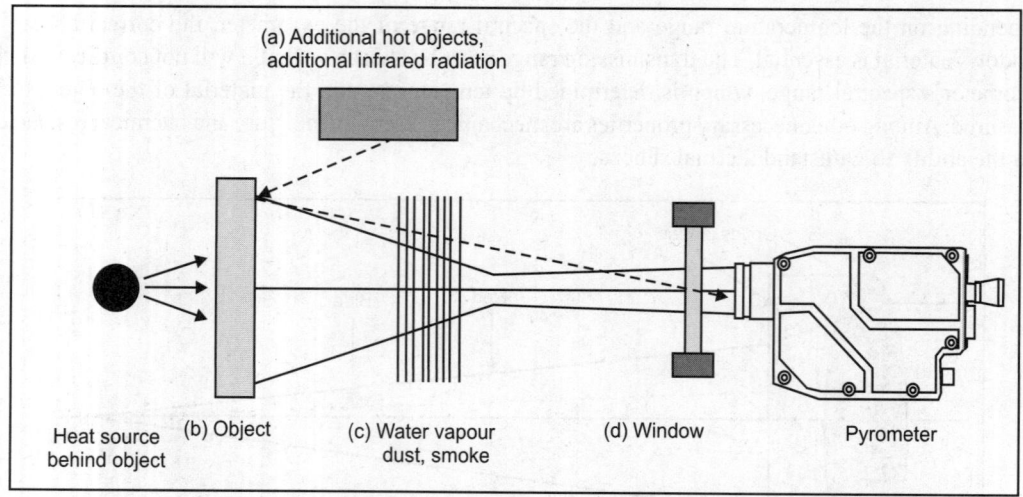

Fig. 22.25. Sources of interference.

Trouble-Shooting

Additional infrared radiation such as daylight, indoorlighting or an infrared source can be blocked with optical filters because of their predominantly short wavelength characteristics. Quality pyrometers with silicon, germanium or InGaAs detectors are equipped with daylight filters so that daylight or artificial light have no effect on the measurement. Exceptions are pyrometers with InGaAs detectors whose temperature range begins at under 300°C. In these cases a shade has to be used to prevent temperature errors. The influence of radiation from infrared radiators or heaters, and certain kinds of furnaces (wavelengths up to 4 µm), can be avoided by using pyrometers which work in the long wavelength range (for example in the area of 8 to 14 µm).

The radiation from a furnace wall or a hot enclosure have the same wavelength range as the radiation coming from the object and cannot be filtered out. One must use mechanical devices to block out the unwanted radiation. Alternatively, the temperature can be mathematically corrected. So long as the temperature of these other hot objects (i.e. the furnace wall) is constant, the input of a certain temperature value into the equation will suffice. However, if it changes, it must be measured with an additional sensor. These values are then processed in the calculating unit together with the signal from the object. When the measurement is done through a window, the emission coefficient must be adjusted to compensate for the degree by which the radiation has been weakened. The influence of water vapour and carbon monoxide in the air can be eliminated by the correct choice of the spectral range. Influences that change at various times, such as dust, smoke and vapour, call for the use of a 2-colour pyrometer. With transparent objects one must use a pyrometer which is designed to work in a wavelength band for which the object is impermeable.

When the area behind the object to be measured is cooler than the object itself, the transparency of the object can be taken into account by a correction of the emissivity. When the spot size is not completely filled the location of the pyrometer must be changed. When this is not possible different optics must be used. A 2-colour pyrometer will permit a measurement with an insufficiently filled spot size so long as the background is cold.

ACCESSORIES

Industrial demands require the availability of special accessories. They have been developed to solve problems and to ease difficulties in the application of measuring devices. An air purge unit protects the optics from dust and other suspended particles, as well as from condensation. Its construction in the shape of a round nozzle creates a coneshaped air cushion in front of the lens. Thus, dust cannot settle on the lens. When operating this air purge it is important to use dry and oil-free compressed air. In normal circumstances a pressure of 0.2 bar is sufficient. A radiation shield is used when most of the heat radiation comes from the front.

A cooling plate is a water-cooled plate. It removes the radiation from the front and does not heat up itself. It allows the use of pyrometers in conditions of 10 to 20 degrees above the normal maximum allowable temperature for pyrometers. Cooling jackets are available as cooling coils or as fully jacketed cooling systems. Coils allow for the operation of pyrometers in high ambient temperatures. Fully jacketed cooling systems permit pyrometers to be used in surrounding temperatures of up to 100°C with air cooling, and up to 250°C with water cooling.

The pyrometer can be firmly set into position with angle brackets. Adjustable positioning devices are used to firmly fix pyrometers with variable alignment axes. Flange systems permit the attachment of pyrometers to furnaces, containers or pipes. With a mounting tube, pyrometers may be built into containers (for example, asphalting or spray booths). A lamination slide is used as protection from incoming particles when measurements are taken in an upward angle. The slide is placed into a mounting tube. A ball and socket mounting is used to hold the pyrometer in place and allow quick adjustments of angle and direction.

Ceramic tubes are available in open or closed form. A closed ceramic tube is used to measure the average inner temperature of a furnace or to measure the temperature during smelting (e.g. glass). An open ceramic tube is used to measure the surface of an object inside a furnace. With the help of scanning optics the spot size is moved back and forth across the object to be measured. A moving mirror oscillates around the centre position. With the scanner one can measure the temperature of moving objects such as in the manufacture of wires.

The scanner should always be used in connection with the maximum value storage unit. This unit stores the highest temperature value of the object during the scanning process (with this proviso; the surrounding temperature is lower than that of the object to be measured). Scanners may either be integral or be attached to the front of the optics. A pyrometer with scanner may also be used as a line scanner so long as the position of the mirror is known. Indicators are designed to display the measured temperature. They can be integrated into the pyrometer but they are also available as external equipment that will display the temperature remotely from the pyrometer, such as in a control room, or a switch box. Indicators can be either analogue or digital, some with built-in maximum value storage functions and limit switches (to regulate heaters, etc.).

Recorders and printers provide graphic evidence of the measured temperature. Where there are swings in temperature, maximum value storage units allow the highest temperature value to be recorded and stored. Their fast response times ensure that even the quickest changes in temperature are registered. These units have proven invaluable during metal heating processes (for instance, during forging).

When scale develops, temperature variations occur on the surface being measured. With a maximum value storage unit the highest measured value is kept on record as it corresponds to the temperature of the measured object.

By using a double storage system one obtains a firm and steady temperature indication. This system is used most often in combination with scanning optics and limit switches.

When there are temperature swings the average value calculating unit determines the average value and supplies a stable output signal which is then easily fed into a controller.

Limit switches come into play when certain temperature values are exceeded or are too low. The converter changes the output signal of 2-wire equipment from 4 to 20 mA into 0 to 20 mA.

Calibrators check the accuracy of the pyrometers. These converters change a RS 485 signal into a RS 232 signal-gateways allow for conversion of RS 485 signals to several bus systems.

Chapter 23
Electrical Properties of Materials

INTRODUCTION

Mechanical engineering and electrical engineering are two broad technical areas which, though nominally distinct, overlap in such a comprehensive fashion that it is often impossible to designate a problem or project as specifically 'electrical' or 'mechanical'. A mechanical engineer simply cannot ply his trade without comprehensive knowledge of things electrical. Similarly, in time of trouble the electrical engineer may discover that the defects in his electrical equipment are mechanical defects.

Consider first some mechanical aspects of electrical equipment. If an electric motor is down for maintenance the reason may be either bearings or a burnout, both mechanical failures. Breakage of electric power lines caused by ice accumulation or wind vibration is mechanical failure. Fracture of the bakelite parts of switchgear is mechanical failure. So is evaporation of the tungsten filament when an incandescent lamp fails. The dissipation of heat from electronic microcomponents is a mechanical design problem, as are the glass-to-metal seals required in all vacuum tubes.

The uses of electrical equipment for nonelectrical applications are almost without number. Most welding equipment is electrical. Most of the nondestructive testing methods used in manufacturing operations are electrical methods—ultrasonic, X-ray, magnetic flaw detection, eddy-current testing. An electronic induction heater used for brazing and heat-treating of metals is similar in design and components to the frequency generator of a radio transmitting station. The electrical characteristics of materials, then, are not of peripheral importance, or of interest only to electrical specialists. Ignorance of these electrical properties may prove a severe occupational handicap. The following is a case in point.

A weld shop decided to install a common ground for ten 300 amp welding machines. Without making any electrical calculations, it was decided to use a 5/8 inch diameter steel bar for the ground, simply because such a bar would be 'plenty big enough'. It wasn't, and it had to be replaced immediately after it was installed, much to the embarrassment of the supervisor responsible.

ELECTRICAL RESISTANCE

The one-dimensional flow of electricity through a resistance and the similar flow of heat by conduction are mathematically identical. For electric current

$$E = IR, \text{ Ohm's law}$$

$$R = \frac{\sigma l}{A}$$

where, σ = the specific resistance of the resistor material in some suitable units,

L = length of the conductor
A = cross section of the conductor

For heat flow by one-dimensional conduction, $Q = (KA\,\Delta t)/L$. If the formula for heat flow is rearranged, it becomes identical mathematically with Ohm's law:

$$\Delta t = Q\left(\frac{L}{KA}\right)$$

Here Δt, the temperature differential, is the potential causing heat flow and corresponding to E, Q Btu/hr is the flow, and L/KA is the heat-flow resistance R, where L/K corresponds to the specific resistance.

For purposes of mechanical engineering, the most convenient unit for specific resistance is ohms per cubic inch, because the conductors involved in mechanical engineering may be of rectangular or irregular shape. Most resistance calculations in electrical engineering are concerned with wire and cable of circular cross section, for which the circular mil-foot is a convenient unit for specific resistance, Finally, for scientific work, the unit or ohm-centimeter is used.

If L is given in inches, and A in square inches, then the units of σ are ohm-inches (ohms per cubic inch). If the circular mil-foot is used, then L must be in feet, and A must be in circular mils. The area of a circle with diameter n mils (thousandths of an inch) is simply n^2 circular mils. This avoids the use of π in calculations. A square, inch of wire contains 1,273,240 circular mils.

In Table 23.1 of specific resistances, there are some uncertainties, since such factors as the purity of the material, the amount of cold-working, and the presence of alloying elements are not specified. Such factors may have a powerful influence on resistance.

Table 23.1. Specific resistance of materials at 20°C.

Material	Microhm-inches	Ohms/circ. mil-foot
Silver	0.6	9.6
Copper	0.7	10.4
Aluminum	1.12	17.1
Mercury	3.8	–
Nickel	2.7	41
Iron	4.0	60
Mild steel	5.0	–
302 stainless steel	29.0	–
Tungsten	2.2	33.3
Carbon	1300	–
Silicon	450	–

Four methods are available for changing the properties of a material, including its electrical resistivity:

1. Alloying: Alloying increases both the strength of a metal and its electrical resistance, but it reduces the electrical resistance of a semiconductor.
2. Plastic deformation. This increases the strength and resistivity of a metal, and it decreases its ductility.
3. Heat treatment: Depending on the heat treatment, properties may be improved or harmed.
4. Irradiation: The material is bombarded with high-energy particles.

The effect of alloying on electrical resistance may be noted in the table of specific resistances by comparing resistance values for pure iron, mild steel, and stainless steel. Mild steel is iron alloyed with about 0.2 per cent carbon and 0.3 per cent of silicon and of manganese, or a total of less than 1 per cent alloying additions. The effect, however, is a 20 per cent increase in resistance. Type 302 stainless steel contains about 29 per cent of alloying additions, chiefly chromium and nickel. As a result the resistance is increased by a factor of 7 over that of pure iron. For the same reasons, brasses have about 4 times the resistance of pure copper. About 0.1 per cent of phosphorus in copper will double the electrical resistance of copper. Silicon and aluminum additions greatly increase the resistance of steel and are used when high-resistance steels are desired, as in the steel cores of transformers. The effect of alloying elements on specific resistance is so powerful that the purity of metals and semiconductors is actually evaluated by means of resistance measurements.

The resistance of most pure metals increases by a factor of 0.4 per cent per degree centigrade, or 0.23 per cent per degree Fahrenheit. This statement is not true of alloys of magnesium, nickel, mercury, or of the rare earth metals, all of which may have temperature coefficients of resistance greater or less than this value.

All substances conduct electrically charged particles. According to the Ohm's law equation, $E = IR$, a nonconductor would ideally have an infinite resistance. No known material has this characteristic. However, three kinds of electrically conductive materials may be distinguished:

1. Conductors.
2. Semiconductors.
3. Insulators.

Conductors are metals and therefore have low impedance to the flow of electrons and increasing resistance to electron flow with increasing temperature. The specific resistance of conductors is in the range of 1×10^{-6} to about 1×10^{-14} ohm-cm. (Specific resistance in ohm-cm is about 2.4 times resistance expressed in ohm-inches.) A semiconductor is partially insulating and partially conducting, with a specific resistance in the range of about 10^{-2} to 10^6 ohm-cm. All semiconductors have less resistance at higher temperatures and in less pure states. An insulator or dielectric has a specific resistance in the range of 10^6 to 10^{20} ohm-cm. Of all the properties of materials, none has a wider range than specific resistance — roughly 10^{40}.

Germanium is a typical semiconductor. At room temperature it has a specific resistance of about 60 ohm-cm. When doped with 0.0001 per cent of arsenic, its resistance falls drastically to about 0.1 microhm-cm. The decrease in resistance is explained by the valence electrons of the two materials: germanium has 4 and arsenic 5 valence electrons. The extra electron of arsenic becomes free for conduction, greatly increasing the conduction. Other elements with 5 valence electrons would have the same effect on germanium, such as phosphorus. Such elements are called donors, and their presence in a semiconductor produces what is called an n-type (for negative) semiconductor. Germanium could be doped with an element such as aluminum, which has only three valence electrons. Such an element produces electron deficiencies called holes and is called an acceptor. The resulting semiconductor is a p-type (for positive).

Metals, which are electrical conductors, conduct as electrons move through the crystal lattice under the attraction of an applied voltage. As the electrons move along the conductor, they meet interference from ions in the space lattice. This impedance to flow is the ohmic resistance of the material. If the metal conductor is heated to a higher temperature, the ions of the space lattice vibrate over greater amplitudes, thus producing a greater collision cross section for the moving electron. The effect is an increased resistance. In a perfect crystal without imperfections, at absolute zero, there should be no interference to electron flow and no resistance. This condition is the superconducting condition, to be discussed presently.

The resistance of a conductor is expressed as ohms or microhms (millionths of an ohm). Conductivity is the reciprocal of resistance, with the units of mhos (mhos = 1/ohms). In certain applications, such as water treatment and water analysis, the conductivity is measured instead of the resistance. Figure 23.1 shows the approximate specific resistance of some refractory oxides. The resistance of these insulating materials decreases markedly at higher temperatures, as in the case of semiconductors. The specific resistance of any ceramic material is sensitive to the presence of impurities such as foreign oxides.

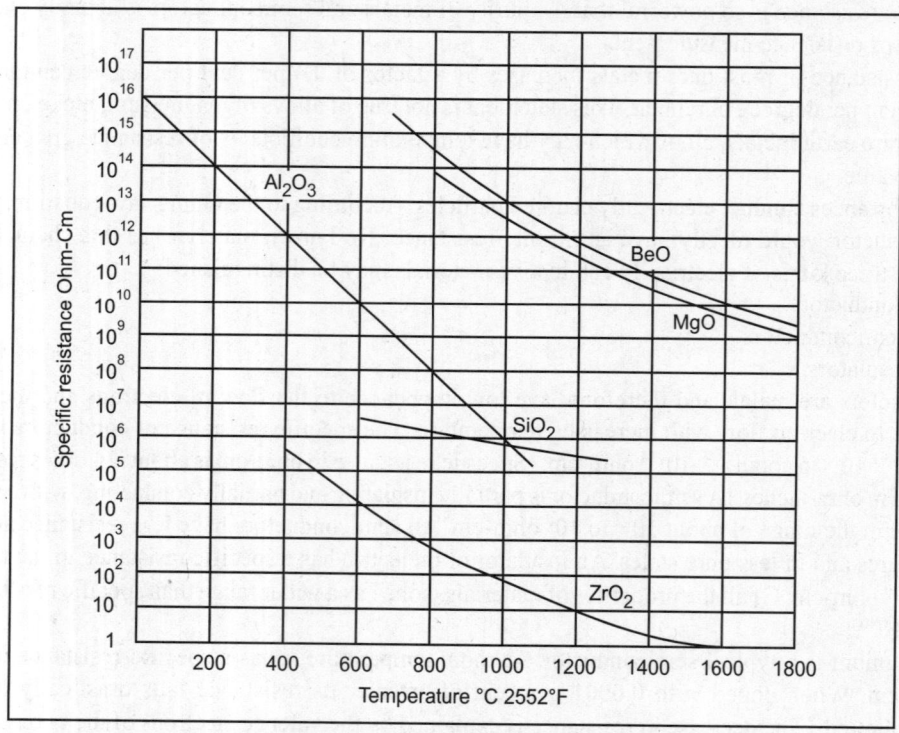

Fig. 23.1. Typical electrical resistance of refractories.

For the transport of heavy currents in welding and the process industries, carbon and graphite are commonly used. Of the three phases of carbon, diamond is an insulator, and carbon and graphite are semiconductors. Graphite has about one-quarter the resistance of carbon, and it is the preferred material for electrodes in carbon arc welding and in arc-melting furnaces.

The specific resistance of carbon ranges from about 0.0010 to 0.004 ohm-inch at 20°C, decreasing at higher temperatures. The electrical resistance of the common plastics and rubbers ranges between 10^{15} and 10^{20} ohm-inches.

APPLICATIONS OF RESISTANCE MATERIALS

Resistance wire is special wire for the purpose of converting electric energy into heat. Most such wire is either nickel or nickel-chromium alloy, with the properties of oxidation resistance and high electrical resistance in the range of 200–800 ohms per circular mil-foot. One such alloy with the trade name Constantan has virtually a constant resistance in the temperature range of 0–900°F. For heavy-duty heating, as in the case of electrically heated industrial furnaces, rods or tubes of silicon carbide may be used as heating elements because of their great resistance to high temperature effects. Silicon carbide has only limited resistance change with temperature. Incandescent lamps use a tungsten filament wire which may range in diameter from 0.001 to 0.060 in. Both tungsten and molybdenum resistors are employed as heating elements in very-high temperature furnaces (3000°F and higher).

For power transmission cables aluminum has become competitive with copper. Although the resistivity of aluminum is higher, aluminum is only one-third the specific weight of copper. For equal resistance, the weight of aluminum is 54 per cent that of copper. For short cables, such as welding cables, the rule of thumb is that an aluminum cable should be one gauge heavier than the required copper cable.

Thermistors are semiconductor crystals with a high negative temperature coefficient of resistance of perhaps 2–3 per cent per degree Fahrenheit. Thermistors are used as thermal switches. For example, a thermistor may be used within an electric motor winding to operate a relay when the motor becomes too hot.

Electrical contacts present special problems. They must be constructed of low-resistance metals, but in addition they must meet the service conditions of arcing, wear, overheating, and tendency to weld. Copper, alloys, carbon, and the platinum metals are the most frequently used materials in these applications. Copper oxidises readily, and its oxide is an insulator. Frequently silver is plated over the copper contact because silver oxide is more readily reduced to metallic silver by arcing than the oxides of other metals. Platinum, palladium, and iridium are perhaps the best contactor materials for low-voltage, low-current conditions and may provide a service life of more than a billion interruptions of current.

SUPERCONDUCTIVITY

The resistance of a single crystal of pure metal without imperfections in its space lattice should be zero at absolute zero. At temperatures below 10°K, the specific resistance or certain conductors falls off rapidly to zero. Such conductors are termed superconductors. Superconductivity is not yet well understood, but as a technology it is about to come out of the laboratory to be turned over to the engineering groups. The best electrical conductors, gold, silver, and copper, are not superconductors; that is, their resistance does not reach zero at absolute zero.

The temperature below which the electrical resistance disappears is termed the critical temperature. But if the magnetic field about the conductor exceeds a certain critical value, superconductivity is lost. Diamagnetism accompanies the superconducting condition, and the thermal conductivity is very low, though not zero.

Technetium has the highest critical temperature, 11.2°K, followed by niobium (columbium) at 9.2°K and lead at 7.2°K. The critical temperature of the other superconducting metals is generally in the range of 0.35°–5.0°K. In general, a superconducting metal will be a poor conductor at room temperature, and will not be ferromagnetic. Certain chemical compounds are also superconducting, with transition temperatures as high as 18°K. Superconductivity at considerably higher temperatures may be a development of the near future.

Applications of superconductivity have been considered in the following areas:
1. Loss less power distribution.
2. Space satellites.
3. Computers.
4. Magnetohydrodynamic generation of electric power.

The benefits of power transmission without I^2R loss are obvious, but they present equally obvious difficulties in refrigerating a long transmission line. The development of magnetohydrodynamic (MHD) power generation is already well under way. The use of superconductivity for switching circuits is found in cryotrons or cold switches. If a superconductor has a coil wound about it, a sufficiently high current passed through the coil will create a magnetic field which will destroy superconductivity in the conductor. This is an example of a simple cryotron switch.

MAGNETISM

The theory of magnetism is a rather complex subject which is still being unravelled by physicists, and only its simpler aspects can be discussed here. Three kinds of magnetism must be noted.

Ferromagnetism

This is the type of magnetism shown by materials which are strongly attracted to a magnet. Ferromagnetism is a property of iron, cobalt, nickel, Fe_3O_4, gadolinium, dysprosium, terbium, and certain metal alloys and ceramic alloys. Ferromagnetism, like super-conductivity, is found only below a certain critical temperature, which in the case of ferromagnetism is called the Curie temperature. The Curie temperature of gadolinium and dysprosium is below room temperature; that of iron is 1435°F. Above the Curie temperature ferromagnetie materials become paramagnetic. Unlike paramagnetism and diamagnetism, Ferromagnetism is a property only of solids.

Paramagnetism

Paramagnetic materials, which may be solid, liquid, or gas (oxygen exhibits strong paramagnetism, for example), are weakly magnetic and orient themselves parallel to a strong magnetic field. Unlike ferromagnetism, paramagnetism is not limited by temperature.

Diamagnetism

This is a weakly negative type of magnetism; that is, diamagnetic materials are repelled from the strongest part of a magnetic field to the weakest. The rare gases and the metals bismuth, beryllium, copper, and zinc are examples of diamagnetic materials.

An electron may be considered as a spinning negative electric charge. Since any such spinning charge is magnetic, an electron is in effect a minute magnet. There are two possible rotations of spin, clockwise and counter-clockwise. In any completely filled energy level of the atom, each electron pairs with another electron of opposite spin. The electron pair is nonmagnetic, since the magnetism of one spin cancels that of the opposite spin. When all the electrons in an atom are thus paired, there can be no paramagnetism, and diamagnetism results. An unpaired electron will produce a paramagnetic condition. Thus any atom such as a silver atom (one atom in the outermost populated energy level) must be paramagnetic. There are other electron configurations which can produce paramagnetism, but these will not be discussed.

The three types of magnetism may also be defined in terms of permeability. Permeability measures the relative ease with which magnetic flux or magnetism may be developed in a material, or it is the relative conductivity of a material for magnetic lines of force. A vacuum is assigned a permeability of 1. Diamagnetic materials have a permeability of less than 1; paramagnetic materials have a permeability greater than 1. The maximum permeability of the common ferromagnetic steels ranges up to about 20,000, though special alloys may be permeabilities exceeding 10,00,000.

Suppose that a material is enclosed in a wire coil and that the coil carries an electric current. This will produce a magnetising effect on the material within the magnetic field of the coil. The magnetising effect will be proportional to the ampere-turns of the coil. The flux density B (lines of magnetic force per unit cross-sectional area) in the magnetised material will be some function of the amp-turns per unit length H:

$$B = f(H)$$

For both diamagnetic and paramagnetic materials, $B = \mu H$, where μ is the permeability (see Fig. 23.2).

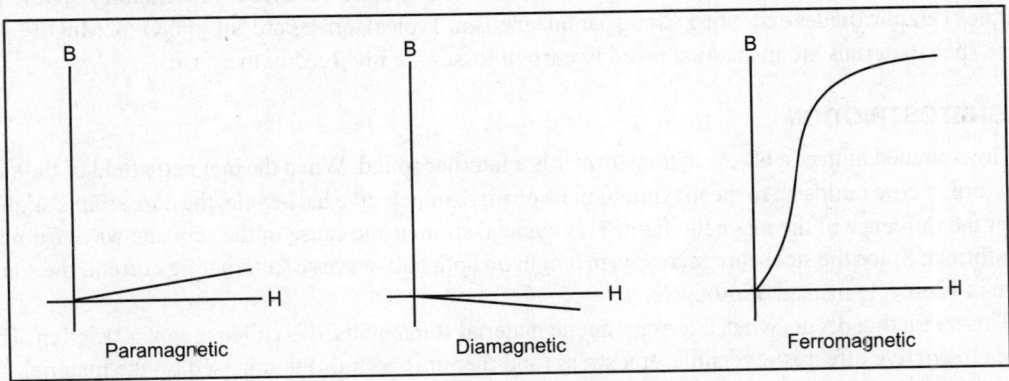

Fig. 23.2. Flux density and magnetising force.

As Fig. 23.2 shows, the relationship between B and H for a ferromagnetic material is nonlinear, and the permeability, B/H, is not a constant. There is a limit to the flux density of any ferromagnetic material; when this point is reached the material is said to be saturated. Magnetic amplifiers and saturable reactors use this phenomenon of saturation for their operation.

Soft steels are used in such electromagnetic equipment as motors, transformers, and relays. The steel is magnetised when current is switched to the magnetising coil. Such steels instantly lose their magnetism when the current is switched off. Hard steels and nickel-steel alloys are used for permanent magnet applications.

The steel core of a transformer presents special problems which are solved by the use of laminations of so-called 'electric' steels. The purpose of a transformer is the induction of a voltage or current in the secondary winding. Unfortunately the steel core is also a secondary, and a current is likewise induced in it. This current is termed an eddy current, and it represents an I^2R loss of power, usually referred to as an iron loss, just as the I^2R losses in the transformer windings are called copper losses. Soft steels have a relatively low specific resistance and would produce large eddy currents and powerful heating effects in a transformer core. To reduce such eddy currents, the core is laminated to increase the resistance by reducing the cross section carrying current, and the steel used is a silicon steel. Up to about 5 per cent silicon is added. The silicon atoms replace iron atoms in the bcc space lattice. The effect is to produce distortions in the space lattice and thus to Increase the specific resistance of the steel (by a factor of about 5 times for 3 per cent silicon). Electric steels, however, have a lower saturation induction. Carbon and nitrogen reduce permeability in such steels and are therefore kept to as low values as possible; the permeability is improved if the steel is coarse-grained.

The following steels are not ferromagnetic:

1. Type 300 stainless steels.

2. Steels containing about 12 per cent manganese (Hadfield, manganese steels).
3. Any steel above its Curie temperature.

The paramagnetic manganese and stainless steels are termed austenitic and have pronounced work-hardening characteristics.

Certain nickel-iron alloys containing about 50 per cent nickel, such as Perminvar, have a constant permeability. The most popular permanent magnet materials are the *Alnicos*. These are Iron-nickel aluminum alloys containing about one-quarter nickel. Like all permanent magnet materials, they are very hard.

Since World War II the ferrites have come into extensive use for electronic circuitry. These are complex ceramic oxides exhibiting strong paramagnetism. Typical ferrites are $NiO \cdot Fe_2O_3$ or $MnO \cdot Fe_2O_3$. Since such materials are insulators, no eddy current losses are involved in their use.

MAGNETOSTRICTION

The low-pitched hum of a 60-cycle transformer is a familiar sound. When the magnetic field of the steel transformer core builds up to the maximum in its positive or negative half-cycle, the core strains slightly under the influence of the magnetic field. This cyclical strain is the cause of the acoustic wave from the transformer. Since the steel core increases in length on both half-waves of alternating current, the sound wave is 120-cycle instead of 60-cycle.

This strain that occurs when a ferromagnetic material is magnetised is called magnetostriction. That magnetostrictive effect is reversible. If a stress (and therefore a strain) is imposed on the material, the magnetisation of the material will be altered. Magnetostriction produces a positive strain (elongation) in iron and a negative strain (shortening) in cobalt and nickel. The effect is greatest in nickel, of the order of 30 millionths of an inch per inch maximum.

The famous antisubmarine Sonar was an early application of magnetostriction. Similar devices are now applied to ultrasonic inspection of welds and castings, ultrasonic detection and counting in automatic conveying, ultrasonic cleaning, ultrasonic welding, depth soundings in oceanography, phonograph pickups, and ultrasonic homogenisation of milk, peanut butter, and other food products.

PIEZOELECTRICITY

Piezoelectricity is analogous to magnetostriction. Certain ceramic materials such as quartz and titanates produce the piezoelectric effect. When a crystal of such material is compressed; a small voltage is generated across the opposite faces of the crystal, and conversely, a potential difference across the opposite faces will cause the crystal to expand or contract. Piezoelectricity is the preferred method of instrumentation for recording pressures in engine cylinders and gun barrels. For this purpose a small mounted crystal is screwed into the wall of the cylinder as a spark plug is, and the pressure is read out as a voltage on an amplifier.

Although piezoelectricity as a method of instrumentation is competitive with magnetostriction in general, the piezoelectric effect is not capable of the high power that can be produced by the magnetostrictive effect. Ultrasonic cleaning, for example, requires considerable power in the hundreds of watts, and the transducers to supply such power must be magnetostrictive.

Piezoelectric instrumentation is not suited to constant or slowly changing forces because of electrical leakage. An excellent application is its use in phonograph pickups, where varying small movements of the needle are converted into shear or bending stress.

PHOTOCONDUCTIVITY

The photoconductive effect occurs when a semiconductor is irradiated with a sufficiently high photon energy to cause a pronounced reduction in its electrical resistance. There are, many photoconductive materials, but the more commonly used ones include selenium, silicon, cadmium sulphide, lead telluride, lead sulphide, and thallium sulphide. The photoconductive material is usually a deposited thin film on a substrate material. Such materials may be used as detectors or switches to record the presence of visible light, ultraviolet, or X-radiation. Cadmium sulphide is preferred for X-ray detection.

Photoconductive devices are found in photographic exposure meters, photoelectric colorimeters, light-activated burglar alarms, electric door opening mechanisms, and counting devices on conveyor belts.

THERMOELECTRICITY

If two dissimilar metals are joined and this junction is then heated, a small voltage in the millivolt range is produced, known as the thermoelectric effect. This is a method of producing direct-current electric power directly from heat. Currently the thermoelectric effect is being developed for a variety of uses. There are actually three thermoelectric effects, but only the following two have industrial applications:

Seebeck Effect

If the two junctions of two dissimilar metals are held at different temperatures, a voltage is produced that is closely proportional to the temperature difference. This seebeck arrangement of wiring is known as a thermocouple and has been in use for the last hundred years as a temperature-measuring device.

Peltier Effect

If current flows through two junctions of two dissimilar metals, one junction will be heated and the other cooled. In terms of practical use, the Peltier effect indicates that one junction is a tiny furnace and the other a tiny refrigerator.

Since Seebeck's discovery there have been repeated attempts to produce electricity directly from heat by his method. So long as metal conductors were employed, these attempts failed because of the tiny currents produced and the abysmal efficiencies—less than 1 per cent. But more recently, advances in solid-state physics have led to the use of semiconductor thermoelectric devices with efficiencies closer to 10 per cent. Bismuth telluride and lead telluride are the favoured semiconductors for this purpose. Thermoelectric power generators with up to 5 kw capacity are now coming into use, and the thermoelectric refrigerator is nearing the end of its research and development stage. Figure 23.3 is a diagram of a semiconductor thermoelectric device, which operates in the following manner.

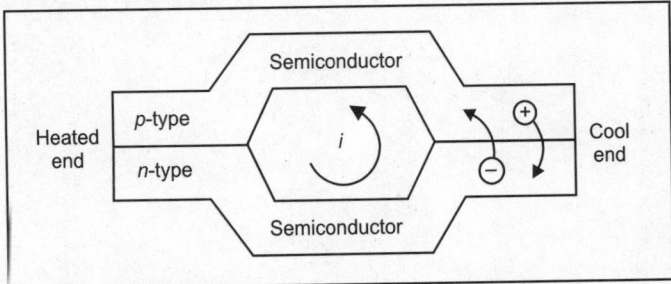

Fig. 23.3. Semiconductor thermoelectric device.

The heat energy applied at one end raises electrons to the conduction band. For each electron thus transferred, a hole is left behind. The electrons travel to the cold junction through the n-type material, while the holes travel to the cold junction through the p-type material. The two unite at the cold junction, the electrons dropping into the holes and releasing energy to the cold junction. Since the charges carried by the holes and electrons are opposed to each other, there is a flow of electric current as indicated in the diagram. At the hot junction both holes and electrons are moving away from the junction. To make up for the loss of these charges, electrons are raised to the conduction band to create new pairs of electrons and holes. Since energy is required for this operation, heat is absorbed at the hot junction.

For temperature-indicating thermocouples, only four combinations are in common use, although other combinations must be used for very high temperature work:

1. Copper-constantan, 300°–700°F, 2 per cent accuracy.
2. Iron-constantan, 0°–1200°F, 4 per cent accuracy.
3. Chromel-alumel, 1000°–2200°F, 4 per cent accuracy.
4. Platinum-platinum plus 4 per cent rhodium. 2000°–3000°F, 5 per cent accuracy.

Chapter 24

Magnetic Properties of Materials

INTRODUCTION

Modern technology would be unthinkable without magnetic materials and magnetic phenomena. Magnetic tapes or disks (for computers, video recorders, etc.) motors, generators, telephones, transformers, permanent magnets, electromagnets, loudspeakers, and magnetic strips on credit cards are only a few examples of their applications. To a certain degree, magnetism and electric phenomena can be considered to be siblings since many common mechanisms exist such as dipoles, attraction, repulsion, spontaneous or forced alignment of dipoles, field lines, field strengths, etc. Thus, the governing equations often have the same form. Actually, electrical and magnetic phenomena are linked by the famous Maxwell equations, which were mentioned already.

At least five different kinds of magnetic materials exist. They have been termed para-, dia-, ferro-, ferri-, and antiferromagnetics. A qualitative as well as a quantitative distinction between these types can be achieved in a relatively simple way by utilising a method proposed by Faraday.

The magnetic material to be investigated is suspended from one of the arms of a sensitive balance and is allowed to reach into an inhomogeneous magnetic field (Fig. 24.1). Diamagnetic materials are expelled from this field, whereas para-, ferro-, antiferro-, and ferrimagnetics are attracted in different degrees. It has been found empirically that the apparent loss or gain in mass, that is, the force, F, on the sample exerted by the magnetic field, is:

$$F = V\chi\mu_0 H \frac{dH}{dx}, \qquad \ldots (24.1)$$

where, V is the volume of the sample, μ_0 is a universal constant called the permeability of free space (1.257×10^{-6} H/m or Vs/Am), and χ is the susceptibility, which expresses how responsive a material is to an applied magnetic field. Characteristic values for χ are given in Table 24.1. The term dH/dx in Eq. 24.1 is the change of the magnetic field strength H in the x-direction. The field strength H of an electromagnet (consisting of helical windings of a long, insulated wire as seen in the lower portion of Fig. 24.1) is proportional to the current, I, which flows through this coil, and on the number, n, of the windings (called turns) that have been used to make the coil. Further, the magnetic field strength is inversely proportional to the length, L, of the solenoid. Thus, the magnetic field strength is expressed by:

$$H = \frac{In}{L} \qquad \ldots (24.2)$$

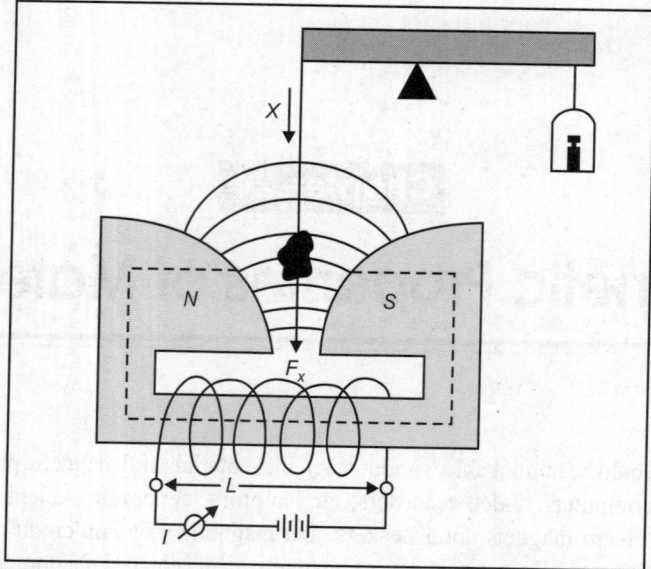

Fig. 24.1. Measurement of the magnetic susceptibility in an nonhomogeneous magnetic field. The magnetic field lines (dashed) follow the iron core.

The field strength is measured (in SI units) in 'Amp-turns per meter' or shortly, in A/m. The magnetic field can be enhanced by inserting, say, iron, into a solenoid, as shown in Fig. 24.1. The parameter which expresses the amount of enhancement of the magnetic field is called the permeability μ. The magnetic field strength within a material is known by the names magnetic induction (or magnetic flux density) and is denoted by B. Magnetic field strength and magnetic induction are related by the equation:

$$B = \mu \mu_0 H \qquad \ldots (24.3)$$

The SI unit for B is the tesla (T) and that of μ_0 is henries per meter (H/m or Vs/Am). The permeability (sometimes called relative permeability, μ_r) in Eq. 24.3 is unitless and is listed in Table 24.1 for some materials. The relationship between the susceptibility and the permeability is:

$$\mu = 1 + \chi \qquad \ldots (24.4)$$

For empty space and, for all practical purposes, also for air, one defines $\chi = 0$ and thus $\mu = 1$ (Eq. 24.4). The susceptibility is small and negative for diamagnetic materials. As a consequence, χ is slightly less than 1 (Table 24.1). For para- and antiferromagnetic materials, χ is again small, but positive. Thus, μ is slightly larger than 1. Finally, χ and μ are large and positive for ferro- and ferrimagnetic materials. The magnetic constants are temperature-dependent, except for diamagnetic materials, as we will see later. Further, the susceptibility for ferrimagnetic materials depends on the field strength, H.

The magnetic field parameters at a given point in space are, as explained above, the magnetic field strength H and the magnetic induction B. In free (empty) space, B and $\mu_0 H$ are identical, as seen in Eq. 24.3. Inside a magnetic material the induction B consists of the free-space component ($\mu_0 H$) plus a contribution to the magnetic field ($\mu_0 M$) which is due to the presence of matter [(Fig. 24.2(a)], that is,

$$B = \mu_0 H + \mu_0 M \qquad \ldots (24.5)$$

where, M is called the magnetisation of the material. Combining (Eqs 24.3 through 24.5 yields:

$$M = \chi H \qquad \ldots (24.6)$$

H, B, and M are actually vectors. Specifically, outside a material, H (and B) point from the north to the south pole. Inside of a ferro- or paramagnetic material, B and M point from the south to the north [Figs 24.2(a) and 24.2(b)]. However, we will mostly utilise their moduli in the following sections and thus use light-face italic letters.

Table 24.1. Magnetic constants of some materials at room temperature.

Material	χ (SI) unitless	χ (cgs) unitless	μ unitless	Type of magnetism
Bi	-165×10^{-6}	-13.13×10^{-6}	0.99983	
Ge	-71.1×10^{-6}	-5.66×10^{-6}	0.99993	
Au	-34.4×10^{-6}	-2.74×10^{-6}	0.99996	Diamagnetic
Ag	-25.3×10^{-6}	-2.016×10^{-6}	0.99997	
Be	-23.2×10^{-6}	-1.85×10^{-6}	0.99998	
Cu	-9.7×10^{-6}	-0.77×10^{-6}	0.99999	
Superconductors	-1.0	$\sim -8 \times 10^{-2}$	0	
β-Sn	$+2.4 \times 10^{-6}$	$+0.19 \times 10^{-6}$	1	
Al	$+20.7 \times 10^{-6}$	$+1.65 \times 10^{-6}$	1.00002	Paramagnetic
W	$+77.7 \times 10^{-6}$	$+6.18 \times 10^{-6}$	1.00008	
Pt	$+264.4 \times 10^{-6}$	$+21.04 \times 10^{-6}$	1.00026	
Low carbon steel	Approximately the same as μ		5×10^3	
Fe-3%Si (grain-oriented)	because of $\chi = \mu - 1$		4×10^4	Ferromagnetic
Ni-Fe-Mo (supermalloy)			10^6	

Note: The table lists the unitless susceptibility, χ in SI and CGS units. Other sources may provide mass, atomic, molar, volume or gram equivalent susceptibilities in cgs or mks units.

B was called above to be the magnetic flux density in a material, that is, the magnetic flux per unit area. The magnetic flux ϕ is then defined as the product of B and area A, that is, by:

$$\phi = B A \qquad \ldots (24.7)$$

Finally, we need to define the magnetic moment μ_m (also a vector) through the following equation:

$$M = \frac{\mu_m}{V}, \qquad \ldots (24.8)$$

which means that the magnetisation is the magnetic moment per unit volume.

A short note on units should be added. This chapter uses SI units throughout. However, the scientific literature on magnetism (particularly in the United States) is still widely written in electromagnetic CGS (emu) units. The magnetic field strength in CGS units is measured in Oersted and the magnetic induction in Gauss.

MAGNETIC PHENOMENA AND THEIR INTERPRETATION

We stated in the last section that different types of magnetism exist which are characterised by the magnitude and the sign of the susceptibility (Table 24.1). Since various materials respond so differently in a magnetic field, we suspect that several fundamentally different mechanisms must be responsible for the magnetic properties.

We shall now attempt to unfold the multiplicity of the magnetic behaviour of materials by describing some pertinent experimental findings and giving some brief interpretations.

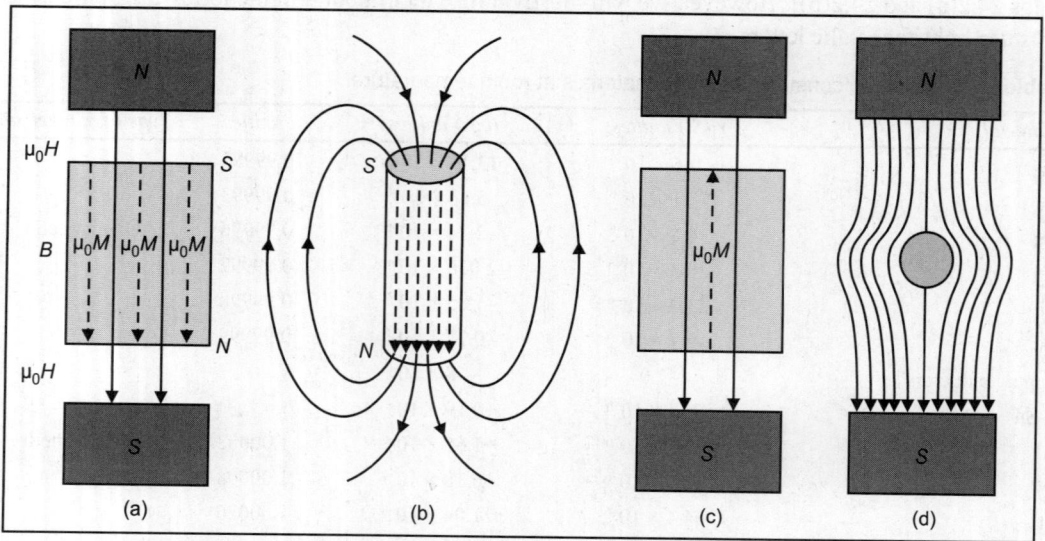

Fig. 24.2. Schematic representation of magnetic field lines in and around different types of materials. (a) para- or ferromagnetics. The magnetic induction (B) inside the material consists of the free-space component ($\mu_0 H$) plus a contribution by the material ($\mu_0 M$) (Eq. 24.5). (b) The magnetic field lines outside a material point from the north to the south poles, whereas inside of para- or ferromagnetics, B and $\mu_0 M$ point from south to north in order to maintain continuity. (c) In diamagnetics, the response of the material counteracts (weakens) the external magnetic field. (d) In a thin surface layer of a superconductor, a supercurrent is created (below its transition temperature) which causes a magnetic field that opposes the external field. As a consequence, the magnetic flux lines are expelled from the interior of the material.

Diamagnetism

Ampere postulated more than one hundred years ago that so-called molecular currents are responsible for the magnetism in solids. He compared these molecular currents to an electric current in a loop-shaped piece of wire which is known to cause a magnetic moment. Today, we replace Ampere's molecular currents by orbiting valence electrons.

To understand diamagnetism, a second aspect needs to be considered. As already explained a current is induced in a wire loop whenever a bar magnet is moved toward (or from) this loop.

The current thus induced causes, in turn, a magnetic moment that is opposite to the one of the bar magnet (Fig. 24.3). (This has to be so in order for mechanical work to be expended in producing the current, i.e. to conserve energy; otherwise, a perpetual motion would be created!) Diamagnetism may then be explained by postulating that the external magnetic field induces a change in the magnitude of the atomic currents, i.e. the external field accelerates or decelerates the orbiting electrons, so that their magnetic moment is in the opposite direction to the external magnetic field. In other words, the responses of the orbiting electrons counteract the external field [Fig. 24.2(c)].

Superconductors have extraordinary diamagnetic properties. They completely expel the magnetic flux lines from their interior when in the superconducting state (Meissner effect). In other words, a superconductor behaves in a magnetic field as if B would be zero inside the material [Figure 24.2(d)], Thus, with Eq. 24.5 one obtains:

$$H = -M, \qquad \qquad \ldots (24.9)$$

which means that the magnetisation is equal and opposite to the external magnetic field strength. The result is a perfect diamagnet. The susceptibility,

$$\chi = \frac{M}{H}, \qquad \qquad \ldots (24.10)$$

in superconductors is therefore -1 compared to about -10^{-5} in the normal state (see Table 24.1). This strong diamagnetism can be used for frictionless bearings, that is, for support of loads by a repelling magnetic force. The often-demonstrated levitation effect in which a magnet hovers above a superconducting material also can be explained by these strong diamagnetic properties of superconductors.

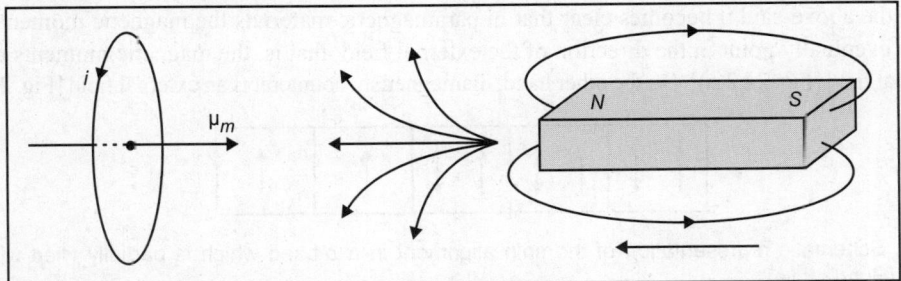

Fig. 24.3. Induction of a current in a loop-shaped piece of wire by moving a bar magnet toward the wire loop. The current in the loop causes a magnetic field that is directed opposite to the magnetic field of the bar magnet.

Paramagnetism

Paramagnetism in solids is attributed to a large extent to a magnetic moment that results from electrons which spin around their own axis [Fig. 24.4(a)]. The spin magnetic moments are generally randomly oriented so that no net magnetic moment results. An external magnetic field tries to turn the unfavourably oriented spin moments in the direction of the external field, but thermal agitation counteracts the alignment. Thus, spin paramagnetism is slightly temperature-dependent. It is generally weak and is observed in some metals and in salts of the transition elements.

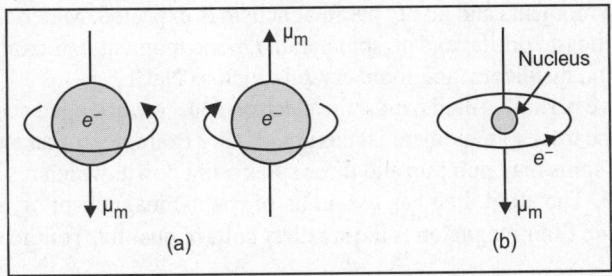

Fig. 24.4. (a) Schematic representation of electrons which spin around their own axis. A (para)magnetic moment μ_m results; its direction depends on the mode of rotation. Only two spin directions are shown (called 'spin up' and 'spin down'), (b) An orbiting electron is the source for electron-orbit paramagnetism.

Free atoms (dilute gases) as well as rare earth elements and their salts and oxides possess an additional source of paramagnetism. It stems from the magnetic moment of the orbiting electrons [Fig. 24.4(b)]. Without an external magnetic field, these magnetic moments are, again, randomly oriented and thus mutually cancel one another. As a result, the net magnetisation is zero. However, when an external field is applied, the individual magnetic vectors tend to turn into the field direction which may be counteracted by thermal agitation. Thus, electron-orbit paramagnetism is also temperature-dependent. Specifically, paramagnetics often (not always!) obey the experimentally found Curie-Weiss law:

$$\chi = \frac{C}{T - \theta} \qquad \ldots (24.11)$$

where, C and θ are constants (given in Kelvin), and C is called the Curie Constant. The Curie-Weiss law is observed to be valid for rare earth elements and salts of the transition elements, for example, the carbonates, chlorides, and sulphates of Fe, Co, Cr, Mn.

From the above-said it becomes clear that in paramagnetic materials the magnetic moments of the electrons eventually point in the direction of the external field, that is, the magnetic moments enhance the external field [Fig. 24.2(a)]. On the other hand, diamagnetism counteracts an external field [Fig. 24.2(c)].

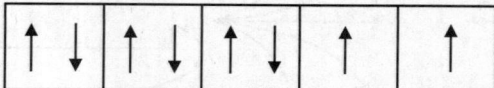

Fig. 24.5. Schematic representation of the spin alignment in a d-band which is partially filled with eight electrons (Hund's rule).

Thus, para- and diamagnetism oppose each other. Solids that have both orbital as well as spin paramagnetism are consequently paramagnetic (since the sum of both paramagnetic compounds is commonly larger than the diamagnetism). Rare earth metals are an example of this.

In many other solids, however, the electron orbits are essentially coupled to the lattice. This prevents the orbital magnetic moments from turning into the field direction. Thus, electron-orbit paramagnetism does not play a role, and only spin paramagnetism remains. The possible presence of a net spin-paramagnetic moment depends, however, on whether or not the magnetic moments of the individual spins cancel each other. Specifically, if a solid has completely filled electron bands, then a quantum mechanical rule, called the Pauli principle, requires the same number of electrons with spins up and with spins down [Figure 24.4(a)]. The Pauli principle stipulates that each electron state can be filled only with two electrons having opposite spins. The case of completely filled bands thus results in a cancellation of the spin moments and no net paramagnetism is expected. Materials in which this occurs are therefore diamagnetic (no orbital and no spin paramagnetic moments). Examples of filled bands are intrinsic semiconductors, insulators, and ionic crystals such as NaCl.

In materials that have partially filled bands, the electron spins are arranged according to Hund's rule in such a manner that the total spin moment is maximised. For example, for an atom with eight valence d-electrons, five of the spins may point up and three spins point down, which results in a net number of two spins up; Fig. 24.5. The atom then has two units of (para-) magnetism or, as it is said, two Bohr magnetons per atom. The Bohr magneton is the smallest unit (or quantum) of the magnetic moment and has the value:

$$\mu_B = \frac{eh}{4\pi m} = 9.274 \times 10^{-24} \left(\frac{J}{T}\right) \equiv \left(A \cdot m^2\right). \qquad \ldots (24.12)$$

Ferromagnetism

Figure 24.6 depicts a ring-shaped solenoid consisting of a newly cast piece of iron and two separate coils which are wound around the iron ring. If the magnetic field strength in the solenoid is temporally increased (by increasing the current in the primary winding), then the magnetisation (measured in the secondary winding with a flux meter) rises slowly at first and then more rapidly, as shown in Fig. 24.7 (dashed line). Finally, M levels off and reaches a constant value, called the saturation magnetisation, M_s. When H is reduced to zero, the magnetisation retains a positive value, called the remanent magnetisation, or remanence, M_r. It is this retained magnetisation which is utilised in permanent magnets. The remanent magnetisation can be removed by reversing the magnetic field strength to a value H_c, called the coercive field. Solids having a large combination of M_r and H_c are called hard magnetic materials (in contrast to soft magnetic materials, for which the area inside the loop of Fig. 24.7 is very small). A complete cycle through positive and negative H-values as shown in Fig. 24.7 is called a hysteresis loop. It should be noted that a second type of hysteresis curve is often used in which B (instead of M) is plotted versus H. No saturation value for B can be observed (Eq. 24.3). Removal of the residual induction requires a field that is called coercivity, but the terms coercive field and coercivity are often used interchangeably. The area within a hysteresis loop (B times H or M times $\mu_0 H$) is proportional to the energy per unit volume, which is dissipated once a full field cycle has been completed.

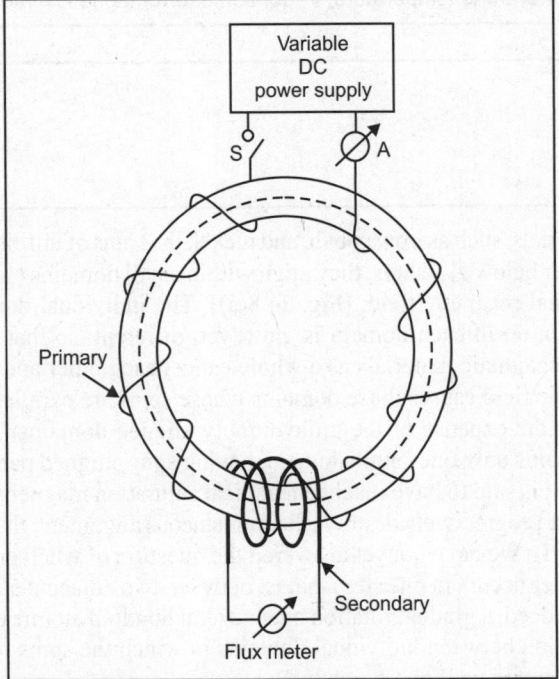

Fig. 24.6. A ring-shaped solenoid with primary and secondary windings. The magnetic flux lines are indicated by a dashed circle. Note that a current can flow in the secondary circuit only if the current (and therefore the magnetic flux) in the primary winding changes with time. An on-off switch in the primary circuit may serve this purpose. A flux meter is an ampmeter without retracting springs.

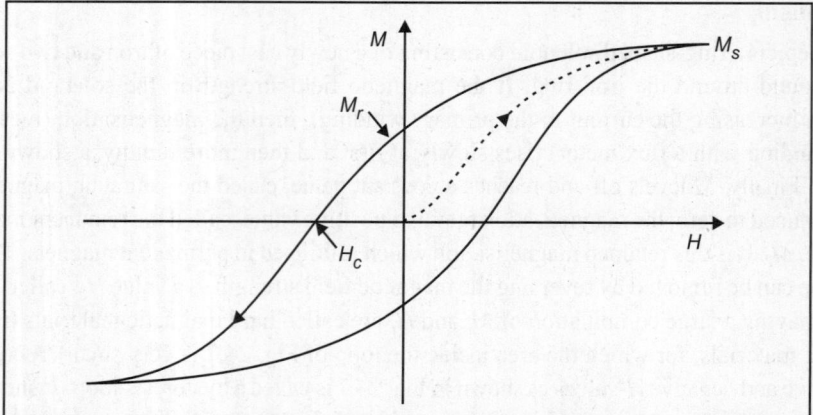

Fig. 24.7. Schematic representation of a hysteresis loop of a ferromagnetic material. The dashed curve is for a newly cast piece of iron (called virgin iron).

The saturation magnetisation is temperature-dependent. Above the curie temperature. T_c, ferromagnetics become paramagnetic. Table 24.2 lists curie temperatures for some elements.

Table 24.2. Curie temperature, T_c, for some ferromagnetic materials.

Metal	T_c (K)
Fe	1043
Co	1404
Ni	631
Gd	289

In ferromagnetic materials, such as iron, cobalt, and nickel, the spins of unfilled d-bands spontaneously align parallel to each other below T_c, that is, they align within small domains (1–100 µm in size) without the presence of an external magnetic field; [Fig. 24.8(a)]. The individual domains are magnetised to saturation. The spin direction in each domain is, however, different, so that the individual magnetic moments for virgin ferromagnetic materials as a whole cancel each other and the net magnetisation is zero. An external magnetic field causes those domains whose spins are parallel or nearly parallel to the external field to grow at the expense of the unfavourably aligned domains [Fig. 24.8(b)]. When the entire crystal finally contains only one single domain, having spins aligned parallel to the external field direction then the material is said to have reached technical saturation magnetisation, M_s [Fig. 24.8(c)]. An increase in temperature progressively destroys the spontaneous alignment; thus reducing the saturation magnetisation, Fig. 24.8(d). We have not yet answered the question of whether or not the flip from one spin direction into the other occurs in one step, that is, between two adjacent atoms or over an extended range of atoms instead. Indeed, a gradual rotation over several hundred atomic distances is energetically most favourable. The region between individual domains in which the spins rotate from one direction into the next is called a domain wall or a bloch wall.

Antiferromagnetism

Antiferromagnetic materials exhibit, just as ferromagnetics, a spontaneous alignment of spin moments below a critical temperature (called the Néel temperature). However, the responsible neighboring atoms in antiferromagnetics are aligned in an antiparallel fashion (Fig. 24.9). Actually, one may consider an antiferromagnetic crystal to be divided into two interpenetrating sublattices, A and B, each of which has a spontaneous alignment of spins. Figure 24.9 depicts the spin alignments for two manganese compounds. (Only the spins of the manganese ions contribute to the antiferromagnetic behaviour.) Figure 24.9(a) implies that the ions in a given plane possess parallel spin alignment, whereas ions in the adjacent plane have antiparallel spins with respect to the first plane. Thus, the magnetic moments of the solid cancel each other and the material as a whole has no net magnetic moment.

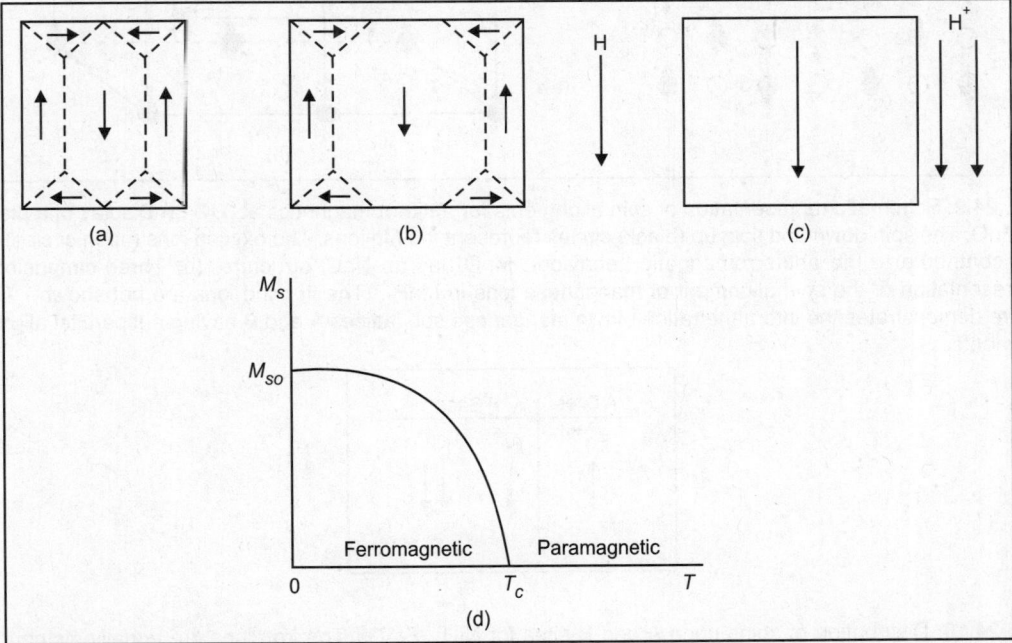

Fig. 24.8. (a) Schematic representation of individual magnetic domains whose spins are spontaneously aligned in one direction, (b) and (c). Same as above but after an external magnetic field of increasing strength has been applied, (d) Temperature-dependence of the saturation magnetisation of ferromagnetic materials.

Most antiferromagnetics are found among ionic compounds such as $MnO \cdot MnF_2$, FeO, NiO, and CoO. They are generally insulators or semiconductors. Additionally, α-manganese and chromium are antiferromagnetic. Antiferromagnets are a crucial component of giant magnetoresistance heads in hard disk drives. Their constant θ in the Curie-Weiss law (Eq. 24.11) is negative.

Ferrimagnetism

Ferrimagnetic materials such as $NiO \cdot Fe_2O_3$ or $FeO \cdot Fe_2O_3$ are of great technical importance. They exhibit a spontaneous magnetic moment (Fig. 24.8) and hysteresis (Fig. 24.7) below a Curie temperature, just as iron, cobalt, and nickel do. In other words, ferrimagnetic materials possess, similar to ferromagnetics, small domains in which the electron spins are spontaneously aligned in parallel. The main difference to ferromagnetics is, however, that ferrimagnetics are ceramic materials (oxides); they are therefore poor electrical conductors. Poor conduction is often desired for high-frequency applications (e.g. to prevent eddy currents in cores of coils).

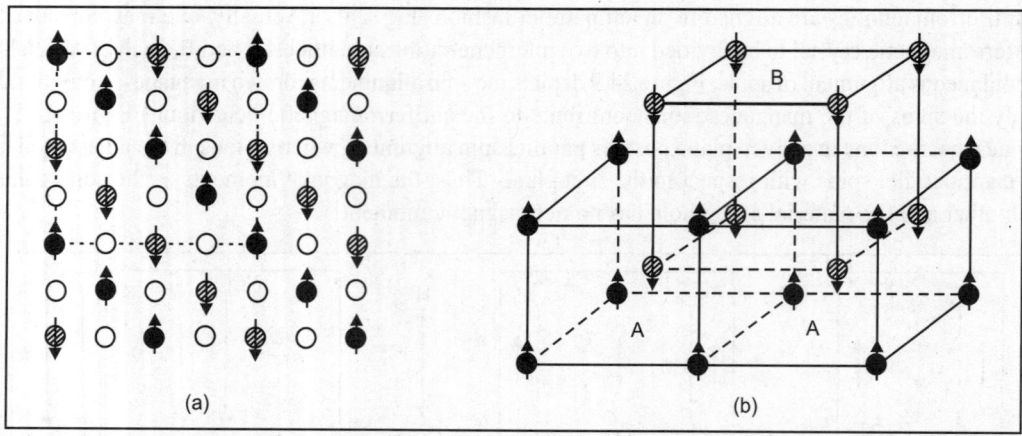

Fig. 24.9. Schematic representation of spin alignments for antiferromagnetics at 0 K. (a) Display of a plane of MnO. The spin down and spin up (black) circles represent the Mn ions. The oxygen ions (open circles) do not contribute to the antiferromagnetic behaviour. MnO has an NaCl structure. (b) Three-dimensional representation of the spin alignment of manganese ions in MnF_2. (The fluorine ions are not shown.) This figure demonstrates the interpenetration of two manganese sub lattices A and B having antiparallel aligned moments.

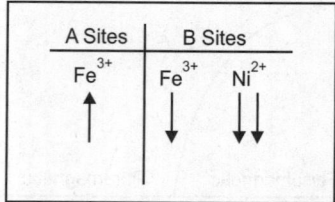

Fig. 24.10. Distribution of spins upon A and B sites for $NiO \cdot Fe_2O_3$. The iron ions are equally distributed among the A and B sites. The nickel ions are only situated on the B sites.

To explain the spontaneous magnetisation in ferrimagnetics. Néel proposed that two sublattices, say A and B, should exist in these materials (just as in antiferromagnetics), each of which contains ions whose spins are aligned parallel to each other. Again, the spins of the ions on the A sites are antiparallel to the spins of the ions on the B sites. The crucial point is that each of the sublattices contains a different amount of magnetic ions. This causes some of the magnetic moments to remain uncancelled. As a consequence, a net magnetic moment results. Ferrimagnetic materials can thus be described as imperfect antiferromagnetics.

We will now discuss as an example nickel ferrite, $NiO \cdot Fe_2O_3$. The Fe^{3+} ions are equally distributed between the A and B sites (Fig. 24.10), and since ions on the A and B sites exhibit spontaneous magnetisation in opposite directions, we expect overall cancellation of spins for the iron ions.

In contrast to this, all nickel ions are accommodated on the B sites only (Fig. 24.10). Two electrons have been stripped in the Ni^{2+} ion (i.e. the two 4s-electrons) so that the eight d-electrons per atom remain. They are arranged according to Hund's rule (Fig. 24.5) to yield two net magnetic moments. In other words, nickel ferrite has two uncancelled spins and therefore two Bohr magnetons per formula unit. This is essentially observed by experiment.

The crystallography of ferrites is rather complex. It suffices to, know that there are two types of lattice site which are available to be occupied by the metal ions. (As before, oxygen ions do not contribute to the magnetic moments.) The unit cell of cubic ferrites rites contains a total of 56 ions. Some of the metal ions are situated inside a tetrahedron formed by the oxygen ions. These are the above-mentioned A sites. Other metal ions are arranged in the center of an octahedron formed by the oxygen ions and are said to be on the B sites. This distribution is called an inverse spinel structure.

APPLICATIONS

Electrical Steels (Soft Magnetic Materials)

Electrical steel is used to multiply the magnetic flux in the core of electromagnets. These materials are therefore widely incorporated in many electrical machines which are in daily use. Among their applications are cores of transformers, electromotors, generators, and electromagnets.

In order to make these devices as energy efficient and economical as possible, one needs to find magnetic materials that have the highest possible permeability (at the lowest possible price). Furthermore, magnetic core materials should be capable of being cations easily magnetised or demangnetised. In other words, the area within the hysteresis loop (or the coercive force, H_c) should be as small as possible (Fig. 24.7). We remember that materials whose hysteresis lops are narrow are called soft magnetic materials. Electrical steels are classified by some of their properties, for example, by the amount of their core losses by their composition, by their permeability, and whether or not they are grainoriented. We shall discuss these different properties momentarily.

The energy losses encountered in electromotors (efficiency between 50 and 90 per cent) or in transformers (efficiency 95–99.5 per cent) are estimated in the United States to be as high as 3×10^{10} KWh per year, which is equivalent to the energy consumption by about 3 million households.

The core loss is the energy that is dissipated in the form of heat within the core of electromagnetic devices when the core is subjected to an alternating magnetic field. Several types of losses are known, among which the eddy current loss and the hysteresis loss contribute most. Typical core losses are between 0.3 and 3 watts per kilogram of core material

Let us first discuss eddy current losses. Consider a transformer whose primary and secondary coils are wound around the legs of a rectangular iron yoke [Fig. 24.11(a)]. An alternating electric current in the primary coil causes an alternating magnetic flux, ϕ, in the core, which in turn induces in the secondary coil an alternating electromotive force, V_e, proportional to $d\phi/dt$ (Eq. 24.7):

$$V_e \propto \frac{d\phi}{dt} = -A\frac{dB}{dt}. \qquad \ldots (24.13)$$

Concurrently, an alternating emf is induced within the core itself, as shown in Fig. 24.11(a). This emf gives rise to the eddy current I_e. The eddy current is larger, the larger the permeability, μ [because $B = \mu \mu_0 H$; (Eq. 24.3)]. Further, I_e increases the larger the conductivity, σ, of the core material, the higher the applied frequency, and the larger the cross-sectional area, A, of the core. [A is perpendicular to the magnetic flux ϕ; Fig. 24.11(a).]

In order to decrease the eddy current, several remedies are possible. First, the core can be made of an insulator in order to decrease σ. Ferrites are thus effective but also expensive materials to build magnetic cores. They are indeed used for high-frequency applications. The most widely applied method to reduce eddy currents is the utilisation of cores made out of thin sheets that are electrically insulated from each other [Fig. 24.11(b)]. In this way, the cross-sectional area A is split into; several smaller areas, A', which in turn decreases V_e (Eq. 24.12). Despite the lamination, a residual eddy current loss still exists which is caused by current losses within the individual laminations, and by interlaminar losses that may arise if the laminations are not sufficiently insulated from each other. These losses are, however, less than 1 per cent of the total energy transferred.

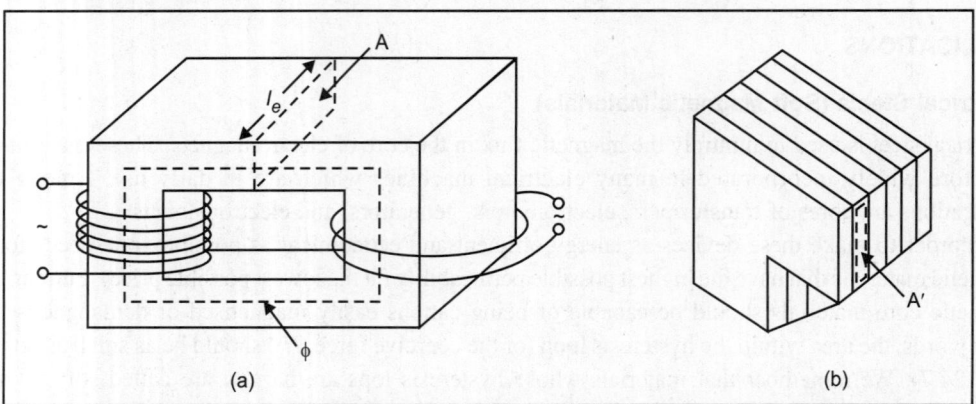

Fig. 24.11. (a) Solid transformer core with eddy current I_e in a cross-sectional area A. Note the magnetic flux lines ϕ, (b) Cross section of a laminated transformer core. The area A′ is smaller than area A in (a).

Hysteresis losses are encountered when the magnetic core is subjected to a complete hysteresis cycle (Fig. 24.7), The electrical energy thus dissipated into heat is proportional to the area enclosed by a B/H loop. Proper materials selection and rolling of the materials with subsequent heat treatment greatly reduces the area of a hysteresis loop.

Grain orientation

The permeability of electrical steel can be substantially increased and the hysteresis losses can be decreased by making use of favourable grain orientations in the material. This needs some explanation. The magnetic properties of crystalline ferromagnetic materials depend on the crystallographic direction in which an external field is applied, an effect which is called magnetic anisotropy. Let us use iron as an example. Figure 24.12 shows magnetisation curves of single crystals for three crystallographic, directions. We observe that, if the external field is applied in the <100> direction, saturation is achieved with the smallest possible field strength, The <100> direction is thus called the easy direction.

A second piece of information also needs to be considered. Metal sheets, which have been manufactured by rolling and heating, often possess a texture; that is, they have a preferred orientation of the grains. It just happens that in α-iron and α-iron alloys the <100> direction is parallel to the rolling direction. This property is exploited when utilising electrical steel. Grain-oriented electrical steel is produced by initially hot-rolling the alloy followed by two stages of cold reduction with intervening anneals. During the rolling, the grains are elongated and their orientation is altered as described above. Finally, the sheets are recrystallised, whereby some crystals grow in size at the expense of others (occupying the entire sheet thickness). This process is called secondary recrystallisation.

In summary, the magnetic properties of grain-oriented steels are best in the direction parallel to the direction of rolling. Electrical machines having core material of grain-oriented steel need less iron and are therefore smaller. The price increase due to tile more elaborate fabrication procedure is often compensated for by the savings in material.

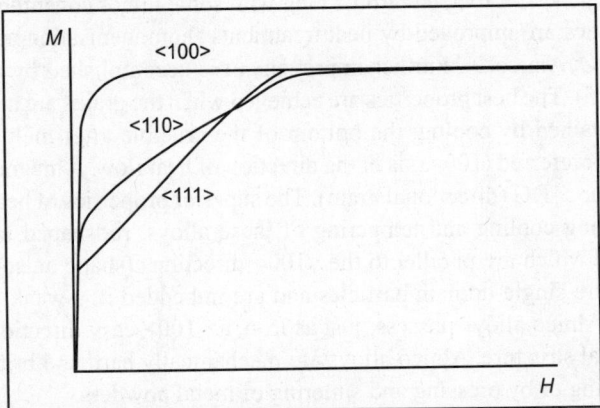

Fig. 24.12. Schematic magnetisation curves for rod-shaped iron single crystals of different orientations (virgin curves). The magnetic field was applied in three different crystallographic directions. (Compare with Fig. 24.7, which refers to polycrystalline materials.)

Composition of core materials

The least expensive core material is commercial low carbon steel (0.05 per cent C). It possesses a relatively small permeability and has about ten times higher core losses than grain-oriented silicon iron. Low carbon steel is used where low cost is more important than the efficient operation of a device. Iron-silicon alloys containing between 1.4 and 3.5 per cent Si and very little carbon have a higher permeability and a lower conductivity than low carbon steel. Grain-oriented silicon 'steel' is the favoured commercial product for highly efficient-high flux multiplying core applications such as transformer sheets. The highest permeability is achieved for certain multicomponent nickel-based alloys such as Permalloy, Supermalloy, or Mumetal. The latter can be rolled into thin sheets and is used to shield electronic equipment from stray magnetic fields.

Amorphous ferromagnets (metallic glasses) consisting of iron, nickel, or cobalt with boron, silicon, or phosphorous have, when properly annealed below the crystalline temperature, a considerably higher permeability and a lower coercivity than commonly used grain-oriented silicon. Further, the electrical resistivity of amorphous alloys is generally larger than their crystalline counterparts, which results in smaller eddy-current losses. However, amorphous ferromagnetic possess a somewhat lower saturation induction (which sharply decreases even further at elevated temperatures), and their core losses increase rapidly at higher flux densities (e.g. above 1.4 T). Thus, their application is limited to magnetic sensors, magnetorestrictive transducers, and transformers.

Permanent Magnets (Hard Magnetic Materials)

Permanent magnets are devices that retain their magnetic field indefinitely. They are characterised by a large remanence B_r (or M_r), a relatively large coercivity H_c, and a large area within the hysteresis loop. They are called hard magnetic materials. Another parameter which is used to characterise hard magnetic materials is the maximum energy product, $(BH)_{max}$, which is related to the maximum area within a hysteresis loop. The values of B_r, H_c, and $(BH)_{max}$ for some materials which are used as permanent magnets are listed. Today, many permanent magnets are made of Alnico alloys, which contain various amounts of aluminum, nickel, cobalt, and iron, along with some minor constituents such as copper and titanium. Their properties are improved by heat treatments (homogenisation at 1250°C, fast cooling, and tempering at 600°C; Alnico 2). Further improvement is accomplished by cooling the alloys in a magnetic field (Alnico 5). The best properties are achieved when the grains are made to have a preferred orientation. This is obtained by cooling the bottom of the crucible after melting, thus forming long columnar grains with a preferred ⟨100⟩ axis in the direction of heat flow. A magnetic field parallel to the <100> axis yields Alnico 5-DG (directional grain). The superior properties of heat-treated Alnico stems from the fact that, during cooling and tempering of these alloys, rodshaped iron and cobalt-rich α-precipitates are formed which are parallel to the <100> directions (shape anisotropy). These strongly magnetic precipitates are single-domain particles and are imbedded in a weakly magnetic nickel and aluminum matrix (α). Alnico alloys possess, just as iron, a <100> easy direction (see Fig. 24.12) and have also a cubic crystal structure. Alnico alloys are mechanically hard and brittle and can, therefore, only be shaped by casting or by pressing and sintering of metal powders.

The newest hard magnetic materials contain rare-earth elements and are made mainly of iron with neodymium and boron. They were discovered in 1983 and possess a superior coercivity and, thus, a much larger $(BH)_{max}$. Their disadvantages are a relatively low Curie temperature and poor corrosion resistance. Neomagnets allow motors, speakers, and magnetic resonance imaging devices (MRI; for medical applications) to do the same job for less magnetic material.

For example, a magnetic resonance imaging system that would require 21 tons of ferrites and a system weight of 70 tons uses only 2.6 tons of neomagnets and a system weight of 24 tons. Without rare-earth magnets, motors of the same power rating would be at least five times heavier and would be less efficient than those using electromagnets.

Ceramic ferrite magnets, such as barium or strontium ferrite ($BaO \cdot 6Fe_2O_3$ or $SrO \cdot 6Fe_2O_3$), are brittle and relatively inexpensive. They crystallise in the form of plates with the hexagonal c-axis (which is the easy axis) perpendicular to the plates. Some preferred orientation is observed because the flat plates arrange parallel to each other during pressing and sintering. Ferrite powder is often imbedded in plastic materials, which yields flexible magnets. They are used, for example, in the gaskets of refrigerator doors. Ferrites account for about 90 per cent of the premanentmagnet market mainly because of their price advantage.

High carbon steel magnets with or without cobalt, tungsten, or chromium are only of historic interest. Their properties are inferior to other magnets. It is believed that the permanent magnetisation of quenched steel stems from the martensite-induced internal stress which impedes the domain walls from moving through the crystal.

Magnetic Recording

Magnetic recording tapes, disks, drums, and magnetic strips on credit cards consist of small, needlelike magnetic oxide particles about 0.1×0.5 µm^2 in size which are imbedded in a nonmagnetic binder. The particles are too small to sustain a domain wall. They therefore consist of a single magnetic domain which is magnetised to saturation along the major axis. The elongated particles are aligned by a field during manufacturing so that their long axes are parallel with the length of the tape or the track. The most popular magnetic material has been ferrimagnetic γ-Fe_2O_3. It coercivity is 20–28 kA/m (250–350 Oe), More recently, ferromagnetic chromium dioxide has been used, having a coercivity between

40–80 kA/m (500–1000 Oe) and a particle size of 0.05 by 0.4 μm². High coercivity and high remanence prevent self-de-magnetisation and accidental erasure; they provide strong signals and permit thinner coatings. A high H_c also allows tape duplication by 'contact printing'. However, CrO_2 has a relatively low Curie temperature (128°C compared to 600°C for γ-Fe_2O_3). Thus, chromium dioxide tapes which are exposed to excessive heat (glove compartment!) may lose their stored information.

Thin magnetic films consisting of Co–Ni–P or Co–Cr–Ta are frequently used in hard-disk devices. They are laid down on an aluminum substrate and are covered by a 40-nm-thick carbon layer for lubrication and corrosion resistance. The coercivities range between 60–120 kA/m (750–1500 Oe). Thin film magnetic memories can be easily fabricated (vapour deposition, sputtering, or, electroplating), they can be switched rapidly, and they have a small unit size. Thin-film recording media are not used for tapes, however, because of their rapid wear.

The hysteresis loop of materials used for magnetically storing, information generally has a nearly square shape as shown in Fig. 24.13. If a sufficiently high magnetic field has been applied, then the material becomes magnetically saturated. An opposite directed magnetic field turns the spins in the reverse direction.

These two spin orientations constitute the necessary values (0 and 1) for the binary system on which all computers operate.

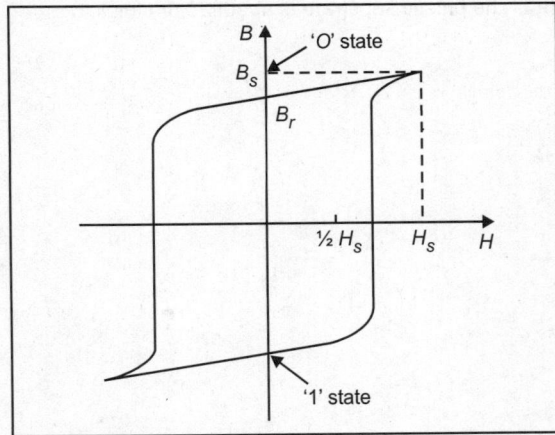

Fig. 24.13. Square-shaped hysteresis loop for magnetic storage devices. A stray magnetic field whose value is only, say, 1/2 H_s does not switch the spins in a given magnetic domain in the opposite direction.

The recording head of a tape machine consists of a laminated electromagnet made of permalloy or soft ferrite which has an air gap about 0.3 μm wide (Fig. 24.14). The tape is passed along this electromagnet whose fringing field redirects the spin moments of the particles in a certain pattern proportional to the current which is applied to the recording head. This leaves a permanent record of the signal. In the playback mode, the moving tape induces an alternating emf in the coil of the same head. The emf is amplified, filtered, and fed to a loudspeaker.

Magnetic disks (for random access) or tapes (sequential access, used mainly for music or video recordings) are the choices for long-term, large-scale information storage, particularly since no electric energy is needed to retain the information. This is in contrast to many (not all!) semiconductor storage devices which need a constant energy supply to hold the information. A third storage mechanism, called optical storage, such as in compact-disk (CD) players, also does not need a constant energy supply to keep the information. It should be noted in closing that magnetic tapes make contact with the recording (and playback) head and are therefore subject to wear.

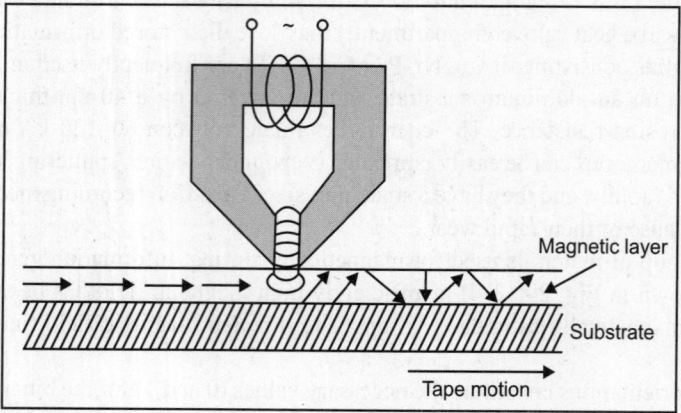

Fig. 24.14. Schematic arrangement of a recording (playback) head and a magnetic tape (recording mode). The gap width is exaggerated. The plastic substrate is about 25 μm thick.

Chapter 25

Optical Properties of Materials

INTRODUCTION

The most apparent properties of metals, their luster and their colour, have been known to mankind since materials were known. Because of these properties, metals were already used in antiquity for mirrors and jewelry. The colour was utilised 4000 years ago by the ancient Chinese as a guide to determine the composition of the melt of copper alloys: the hue of a preliminary cast indicated whether the melt, from which bells or mirrors were to be made, already had the right tin content.

The German poet Goethe was probably the first one who explicitly spelled out 200 years ago in his Treatise on colour that colour is not an absolute property of matter (such as the resistivity), but requires a living being for its perception and description. Goethe realised that the perceived colour of a region in the visual field depends not only on the properties of light coming from that region, but also on the light coming from the rest of the visual field. Applying Goethe's findings, it was possible to explain qualitatively the colour of, say, gold in simple terms. Goethe wrote: 'If the colour blue is removed from the spectrum, then blue, violet, and green are missing and red and yellow remain.' Thin gold films are bluish-green when viewed in transmission. These colours are missing in reflection. Consequently, gold appears reddish-yellow. On the other hand, Newton stated quite correctly in his 'Opticks' that light rays are not coloured. The nature of colour remained, however, unclear.

This chapter treats the optical properties from a completely different point of view. Measurable quantities such as the index of refraction or the reflectivity and their spectral variations are used to characterise materials. In doing so, the term 'colour' will almost completely disappear from our vocabulary. Instead, it will be postulated that the interactions of light with the electrons of a material are responsible for the optical properties. At the beginning of the 20th century, the study of the interactions of light with matter (black-body radiation, etc.) laid the foundations for quantum theory. Today, optical methods are among the most important tools for elucidating the electron structure of matter. Most recently, a number of optical devices such as lasers, photodetectors, waveguides, etc. have gained considerable technological importance. They are used in telecommunication, fiber optics, CD players, laser printers, medical diagnostics, night viewing, solar applications, optical computing, and for optoelectronic purposes. Traditional utilisations of optical materials for windows, antireflection coatings, lenses, mirrors, etc. should be likewise mentioned.

We perceive light intuitively as a wave (specifically, an electromagnetic wave) that travels in undulations from a given source to a point of observation. The colour of the light is related to its wavelength. Many crucial experiments, such as diffraction, interference, and dispersion, dearly confirm the wavelike nature of light. Nevertheless, at least since the discovery of the photoelectric effect in 1887 by Hertz, and its interpretation in 1905 by Einstein, do we know that light also has a particle nature. (The photoelectric effect describes the emission of electrons from a metallic surface after it has been illuminated by light of appropriately high energy, e.g. by blue light.) Interestingly enough, Newton, about 300 years ago, was a strong proponent of the particle concept of light. His original ideas, however, were in need of some refinement, which was eventually provided in 1901 by quantum theory. We know today (based on Planck's famous hypothesis) that a certain minimal energy of light, that is, at least one light quantum, called a photon, with the energy:

$$E = vh = \omega \hbar \qquad \ldots (25.1)$$

needs to impinge on a metal in order that a negatively charged electron may overcome its binding energy to its positively charged nucleus, and can escape into free space. (This is true regardless of the intensity of the light.) In Eq. 25.1, h is the Planck constant and v is the frequency of light given as the number of vibrations (cycles) per second or hertz (Hz). Frequently, the reduced Planck constant:

$$\hbar = \frac{h}{2\pi} \qquad \ldots (25.2)$$

is utilised in conjunction with the angular frequency, $\omega = 2\pi v$. In short, the wave-particle duality of light (or more generally, of electromagnetic radiation) has been firmly established at about 1924. The speed of light, c, and the frequency are connected by the equation:

$$c = v\lambda, \qquad \ldots (25.3)$$

where, λ is the wavelength of the light.

Light comprises only an extremely small segment of the entire electromagnetic spectrum, which ranges from radio waves via microwaves, infrared, visible, ultraviolet, X-rays, to γ rays. Many of the consideration which will be advanced in this chapter are therefore also valid for other wavelength ranges, i.e. for radio waves or X-rays.

OPTICAL CONSTANTS

When light passes from an optically 'thin' medium (e.g. vacuum, air) into an optically dense medium one observes that in the dense medium, the angle of refraction β (i.e. the angle between the refracted light beam and a line perpendicular to the surface) is smaller than the angle of incidence, α. This well-known phenomenon is used for the definition of the refractive power of a material and is called the Snell law:

$$\frac{\sin \alpha}{\sin \beta} = \frac{n_{\text{med}}}{n_{\text{vac}}} = n. \qquad \ldots (25.4)$$

Commonly, the index of refraction for vacuum n_{vac} is arbitrarily set to be unity. The refraction is caused by the different velocities, c, of the light in the two media:

$$\frac{\sin \alpha}{\sin \beta} = \frac{c_{\text{vac}}}{n_{\text{med}}}. \qquad \ldots (25.5)$$

Thus, if light passes from vacuum into a medium, we find:

$$n = \frac{c_{\text{vac}}}{n_{\text{med}}} = \frac{c}{v} \qquad \ldots (25.6)$$

where, $v = c_{\text{med}}$ is the velocity of light in the material.

The magnitude of the refractive index depends on the wavelength of the incident light. This property is called dispersion. In metals, the index of refraction varies also with the angle of incidence. This is particularly true when n is small.

The index of refraction is generally a complex number, designated as $\hat{n}$, which is comprised of a real and an imaginary part n_1 and n_2, respectively, i.e.

$$\hat{n} = n_1 - i\, n_2 \qquad \ldots (25.7)$$

In the literature, the imaginary part of $\hat{n}$ is often denoted by k. Equation 25.7 is then written as:

$$\hat{n} = n - i\, k. \qquad \ldots (25.8)$$

We will call n_2 or k the damping constant. (In some books, n_2 and k are named absorption constant, attenuation index, or extinction coefficient.) The square of the (complex) index of refraction is equal to the (complex) dielectric constant:

$$\hat{n}^2 = \hat{\varepsilon} = \varepsilon_1 - i\, \varepsilon_2, \qquad \ldots (25.9)$$

which yields, with (Eq. 25.8),

$$\hat{n}^2 = n^2 - k^2 - 2nki = \varepsilon_1 - i\, \varepsilon_2. \qquad \ldots (25.10)$$

Equating individually the real and imaginary parts in Eq. 25.10 yields:

$$\varepsilon_1 = n^2 - k^2 \qquad \ldots (25.11)$$

and

$$\varepsilon_2 = 2nk. \qquad \ldots (25.12)$$

ε_1 is called polarisation whereas ε_2 is known by the name absorption. Values for n and k for some materials are given in Table 25.1. For insulators, k is nearly zero, which yields for dielectrics $\varepsilon_1 \approx n^2$ and $\varepsilon_2 \to 0$.

Table 25.1. Optical constants for some materials ($\lambda = 600$ nm).

	n	k	$R\,\%$[b]
Metals			
Copper	0.14	3.53	95.6
Silver	0.05	4.09	98.9
Gold	0.21	3.24	92.9
Aluminum	0.97	6.0	90.3
Ceramics			
Silica glass (Vycor)	1.46	a	3.50
Soda-lime glass	1.51	a	4.13
Dense flint glass	1.75	a	7.44
Quartz	1.55	a	4.65
Al_2O_3	1.76	a	7.58
Polymers			
Polyethylene	1.51	a	4.13
Polystyrene	1.60	a	5.32

(Contd ...)

	n	k	$R \%^b$
Polytetrafluoroethylene	1.35	a	2.22
Semiconductots			
Silicon	3.94	0.025	35.42
GaAs	3.91	0.228	35.26

[a]The damping constant for dielectrics is about 10^{-7}; see Table 25.2.
[b]The reflection is considered to have occurred on one reflecting surface only.

When electromagnetic radiation (e.g. light) passes from vacuum (or air) into an optically denser material then the amplitude of the wave decreases exponentially with increasing damping constant k and for increasing distance, z, from the surface, as shown in Fig. 25.1. Specifically, the intensity, I, of the light (that is the square of the electric field strength ξ) obeys the following equation (which can be derived from the Maxwell equations):

$$I = \xi^2 = I_0 \exp\left(-\frac{4\pi\nu k}{c} z\right). \qquad \ldots (25.13)$$

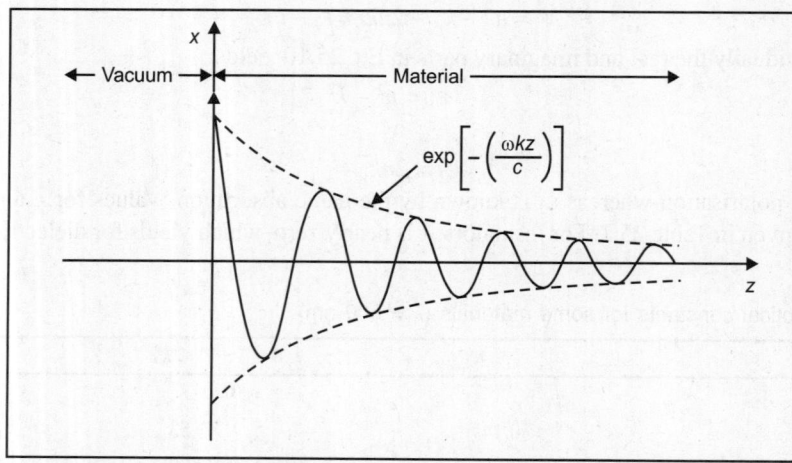

Fig. 25.1. Exponential decrease of the amplitude of electromagnetic radiation in optically dense materials such as metals.

We define a characteristic penetration depth, W, as that distance at which the intensify of the light wave, which travels through a material, has decreased to $1/e$ or 37 per cent of its original value, i.e. when:

$$\frac{I}{I_0} = \frac{1}{e} = e^{-1}. \qquad \ldots (25.14)$$

This definition yields, in conjunction with (Eq. 25.13),

$$z = W = \frac{c}{4\pi\nu k} = \frac{\lambda}{4\pi k}. \qquad \ldots (25.15)$$

Table 25.2 presents experimental values for k and W for some materials obtained by using sodium vapour light ($\lambda = 589.3$ nm).

The inverse of W is sometimes called the (exponential) attenuation or the absorbance, α, which is, by making use of Eqs 25.15 and 25.12:

$$\alpha = \frac{4\pi k}{\lambda} = \frac{4\pi v k}{c} = \frac{2\pi \varepsilon_2}{\lambda n}. \qquad \ldots (25.16)$$

It is measured, for example, in cm^{-1}. The energy loss per unit length (given, for example, in decibels, dB, per centimeter) is obtained by multiplying the absorbance, α, with 4.34, see Problem 25.7. (1 dB = 10 log I/I_0).

Table 25.2. Characteristic penetration depth, W, and damping constant, k, for some materials ($\lambda = 589.3$ nm).

Material	Water	Flint glass	Graphite	Gold
W (cm)	32	29	6×10^{-6}	1.5×10^{-6}
k	1.4×10^{-7}	1.5×10^{-7}	0.8	3.2

The ratio between the reflected intensity I_R and the incoming intensity I_0 of the light is the reflectivity:

$$R = \frac{I_R}{I_0}. \qquad \ldots (25.17)$$

Quite similarly, one defines the ratio between the transmitted intensity, I_T, and the impinging light intensity as the transmissivity:

$$T = \frac{I_T}{I_0}. \qquad \ldots (25.18)$$

The reflectivity is connected with n and k (assuming normal incidence) through:

$$R = \frac{(n-1)^2 + k^2}{(n+1)^2 + k^2}. \qquad \ldots (25.19)$$

Beer equation: The reflectivity is a unitless material constant and is often given in per cent of the incoming light (Table 25.1). R is, like the index of refraction, a function of the wavelength of the light. For insulators ($k \approx 0$) one finds that R depends solely on the index of refraction:

$$R = \frac{(n-1)^2}{(n+1)^2}. \qquad \ldots (25.20)$$

Metals are characterised by a large reflectivity. This stems from the fact that light penetrates metals only a short distance, as shown in Fig. 25.2 and Table 25.2. Thus, only a small part of the impinging energy is converted into heat. The major part of the energy is reflected (in some cases as much as 99 per cent, Table 25.1). In contrast to this, visible light penetrates into glass (and many other dielectrics) much farther than into metals, that is, approximately seven orders of magnitude more; see Table 25.2. As a consequence, very little light is reflected by glass. Nevertheless, a piece of glass about 1 or 2 m thick eventually dissipates a substantial part of the impinging light into heat. (In practical applications, one does not observe this large reduction in light intensity because windows are, as a rule, only a few millimeters thick.) It should be noted that window panes, lenses, etc. reflect the light on the front as well as on the back side.

An energy conservation law requires that the intensity of the light impinging on a material, I_0, must be equal to the reflected intensity. I_R, plus the transmitted intensity, I_T, plus that intensity which has been extinct, I_E, for example, transferred into heat, that is,

$$I_0 = I_R + I_T + I_E. \qquad \ldots (25.21)$$

Dividing Eq. 25.21 by I_0 and making use of Eqs 25.17 and 25.18 yields:

$$R + T + E = 1 \qquad \ldots (25.22)$$

(It has been assumed for these considerations that the light which has been scattered inside the material may be transmitted through the sides and is therefore contained in I_T and I_E.)

The reflection losses encountered in optical instruments such as lenses can be significantly reduced by coating the surfaces with a thin layer of a dielectric material such as magnesium fluoride. This results in the well-known blue hue on lenses for cameras.

Metals are generally opaque in the visible spectral region because of their comparatively high damping constant and thus high reflectivity. Still, very thin metal films (up to about 50 nm thickness) may allow some light to be transmitted. Dielectric materials, on the other hand, are often transparent. Occasionally, however, some opacifiers are inherently or artificially added to dielectrics which cause the light to be internally deflected by multiple scattering. Finally, if the diffuse scattering is not very severe, dielectrics might appear translucent, that is, objects viewed through them are vaguely seen, but not clearly distinguishable. Scattering of light may occur, for example, due to residual porosity in ceramic materials, or on grain boundaries (which have a small variation in refractive index compared to the matrix), or on finely dispersed particles, or on boundaries between crystalline and amorphous regions in polymers, to mention only a few mechanisms.

There exists an important equation which relates the reflectivity of light at low frequencies (infrared spectral region) with the direct-current conductivity, σ:

$$R = 1 - 4\sqrt{\pi \varepsilon_0 \frac{v}{\sigma}}. \qquad \ldots (25.23)$$

This relation, which was experimentally found at the end of the 19th century by Hagen and Rubens, states that materials having a large electrical conductivity (such as metals) also possess essentially a large reflectivity (and vice versa).

ABSORPTION OF LIGHT

If light impinges on a material, it is either re-emitted in one form or another (reflection, transmission) or its energy is extinct, for example, transformed into heat. In any of these cases, some interaction between light and matter will take place, as was explained in the preceding section. One of the major mechanisms by which this interaction occurs is called absorption of light.

The classical description of absorption and re-emission of light was developed at the turn of the 20th century by P. Drude, a German physicist. (Drude postulated that some electrons in a metal (essentially the valence electrons) can be considered to be free, that is, they can be separated from their respective nuclei. He further assumed that the free electrons within the crystal can be accelerated by an external electric field. This preliminary Drude model was refined by considering that the moving electrons on their path collide with certain metal atoms in a non ideal lattice. If an alternating electric field (as through interaction with light) is envolved then the free electrons are thought to perform oscillating motions. These vibrations are restrained by the above-mentioned interactions of the electrons with the atoms of a nonideal lattice. Thus, a friction force is introduced which takes this interaction into consideration. The calculation of the frequency dependence of the optical constants is accomplished by using the classical equations for vibrations whereby the interactions of electrons with atoms are taken into account by a damping term which is assumed to be proportional to the velocity of the electrons. The Newtonian-type equation (Force = mass times acceleration) is essentially identical to that of Eq. 25.9) except that the direct-current excitation force $e\xi$ is now replaced by a periodic (i.e. sinusoidal) excitation force:

$$F = e\xi_0 \sin(2\pi vt) \qquad \ldots (25.24)$$

where, v is the frequency of the light, t is the time, and ξ_0 is the maximal field strength of the light wave. In short, the equation describing the motion of free electrons which are excited to perform forced, periodic vibrations under the influence of light can be written as:

$$m\frac{dv}{dt} + \gamma v = e\xi_0 \sin(2\pi vt) \qquad \ldots (25.25)$$

where, γ is the damping strength which takes the damping of the electron motion into account.

The solution of this equation, which shall not be attempted here, yields the frequency dependence (or dispersion) of the optical constant.

The free electron theory describes, to a certain degree, the dispersion of the optical constants quite well. This is schematically shown in Fig. 25.2, in which the spectral dependence of the reflectivity is plotted for a specific case. The Hagen-Rubens relation (shown in Eq. 25.23) reproduces the experimental findings only up to about $v = 10^{13}$ s^{-1}. In contrast to this, the Drude theory correctly reproduces the frequency dependence of R even in the visible spectrum. Proceeding to yet higher frequencies, however, the experimentally found reflectivity eventually rises and then decreases again. Such an absorption band cannot be explained by the free electron theory. For its interpretation, a different concept needs to be applied; see below. By making use of the Drude theory, one can obtain the number of free electrons per unit volume, N_f, from optical measurements:

$$N_f = \frac{(1 - n^2 + k^2)v^2 m \, 4\pi^2 \varepsilon_0}{e^2} \qquad \ldots (25.26)$$

where, m is the mass of the electrons, e their charge, and ε_0 is the permittivity of empty space. The number of free electrons is a parameter which is of great interest because it is contained in several nonoptical equations (Hall effect, electromigration, superconductivity, etc.).

The Drude theory also provides the plasma frequency which is that frequency at which all electrons perform collective, fluid:

$$v_1 = \sqrt{\frac{e^2 Nf}{4\pi^2 \varepsilon_0 m}}. \qquad \ldots (25.27)$$

A selection of plasma frequencies is given in Table 25.3 and a value for v_1 is shown in Fig. 25.2.

Table 25.3. Experimentally found plasma frequencies for some materials.

	Cs	K	Na	Au	Ag	Cu
$v_1 \times 10^{14}$ (1/s)	6.81	9.52	14.3	21.3	22.5	22.5

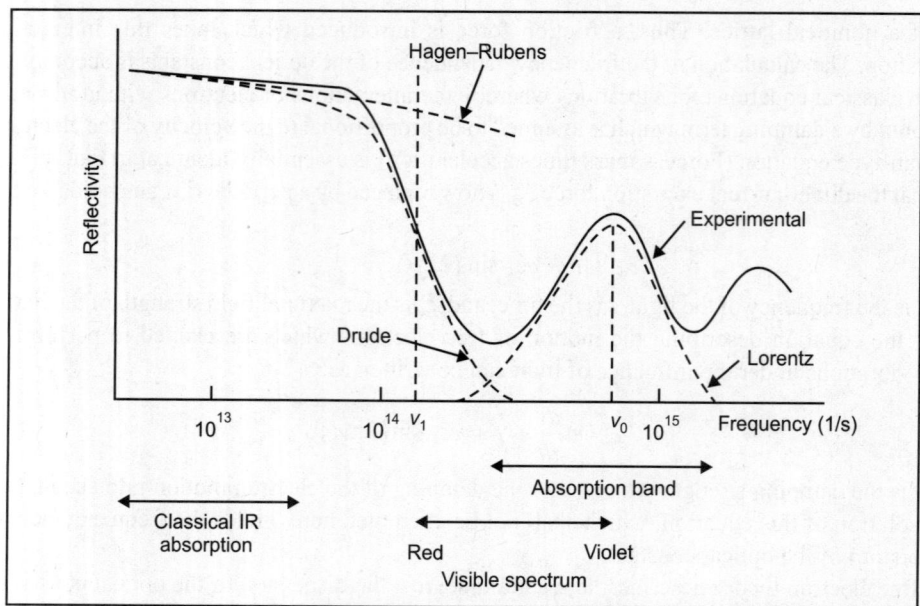

Fig. 25.2. Schematic frequency dependence of the reflectivity of metals, experimentally (solid line) and calculated according to three models. The spectral dependence of the reflectivity is often quite similar to that of the absorption, ε_2. The plasma frequency is marked by v_1.

Lorentz postulated in contrast to Drude that the electrons should be considered to be bound to their nuclei and that an external electric field displaces the negatively charged electron cloud against the positively charged atomic nucleus. In other words, he represented each atom as an electric dipole. If one shines light onto a solid, that is, if one applies an alternating electric field to the atoms, then the dipoles are thought to perform forced vibrations. Thus, a dipole is considered to be have similarly as a mass which is suspended on a spring (Fig. 25.3), i.e. the equations for a harmonic oscillator may be applied. The displacement of the positive and the negative charge is counteracted by a restoring force $\kappa \cdot x$ which is proportional to the displacement, x. Then the vibration equation becomes:

$$m\frac{dv}{dt} + \gamma' v + kx = e\xi_0 \sin(2\pi vt) \qquad \ldots (25.28)$$

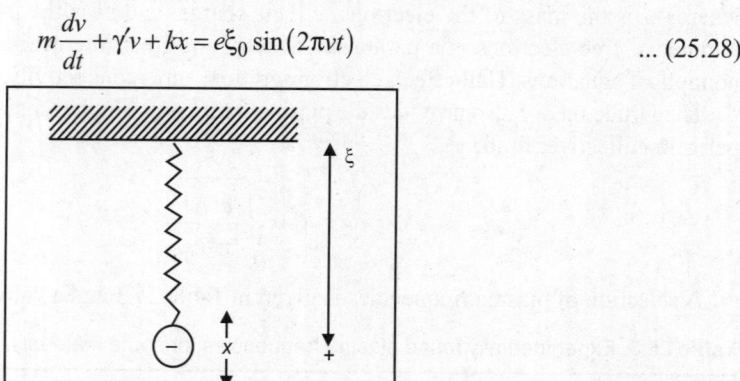

Fig. 25.3. Quasi-elastic bound electron in an external electron field (harmonic oscillator).

The factor κ is the spring constant which determines the binding strength between the atom and an electron. Each vibrating dipole (such as an antenna) loses energy by radiation. Thus, $\gamma' v$ represents the damping of the oscillator by radiation (γ' = damping constant). An oscillator is known to absorb a maximal amount of energy when excited near its resonance frequency as shown in Fig. 25.2. Thus,

$$v_0 = \frac{1}{2\pi}\sqrt{\frac{\kappa}{m}}. \qquad \ldots (25.29)$$

Very often, the electrons oscillate with more than one frequency v_0. In this case, more than one absorption band is observed as depicted in Fig. 25.2.

Thirty or forty years ago, many scientists considered the electrons in metals to behave at low frequencies as if they were free and at higher frequencies as if they were bound. In other words, electrons in a metal under the influence of light were described to behave as a series of classical free electrons and a series of classical harmonic oscillators. Insulators, on the other hand, were described by harmonic oscillators only. Quantum mechanics provides a deeper understanding of the absorption of light. To explain this, one needs to make use of the electron band diagrams introduced.

When light, having sufficiently large energy impinges on a solid, the electrons in the crystal are thought to absorb the energy of the photons and in turn are excited into higher energy states, provided that unoccupied higher energy states are available. This is shown in Fig. 25.4(a) for the specific case of a semiconductor or an insulator in which essentially a completely filled valence band and an empty conduction band are encountered. In order that electrons may be excited into a higher energy state, the light (photon) has to have an energy, $h\nu$, which is equal to or larger than the band gap. This process is called interband transition since an electron transfer from one band to a higher band is involved. The smallest possible energy at which photons can be absorbed to yield interband transitions is called the threshold energy for photon absorption. The threshold energy is understandably larger, the larger the band gap energy. Thus, the onset for interband absorption in insulators occurs at relatively high energies. For example, the gap energy for fused silica 'glass' (SiO_2) is characteristically about $6.2\ eV$. Thus, silica does not absorb light in the visible region by the process of interband transitions and is therefore essentially transparent in this spectral range. However, silica eventually absorbs light in the ultraviolet, that is, at energies larger than $6.2\ eV$ (or at wavelengths smaller than 200 nm).

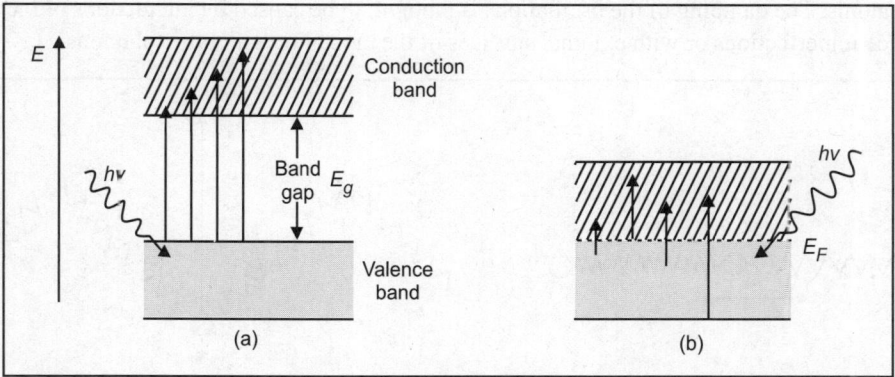

Fig. 25.4. Schematic representation of the absorption of light and excitation of electrons into a higher energy state by (a) interband transitions, as encountered for insulators and semiconductors (as well as in metals, which is not shown), and (b) intraband transitions, as observed in metals only.

Semiconductors, such as silicon, on the other hand, having gap energies in the neighborhood of 1 eV, start to absorb light already in the near *IR* region and are therefore opaque in the visible spectral range. They transmit, however, far-infrared wave lengths (equivalent to say, 1 eV and smaller). Interband transitions are equivalent to the behaviour of bound electrons in classical physics.

Metals, finally, have partially filled electron bands. Evidently, interband transitions into higher bands also take place in this case. Interestingly enough, a second absorption mechanism, involving transitions within the same band, additionally occurs. This process is called intra band transition; Fig. 25.4(b). No threshold energy for intra band transitions exists that is even very small photon energies can be absorbed. This causes a lift of electrons into higher energy states already at small energies. Specifically an electron residing just below the Fermi energy can be excited by a photon to an energy state barely above E_F and larger energies. In other words, metals absorb light across the entire spectral region and are therefore opaque in the visible, as well as, in the IR or UV ranges. Intraband transitions are equivalent to the behaviour of free electrons in classical physics.

It should be mentioned in passing that quantum mechanics provides a further refinement to the above-stated facts, During the absorption of light by intraband transitions, an additional mechanism may take place. It involves lattice vibration quanta, called phonons. The same is also true for many (but not all) interband transitions, particularly in semiconductors. Whenever this occurs, a phonon is said to have been exchanged with the lattice, which causes the solid to receive thermal energy. Electron transitions that involve phonons are called indirect transitions. For its understanding, a more complete band structure needs to be considered, which is beyond the scope of this book.

So far we have discussed only the absorption of photons by electrons. However, in the infrared region another absorption mechanism may become effective. It involves the light-induced vibrations of lattice atoms, that is, the excitation of phonons by photons. The individual atoms are thought to be excited by light of an appropriate frequency to perform oscillations about their point of rest. Now, the individual atoms are surely not vibrating independently; instead they interact with their neighbours to a large degree. For simplicity, one usually models the atoms to be interconnected by elastic springs; Fig. 25.5. Thus, the interaction of light with the lattice atoms can be mathematically represented in quite a similar manner as above when we calculated the classical electron theory for bound electrons. In other words, an equation similar to Eq. 25.28 can be used whereby κ now represents the binding strength between atoms. The damping of the oscillations is thought: to be caused by interactions of the phonons with lattice imperfections or with external surfaces of the crystal or with other phonons.

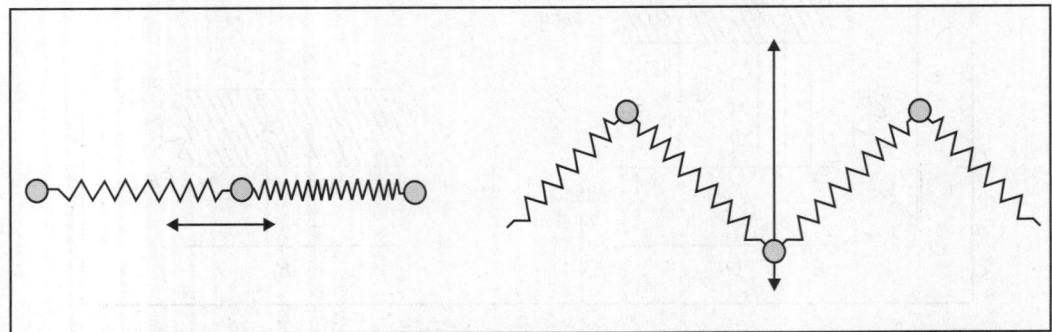

Fig. 25.5. One-dimensional representations of possible vibration modes of atoms which have been excited by IR electromagnetic radiation (heat).

The oscillations possess a resonance frequency, v_0, which depends on the mass of the atoms and on their degree of mutual interaction. The absorption of light is particularly strong at the resonance frequency. Thus, an absorption peak is observed at or near v_0. Phonon absorption causes the lattice to heat up.

We consider as an example fused silica (quartz), which is essentially transparent for wavelengths between 0.2 Mm (in the UV) and 4.28 μm (in the IR). Fused quartz has, however, two pronounced absorption peaks, one near 1.38 μm (similarly as seen in Fig. 25.7) and the other near 2.8 μm. (Window glass has a comparable absorption spectrum with the exception that the UV cutoff wavelength is already near 0.38 μm.) In recently developed sol-gel silica 'glasses,' the absorption peaks near 1.38 and 2.8 μm are virtually suppressed, which causes this material to be transparent from 0.16 to 4 μm. The absorption spectrum for the commercially important borosilicate/phosphosilicate glass, used for optical fibers, is shown in Fig. 25.6. The just-mentioned absorption peak near 1.38 μm is discernable.

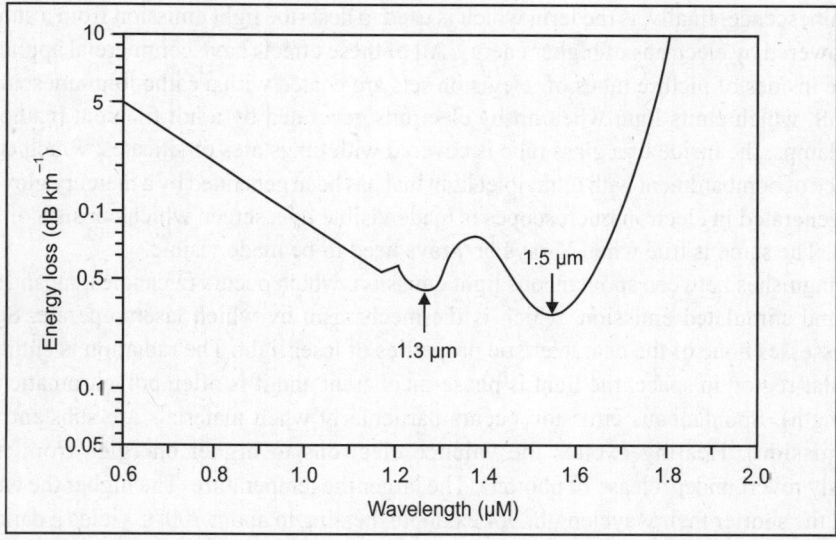

Fig. 25.6. Energy loss spectrum of highly purified glass for fibre-optic applications which features a phosphosilicate core surrounded by a borosilicate cladding. Two communication channels near 1.3 μm and 1.5 μm are indicated.

Ordinary window glass, when used for telecommunication purposes, that is, when drawn into a fibre, has a transmission loss of 1000 dB/km [for a definition of dB, see Eq. 28,16]. High quality optical glass fibers have a loss of 100 dB/km. In 1970, Corning glass developed a glass fiber that brought the losses down to 20 dB/km. Finally, in 1982, the loss was again reduced to 0.02 dB/km, near where it stands today. In summary, the absorption of light (or generally of electromagnetic radiation) occurs by several mechanisms which cause either the atoms to oscillate about their equilibrium positions (far-IR spectral region) or cause electrons to be excited into higher energy states within the same band (intraband transitions) or between two or more bands (interband transitions). Additionally, other absorption processes have been observed (e.g. involving excitons, solitons, etc.) which shall not be covered here.

EMISSION OF LIGHT

An electron, once excited must eventually revert back into a lower, empty energy state. This occurs, as a rule, spontaneously within a fraction of a second and is accompanied by the emission of a photon and/or the dissipation of heat, that is, phonons. The emission of light due to reversion of electrons from a higher energy state is called luminescence. If the electron transition occurs within nanoseconds or faster. The process is called fluorescence. In some material, the emission takes place after microsecond, or milliseconds. This slower process is referred to as phosphorescence. A third process, called afterglow, which is even slower (seconds), occurs when excited electrons have been temporarily trapped, for example, in impurity states from which they eventually return after some time into the valence band. Commonly used phosphorescing materials consist, for example, of metal sulphides (such as ZnS), tungstates, oxides, and many organic substances.

Photoluminescence is observed when photons impinge on a material which in turn re-emits light of a lower energy. Electroluminescing materials emit light as a consequence of an applied voltage or electric field. Thermoluminescence is experienced when heating a substance, such as wax in a candle. Cathodoluminescence, finally, is the term which is used to describe light emission from a substance that has been showered by electrons of higher energy. All of these effects have commercial applications. For example, the insides of picture tubes of television sets are coated with a cathodoluminescing material, basically ZnS, which emits light when hit by electrons generated by a hot filament (cathode ray). In fluorescent lamps, the inside of a glass tube is covered with tungstates or silicates, which emit light as a consequence of bombardment with ultraviolet light that has been generated by a mercury glow discharge. The image generated in electron microscopes is made visible by a screen which consists of a phosphor such as ZnS. The same is true when X-rays or γ-rays need to be made visible.

One distinguishes between spontaneous light emission, which occurs in candles, incandescent light bulbs, etc. and stimulated emission, which is the mechanism by which lasers operate. Spontaneous emission possesses none of the characteristic properties of laser light. The radiation is emitted through a wide angular region in space, the light is phase-incoherent and it is often polychromatic (more than one wavelength). Spontaneous emission occurs particularly when materials are substantially heated (thermal emission). Heating excites the valence electrons to higher energies from which they spontaneously revert under release of photons. The larger the temperature. The higher the energy of the photons and the shorter their wavelength. For example, heating to about 700°C yields a dark red colour whereas heating near 1600°C results in orange hues. At still higher temperatures, the emitted light appears to be white since large portions of the visible spectrum are emitted.

The situation changes considerably when stimulated emission is induced. Consider two energy levels E_1 and E_2, and let us assume for a moment that the higher energy level, E_2, contains more electrons than the lower level, E_1, that is, let us assume a population inversion of electrons [Fig. 25.7(a)]. We further assume that, by some means, the electrons in E_2 are made to stay there for an appreciable amount of time. Nevertheless, one electron will eventually revert to the lower state. As a consequence, a photon with energy $E_{21} = h\nu_{21}$ is emitted [Fig. 25.7(b)].

This photon might stimulate a second electron to descend in step to E_1, thus causing the emission of another photon that vibrates in phase with the first one.

The two photons are consequently phase-coherent [Fig. 25.7(c)]. They might stimulate two more electrons to descend in step [Fig. 25.7(d)] and so on until an avalanche of photons is created. In short, stimulated emission of light occurs when electrons are forced by incident radiation to add more photons to an incident beam. The acronym LASER can now be understood; it stands for light amplification by stimulated emission of radiation.

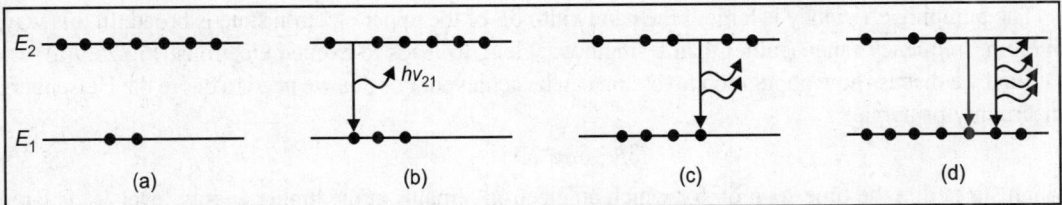

Fig. 25.7. Schematic representation of stimulated emission between two energy levels E_2 and E_1. The dots symbolise electrons.

Laser light is highly monochromatic (one colour only) because it is generated by electron transitions between two narrow energy levels. (As a consequence, laser light can be focused with a lens to a spot less than 1 μm in diameter which cannot be done with 'white' light because of dispersion.) Another outstanding feature of laser light is its strong collimation, i.e. the parallel emergence of light from a laser window. (The cross section of a laser beam transmitted to the moon is only 3 km in diameter.) We understand the reason for the collimation best by knowing the physical setup of a laser.

The lasing material is embodied in a long, narrow container called the cavity; the two faces at opposite ends of this cavity must be absolutely parallel to each other. One of the faces is silvered and acts as a perfect mirror, whereas the other face is silver-coated by a thin film only and thus transmits some of the light (Fig. 25.8). The laser light is reflected back and forth by these mirrors, thus increasing the number of photons during each pass. After the laser has been started, the light is initially emitted in all possible directions (left part of Fig. 25.8). However, only photons that travel strictly parallel to the cavity axis will remain in action, whereas the photons traveling at an angle will eventually be extinct in the cavity walls (center part in Fig. 25.8). A fraction of the photons escape through the partially transparent mirror. They constitute the emitted beam.

We now need to explain how the electrons arrive at the higher energy level, that is, we need to discuss how they are pumped from E_1 into E_2. One of the methods is, of course, optical pumping, i.e. the absorption of light stemming from a polychromatic light source. (Xenon flashlamps for pulsed lasers, or tungsten-iodine lamps for continuously operating lasers, are often used for optical pumping. The lamp is either wrapped in helical form around the cavity, or the lamp is placed in one of the focal axes of a specularly reflecting elliptical cylinder, whereas the laser rod is placed along the second focal axis.) Other pumping methods involve electron/gas-ion collisions in an electric discharge, chemical reactions, nuclear reactions or external electron beam injection.

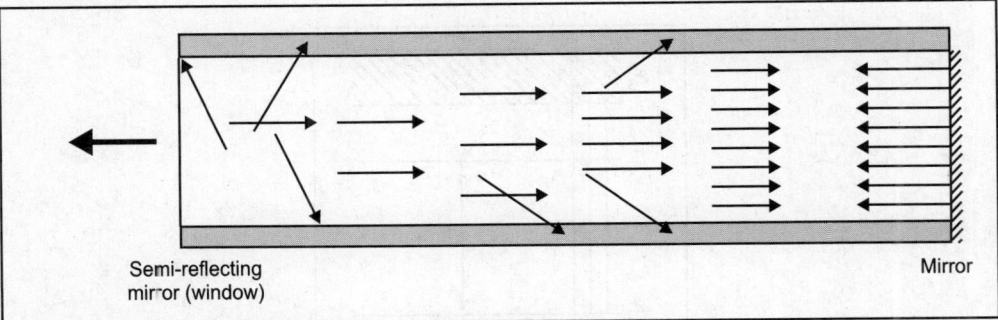

Fig. 25.8. Schematic representation of a laser cavity (containing, for example, a mixture of example, a mixture of helium and neon gases) and the buildup of laser oscillations. The stimulated emission eventually dominates over the spontaneous emission. The light leaves the cavity at the left side.

The pumping efficiency is large if the bandwidth δE of the upper electron state is broad. In this way, an entire frequency range (rather than a single wavelength) leads to excited electrons [Fig.25.9(a)].

Next we discuss how population inversion can be achieved. For this we need to quote the Heisenberg uncertainty principle:

$$\delta E \cdot \delta t \propto h, \qquad \ldots (25.30)$$

which states that the time span δt, for which an electron remains at the higher energy level E_2, is large when the bandwidth δE of E_2 is narrow. In other words, a sharp energy level (δE small, δt large) supports the population inversion; Fig. 25.9(b). On the other hand, a large pumping efficiency requires a large δE [Fig. 25.9(a)], which results in a small δt and a small population inversion. Thus, high pumping efficiency and large population inversion mutually exclude each other in a two-level configuration. In essence, a two-level configuration as depicted in Fig. 25.9 does not yield laser action.

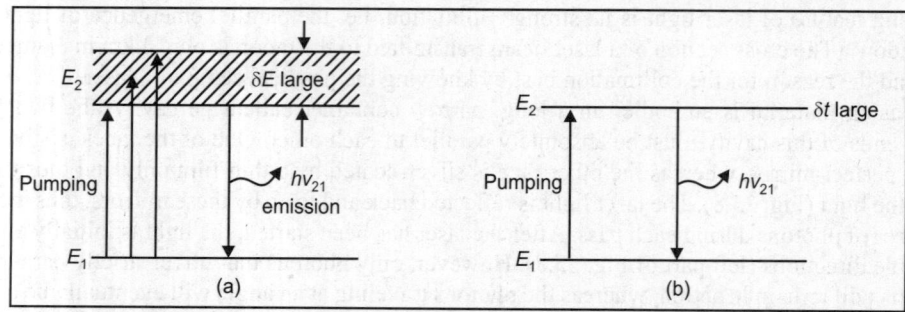

Fig. 25.9. Examples of possible energy states in a two-level configuration. (a) δE large, i.e. large pumping efficiency but little or no population inversion. (b) potentially large population inversion (δt large) but small pumping efficiency.

The three level laser (Fig. 25.10) provides improvement. There, the 'pump band' E_3 is broad, which enables a good pumping efficiency. The electrons revert after about 10^{-14} s into an intermediate level, E_2, via a nonradiative, phonon-assisted process. Since E_2 is sharp, and not strongly coupled to the ground state, the electrons remain much longer, i.e. for some micro- or milliseconds on this level. This provides the required population inversion. An even larger population inversion is achieved by a four-level laser in which the energy level E_1 is rapidly emptied by electron transitions into a lower level E_0. Pumping occurs then between E_0 and E_3.

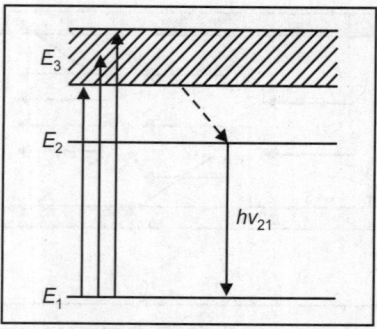

Fig. 25.10. Three-level laser. The nonradiative, phonon-assisted decay is marked by a dashed line. Lasing occurs between levels E_2 and E_1. High pumping efficiency to E_3. High population inversion at E_2.

Laser materials can be selected from hundreds of substances to suit a specific purpose. Laser materials include crystals (such as ruby), glasses (such as neodymium-doped glass), gases (such as helium, argon, xenon), metal vapours (such as cadmium, zinc or mercury), molecules (such as carbon dioxide) or liquids (solvents which contain organic dye molecules). Lasers can be operated in a continuous mode (CW) or with a higher power output, in the pulsed mode.

Semiconductor lasers are widely used for laser printers, CD players, distance measurements (land surveying), and particularly for optical telecommunication purposes. The 'cavity' for a semiconductor laser consists of a combination of heavily doped (10^{18} cm^{-3}) n- and p-type semiconductors such as GaAs. The p-n junction is forward-biased. This causes electrons to be excited from the valence band into the conduction band if the applied voltage is equal to or larger than the gap energy. In this case, one observes a population inversion of electrons in the junction region between the p- and n-layers. Two opposite end faces of this p-n junction are made parallel and are polished or cleaved along crystal planes. The other faces are left untreated to suppress lasing in unwanted directions (Fig. 25.11). A reflective coating of the window is usually not necessary since the reflectivity of the semiconductor is already 35 per cent (Table 25.1). Semiconductor lasers are small and can be quite efficient. The wavelength of a binary GaAs laser is about 0.87 µm. This is, however, not the most advantageous wavelength for telecommunication purposes because some glasses attenuate light of this wavelength appreciably. In general, the optical absorption in glass is quite wavelength-dependent, as shown, for example, in Fig. 25.6, where a minimum in absorption at 1.3 µm is seen. Fortunately, the bandgap energy, i.e. the wavelength at which a laser emits light, can be adjusted to a certain degree by utilising ternary or quaternary compound semiconductors. Among them, $In_{1-x}Ga_xAs_yP_{1-y}$ plays a considerable role for telecommunication purposes, because the useful emission wavelengths of these compounds can be varied between 0.886 and 1.55 µm (which corresponds to gap energies from 1.4 to 0.8 eV). In other words, the above-mentioned desirable wavelength of 1.3 µm can be conveniently obtained by utilising a properly designed indium-gallium-arsenide-phosphide laser.

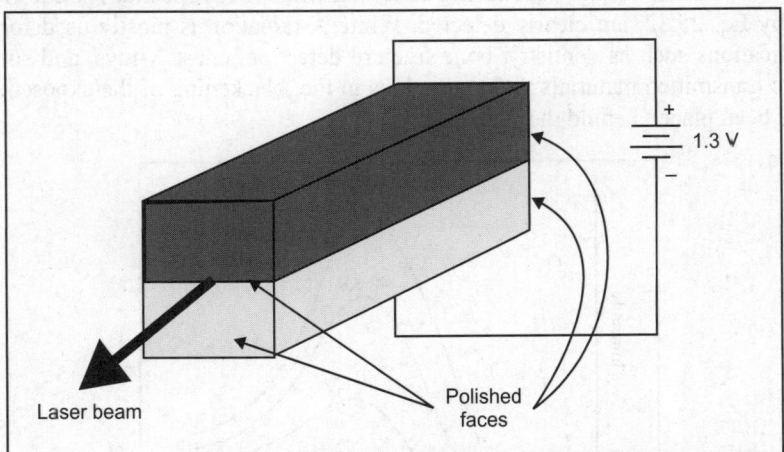

Fig. 25.11. Schematic setup for a semiconductor laser (Homo-junction laser).

Light-emitting diodes (LEDs) are of great technical importance as inexpensive, rugged, small, and efficient light sources for display purposes. The LED consists, like the semiconductor laser, of a forward-biased p-n junction. The above-mentioned special facing procedures are, however, omitted during the manufacturing process. Thus, the LED does not operate in the lasing mode. The emitted light is therefore neither phase-coherent nor collimated. It is, of course, desirable that the light emission occurs in the visible spectrum. Certain III/V compound semiconductors, such as $Ga_xAs_{1-x}P$, GaP, and $Ga_xAl_{1-x}As_6$. fulfill this requirement. The light is emitted in the red, green, yellow, or orange part of the spectrum; blue colour is achieved when using Ga-N-8%In, silicon carbide or zinc selenide. The radiation may leave the device through a window that has been etched through the metallic contact (surface emitter). For efficiencies of LEDs.

The emission of electromagnetic radiation of higher energies than that characteristic for UV light is called X-rays. (Still higher energetic radiation are γ-rays). X-rays were discovered in 1895 by Wilhelm Conrad Röntgen, a German scientist. In 1901, he received the first Nobel Prize in physics for this discovery. The wavelength of X-rays is in the order of 10^{-10} m. For its production, a beam of electrons emitted from a hot filament is accelerated in a high electric field towards a metallic (or other) electrode. On impact, the energy of the electrons is lost either by white X-radiation, that is, in the form of a continuous spectrum (within limits), or by essentially monochromatic X-rays (called characteristic X-rays) that are specific for the target material. The white X-rays are emitted as a consequence of the deceleration of the electrons in the electric field of a series of atoms, whereas each interaction with an atom may lead to photons of different energies. The maximal energy that can be emitted this way (assuming only one interaction with an atom) is proportional to the acceleration voltage, V, and the charge of the electron, e, that is:

$$E_{max} = eV = h\nu = \frac{hc}{\lambda} \qquad \ldots (25.31)$$

(See equations 25.1 and 25.3) From this equation the minimum wavelength, λ (in nm), can be calculated using the values of the constants as listed and inserting V in volts, that is:

$$\lambda = \frac{1240}{V}. \qquad \ldots (25.32)$$

Figure 25.12 depicts the voltage dependence of several white X-ray spectra, The cutoff wavelengths, as calculated by Eq. 25.32, are clearly detected. White X-radiation is mostly used for medical and industrial applications such as dentistry, bone fracture detection, chest X-rays, and so on. Different densities of the transmitted materials yield variations in the, blackening of the exposed photographic film which has been placed behind the specimen.

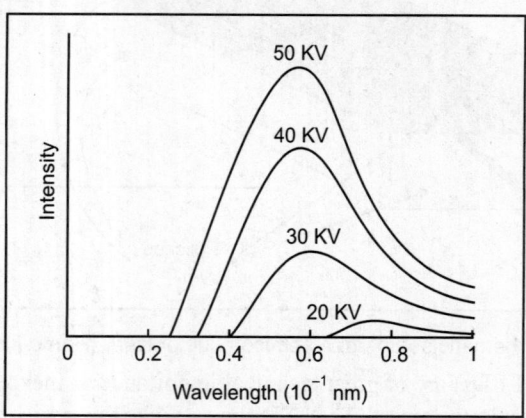

Fig. 25.12. Schematic representation of the wavelength dependence of the intensity of white X-ray emission for selected acceleration voltages.

The wavelength of characteristic X-rays depends on the material on which the accelerated electrons impinge. Let us assume that the impinging electrons possess a high enough energy to excite inner electrons, for example, electrons from the K-shell, to leave the atom. As a consequence, an L electron may immediately revert into the thus created vacancy while emitting a photon having a narrow and characteristic wavelength. This mechanism is said to produce K_α X-rays (Fig. 25.13). Alternately and/or simultaneously, an electron from the M shell may revert to the K shell. This is termed to produce K_β-radiation.

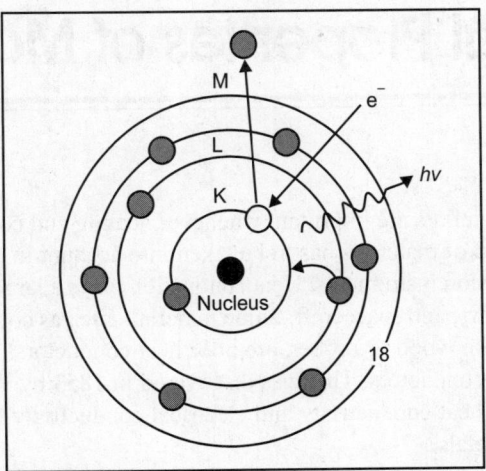

Fig. 25.13. Schematic representation of the emission of characteristic X-radiation by exciting a K-electron and refilling the vacancy thus created by a L-electron.

For the case of copper, the respective wavelengths are 0.1542 nm and 0.1392 nm. (As a second example, aluminum yields K_α and K_β-radiations having characteristic wavelengths of 0.8337 nm and 0.7981 nm.) Characteristic (monochromatic) X-radiation is frequently used in materials science, for example, for investigating the crystal structure of materials. For this, only one of the possible wavelengths is used by eliminating the others utilising appropriate filters, made, for example, of nickel foils which strongly absorb the K_β-radiation of copper while the stronger K_α-radiation is only weakly absorbed. The characteristic X-radiation is superimposed on the often weaker, white X-ray spectrum.

Chapter 26

Thermal Properties of Materials

INTRODUCTION

The thermal properties of materials are important whenever heating and cooling devices are designed. Thermally induced expansion of materials has to be taken into account in the construction industry as well as in the design of precision instruments. Heat conduction plays a large role in thermal insulation, for example, in homes, industry, and spacecraft. Some materials such as copper and silver conduct heat very well; other materials, like wood or rubber, are poor heat conductors. Good electrical conductors are generally also good heat conductors. This was discovered in 1853 by Wiedemann and Franz, who found that the ratio between heat conductivity and electrical conductivity (divided by temperature) is essentially constant for all metals.

The thermal conductivity of materials varies only within five orders of magnitude (Fig. 26.1). This is in sharp contrast to the variation in electrical conductivity, which spans about twenty-five orders of magnitude. The thermal conductivity of metals and alloys can be readily interpreted by making use of the electron theory. The electron theory postulates that free electrons perform random motions with high velocity over a large number of atomic distances. In the hot part of a metal bar they pick up energy by interactions with the vibrating lattice atoms. This thermal energy is eventually transmitted to the cold end of the bar.

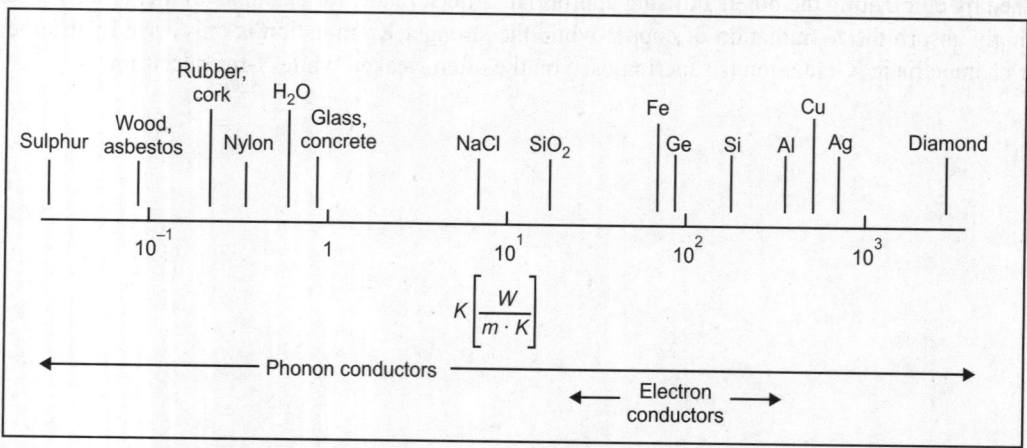

Fig. 26.1. Room-temperature thermal conductivities for some materials.

In electric insulators, in which no free electrons exist, the conduction of thermal energy must occur by a different mechanism. This new mechanism was found by Einstein at the beginning of the 20th century. He postulated the existence of phonons or lattice vibration quanta, which are thought to be created in large numbers in the hot part of a solid and partially eliminated in the cold part. The transfer of heat in dielectric solids is thus linked to a flow of phonons from hot to cold. Figure 26.1 indicates that in a transition region both electrons as well as phonons may contribute, in various degrees, to thermal conduction.

Actually, phonon-induced thermal conduction occurs even in metals, but its contribution is negligible compared to that of electrons.

Other thermal properties are the specific heat capacity, and a related property, the molar heat capacity. Their importance can best be appreciated by the following experimental observations: Two substances with the same mass but different values for the specific heat capacity require different amounts of thermal energy to reach the same temperature. Water, for example, which has a relatively high specific heat capacity, needs more thermal energy to reach a given temperature than, say, copper or lead of the same mass. Specifically, it takes 4.18 J to raise 1 g of water by 1 K. But the same heat raises the temperature of 1 g of copper by about 11 K. In short, water has a larger heat capacity than copper. (The large heat capacity of water is, incidentally, the reason for the balanced climate in coastal regions and the heating of North European countries by the warm water of the Gulf stream.) We need to define the various versions of heat capacities for clarification.

The heat capacity, C', is the amount of heat, dQ, that needs to be transferred to a substance in order to raise its temperature by a certain temperature interval. The unit for the heat capacity is J/K.

The heat capacity is not defined uniquely, that is, one needs to specify the conditions under which the heat is added to the system. Even though several choices for the heat capacities are possible, one is generally interested in only two: the heat capacity at constant volume C'_v and the heat capacity at constant pressure C'_p. The former is the most useful quantity because C'_v is obtained immediately from the energy, E, of the system. The heat capacity at constant volume is defined as:

$$C'_v = \left(\frac{\partial E}{\partial T}\right)_v \qquad \ldots (26.1)$$

On the other hand, it is much easier to measure the heat capacity of a solid at constant pressure than at constant volume. Fortunately, the difference between C'_p and C'_v for solids vanishes at low temperatures and is only about 5 per cent at room temperature.

The specific heat capacity is the heat capacity per unit mass:

$$c = \frac{C'}{m} \qquad \ldots (26.2)$$

where, m is the mass of the system. Again, one can define it for constant volume or constant pressure. It is a material constant and is temperature-dependent. Characteristic values for c_p are given in Table 26.1. The unit of the specific heat capacity is J/g·K. We note from Table 26.1 that the c_p values for solids are considerably smaller than the specific heat capacity of water. Combining Eqs. 26.1 and 26.2 yields:

$$\Delta E = \Delta T m\, c_v \qquad \ldots (26.3)$$

which expresses that the thermal energy (or heat) which is transferred to a system equals the product of mass, increase in temperature, and specific heat capacity.

Table 26.1. Experimental thermal parameters of various substances at room temperature and ambient pressure.

Substance	Specific heat capacity, (c_p) (J/g·K)	Molar (atomic) mass (g/mol)	Molar heat capacity (C_p) (J/mol·K)	Molar heat capacity (C_v) (J/mol·K)
Al	0.897	27.0	24.25	23.01
Fe	0.449	55.8	25.15	24.68
Ni	0.456	58.7	26.8	24.68
Cu	0.385	63.5	24.48	23.43
Pb	0.129	207.2	26.85	24.68
Ag	0.235	107.9	25.36	24.27
C (graphite)	0.904	12.0	10.9	9.20
Water	4.184	18.0	75.3	–

A further useful material constant is the heat capacity per mole. It compares materials that contain the same number of molecules or atoms. The molar heat capacity is obtained by multiplying the specific heat capacity c_v (or c_p) by the molar mass, M (see Table 26.1):

$$C_v = \frac{C_v'}{n} = c_v \cdot M \qquad \ldots (26.4)$$

where, n is the amount of substance in mol.

We see from Table 26.1 that the room-temperature molar heat capacity at constant volume is approximately 25 J/mol·K for most solids. This was experimentally discovered in 1819 by Dulong and Petit. The experimental molar heat capacities for some materials are depicted in Fig. 26.2 as a function of temperature. We notice that some materials, such as carbon, reach the Dulong–Petit value only at high temperatures. Some other materials such as lead reach 25 J/mol·K at relatively low temperatures.

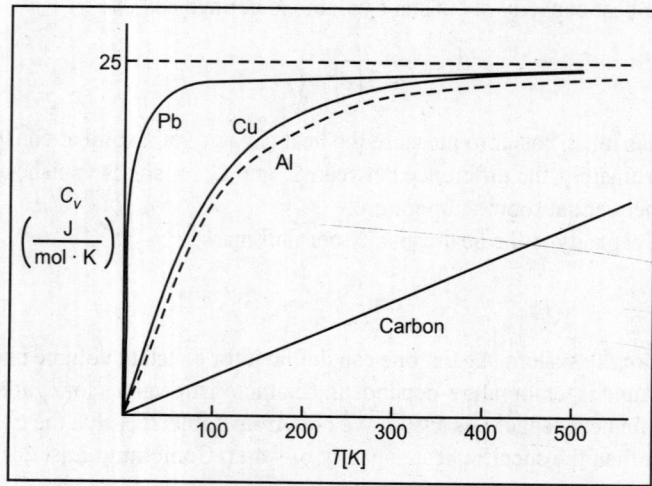

Fig. 26.2. Temperature dependence of the molar heat capacity C_v for some materials.

All heat capacities are zero at $T = 0$ K. The C_v values near $T = 0$ K climb in proportion to T^3 and reach 96 per cent of their final value at a temperature θ_D, which is defined to be the Debye temperature.

θ_D is an approximate dividing point between a high-temperature region, where classical models can be used for the interpretation of C_v, and a low-temperature region, where quantum theory needs to be applied. Selected Debye temperatures are listed in Table 26.2.

Table 26.2. Debye temperatures of some materials.

Substance	θ_D (K)
Pb	95
Au	170
Ag	230
W	270
Cu	340
Fe	360
Al	375
Si	650
C	1850
GaAs	204
InP	162

INTERPRETATION OF THE HEAT CAPACITY BY VARIOUS MODELS

The classical (atomistic) theory for the interpretation of the heat capacity postulates that each atom in a crystal is bound to its site by a harmonic force similar to a spring. A given atom is thought to be capable of absorbing thermal energy, and in doing so it starts to vibrate about its point of rest. The amplitude of the oscillation is restricted by electrostatic repulsion forces of the nearest neighbours.

The extent of this thermal vibration is therefore not more than 5 or 10 per cent of the interatomic spacing, depending on the temperature. In short, we compare an atom with a sphere which is held at its site by two springs [Fig. 26.3(a)].

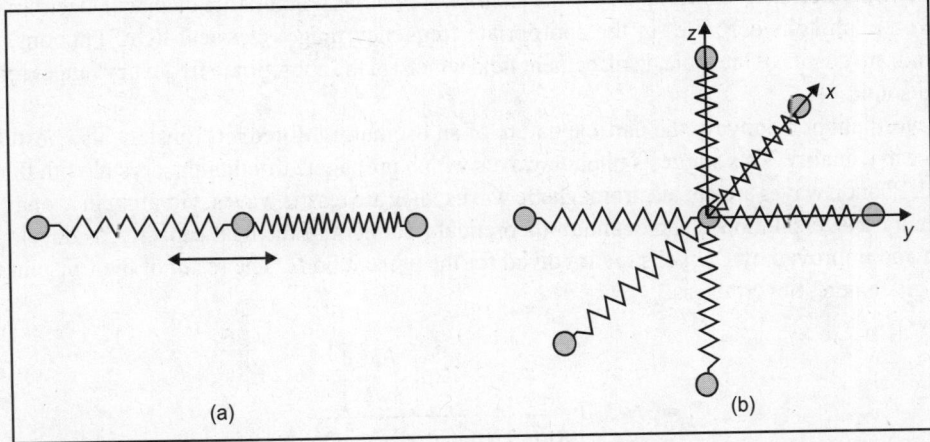

Fig. 26.3. (a) A one-dimensional harmonic oscillator, and (b) a three-dimensional harmonic oscillator.

The thermal energy that a harmonic oscillator of this kind can absorb is proportional to the absolute temperature of the environment. The proportionality factor has been found to be the Boltzmann constant k_B. The average energy of the oscillator is then:

$$E = k_B T. \qquad \ldots (26.5)$$

Now, solids are three-dimensional. Thus, a given atom in a cubic crystal also responds to the harmonic forces of lattice atoms in the other two directions. In other words, it is postulated that each atom in a cubic crystal represents three oscillators [Fig. 26.3(b)], each of which absorbs the thermal energy $k_B T$. Therefore, the average energy per atom is:

$$E = 3k_B T. \qquad \ldots (26.6)$$

We consider now nN_0 atoms, where, N_0 is the Avogadro number. Then the total internal energy of, these atoms is:

$$E = 3nN_0 k_B T. \qquad (26.7)$$

Finally, the molar heat capacity is given by combining Eqs. 26.1, 26.4, and 26.7, which yields:

$$C_v = 3N_0 k_B. \qquad \ldots (26.8)$$

Inserting the numerical values for N_0 and k_B into Eq. 26.8 yields

$$C_v = 24.95 \text{ J/mol} \cdot \text{K}$$

i.e. about 25 J/mol · K which is quite in agreement with the experimental findings at high temperatures (Fig. 26.2).

It is satisfying to see that a simple model involving three harmonic oscillators per atom can readily explain the experimentally observed heat capacity. However, one shortcoming is immediately evident: the calculated molar heat capacity turned out to be temperature-independent, according to Eq. 26.8, and also independent of the material. This discrepancy with the observed behaviour (Fig. 26.2) was puzzling to scientists at the turn of the 20th century and had to await quantum theory to be explained) properly. Einstein postulated in 1907 that the energies of the above-mentioned classical oscillators should be quantised, i.e. he postulated that only certain vibrational modes should be allowed, quite in analogy to the allowed energy states of electrons. These lattice vibration quanta were called phonons.

The term phonon stresses an analogy with electrons or photons. Photons are quanta of electromagnetic radiation, i.e. photons describe (in the appropriate frequency range) classical light. Phonons, on the other hand, are quanta of the ionic displacement field which (in the appropriate frequency range) represent classical sound.

The word phonon conveys the particle nature of an oscillator. Moreover, Einstein also postulated a particle-wave duality. This suggests phonon waves which propagate through the crystal with the speed of sound. Phonon waves are not electromagnetic waves; they are elastic waves, vibrating in a longitudinal and/or in a transversal mode. The quantum theoretical treatment of the heat capacity, as developed by Einstein and improved by Debye is too involved for the present book. The result of the Einstein theory may be given here, nevertheless:

$$C_v = 3N_0 k_B \left(\frac{\hbar w}{k_B T}\right)^2 \frac{\exp\left(\frac{\hbar w}{k_B T}\right)}{\left(\exp\left(\frac{\hbar w}{k_B T}\right) - 1\right)^2}. \qquad \ldots (26.9)$$

We discuss C_v for two special temperature regions. For large temperatures the approximation $e^x \simeq 1 + x$ can be applied, which yields $C_v \cong 3N_0kB$, i.e. we obtain the classical Dulong–Petit value. For $T \to 0$, C_v approaches zero, again in agreement with experimental observations. Thus, the temperature dependence of C_v is now in qualitative accord with the experimental findings. One minor discrepancy, however, has to be noted. At very small temperatures the experimental C_v decreases by T^3, as stated above. The Einstein theory predicts, instead, an exponential decrease. The Debye theory which we shall not discuss here alleviates this discrepancy by postulating that the individual oscillators interact with each other.

At very high and very low temperatures, the phonon theory does not yield a complete description of the observed behaviour. The reason for this is that at those temperatures the free electrons (if present) provide a noticeable contribution to C_v. The electron contribution yields (for monovalent metals) the following expression:

$$C_v^{el} = \frac{\pi^2 N_0 k_B^2 T}{2E_F} \qquad \ldots (26.10)$$

where, E_F is the Fermi energy. We notice a linear relationship between heat capacity and temperature. Figure 26.4 summarises the experimentally observed C_v-values as well as the contributions of electron theory, phonon theory, and classical considerations as outlined above.

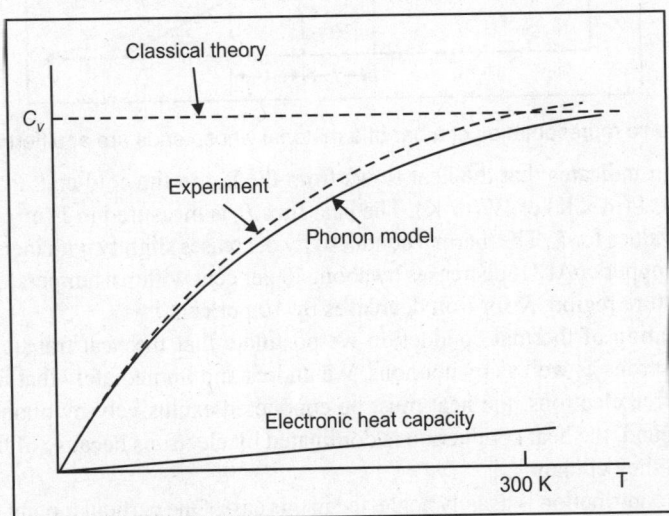

Fig. 26.4. Schematic representation of the temperature dependence of the molar heat capacity, experimental and according to three models.

THERMAL CONDUCTION

Heat conduction (or thermal conduction) is the transfer of thermal energy from a hot body to a cold body when both bodies are brought into contact. For best visualisation we consider a bar of a material of length x whose ends are held at different temperatures (Fig. 26.5). The heat that flows through a cross section of the bar divided by time and area (i.e. the heat flux, J_Q) is proportional to the temperature gradient dT/dx.

The proportionality constant is called the thermal conductivity K (or λ). We thus write:

$$J_Q = -K \frac{dT}{dx}. \qquad \ldots (26.11)$$

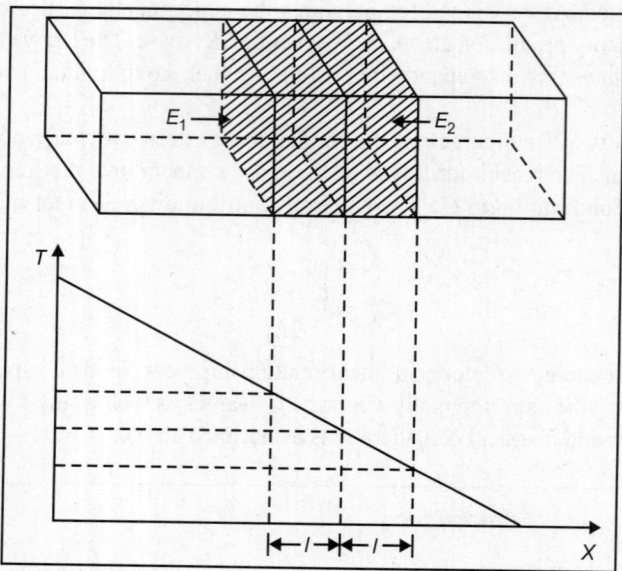

Fig. 26.5. Schematic representation of a bar of a material whose ends are at different temperatures.

The negative sign indicates that the heat flows from the hot to the cold end. Possible units for the heat conductivity are $J/(m \cdot s \cdot K)$ or $W/(m \cdot K)$. The heat flux J_Q is measured in $J/(m^2 \cdot s)$. Table 26.3 gives some characteristic values for K. The thermal conductivity decreases slightly with increasing temperature. For example, K for copper or Al_2O_3 decreases by about 20 per cent within a temperature span of 1000°C. In the same temperature region, K for iron decreases by 10 per cent.

For the interpretation of thermal conduction we postulate that the heat transfer in solids may be provided by free electrons as well as by phonons. We understand immediately that in insulators, which do not contain any free electrons, the heat must be conducted exclusively by phonons. In metals and alloys, on the other hand, the heat conduction is dominated by electrons because of the large number of free electrons which they contain.

Thus, the phonon contribution is usually neglected in this case. One particular point should be clarified. Electrons in metals travel in equal numbers from hot to cold and from cold to hot in order that the charge neutrality is maintained.

This is indicated in Fig. 26.5 by two arrows marked E_1 and E_2. Now, the electrons in the hot part of a metal possess and transfer a high energy. In contrast to this, the electrons in the cold end possess and transfer a lower energy. The heat transferred from hot to cold is thus proportional to the difference in the energies of the electrons.

The situation is quite different in phonon conductors. The number of phonons is larger at the hot end than at the cold end. Thermal equilibrium thus involves, in this case, a net transfer of phonons from the hot into the cold part of a material.

Table 26.3. Thermal conductivities at room temperature[a].

Substance	$K(W/m \cdot K) \equiv (J/m \cdot s \cdot K)$
Diamond type IIa	2.3×10^3
SiC	4.9×10^2
Silver	4.29×10^2
Copper	4.01×10^2
Aluminium	2.37×10^2
Silicon	1.48×10^2
Brass (leaded)	1.2×10^2
Iron	8.02×10^1
GaAs	5×10^1
Ni–Silver[b]	2.3×10^1
Al_2O_3 (sintered)	3.5×10^1
SiO_2 (fused silica)	1.4
Concrete	9.3×10^{-1}
Soda-lime glass	9.5×10^{-1}
Water	6.3×10^{-1}
Polyethylene	3.8×10^{-1}
Teflon	2.25×10^{-1}
Snow (0°C)	1.6×10^{-1}
Wood (oak)	1.6×10^{-1}
Sulphur	2.0×10^{-2}
Cork	3×10^{-2}
Glass wool	5×10^{-3}
Air	2.3×10^{-4}

[a] See also Fig. 26.1.
[b] 52% Cu, 15% Ni. 22% Zn.

Returning to the portion of thermal conduction caused by electrons, we consider a volume at the center of the bar depicted in Fig. 26.5 whose faces have the size of a unit area and whose length is $2l$, where, l is the mean free path between two consecutive collisions between an electron and lattice atoms. A simple energy balance, taking in account the electrons of energy E_1 that travel from left to right and electrons having a lower energy, E_2, drifting from right to left, yields for the classical equation for the heat conductivity of metals and alloys:

$$K = \frac{N_v v \, k_B l}{2} \qquad \ldots (26.12)$$

Equation 26.12 thus reveals that the heat conductivity is larger the more electrons, N_v, per unit volume are involved, the larger their velocity, v, and the larger the mean free path l, between two consecutive electron–atom collisions. The connection between thermal conductivity and the heat capacity per volume is:

$$K = \tfrac{1}{3} C_v^{el} v \, l \qquad (26.13)$$

All three variables contained in Eq. 26.13 are temperature-dependent, but while C_v^{el} increases with temperature (Fig. 26.4), l and, to a small degree, also v are decreasing. Thus, K should change very little with temperature, which is indeed experimentally observed. As mentioned above, the thermal conductivity decreases about 10^{-5} W/(m · K) per degree. K also changes at the melting point and when a change in atomic packing occurs.

The question arises as to what velocity the electrons (that participate in the heat conduction process) have? Further, do all of the electrons participate in the heat conduction? We know from there that only those electrons which have an energy close to the Fermi energy, E_F, are able to participate in the conduction process. Thus, the velocity in Eqs. 26.12 and 26.13 is essentially the Fermi velocity, v_F, which can be calculated with:

$$E_F = \tfrac{1}{2} m v_F^2 \quad\quad \ldots (26.14)$$

if the Fermi energy is known.

Second, the number of participating electrons contained in Eq. 26.12 is proportional to the population density at the Fermi energy, $N(E_F)$, that is, in first approximation, by the number of free electrons Nf per volume. Combining Eq. 26.10 (per volume) with Eq. 26.13 yields the quantum mechanical expression for the heat conductivity:

$$K = \frac{\pi^2 N_f k_B^2 T v_F l_F}{6 E_F} \quad\quad \ldots (26.15)$$

where, l_F is now the mean free path of the electrons near the Fermi energy E_F. Both the classical Eq. 26.12 and the quantum mechanical relation (Eq. 26.15) contain similar variables and constants, whereas quantum mechanics deepens our understanding.

Heat conduction in dielectric materials occurs as already explained by a flow of phonons. The hot end possesses more phonons than the cold end, causing a drift of phonons down a concentration gradient. The thermal conductivity can be calculated similarly as above, which leads to the same equation as (26.13):

$$K^{ph} = \tfrac{1}{3} C_v^{ph} v^{ph} l^{ph} \quad\quad \ldots (26.16)$$

In the present case C_v^{ph} is the (lattice) heat capacity per volume of the phonons, v^{ph} is the phonon velocity, and l^{ph} is the phonon mean free path. A typical value for v^{ph} is about 5×10^5 cm/s (sound velocity) with v^{ph} being relatively temperature-independent. In contrast, the mean free path varies over several orders of magnitude, that is, from about 10 nm at room temperature to 10^4 nm near 20 K. The drifting phonons interact on their path with lattice imperfections, with external boundaries, and with other phonons.

These interactions constitute a thermal, resistivity which is quite analogous to the electrical resistivity. Thus, we may treat the thermal resistance, i.e. in terms of interactions between particles (here phonons) and matter, or in terms of the scattering of phonon waves on lattice imperfections.

THERMAL EXPANSION

The length L of a rod increases with increasing temperature. Experiments have shown that in a relatively wide temperature range, the linear expansion ΔL is proportional to the increase in temperature ΔT. The proportionality constant is called the coefficient of linear expansion α_L.

The observations can be summarised in:

$$\frac{\Delta L}{L} = \alpha_L \Delta T \qquad \ldots (26.17)$$

Experimentally observed values for α_L are given in Table 26.4.

Table 26.4. Linear expansion coefficients α_L some solids measured at room temperature.

Substance	$\alpha_L \times 10^{-5}$ [K–1]
Hard rubber	8.00
Lead	2.73
Aluminium	2.39
Brass	1.80
Copper	1.67
Iron	1.23
Glass (ordinary)	0.90
Glass (pyrex)	0.32
NaCl	0.16
Invar (Fe-36% Ni)	0.07
Quartz	0.05

The expansion coefficient has been found to be proportional to the molar heat capacity C_v, i.e. the temperature dependence of α_L is similar to the temperature dependence of C_v. As a consequence, the temperature dependence of α_L for dielectric materials follows closely the $C_v = f(T)$ relationship shown in Fig. 26.4. Specifically, α_L approaches a constant value for $T > \theta_D$ and vanishes as T^3 for $T \rightarrow 0$. The thermal expansion coefficient for metals, on the other hand, decreases at very small temperatures in proportion to T, and depends, in other temperature regions, on the sum of the heat capacities of phonons and electrons (Fig. 26.4). We turn now to a discussion of a possible mechanism that may explain thermal expansion from an atomistic point of view. We postulate, as in the previous sections, that the lattice atoms absorb thermal energy by vibrating about their equilibrium position. In doing so, a given atom responds with increasing temperature and vibrational amplitude to the repulsive forces of the neighbouring atoms. Let us consider for a moment two adjacent atoms only, and let us inspect their potential energy as a function of internuclear separation (Fig. 26.6).

We understand that as two atoms move closer to each other, strong repulsive forces are experienced between them. As a consequence, the potential energy [$U(r)$] curve rises steeply with decreasing r. On the other hand, we know that two somewhat separated atoms also attract each other in some degree. This results in a slight decrease in $U(r)$ with decreasing r.

Now, at low temperatures, a given atom may rest in its equilibrium position r_0, i.e. at the minimum of potential energy. If, however, the temperature is raised, the amplitude of the vibrating atom also increases. Since the amplitudes of the vibrating atom are symmetric about a median position, and since the potential curve is not symmetric, a given atom moves farther apart from its neighbour, that is, the average position of an atom moves to a larger r, say r_T, as shown in Fig. 26.6. In other words, the thermal expansion is a direct consequence of the asymmetry the potential energy curve. The same arguments hold true if all of the atoms in a solid are considered.

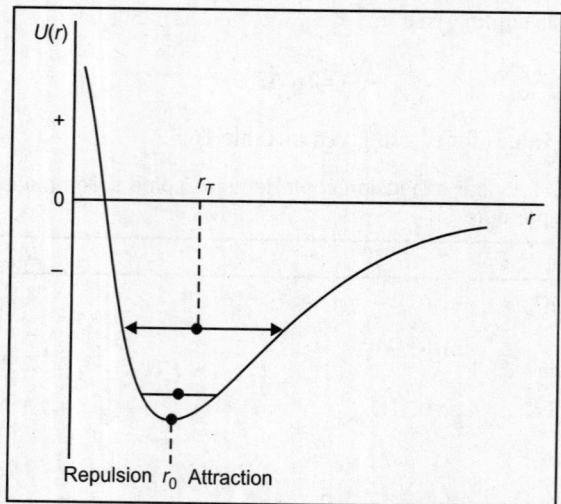

Fig. 26.6. Schematic representation of the potential energy, $U(r)$, for two adjacent atoms as a function of internuclear separation, r.

A few substances are known to behave differently from that described above. They contract during a temperature increase.

This happens, however, only within a narrow temperature region. For its explanation, we need to realise that longitudinal as well as transverse vibrational modes may be excited by thermal energy. The lattice is expected to contract if transverse modes predominate. Interestingly enough, only one known liquid substance, namely water, behaves in a limited temperature range in this manner. Specifically, water has its largest density at 4°C. (Furthermore, the density of ice is smaller than the density of water at the freezing point.) As a consequence, water of 4°C sinks to the bottom of a lake during winter, while ice stays on top. This prevents the freezing of a lake at the bottom and thus enables aquatic life to survive during the winter. This exceptional behaviour of water suggests that the laws of physics do not just 'happen' but rather, they were created by a superior being.

Glossary

Acid steel	:	Steel made in an acid furnace under a siliceous slag.
Age-hardening	:	Hardening of a metal induced in the process of ageing.
Ageing	:	A change in properties that may occur gradually over a period of time in a metal at room temperature or more rapidly at elevated temperature.
Air-hardening	:	Hardening that occurs in some alloy steels during cooling in air from an elevated temperature within a critical range.
Allotriomorphic	:	Without regular shape, e.g. the grains resulting from random nucleation in a cast metal.
Annealing	:	Primarily, the process of heating a metal which is in a metastable or distorted structural state, to a temperature which will remove the instability or distortion, and then cooling it (usually at a slow rate) so that the room-temperature structure is table and/or strain free.
Arc welding	:	Fusion welding using an electric arc as heat source.
Austempering	:	Quenching steel from a temperature above the transformation range to some temperature above the upper limit of martensite formation, and holding it at this temperature until the austenite is completely transformed to bainite.
Austenite	:	The solid solution of carbon and/or other alloying elements in gamma iron.
Austenitic steel	:	Steel which, owing to the influence of alloying elements is retained in the face-centred cubic state at room temperature. Usually nonmagnetic.
Basic steel	:	Steel produced in a basic furnace under a basic slag.
Bessemer process	:	A process for making steel by blowing air through steel by molten pig iron contained in a vessel called a 'converter'.
Bead (Welding)	:	A single run of weld deposited on a surface.
Binary alloy	:	A metal containing one alloying addition.
Blacksmith welding	:	Forge welding by manual hammering of hot metal.
Blank	:	A piece of metal cut from sheet or otherwise formed to act as the starting piece in the shaping of a single component.
Blast furnace	:	A large, vertical, tubular furnace, heated by combustion of metallurgical coke under forced draught, usually for extracting crude metal or matter from the ore which is mixed with the coke.
Blister copper	:	A form of partly refined copper produced in a converter.
Blister steel	:	A crude form of steel produced by absorption of carbon into the surface of wrought iron.
Blowhole	:	A hole produced within a metal during solidification by entrapment of evolved gas.

Blue annealing	:	Subcritical annealing of clean steel in a controlled atmosphere at a temperature which prevents scaling but does not stop oxidation colouring of the surface.
Blue brittleness	:	Brittleness occurring in steel when it is worked in the temperature range of approximately 200°–400°C or when the steel is cold after being worked within this temperature range.
Bright annealing	:	An annealing operation performed in a controlled atmosphere so that oxidation is minimised and the metal surface remains bright.
Brinell hardness	:	A measure of hardness obtained by pressing a ball of known diameter under a predetermined load into the surface of a metal. The load is divided by the superficial area of the resulting impression, giving the Brinell hardness number (BHN). Not reliable for very hard materials.
Brittle fracture	:	Fracture without visible plastic deformation.
Burger's vector	:	The magnitude and direction of the strain component of a dislocation.
Carbon steel	:	Steel which owes its properties mainly to carbon without substantial amounts of other alloy additions.
Carbonising	:	Coking or driving off the volatile matter from fuels such as coal and wood.
Carburising	:	A method of introducing carbon into solid iron-base alloys by heating them in the presence of carbonaceous solids, liquids or gases. Also called 'cementation'.
Case hardening	:	Surface zone hardening of an iron-base alloy component by carburising and heat treatment alone.
Cast iron	:	Alloys of iron and carbon containing, as cast, more than 1.7 per cent carbon (generally between 2.4 and 4.0 per cent carbon). Silicon, manganese, sulphur and phosphorus are usually present in varying amounts. Rarely used in any but the as-cast, or as-cast and heat treated condition.
Cast iron thermit	:	Welding thermit with the addition of ferro-silicon for the thermit fusion welding of cast iron.
Casting	:	The process of pouring a liquid metal into a mould and allowing it to solidity into shape.
Casting stresses	:	Stresses associated with casting strain.
Caustic embrittlement	:	Intercrystalline cracking of stressed low-carbon steel which is in contact with a hot alkaline solution.
Chill	:	A mass of solid metal incorporated into a mould to speed up local solidification.
Chill-cast metal	:	Metal which is relatively rapidly cooled during casting, usually by being cast in a water cooled metal mould.
Close annealing	:	Annealing performed in a container with a closely fitted cover, with or without a suitable packing medium, to minimise oxidation of the surface.
Cold welding	:	Pressure welding in which pressure alone is used.
Cold working	:	Plastic deformation of a metal which results in strain-hardening. Usually involves working at ordinary temperatures, but for low-melting-point metals ordinary temperatures might give hot working.
Corrosion	:	The result of chemical or electrochemical attack on a metal.
Corrosion embrittlement	:	Embrittlement of a metal as a result of intergranular corrosion attack, or stress-accentuated pitting.

Creep	:	Plastic deformation which proceeds continuously under a constant stress.
Creep curve	:	A curve recording the creep characteristics of a metal, either as strain against time at a given stress and temperature; or as stress to produce a given strain in a given time against temperature; or as stress to produce a limiting rate of creep in a given time against temperature.
Crystal boundary	:	The outer limiting surface of a crystal.
Crsytallography	:	The study of the atomic structure of crystals.
Cupping test	:	A test of ductility of a metal made by forming a cup shape from a blank by means of a die former.
Decarburisation	:	Loss of carbon from the surface of steel, usually during hot working, heat treatment or reheating.
Differential quenching	:	Selective quenching of different portions of an article.
Diffusion	:	The movement of atoms between different regions in a solid, liquid or gas.
Ductility	:	Ability to undergo cold plastic deformation, usually as a result of tension.
Electro-galvanising	:	Using electrolysis to deposit a zinc coating.
Elongation	:	The proportionate increase in length of a tensile test piece when stressed. The elongation at fracture is usually expressed as a percentage of the original gauge length.
Etching	:	Treatment of prepared metal surfaces by electrolysis or with acid or other reagents, which by differential attack reveal the structure.
Eutectic point	:	The point in the equilibrium diagram indicating the composition of the eutectic and its freezing temperature.
Extraction	:	The technique for extracting metal from its ore.
Fatigue	:	The tendency to fracture by means of a progressive crack under repeated alternating or cyclic stresses of intensity considerably below the tensile strength.
Fatigue ratio	:	The ratio of the fatigue limit to the tensile strength.
Ferrite	:	The micro-constituent alpha iron, or solid solutions of which alpha iron is the solvent.
Ferro-alloys	:	Alloys of metals with iron, used mainly as alloying additions to steel and iron, e.g. ferro-silicon and ferro-maganese.
Flux	:	An agent which under the influence of heat will combine with an oxide to make it fluid or otherwise controllable. Used in extraction, refining, casting and welding to offset the harmful effects of oxides and oxygen.
Forge welding	:	Any welding process in which the weld is made by hammering or other impulsive pressure while the surfaces to be united are plastic.
Foundry	:	A place for melting and casting metal.
Galvanising	:	Coating with a film of zinc.
Gas carburising	:	Carburising steel by heating in a current of gas rich in carbon compounds such as carbon monoxide and/or hydrocarbons.
Hardenability	:	That property of a heat treatable steel which determines the depth and distribution of hardness after quenching under specified conditions. This should no be confused with the intensity of hardening, which is measured by the actual hardness obtained.
Hardness test	:	A test of hardness, usually by determining the resistance of the material to indentation under standard conditions.

Heat treatment	:	A process in which the metal in the solid state is subjected to one or more temperature cycles, to confer certain desired properties. Heating for the sole purpose of hot working is excluded from the meaning of this definition.
Hot galvanising	:	Coating with zinc by immersion in a bath of molten zinc.
Ingot	:	A cast metal bar or block intended for further treatment such as remelting, for alloying purposes, or mechanical working.
Leaching	:	Extracting a constituent from an agglomerate by mixing the latter in a liquid which will dissolve the constituent. The constituent may later be separated from the liquid.
Light alloy	:	An alloy based mainly on one of the lighter metals such as aluminium or magnesium or more rarely, beryllium.
Malleability	:	Capacity for undergoing deformation in all directions by hammering or squeezing. Often refers only to cold deformation.
Malleable cast iron	:	A white cast iron made malleable by prolonged annealing in an oxidising or a neutral medium.
Martempering	:	Quenching steel from a temperature above the transformation range to some temperature slightly above the upper limit of martensite formation, holding it at that temperature long enough to permit equalisation of temperature without transformation of the austenite, followed by cooling in air. This results in the formation of martensite which may be tempered as desired.
Martensite	:	A constituent formed in steel and other alloys as a result of a shear-type transformation with virtually no diffusion. Normally a product of quenching.
Metallography	:	The study of the constitution and structure of metals and alloys, mainly by microscopical examination.
Mild steel	:	Low-carbon steel containing approximately 0.12 to 0.25 per cent of carbon.
Nitriding	:	The introduction of nitrogen into the surface of certain types of steel by heating it and holding it at a suitable temperature in contact with partially dissociated ammonia or other suitable medium. This process produces a hard case without further heat treatment.
Normalising	:	Heating steel to and, if necessary, holding it at suitable temperature above the transformation range, followed by cooling freely in air in order to modify the grain size, render the structure more uniform, and usually, to improve the mechanical properties.
Nucleation	:	The formation of centres from which individual crystals or grains may grow.
Open annealing	:	Annealing without a protective medium.
Pig iron	:	The product of the iron blast furnace, containing from 2½ to 5 per cent carbon and varying percentages of silicon, manganese, sulphur and phosphorus. Pig iron is a raw material for steelmaking.
Porosity	:	Numbers of gas bubbles entrapped in a solidifying metal.
Recrystallisation	:	A structural change that can occur when a cold worked metal is heated. New crystals grow and absorb the cold worked structure, leaving the metal either completely strain-free and stable or a nearly in that condition as is possible.
Red hardness	:	The relatively high hardness retained up to a low red heat by high-speed tool steels and certain other cutting materials.

Rockwell hardness test	:	A test to determine hardness by indicating on a dial the depth of the impression caused by a loaded indenter in the form of either a diamond cone or a hardened steel ball.
Roll forming	:	The shaping of flat sheet or strip into longitudinally or transversely curved and folded forms by passing the material through successive stages.
Roll welding	:	Forge welding in which pressure is progressively applied to overlapping plates by mechanically operated rolls after heating in a Smith's fire or by water-gas flame or other equivalent means.
Self-hardening steel	:	Air-hardening steel.
Sintering	:	Heating of a previously compacted aggregate of particles at a temperature high enough to cause solid phase welding or partial fusion between the particles.
Slag	:	The reaction products that usually result from the use of a flux in a hot molten or pasty metal. Normally the slag floats to the surface of the molten metal, from whence it may be removed by skimming or draining. In the solidified cold state it generally forms into a hard, porous, dirty-looking mass composed mainly of nonmetallic oxides.
Slush casting	:	A method of casting a hollow component without using a core or cod. The mould is poured and the metal allowed to solidify until it forms a self-supporting skin of the required thickness, after which the remaining liquid metal is decanted out.
Solder	:	A low-melting-temperature alloy, usually composed mainly of lead and/or tin, used in soldering.
Smelting	:	Fusing, melting, or refining an ore using heat that is generated, all or in part, from fuel (e.g. coke) burning within a mixture of the ore and the fuel.
Steel	:	An alloy of iron and carbon which can be hot worked and in which the carbon is in the combined state. It may also contain other elements in controlled amounts.
Tertiary creep	:	The final stage of accelerating creep immediately preceding failure.
Tetravalent	:	Having four valency electrons or being four electrons short in the outer electron 'shell'.
Toughness	:	The capacity of a metal to resist application of high rates of strain.
Yield	:	The stage in the straining of a metal when plastic strain begins to supersede elastic strain as the predominating type.
Zone axis	:	A line parallel to the principal planes in any given zone of a crystal.
Zoning	:	A defect encountered in extrusion, whereby, due to uneven flow in the metal, the grain size varies in different parts of the cross-section of the extruded product.

References

Alvarez, J.L., *Mechanical Properties of Steel*, John Wiley & Sons, New York.
Arceivala, K.J., *Case Hardening of Steel*, Marcel Dekker Inc., New York.
Barsom, K.G., *Heat Treatment of Metals*, Swedish Institute of Metal Research.
Brown, M.H., *Alloying Elements in Steel*, Cambridge University Press, Cambridge.
Cambell, K.E. and Lemer, H.A., *Iron and Steel Alloys*, Academic Press, London.
Coolingwood, R.W., *Temperability of Steel*, John Wiley & Sons, New York.
Downe, S.A., *Hardenability concepts with Applications of Steel*, John Wiley & Sons, New York.
Friedel, J., *Tempering of Steel*, Van Nostrand, London.
Gould, G.W., *Physical Metallurgy Principles*, D. Van Nostrand, New York.
Hillert, M., *Decomposition of Austenite by Diffusional Processes, Intersciences*, New York, London.
Huff, C.B., *Cast Iron and Ductile Iron*, Elsevier Scientific Publishing Co., Amsterdam.
Jackwerth, E., *Heat Treatment Furnaces and Equipments*, Academic Press, London.
Jencks, W.P., *Salt and Fluidised Bed Equipments*, John Wiley & Sons, New York.
Kiessling, R., *Heat Treatment of Non-ferrous Metals*, The Metals Society, London.
Kim, C.K., *Diffusio in Solids, Liquids and Gases*, Marcel Dekker, New York.
Lechevallier, M.W., *Dimensional Stability of Steel*, Academic Press, London.
Lewis, R.L., *Heat Treatment Furnaces*, Chilton Book Co., USA.
Mason, C.F., *Testing of Metals*, Longman Group Ltd., London.
McCaull, J. and Crossland, J., *Hardening of Steel*, Harcourt Brace Jovanovich, New York.
Nyer, E.K., *Normalising of Steel*, Van Nostrand Reinhold, New York.
Phillips, D.J.H., *Testing of Metals*, Applied Science Publishers, London.
Randak, A.M., *Carbon and Tool Steels*, Academic Press, London.
Reid, G.K., *Carburising and Nitriding*, Reinhold Publishing Corporation, New York.
Samson, R.A., *Physicalmetallurgy*, Pergamon Press, Oxford, London.
Scott. H., *Influence of Tempering Temperature on Quenched Steel*, Progress Publishers, Moscow.
Southwood, T.R.E., *Cyaniding and Carbonitriding,*, Swedish Institute of Metal Research, London.
Stumm, W. and Stumm-Zollineger, E., *Distortion in Tool Steel*, Wiley Interscience, New York.
Teal, J.M., *Nature of Metals and Alloys*, Pergamon Press, New York.
Thelning, K.E., *Steel and its Heat Treatments*, Butterworth, U.K.
Wyatt, M., *Nonmetallic Inclusions in Steel*, Reston Publishing Co., Reston, Virginia.

Index

A

Absorption of light, 490
Active-passive cells, 200
Adhesive, 371
Advantages and disadvantages of powder metallurgy (P/M), 249
Advantages of digital signal conversion, 450
Advantages of pyrometers, 432
Aerospace alloys, 272
Age (precipitation hardening), 40
Age-hardenable alloys, 291
Ageing at room temperature (natural ageing), 274
Air-hardening grades, 155
AISI-SAE grades, 154
Alloy cast irons, 234
Alloy identification, 415
Alloy types and response to heat treatment, 309
Alloying elements, 224, 276
Alloying the metal, 176
Alloys containing insoluble constituents required in a fine dispersion, 265
Alloys of metals which are mutually insoluble in the liquid state, 264
Alloys with excessively high melting temperatures, 263
Alloys with poor casting qualities, 264
Alpha aluminium bronzes, 306
Aluminium alloys, 314, 319
Aluminium alloys versus types of steel, 267
Aluminium and aluminium alloy, 267
Aluminium bronze, 297
Annealing, 79, 235, 273, 304
Annealing after welding, 81
Annealing ductile cast iron, 287
Annealing treatments, 279
Anodising, 178
Antiferromagnetism, 476
Application of adhesion, 373
Applications of resistance materials, 462
Applications of SG iron, 286
Arc welding, 386
Atmospheric windows, 441
Atomic size difference, 38
Atomic structure, 1
Atoms and molecules, 1
Ausforming, 134
Austempering, 280
Austempering ductile cast iron 289
Austenitic and ferritic grain size in steels, 117
Austenitising ductile cast iron, 287
Austenitising treatments, 147
Auto tempering, 139

B

Basic soldering techniques, 377
Basic structure of materials, 1
Beryllium copper, 302
Binary phase diagrams, 55
Biohazards, 146
Blending of the raw materials, 262
Block slip model, 22
Boiler steels, 102
Bonds, 6
Box annealing, 126
Braze welding, 384
Brazing, 380
Brazing solder (50Cu: 50Zn), 295
Bright and dark field microscopy, 413
Bright annealing, 126
Bright flames flame pyrometers, 446
Brinell (HBW), 169
Brinell test, 397
Brittle fracture, 326
Broad band pyrometers, 445
Bronze, 295

C

C23000—Red brass (85Cu, 15Zn), 294
C26000—Cartridge brass (70Cu: 30Zn), 294
C28000—Muntz metal (60Cu: 40Zn), 294
Carbide in the structure, 284

Carbonitriding, 151
Carburising, 149
Case hardening, 168
Case hardening steels, 102
Cast alloys, 270
Cast iron, 216
Cast iron alloys, 276
Cast iron 'welding', 384
Casting, 355
Casting and grain structure, 359
Caustic embrittlement, 209
Cavitation, 210
Cemented carbide tipped tools (sintered carbide cutting tools), 258
Cemented carbides, 257
Cermets, 258
Characterisation and testing of metal powders, 250
Chemistry of corrosion, 173
Chilled cast irons, 232
Choice of steel, 171
Chromium coppers, 306
Classification and applications of steels, 96
Classification of copper alloys, 291
Classification of titanium alloys, 307
Clips, 395
Coating the metal, 175
Cohesive fracture, 374
Cold mounting, 252
Cold pressing and sintering, 258
Cold treatment (subzero treatment), 136
Cold work on α', 42
Cold working, 360
Cold working processes, 362
Cold-working grades, 155
Composite materials, 44
Compression test, 403
Concentration cell corrosion, 198
Conditioning the corrosive environment, 176
Conditioning the metal, 175
Conjoint action, 336
Consequences of corrosion, 172
Continuous cooling transformation (CCT) diagrams, 112
Conventional annealing (full annealing) 125
Conventional hardening, 130
Cooling and quenching, 80
Cooling media, 115
Cooling of a hypereutectic white cast iron, 227
Cooling of a hypoeutetic cast iron with 3 per cent carbon, 226
Cooling of an eutectic cast iron, 226
Copper and copper alloys, 290

Copper–nickel–phosphorus alloys, 306
Copper–nickel–zinc alloys, 300
Copper–zinc alloys: the brasses, 292
Corrosion and heat resistant steels, 102
Corrosion fatigue, 209
Corrosion inhibitors, 176
Corrosion of welds, 392
Corrosion prevention, 175
Corrosion prevention measures, 187
Corrosion technology of metals, 172
Corrosion/selection of materials, 212
Covalent bonding, 7
Crack separation modes, 327
Critical cooling rate, 111
Critical temperatures, 88
Crucial mechanisms determining corrosion rates, 186
Crystals, 10
Crystal defects, 26
Cubic law, 182
Cumulative damage, 351
Cyaniding, 150

D

Deep drawing steels, 102
Deoxidisers, 292
Derivation of the phase rule, 55
Description of a wet corrosion process, 185
Design of adhesive joints, 374
Design, resolution and image contrast, 412
Designation system of brasses, 294
Desoldering and resoldering, 379
Desulphurisation, 281
Detection of stray currents, 201
Determination of CCT curves, 112
Determination of TTT diagram, 108
Determining the emissivity of an object, 439
Diamagnetism, 464, 472
Diamond impregnated tools, 259
Die casting alloys, 314
Die casting, 357
Differential interference contrast microscopy, 413
Dimensional and shape stability, 164
Dip brazing, 385
Dislocations, 25
Dislocation multiplication, 29
Disperse materials, 46
Dispersion strengthening or hardening, 39
Distortion during the hardening and tempering of tool steel, 164
Dry corrosion, 177
Dry corrosion reactions, 179

Ductile cast iron, 231, 278
Ductile fracture, 326, 406
Ductility, 282, 399

E

Effect of alloying elements on the properties of ductile iron, 283
Effect of heat on cold-worked metals, 364
Effect of previous deformation, 406
Effect of size and shape of specimens on the compressive strength, 405
Effects of alloying elements on α-β transformation, 309
Effects of retained austenite, 136
Elasticity and plasticity, 334
Electrical properties of materials, 459
Electrical resistance, 459
Electrical steels, 102
Electrical steels (soft magnetic materials), 479
Electrochemical control, 177
Electrochemical series, 190
Electron microscope, 421
Elimination of retained austenite, 136
Elongation, 402
Emission of light, 495
Emissivity errors, 440
Emissivity of various materials, 437
Emittance, emissivity and the N-factor, 447
Energy beam, 388
Engineering uses of aluminium alloys, 267
Erosion-corrosion, 210
Estimation of carbon from microstructures, 93
Eutectoid transformation, 86
Excellent corrosion resistance, 283
Expressions and measures of corrosion rates, 187
External corrosion, 214

F

Fabrication techniques, 416
Factors affecting recrystallisation, 367
Factors affecting the fatigue properties of metals, 351
Factors influencing microstructure, 216
Factors that affect fatigue-life, 342
Factors that affect the properties of the SG cast iron, 285
Factors that control the corrosion rate, 174
Factors that influence galvanic corrosion, 195
Failure of the adhesive joint, 373
Fastener, 393
Fastening systems, 393
Fatigue, 338
Fatigue and fracture mechanics, 342

Fatigue failure, 343
Fatigue fractures, 406
Fatigue life, 338
Fatigue properties of fastened joints, 394
Fatigue tests, 345
Ferrimagnetism, 477
Ferritic iron, 415
Ferritic malleable, 230
Ferritic nitrocarburising, 152
Ferromagnetism, 464, 475
Fibre optics pyrometer, 450
Fibre reinforced materials, 45
Filling up the spot size, 443
Fixed optics, 443
Flame and induction hardening, 149
Flow rate, 253
Flux, 376
Formation and growth of films, 180
Formation of an oxide layer, 178
Forming processes with metals, 355
Four-colour pyrometer, 447
Fracture, 325, 406
Fracture mechanics and fracture toughness, 410
Fracture mechanics, 328
Fracture strength, 325
Fracture toughness, 334
Free cutting (or machining) steels, 103
Friction, 18
Furnace brazing, 382

G

Galvanic compatibility, 196
Galvanic corrosion, 192
Galvanic series, 194
Gas welding, 386
Gibbs' phase rule, 50
Glossary, 513
Grades of grey cast iron, 224
Grain boundary strengthening, 34
Grain orientation, 480
Grain refinement, 37
Grain refinement methods, 319
Grain refinement of light alloys, 318
Grain size control, 117
Grain size measurement, 119
Graphite amount, 285
Graphite structure, 285
Grey cast iron, 220, 227, 277
Griffith's criterion, 328, 333
Growth of metal crystals, 21

Growth of nonporous films, 180
Growth of porous films, 180

H

Hall-Petch relationship, 36
Hard chromium plating, 168
Hardenability, 143
Hardenability of steel, 143
Hardening and tempering, 157, 236
Hardness, 397
Hardness testing, 168
Heat sensitivity considerations, 268
Heat treating iron castings, 279
Heat treating of aluminium and aluminium alloys, 273
Heat treating of copper and copper alloys, 304
Heat treating of titanium and titanium alloys, 309
Heat treatment of cast irons, 235
Heat treatment of SG cast iron, 286
Heat treatment of stainless steel, 75, 79
Heat treatment of steel, 83, 112
Heat treatment of tool steel, 154
Heating methods, 385
Heating to hardening temperature, 159
Heyn's intercept method, 124
High carbon steels, 98
High speed grades, 156
High temperature tempering, 138
High-cycle fatigue, 339
Holding time at hardening temperature, 160
Holding times in connection with tempering, 164
Homogenising, 304
Hot air balloons, 432
Hot mounting, 252
Hot working processes, 368
Hot-bar reflow, 378
Hydrogen attack, 185
Hydrogen embrittlement, 184

I

Ideal diameter, 145
Impact testing, 170
Impurity and homogeneity, 43
Induction hardening, 152
Infrared radiation thermometers/pyrometers, 447
Ingot preheating treatments (homogenising), 273
Inoculation, 282
Insoluble alloying elements, 292
Interatomic forces in crystals, 13
Intercrystalline, 406
Interfacial fracture, 374
Intergranular corrosion, 211

Interpretation of the heat capacity by various models, 505
Ion nitriding, 167
Ionic bonding, 6
Iron–iron carbide equilibrium diagram, 83
Irwin's modification, 329, 333
Isothermal (cycle) annealing, 127
Isothermal transformation diagram, 108

J

Jefferies planimetric method, 124
Jominy end-quench, 145

K

Killed steels, 99

L

Laminated materials, 46
Lasagna cell, 196
Laser, 378
Lead-free electronic soldering, 380
Lever rule, 57
Linear elastic fracture mechanics, 328
Linear law, 182
Linearisation, 453
Localised corrosion, 213
Logarithmic law, 182
Low carbon steels, 98
Low temperature stress relieving, 81
Low temperature tempering, 138
Low-cycle fatigue, 341

M

Machinery steels, 103
Machining, 258, 369
Machining stresses, 164
Macrography, 423
Magnesium alloys, 321
Magnesium treatment, 284
Magnetic phenomena and their interpretation, 471
Magnetic properties of materials, 469
Magnetic recording, 482
Magnetism, 464
Magnetostriction, 466
Main types of sand casting, 356
Malleable cast iron, 228, 278
Manipulative processes, 360
Manufacture of some typical powder metallurgy
    (P/M) components, 256
Martempering, 281
Martempering (marquenching), 133
Martensitic transformation, 44

Mass transport control, 210
Materials and fatigue resistance, 353
Materials selection, 214
Matrix structure, 285
Maximum hardness, 143
Measuring moving objects, 433
Measuring objects which are difficult to access by contact measuring devices, 433
Mechanical and aluminium soldering, 379
Mechanical and nondestructive tests, 396
Mechanisms of adhesion, 373
Medium carbon steels, 98
Medium temperature tempering, 138
Metal ion concentration cells, 199
Metallic bonding, 8
Metallographic examination, 415
Metallography, 411
Metals as crystalline, 21
Micrography, 417
Microscopic method, 251
Microstructures of hypereutectoid steels, 91
Microstructures of hypoeutectoid steels, 89
Milling, 257
Miner's rule, 340
Molecular dynamics simulations, 48
Mottled cast irons, 232
Movement of dislocations, 27

N

Named alloys, 271
Narrow band pyrometers, 445
Natural adhesives, 373
Nature of stray currents, 202
Nernst equation, 190
Ni-hard, 234
Ni-resist, 235
Nitriding, 82, 149, 167
Nitrocarburising, 167
Nodulising, 282
Non-equilibrium cooling of steels, 93
Nonferrous alloys, 416
Nonlinear elasticity and plasticity, 332
Non-luminous flames, 447
Nonreactive adhesives, 371
Normalising, 129
Normalising ductile cast iron, 288
Normalising treatments, 280
Notched bar tests, 409

O

Oblique illumination, 413

Oil impregnated porous bearings (self-lubricating bearings), 256
Optical constants, 486
Optical properties of materials, 485
Optics with variable focus, 443
Optics, lenses and window material, 453
Over-the-bath pyrometer, 432
Oxygen concentration cells, 200

P

Parabolic law, 181
Paramagnetism, 464, 473
Particle porosity and microstructure, 252
Passivation, 178
Pearlitic malleable, 230
Pearlitic-ferritic malleable, 230
Peltier effect, 467
Performance tests, 215
Peritectic transformation, 85
Permanent magnets (hard magnetic materials), 481
Phase diagrams, 49
Phase transport control, 210
Phosphor bronze, 297
Phosphoric iron, 416
Photoconductivity, 467
Physical hazards, 146
Physical vapour deposition (PVD), 82
Piezoelectricity, 466
Pilling-bedworth ratio, 179
Pipe soldering, 378
Pitting and crevice corrosion of stainless steel, 204
Pitting corrosion, 203
Plastic deformation, 137
Polarisation, 191, 196
Polarised light microscopy, 413
Porous metals, 263
Pourbaix diagram of iron, 192
Powder manufacture, 257
Powder metallurgy, 237
Powders preparation, 238
Practical use of reference electrodes, 191
Precipitation hardening, 33, 274, 305
Precipitation heat treating (artificial ageing), 275
Precipitation heat treating cast products, 275
Precipitation heat treating without prior solution heat treatment, 275
Preparing metallographic specimens, 411
Preventing galvanic corrosion, 194
Probabilistic nature of fatigue, 340
Process annealing (intermediate annealing), 129
Process fluid corrosion, 213

Processes involved in welding, 386
Production of cast iron, 216
Production of cast iron alloys, 276
Production of refractory metals, 260
Production of tungsten and molybdenum, 260
Properties of real objects, 435
Properties of SG cast iron, 282
Property variation with microstructure, 95
Protective equipment, 146
Pyrometer, 444
Pyrometry, 430
Pyrometry of gases, 432

Q

Quantitative metallography, 414
Quantum numbers, 3
Quench annealing, 79
Quench cracks, 140
Quenching and tempering ductile cast iron, 288
Quenching, 41, 160, 274

R

Radiation hazards, 146
Rail fastening system, 394
R-curve, 332
Reactive adhesives, 372
Recrystallisation annealing, 129
Resistance welding, 386
Retention of austenite, 134
Reverse or inverse Hall-Petch relation, 37
Rimmed steels, 99
Rockwell (HRC), 168
Rockwell test, 399

S

Sand casting, 356
Scanning electron and transmission electron microscopes, 414
Season cracking, 208
Secondary hardening, 140
Sedimentation method, 251
Seebeck effect, 467
Selective corrosion, 212
Semi-killed steels, 100
Shock resisting grades, 156
Shore scleroscope, 399
Sieve method, 251
Sighting and viewing devices, 452
Silal and nicrosilal, 235
Silver brazing, 383

Simple one-component, 52
Sintered metal friction materials, 262
Sintering characteristics, 255
Size of atoms, 5
Slag content, 415
Slip planes, 24
Smelter industry, 432
S-N curve, 339
Solderability, 379
Soldering, 375
Soldering defects, 380
Solders, 375
Solid solution alloys, 291
Solid solution strengthening or hardening, 38
Solid solution strengthening/alloying, 32
Solidification and microstructures of slowly cooled steels, 89
Solution treating and ageing, 312
Special purpose grades, 156
Specific surface, 253
Spectral intensity, 434
Speed of loading, 405
Spheroidal graphite cast iron, 281
Spheroidise annealing, 127
Spikes and screws, 394
Spot size and measuring distance, 442
Stabilising anneal, 79
Stages in fatigue failure, 344
Stages of heat treatment, 79
Stained glass soldering, 379
Stainless steel finishes, 79
Stainless steel grades, 78
Stainless steel in 3D printing, 79
Steam boilers, 432
Steps in heat treating, 279
Steps in production of SG iron, 281
Stopping fatigue, 343
Strain energy release, 331
Stray currents in transit systems, 201
Stray-current corrosion, 200
Strengthening mechanism of materials, 31
Strengthening mechanisms in amorphous materials, 46
Strengthening mechanisms in metals, 32
Stress corrosion cracking, 206
Stress intensity factor, 330
Stress relieving, 81, 159, 235, 305
Stress-corrosion cracking (SCC), 337
Stress-relief annealing, 128
Stress-relieving treatments, 279
Stress-strain curve, 400
Structural steels, 103

Structure of cold worked metals, 361
Subcritical annealing, 128
Subgrain strengthening, 35
Sub-zero treatment, 166
Superconductivity, 463
Surface coating, 168
Surface hardening, 81, 236
Surface treatment, 167
Susceptible alloys, 204
Synthetic adhesives, 373

T

Temper brittleness (embrittlement), 140
Temperature of ageing, 41
Tempering, 137, 163
Tensile strength, 170
Tensile test, 400
Testing mechanical properties of tool steel, 168
Testing the resistance of the adhesive, 374
Theories of grain refinement, 323
Thermal analysis—heating and cooling curves, 69
Thermal conduction, 507
Thermal expansion, 510
Thermal properties of materials, 502
Thermal stresses, 165
Thermoelectricity, 467
Timed quench (interrupted quench), 131
Time-temperature-transformation curves, 72
Titanium alloys, 307
Tool steels, 103
Torch brazing, 382
Total band pyrometers, 445
Total intensity, 435
Transformation of austenite to bainite, 104
Transformation of austenite to martensite, 105
Transformation of austenite to pearlite, 103
Transformation products of austenite, 103
Transformation stresses, 165
Transformation toughening, 336
Transition temperature, 307
Tuyère pyrometer, 432
Two-colour pyrometer, 445
Type of fracture, 404

Types of adhesives, 371
Types of annealing, 126
Types of cast iron, 220
Types of fracture, 326
Types of grey cast iron, 221
Types of malleable cast iron, 230
Types of metals and applications, 263

U

Uniform corrosion, 203

V

Vacuum brazing, 384
Van der Waals bonding, 8
Various phases in diagram, 84
Vickers (HV), 169
Vickers machine, 397

W

Water-hardening grades, 154
Wavelength of maximum intensity, 435
Weldability, 392
Welding, 386
Welds in aluminium, 390
Welds in copper, 391
Welds in steel, 388
Wet corrosion, 185
White cast iron, 225, 277
White heart malleable, 231
Widmanstatten structures, 94
Window materials, 454
Wrought alloys, 269
Wrought copper–nickel alloys and nickel silvers, 299
Wrought phosphor bronzes, 299

X

X-ray diffraction techniques, 414

Z

Zinc alloys, 314
Zinc-aluminum (ZA) alloys, 316
Zirconium copper, 306